Ultrasonography in Reproductive Medicine and Infertility

Ultrasonography in Reproductive Medicine and Infertility

Edited by

Botros R. M. B. Rizk

Professor and Head, Division of Reproductive Endocrinology and Infertility, Department of Obstetrics and Gynecology, and Medical and Scientific Director of USA IVF Program, University of South Alabama, Mobile, Alabama, USA

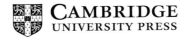

CAMBRIDGE
UNIVERSITY PRESS

CAMBRIDGE UNIVERSITY PRESS
Cambridge, New York, Melbourne, Madrid, Cape Town,
Singapore, São Paulo, Delhi, Dubai, Tokyo

Cambridge University Press
The Edinburgh Building, Cambridge CB2 8RU, UK

Published in the United States of America by
Cambridge University Press, New York

www.cambridge.org
Information on this title: www.cambridge.org/9780521509763

First published 2010

Printed in the United Kingdom at the University Press, Cambridge

*A catalogue record for this publication is available from the
British Library*

ISBN 978-0-521-50976-3 Hardback

This book is dedicated to my very dear wife and life partner Mary for her love, support and sacrifice and to my children Christopher, Christine, David, and Danielle who inspire me every morning.

Contents

Section 4: Early pregnancy after infertility treatment

Contributors

Mona Aboulghar, MD, MBCH
Assistant Professor, Department of Obstetrics and Gynecology, Cairo University; IVF Consultant, The Egyptian IVF Center, Maadi, Cairo, Egypt

Mostafa Abuzeid, MD, FACOG, FRCOG
Director of the Division of Reproductive Endocrinology, Department of Obstetrics and Gynecology, Hurley Medical Center, Flint, Michigan; Practice Director, IVF Michigan, Rochester Hills, Michigan; Professor, Department of Obstetrics and Gynecology, Michigan State University College of Human Medicine, East Lansing, Michigan, USA

Valentine Akande, PhD, MRCOG
Consultant Obstetrician and Gynecologist, Bristol Centre for Reproductive Medicine and Division of Women's Health, Southmead Hospital, Bristol, United Kingdom

Carolyn J. Alexander, MD
Associate Residency Program Director, Division of Reproductive Endocrinology and Infertility; Assistant Professor, David Geffen School of Medicine at UCLA, Department of Obstetrics and Gynecology, Cedars-Sinai Medical Center, Los Angeles, California, USA

Gautam N. Allahbadia, MD, DNB, FNAMS, FCPS, DGO, DFP, FICMU, FICOG
Medical Director, Deccan Fertility Clinic and Keyhole Surgery Center, Rotunda – The Center for Human Reproduction, Mumbai, India

Vicki Arguello, RDMS
Senior Ultrasonographer, Department of Obstetrics and Gynecology, University of South Alabama Mobile, Alabama, USA

Nabil Aziz, MB ChB, MRCOG, MD
Consultant in Gynecology and Reproductive Medicine, Liverpool Women's Hospital and The University of Liverpool, Liverpool, United Kingdom

Osama M. Azmy, MD
Professor of Reproductive Health, National Research Center, Cairo, Egypt

Shawky Z. A. Badawy, MD, EACOG
Professor and Chair, Department of Obstetrics and Gynecology, State University of New York, Upstate Medical University, Syracuse, New York, USA

Susan L. Baker, MD, FACOG
Associate Professor, Division of Maternal and Fetal Medicine, Department of Obstetrics and Gynecology Department, University of South Alabama, Mobile, Alabama, USA

Tony Bazi, MD
Assistant Professor, Department of Obstetrics and Gynecology, American University of Beirut Medical Center, Beirut, Lebanon

Nicole Brooks, DO, FACOG
Assistant Professor, Assistant residency Program Director, Department of Obstetrics and Gynecology, University of South Alabama, Mobile, Alabama, USA

Robin Brown, RDMS
Senior Ultrasonographer, Department of Obstetrics and Gynecology, University of South Alabama, Mobile, Alabama, USA

William W. Brown, III, MD
Director, Ambulatory Obstetrics and Gynecology, Denver Community Health Services; Assistant Professor, Department of Obstetrics and Gynecology, University of Colorado School of Medicine, Colorado, USA

Maria Cerrillo
IVI Madrid, Rey Juan Carlos University, Madrid, Spain

Rebecca Chilvers, MD
Division of Reproductive Endocrinology and Infertility, Department of Obstetrics and Gynecology, University of Texas Medical Branch, Galveston, Texas, USA

Angela Clough
Senior Ultrasonographer, Guy's and St Thomas' Hospital Assisted Conception Unit, London, United Kingdom

Willie Cotten, RDMS
Ultrasonographer, Department of Obstetrics and Gynecology, University of South Alabama Mobile, Alabama, USA

Alan H. DeCherney, MD

Branch Chief of Reproductive Biology and Medicine Branch, National Institute of Child Health & Human Development, Bethesda, Maryland, USA

Aygul Demirol, MD

Associate Professor, Medical Director, Gurgan Clinic Women's Health, Infertility and IVF Center, Ankara, Turkey

Richard Palmer Dickey, MD, PhD, FACOG

Clinical Professor and Chief, Section of Reproductive Endocrinology and Infertility, Department of Obstetrics and Gynecology, Louisiana State University, New Orleans, Louisiana; Medical Director, The Fertility Institute of New Orleans, Mandeville, Louisiana, USA

Essam S. Dimitry, MBBCH, FRCOG, MPhil

Consultant Gynecologist, Heatherwood Hospital, Ascot, United Kingdom

Maria Dimitry, MBBS, BSc

Lister Hospital, Stevenage, United Kingdom

Tiffany Driver, RDMS

Ultrasonographer, Department of Obstetrics and Gynecology, University of South Alabama, Mobile, Alabama, USA

Alaa El-Ebrashy, MD

Professor of Obstetrics and Gynecology, Assistant Director of Fetal Medicine Unit, Cairo University, Cairo, Egypt

Kareem El-Nahhas, MSc

Research Fellow of Reproductive Health, Reproductive Health Research Department, National Research Center, Cairo, Egypt

Amr Etman, MD

Department of Obstetrics and Gynecology, Upstate Medical University, Syracuse, New York, USA

Aimee Eyvazzadeh, MD, MPH

Department of Obstetrics and Gynecology, University of Michigan, Ann Arbor, Michigan, USA

Juan A. Garcia-Velasco, MD

Vice President for Scientific Affairs, University of South Alabama, Alabama, USA Director, IVI Madrid, Assistant Professor of Obstetrics and Gynecology, Rey Juan Carlos University, Madrid, Spain

Tarek A. Gelbaya, MD

Department of Reproductive Medicine, St. Mary's Hospital, Manchester, United Kingdom

Seth Granberg, MD

Professor, Department of Obstetrics and Gynecology, Akershus University Hospital, Lørenskog, Norway

Timur Gurgan, MD

Professor and Chief, Division of Reproductive Medicine and Infertility, Department of Obstetrics and Gynecology, Faculty of Medicine, Hacettepe University, Ankara, Turkey

Levent Gurkan, MD

Department of Urology, Universal Hospitals Group, Istanbul, Turkey

Suleyman Guven, MD

Associate Professor, Department of Obstetrics and Gynecology, School of Medicine, Karadeniz Technical University, Trabzon, Turkey

Lars Hamberger, MD, PhD, FRCOG

Professor, Department of Obstetrics and Gynecology University of Gothenburg, University of Gothenburg, Gothenburg, Sweden

Andrew C. Harbin, MD

Department of Urology, Tulane University School of Medicine, New Orleans, Louisiana, USA

Wayne J. G. Hellstrom, MD, FACS

Professor, Department of Urology, Tulane University School of Medicine, New Orleans, Louisiana, USA

Micah J. Hill, DO

Eunice Kennedy Shriver National Institute of Child Health and Human Development, Program in Reproductive and Adult Endocrinology, Bethesda, Maryland, USA

James Hole, DO

Assistant Professor, Division of Maternal Fetal Medicine, Department of Obstetrics and Gynecology University of South Alabama, Mobile, Alabama, USA; Director of Antenatal Testing, Wellspan Maternal-Fetal-Medicine; Assistant Clinical Professor of OB/GYN, Penn State University College of Medicine, Hershey, Pennsylvania, USA

Yakoub Khalaf MSc, MD, MRCOG

Consultant and Senior Lecturer in Reproductive Medicine and Surgery; Medical Director, The Assisted Conception Unit, Guy's and St Thomas' Hospital Foundation Trust, London, United Kingdom

John C. LaFleur, MD

Assistant Professor, Assistant Clerkship Director, Department of Obstetrics and Gynecology, University of South Alabama, Mobile, Alabama, USA

Deborah Levine, MD

Associate Chief of Academic Affairs, Departments of Radiology and Obstetrics and Gynecology, Beth Israel Deaconess Medical Center, Boston, Massachusetts, USA

Iwan Lewis-Jones, MB ChB, MD

Consultant Andrologist, Liverpool Women's Hospital, Liverpool, United Kingdom

Edward A. Lyons, OC, FRCP(C), FACR
Professor of Radiology, Obstetrics and Gynecology and Anatomy, University of Manitoba, Canada; President, Canadian Association of Radiologists, Manitoba, Canada

Diana M. Marcus, MD
Department of Obstetrics and Gynecology, University College Hospital, London, United Kingdom

Samuel F. Marcus, MD, FRCS, FRCOG
Consultant of Obstetrics and Gynecology, Lead Clinician Fertility Services, Queen Elizabeth Hospital, London, United Kingdom

Mohamed F. M. Mitwally, MD, HCLD, FACOG
Reproductive Endocrinologist, TCART, Toronto, Canada; President CAREM (Canadian American Reproductive Medicine Incorp), Windsor, Ontario, Canada

Hany F. Moustafa, MD
Research Fellow, Division of Reproductive Endocrinology and Infertility, Department of Obstetrics and Gynecology, University of South Alabama, Mobile, Alabama, USA

Manubai Nagamani, MD
Professor and Division Chief, Division of Reproductive Endocrinology and Infertility, Department of Obstetrics and Gynecology, University of Texas Medical Branch, Galveston, Texas, USA

Luciano G. Nardo, MD
Consultant in Reproductive Medicine and Surgery, Department of Reproductive Medicine Manchester, United Kingdom

Mary G. Nawar, MD, MRCOph
Department of Obstetrics and Gynecology, University of South Alabama, Mobile, Alabama, USA

Moshood Olatinwo, MD
Assistant Professor, Department of Obstetrics and Gynecology, University of South Alabama Mobile, Alabama, USA

Lia Ornat, MD
IVI Madrid, Rey Juan Carlos University, Madrid, Spain

Sheri Owens, MD
Assistant Professor and Clerkship Director, Department of Obstetrics and Gynecology, University of South Alabama, Mobile, Alabama, USA

Kathy B. Porter, MD, MBA
Professor and Chair, Department of Obstetrics and Gynecology; Director, Division of Maternal fetal Medicine, University of South Alabama, Mobile, Alabama, USA

Jose M. Puente, MD
IVI Madrid, Rey Juan Carlos University, Madrid, Spain

Elizabeth Puscheck, MD, FACOG
Professor, Director of IVF, Director of Gynecologic Ultrasonography, Division of Reproductive Endocrinology and Infertility, Wayne State University, Detroit, Michigan, USA

Botros Rizk, MD, MA, FRCOG, FRCS(C), HCLD, FACOG, FACS
Professor and Head, Division of Reproductive Endocrinology and Infertility, Department of Obstetrics and Gynecology, Medical and Scientific Director of USA IVF Program, University of South Alabama, Mobile, Alabama, USA

Christine B. Rizk
John Emory Scholar, Emory University, Atlanta, Georgia, USA

Christopher B. Rizk
Rice University, Houston, Texas, USA

Hassan N. Sallam, MD, FRCOG, PhD
Director, The Suzanne Mubarak Regional Centre for Women's Health and Development; Professor and Chair, Department of Obstetrics and Gynecology, Director of Research in the Faculty of Medicine, University of Alexandria, Alexandria, Egypt

Dimitrios Siassakos MSc DLSHTM, MRCOG
Division of Women's Health, Southmead Hospital, Bristol, United Kingdom

Youssef Simaika, MRCOG
Consultant Gynecologist, Coptic Hospital, Cairo, Egypt

Stuart J. Singer, MD
Division of Interventional Radiology, Department of Radiology, Syracuse, New York, USA

Brad Steffler, MD
Associate Professor, Chief of Interventional Radiology, Department of Radiology, University of South Alabama, Mobile, Alabama, USA

Annika Strandell, MD, PhD
Associate Professor, Department of Obstetrics and Gynecology, University of Gothenburg, Gothenburg, Sweden

Sherri K. Taylor, MD
Assistant Professor, Department of Obstetrics and Gynecology, University of South Alabama Mobile, Alabama, USA

Antoine Watrelot, MD
Centre de Recherche et d'Etude de la Stérilité (CRES), Le Britannia-20, Boulevard Eugène Deruelle, Lyon, France

Matts Wikland, MD, PhD
Fertility Centre Scandinavia, Carlanders Hospital, Gothenburg, Sweden

Tony G. Zreik, MD, MBA
Associate Professor, Department of Obstetrics and Gynecology, Lebanese American University School of Medicine, Beirut, Lebanon; Clinical Assistant Professor, Department of Obstetrics and Gynecology and Reproductive Sciences, Yale University School of Medicine, New Haven, Connecticut, USA

Foreword

In his third book, Dr. Botros Rizk has assembled a comprehensive overview of ultrasonography's multiple uses in reproductive medicine. It stresses the recent advances in ultrasonography, in particular its improved image clarity, and its impact on the success of gynecologists and urologists in the treatment of infertility and reproductive failure. A select group of international experts provides a very practical, clinically relevant guide to the diagnostic use of ultrasonography in unraveling the complex clinical conditions that prevent conception. With depth and precision, this book will be of substantial benefit to the generalist as well as the subspecialist engaged in the assessment and treatment of such patients. Written in an easily understood style with frequent clinical examples, the reader will return again and again to this volume for invaluable assistance in the effective use of ultrasonography in the treatment of reproductive failure.

Ronald Franks

Preface

Ultrasonography is both an art and a science that the authors and readers of this book practice and enjoy every day. This ultrasonography book is written for every gynecologist, infertility specialist, ultrasonographer and radiologist who perform ultrasonography daily in the pursuit of precise diagnoses and planned management.

The practice and development of reproductive medicine have been revolutionized by advances in gynecological ultrasonography. In fact, evaluation of male and female infertility has been redefined by the use of ultrasonography and the practice of assisted reproductive technology (ART) has been reinvented. Ultrasound images for every gynecological disease or abnormality encountered during the reproductive years are at your fingertips in this book, which is written by an international group of authorities and leaders of gynecological ultrasound from four continents and eleven countries. The authors have compiled hundreds of original ultrasound images to enrich your experience.

The book has a simple layout in four sections. The first section covers the different imaging techniques such as sonohysterography and hysterosalpingography. The physics of ultrasound as well as the principles of Doppler are clearly explained.

The second section covers most aspects of female and male infertility; common gynecological diseases such as endometriosis, adenomyosis, uterine fibroids and polycystic ovary syndrome are elegantly captured in a series of original images. Male infertility is described in two chapters addressing scrotal and transrectal ultrasonography. Acute and chronic pelvic pain are visualized in a series of cases that are readily imprinted in readers' minds. The third section takes the reader through in vitro fertilization (IVF) step by step. The optimization processes prior to IVF of assessment of the ovarian reserve and hydrosalpinges are also described. The use of ultrasonography for oocyte retrieval and embryo transfer are illustrated in an extensive series of ultrasound images. The final section deals with pregnancy after infertility treatment. It highlights pregnancy failures in the first trimester as well as the variety of ectopic pregnancies encountered. The congenital anomalies after IVF have attracted the attention of both the media and the obstetrician and are elegantly demonstrated. Finally, the most common and serious complications of IVF, namely multiple pregnancies and ovarian hyperstimulation syndrome, are covered in the concluding chapters.

I sincerely wish you, our readers, an enjoyable book that enhances your personal expertise every day.

Acknowledgments

It is a special pleasure to give thanks to whom thanks are due. My interest in ultrasonography started when I shadowed my mother, Dr. Isis Mahrous Rofail, in her gynecology office in Cairo, Egypt in the early 1980s. Every time we performed an ultrasound of a uterine fibroid or a pelvic mass, it complimented clinical acumen. During the first year of my residency in England, I had the greatest pleasure of working with Dr. Dudley Mathews. As the most senior consultant, he took it upon himself to see the majority of patients to allow me to spend time with my patients and to learn how to perform ultrasound well. That year was the most exciting of the last 25 years. During my fellowship in London – training under Professor Robert Edwards, an icon in physiology and reproduction, and Professor Stuart Campbell, an icon in ultrasound and gynecology – each day brought new and exciting discoveries. Professor Campbell opened the floodgates for new ideas in ultrasonography and every month brought in a new ultrasound machine to test. He pioneered transabdominal ultrasound oocyte retrieval, which replaced laparoscopic oocyte retrieval as had been established by the late Patrick Steptoe. When I moved to Alabama years later, I was pleasantly surprised to find that my former mentor in London, Professor Campbell, had initiated advanced ultrasonography in Obstetrics and Gynecology there on the invitation of our Former Chair of Gynecology, Dr. Hiram W. Mendenhall. Dr. Mendenhall had learnt advanced sonography under Professor Campbell at Kings College Hospital London. Our Unit has been a leader in the field since that time.

A special thanks go to every one of our ultrasonographers who have contributed to the images in this book: Vicki Arguello, Robin Brown, Tiffany Driver, Willie Cotten, Lucy Baldwin, Shelley Zimbleman, and Amy Bower. I am very indebted to Mr. Nick Dunton, the senior acquisition editor of Cambridge University Press, for the skill with which he has addressed every stage and to Nisha Doshi, Katy James and Rachael Lazenby for their outstanding production of a highly illustrated book.

Botros Rizk, MD, MA, FRCOG, FRCS(C), HCLD, FACOG, FACS Professor and Head, Reproductive Endocrinology and Infertility, Department of Obstetrics and Gynecology, University of South Alabama, Alabama

The future of imaging and assisted reproduction

Alan H. DeCherney and Micah J. Hill

Introduction

The clinician has many tools in evaluating the patient with diseases of the reproductive tract: patient history, a thorough examination, an array of serum tests, and several imaging studies. In order to obtain and interpret the appropriate tests, the clinician requires a basic understanding of how each radiologic modality functions and which test will best serve the patient. An intimate knowledge of the anatomy is required to appropriately interpret and apply the results of the test. This chapter reviews the basic principles of radiologic tests, reviews basic female anatomy, and provides information for appropriate imaging modalities for each part of the female genital tract.

Technology

Radiographs comprise the majority of radiologic examinations, although they are used less frequently in evaluating the female genital tract. Radiographic examinations are performed by passing x-ray beams through the patient and detecting them on film or with detectors. These beams are either absorbed or scattered, depending on the type of tissue the radiation is passing through. Air and water typically show as black on the film. Bone and calcium deposits appear white. Fat and muscle appear as a faded white or gray color. Contrast agents also typically appear white. Radiographs provide only a two-dimensional view of tissue, often necessitating multiple films from multiple angles to provide a three-dimensional impression.

An extension of x-ray imaging used in reproductive medicine is hysterosalpingography (HSG). As the internal anatomy of the pelvis is primarily soft tissue, it appears black or gray on regular x-ray film. HSG utilizes a steady stream of x-rays (fluoroscopy) to capture images of the pelvis. As contrast material is injected into the uterus, a stream of images captures the contrast material, which reflects the internal anatomy of the uterus and fallopian tubes. HSG was initially described by Rindfleisch in 1910 [1] when early testing was performed with oil-soluble media. As this was accompanied by the risk of oil embolus and granuloma formation, water-soluble contrast materials are more commonly used today.

Computed tomography (CT) is performed using a rotating beam of x-rays which pass through the patient. The transmitted x-rays are measured at thousands of points and a computer then creates an image based upon these data. A helical or spiral CT moves the x-ray tube and moves the patient table at the same time. The colors displayed in a CT image are similar to those on plain radiographs: air shows black, bone and contrast materials show white, and fat shows dark gray while soft tissue shows a lighter gray. CT scans present the images as "slices" or transverse two-dimensional images of the body. In CT imaging the density of tissue or fluid can be expressed using Hounsfield units.

Magnetic resonance imaging (MRI) is obtained by applying magnetic fields to the body. As the magnetic field passes through tissue, the intrinsic spins of hydrogen protons, initially randomly directed, are aligned with the field. Different radiofrequency pulses are then generated by the machine; the hydrogen protons absorb the energy as their spin "flips" to align against the direction of the applied magnetic field. This phenomenon is the resonance part of MRI. When the radiofrequency pulse is turned off, the hydrogen protons return to their natural alignment and energy is released. This produces a signal that is picked up by the coils and transmitted to a computer, which in turn uses the data to generate an image. MRI gradient magnets can be turned on and off in a very specific manner to target the tissue being imaged. MRI produces superior imaging of soft tissue and central nervous system tissue, but is poor for imaging bone and calcium. MRI can even be used to image the heart and blood vessels without the use of intravenous contrast. T1-weighted images produce images in which the fat is white and water is black. T2-weighted images show this reversed, with fat being dark and water being light. With both T1- and T2-weighted images, soft tissue appears gray in color.

Ultrasound images are produced by passing high-frequency sound waves through tissue and reading the echoes. The bladder or a fluid-filled cyst has few echoes and appears dark. Calcium and fat, on the other hand, reflect back high-intensity echoes and appear lighter. Advantages of ultrasound technology include real-time images and lack of ionizing radiation. Doppler modalities of ultrasound allow identification of the direction and magnitude of blood flow. More recently, three-dimensional ultrasound (3D US) has gained application in gynecology. Freehand 3D US images are obtained by manual

Ultrasonography in Reproductive Medicine and Infertility, ed. Botros R. M. B. Rizk. Published by Cambridge University Press. © Cambridge University Press 2010.

movement of the transducer through the region of interest, whereas automated 3D US images are obtained by holding the probe still while the transducer automatically sweeps through the area of interest. 3D US produces a variety of useful views of the organ being imaged, including multiplanar display, volume rendering, and surface rendering.

Positron emission tomography (PET) is unique in that in not only provides imaging of anatomical structures but can also give information on organ function. Small amounts of radiotracer are taken into the body by various routes (intravenous, inhalation, oral consumption) depending upon the organ being imaged. The tracer then gives off energy, which is detected by the PET scanner. Biologic function can be measured by this activity, including blood flow, oxygen consumption, and glucose metabolism.

Uterus

No other reproductive organ involves more imaging tests than the uterus in reproductive medicine. From routine assessment of the cavity for infertility to disease states such as leiomyoma, adenomyosis, and müllerian anomalies, uterine imagining is essential to diagnosing reproductive disease. There are numerous imaging modalities well suited to evaluating the uterus, including conventional ultrasound, three-dimensional ultrasound, saline sonography, hysterosalpingography, magnetic resonance imaging, and computed tomography.

The inferiormost portion of the uterus is the cervix, which is mostly composed of fibrous tissue as opposed to the smooth muscle of the remainder of the uterus. The cervix is usually 2.5–3.5 cm in length and penetrates the vagina at the portio vaginalis. The body of the uterus is essentially a hollow muscular structure that consists of three layers similar to other visceral organs. The innermost layer is the endometrium, which functions as the implantation site for pregnancy. The middle layer, or myometrium, consists of interlacing smooth-muscle fibers and vascular channels. The outer layer is composed of visceral peritoneum and endopelvic fascia and covers the entire uterus with the exception of the vaginal portion of the cervix. The uterine blood supply comes from the uterine branch of the hypogastric artery. The vessels originate at the level of the cervix and course along the outer edge of the uterus up toward the fundus, where they anastamose with the ovarian vessels.

Imaging of the uterine cavity is typically performed with ultrasound technology, whether transvaginal (TVUS), transabdominal, or saline infusion sonography (SIS) or via hysterosalpingography (HSG). Infertility patients have a higher rate of cavitary lesions than patients with abnormal uterine bleeding. In a study of infertility patients, 20% were found to have a cavitary abnormality, including arcuate uterus (15%), polyps (13%), submucosal fibroids (3%), and adhesions (<1%) [2]. Traditional ultrasound may reveal abnormalities of the endometrium or uterine cavity as a thickened endometrial stripe. However, the sensitivity of transvaginal ultrasound in detecting cavitary abnormalities is low. Kelekci et al. showed that transvaginal sonography, SIS, and hysteroscopy had sensitivities and specificities of 56.3% and 72%, 81.3% and 100%, and 87.5% and 100% respectively for detecting cavitary lesions [3].

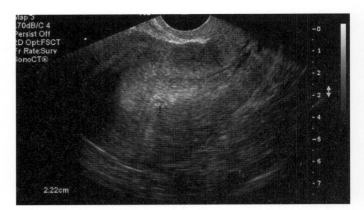

Figure 1.1. Transvaginal ultrasound showing a 22 mm endometrial stripe.

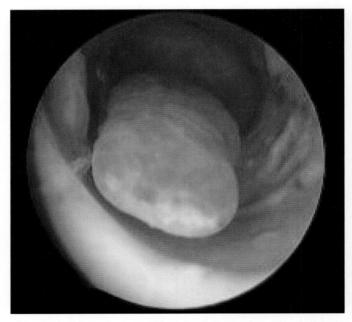

Figure 1.2. Hysteroscopic view of the uterus imaged in Figure 1.1 revealing the TVUS abnormality to be a uterine polyp.

Figure 1.1 shows a transvaginal ultrasound image exhibiting a thickened endometrial stripe of 22 mm. The differential diagnosis on this patient included an endometrial polyp and endometrial hyperplasia. Hysteroscopy (Figure 1.2) revealed an endometrial polyp with complex hyperplasia. While TVUS detected an abnormality, it was unable to provide specificity to the diagnosis. However, the ability of TVUS to suggest that an abnormality was present led to the confirmatory test and treatment, in this case hysteroscopy. Removal of endometrial polyps has been shown to increase pregnancy rates in intrauterine insemination cycles [4] and may decrease miscarriage rates in IVF cycles [5]. The high incidence of cavitary abnormalities in infertility patients and the potential improvements in pregnancy outcomes highlight the importance of a cavitary assessment for these patients. In addition to polyps, uterine synechiae and submucosal fibroids can be detected with these modalities.

The diagnosis of uterine adhesions or synechiae is difficult to make without uterine distension. A thickened endometrial stripe on routine ultrasound may suggest occurrence of synechia in the differential diagnosis. MRI may pick up synechiae as hypointense bands within the cavity. However, synechiae are best seen as areas of nonfilling inside the cavity on HSG or as bands of hyperechoic tissue within the cavity on SIS. While the occurrence of synechia may be strongly suspected on the basis of imaging studies, ultimately hysteroscopy is required for definitive diagnosis and treatment.

Currently, many patients may undergo both HSG and SIS during the course of an infertility evaluation. SIS allows cavity and myometrial assessment and HSG allows cavity and tubal patency assessment. Newer technologies provide the possibility of performing a single test that can assess the uterine cavity, uterine myometrium, and tubal patency. Three-dimensional dynamic magnetic resonance hysterosalpingography (3D dMR-HSG) offers similar tubal diagnostics as HSG with MRI-quality evaluation of the myometrium and other pelvic organs [6]. Another test uses CT technology to offer a similar assessment. Dubbed virtual hysterosalpingography (VHSG) or multi-slice computed tomography hysterosalpingography(MSCT-H), this technology offers similar information on tubal patency to that provided by HSG while providing superior information on the uterine cavity and myometrium [7,8]. These tests have the advantage of causing less patient discomfort and affording more diagnostic information in a single test. However, they are more expensive than either HSG or SIS.

Assessment of uterine leiomyoma is historically achieved with ultrasonography, although CT and MRI also offer detection of uterine fibroids. For intramural fibroids, transvaginal ultrasound offers good diagnostic capabilities. When a submucosal fibroid is suspected, SIS can characterize the size and cavity involvement. Recently, 3D ultrasound was found to have similar diagnostic capability to hysteroscopy. The advantage of 3D ultrasound over 2D imaging is a more accurate measurement of intramural versus submucosal involvement of the leiomyoma [9]. This information may be useful to the surgeon in determining whether to employ a hysteroscopic or an abdominal route to myomectomy.

MRI is superior to CT in imaging of soft tissue, as sensitive in identifying fibroids as TVUS, and is superior to TVUS for mapping fibroids, especially when they are large and multiple [10]. The signal intensity of T2- and T1-weighted images provides additional architectural information [11]. Low T2 signal intensity is associated with hyalinization, whereas increased T2 intensity is associated with edema and myxoid degeneration. Cystic degeneration lacks enhancement and has low T1 intensity with high T2 intensity. Hemorrhagic infarction can appear as a high-intensity T1 signal on the periphery of the lesion and a low-intensity T2 signal inside. Ultrasound remains the most cost-effective screening modality for uterine fibroids. When more information is needed on the location and architecture of a fibroid, MRI is an effective secondary imaging modality.

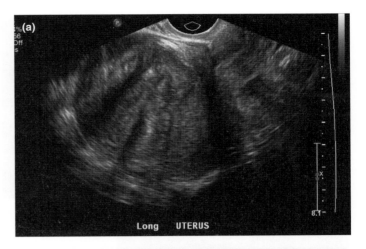

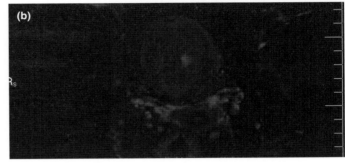

Figure 1.3. (a) Ultrasound shows the appearance of uterine leiomyoma. (b) MRI confirms the suspected diagnosis.

In Figures 1.3 and 1.4, various uterine imaging techniques are shown for a patient with hereditary leiomyomatosis and renal cell cancer (HLRCC), an autosomal dominant syndrome typified by renal cell carcinoma and uterine leiomyomas and an increased risk of leiomyosarcoma. Figure 1.3a shows a very typical appearance of a leiomoyoma on ultrasound, with a heterogeneous swirling pattern in the tissue. On MRI, the lesion was confirmed to be a single and large uterine fibroid as suspected from ultrasound (Figure 1.3b). In HLRCC, the underlying disease is caused by mutations in the fumarate hydratase gene. This gene encodes for an enzyme in the Krebs cycle and affected cells show abnormalities in energy metabolism. Leiomyomas in HLRCC patients show significant uptake of fluorodeoxyglucose (FDG) on PET scan (Figure 1.4). This is in contrast to the majority of leiomyomas which show no FDG activity. Whether PET scan uptake of FDG has any predictive value for the behavior of fibroids is unknown.

In the management of uterine fibroids, radiologic technology is moving from the realm of diagnostics into the realm of treatment. Uterine artery embolization (UAE) is an interventional procedure wherein the uterine vessels are embolized. While it is an effective treatment for some women with menorrhagia, it is not recommended for patients desiring fertility and currently does not have a role in reproductive medicine. MRI-guided focused ultrasound surgery (MRgFUS) identifies

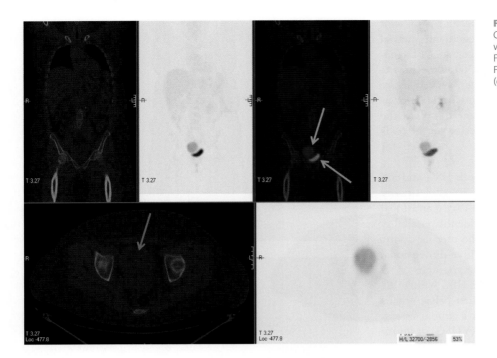

Figure 1.4. PET-CT images of the patient in Figure 3. CT shows the appearance of the fibroid (blue arrow) with less architectural information than the MRI in Figure 1.3. The fibroid shows significant uptake of FDG (orange arrow) and is distinct from the bladder (green arrow).

the fibroids with MRI and utilizes transabdominal ultrasound waves to cause thermoablation [12]. Two case reports have identified successful pregnancies after this treatment [13,14]. While this technology is still investigational, it may represent a viable alternative to the surgical risks and adhesion formation associated with abdominal myomectomy.

Adenomysois is a cause of dysmenorrhea and menorrhagia. Recent data suggest that up to 90% of infertile women with endometriosis have concurrent adenomyosis [15]. Adenomyosis can be identified with either TVUS or MRI, although MRI is more accurate [16]. On ultrasound, adenomyosis appears as an asymmetry and thickening of the uterine walls. Adenomyosis is also suspected when a poorly defined, heterogeneous area is seen with either increased or decreased echogenicity [11]. On MRI, a diagnosis of adenomyosis is made with a thickened junctional zone on T2-weighted images or an area with low T1 and T2 signal intensity and indistinct margins [11]. MRI is the imaging of choice when differentiating between adenomyosis and leiomyosis, although diffuse adenomysois may overlap with fibroids and become difficult to differentiate [17]. MRgFUS has been used to treat one patient with adenomyosis who subsequently had a successful pregnancy [13].

Müllerian anomalies are congenital defects in the development of the uterus and upper vagina. Suspicion of a müllerian anomaly typically arises in response to an abnormal screening test, such as HSG or ultrasound. While HSG and ultrasound are effective at defining normal anatomy, they lack specificity in diagnosing müllerian anomalies. For example, HSG may show a filling defect in the caudal midline of the uterus, but cannot definitively differentiate between a septum, bicornuate, or arcuate uterus. For definitive classification of a müllerian anomaly, MRI is typically indicated. The ability of this test to define soft

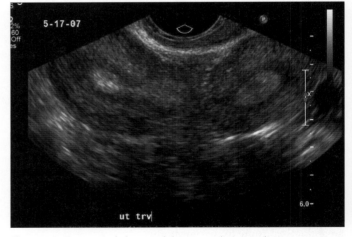

Figure 1.5. Transvaginal ultrasound shows two distinct and separate endometrial stripes approaching the uterine fundus.

tissue (such as endometrium versus myometrium) allows for accurate description of the anomaly.

Figures 1.5–1.10 show patients with congenital anomalies of the uterus. The first is an infertility patient thought to have a bicornuate uterus on routine screening transvaginal ultrasound (Figure 1.5). Routine 2D US can lack specificity if differentiating arcuate, bicornuate, and septated uteri. The diagnosis was confirmed with a 3D ultrasound (Figure 1.6), which provides a much better three-dimensional analysis of the uterus. MRI has historically been the gold standard radiologic test for uterine anomalies and combined laparoscopy and hysteroscopy the definitive test. Figures 1.7–1.10 show various images from patients with uterine septi both preoperatively and postoperatively. In the first patient, screening TVUS

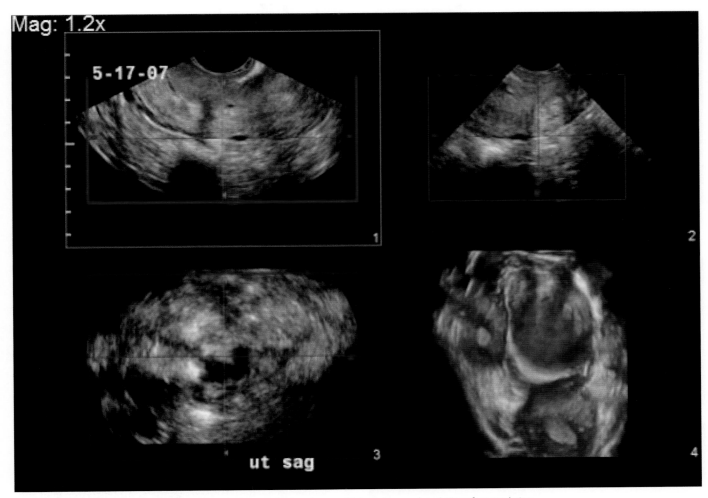

Figure 1.6. Multiplanar display of a septated uterus. Images displayed are sagittal, axial, coronal, and 3D surface rendering.

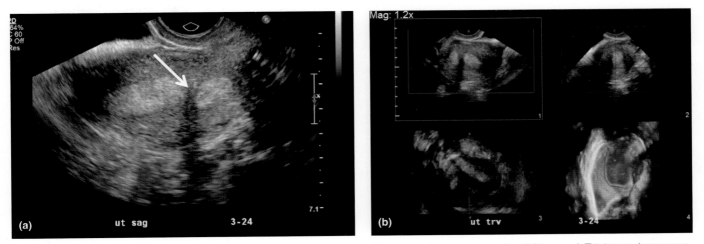

Figure 1.7. 2D and 3D TVUS views of a thick uterine septum. (a) 2D TVUS reviews a defect separating the endometrium (white arrow). This image alone cannot differentiate between septum, bicornuate, and arcuate uterus. (b) Multiplanar images (sagittal, axial, coronal, and 3D rendering) of the septum.

revealed a defect in the endometrium thought to represent a uterine septum (Figure 1.7a) and this was again confirmed with 3D US (Figure 1.7b). MRI further defined this very thick muscular septum (Figure 1.8a,b). Postoperative views of a different patient with a septum in Figure 1.9 show persistence of the septum at the cervix with absence of the septum in the uterine cavity itself. Finally, an intraoperative saline infusion sonogram (Figure 1.10), confirms resection of the septum within the uterine cavity.

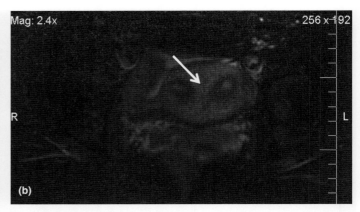
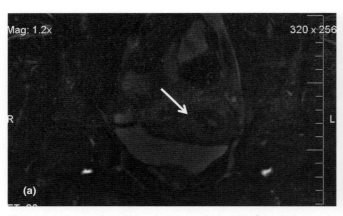

Figure 1.8. A coronal view (a) and axial view (b) by MRI of the thick muscular uterine septum (white arrows).

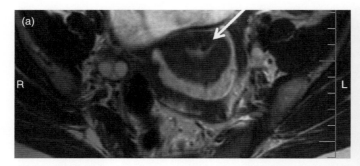

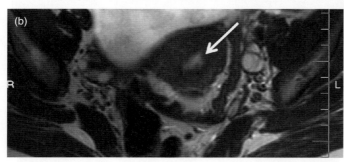

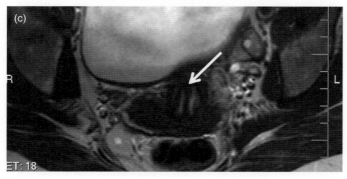

Figure 1.9. Three MRI T2-weighted axial views of the uterus from the fundus (a), mid-uterus (b), and the cervix (c). The patient had undergone resection of a uterine septum. The remaining portion of the septum at the fundus (top white arrow) is typical as the resection is often stopped prior to entry to the myometrium in an effort to avoid perforation. The middle arrow shows no evidence of septum in the main portion of the uterine cavity. The bottom white arrow shows persistence of the septum at the level of the cervix.

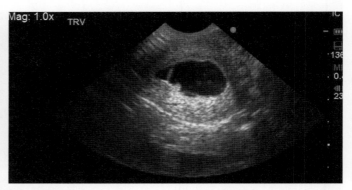

Figure 1.10. Intraoperative SIS showing resection of the septum with a small amount of fundal debris.

Müllerian agenesis appears as the complete absence of uterine tissue between the bladder and the rectum with a blind-ending vaginal pouch. A unicornuate uterus shows normal endometrial and myometrial tissue, but in a banana shape typically bending toward a unilateral side. MRI can also detect the presence of communicating and noncommunicating accessory horns. A didelphic uterus appears as two distinct uteri with normal zonal anatomy and decreased volume. Two distinct cervixes may also be seen (bicolis). A bicornuate uterus appears as two separate uterine fundi with a communicating endometrium at some point in the midline. The joining of the endometrium and often a fundal indentation in the myometrium separates the bicornuate uterus from the didelphic and septated uterus. A uterine septum typically appears as a low-signal intensity T2 band compared with the myometrium. The external surface of the septated uterus is typically convex compared with the bicornuate uterus. Diethylstilbestrol (DES) exposure is seen with a T-shaped hypoplastic uterus and is easily noted on both MRI and HSG. For evaluation of müllerian anomalies, MRI is currently the modality of choice [17]. As renal and skeletal anomalies can occur in conjunction with müllerian anomalies, additional imaging is also warranted.

Currently ultrasound plays a role in monitoring the uterus during ovarian stimulation and early pregnancy, although the role of uterine monitoring may be less important than ovarian monitoring. It appears that the initial endometrial thickness is not predictive of IVF pregnancy outcomes but that the change in endometrial thickness on day 6 of gonadotropins is predictive of pregnancy rates [18].

After any form of ovarian stimulation or the use of assisted reproductive technology, it is incumbent upon the clinician to insure that an intrauterine pregnancy has resulted. In the presence of a positive serum or urine hCG (human chorionic gonadotropin) test, well-defined progression of ultrasound findings should ensue. Absence of these sonographic milestones in concert with aberrant hCG trends may suggest ectopic pregnancy or an abnormal uterine gestation. Early pregnancy is best assessed through transvaginal ultrasound. Imaging that utilizes ionizing radiation is unnecessary and is discouraged.

The first sign of intrauterine pregnancy is the gestational sac, a small hypoechoic area that can be detected at 2–3 mm. A small gestational sac is not diagnostic of intrauterine gestation, as ectopic pregnancy can be associated with an intrauterine pseudogestational sac. Gestational sac size should be measured in three dimensions and averaged to give a mean sac diameter (MSD). The next sonographic finding of a normal gestation is the appearance of the yolk sac, a hyperechoic ring within the gestation sac which should be visible with a MSD of 8 mm. When the MSD is 16 mm, the presence of an embryo with cardiac activity should be seen [19]. Transvaginal ultrasound will detect a singleton fetal pole when the hCG is between 1500 and 2000 (mIU/ml). The specific value should be determined individually at each institution, and is dependent upon the machines used and the experience of the sonographer. Finally, while there are many guidelines and milestones in use for early pregnancy ultrasonography, it should be emphasized that these are typically based upon singleton gestation data. In the USA in 2005, 37% of all live births from ART were multiple gestations [20]. Sonographic and hCG milestones for multiple gestations are not well established.

Ovaries

The ovaries are paired organs suspended bilaterally to the uterus via the utero-ovarian ligaments and to the pelvic sidewall via the infundibulo-pelvic ligaments. The ovary itself is composed of germ cells, stromal cells, and epithelium. Antral follicles are visible as small cysts within the ovary. Stromal cells around the follicles secrete androgens and estrogens. Ovarian stroma appears heterogeneous and mildly hyperechoic on ultrasound, whereas follicles are hypoechoic.

Historically, the diagnosis of polycystic ovary syndrome (PCOS) was based upon ultrasound findings such as a "string of pearls" appearance of the antral follicles. The 2003 revised Rotterdam criteria for PCOS include the "presence of 12 or more follicles in each ovary measuring 2 ± 9 mm in diameter, and/or increased ovarian volume (>10 ml)" [21]. An assessment of ovarian follicles is best made with transvaginal ultrasound. A three-dimensional volumetric measurement can also be obtained easily with ultrasound. These ultrasound findings together with the clinical criteria of anovulation or oligo-ovulation

and hyperandrogenism define PCOS. While the ovarian measurements are important to the Rotterdam criteria, the clinical manifestations of PCOS remain the essential features of the disease.

Ultrasonography of the ovary also has a role in assisted reproductive technologies' (ART) monitoring and prediction of success. Baseline characteristics and changes in follicle size during ovarian stimulation are readily measured via transvaginal ultrasound. Antral follicles are small hypoechoic structures within the ovary and typically measure between 2 and 10 mm. A basal count (BAFC) can be measured in the early follicular phase or after pituitary downregulation. Several studies suggest that the basal antral follicle count is predictive of ovarian response to gonadotropins and correlates with pregnancy rates [22,23]. In a meta-analysis by Hendriks et al., receiver operator curves showed basal antral follicle count (BAFC) as outperforming FSH in predicting poor response to ovarian stimulation [24]. Both tests performed poorly in predicting pregnancy. Ovarian volume also correlates with stimulation parameters and is predictive of cycle cancellation when <20 mm [22]. Many ART programs employ TVUS ovarian monitoring in concert with serum estradiol levels to manage gonadotropin stimulation, hCG injection timing, and oocyte retrieval. Such monitoring gives knowledge of the number of growing follicles and their individual size.

In addition to ART monitoring, basal ovarian ultrasound is often assessed prior to any form of ovarian stimulation. Ovarian cysts may have a negative effect on ovarian stimulation and can occur in up to 18% of patients. In one study, patients with ovarian cysts greater than 10 mm ovulated 81% of the time on clomiphene citrate as compared with 97% in the group without cysts [25]. A screening evaluation of the ovary for cysts over 1 cm may be indicated before ovarian stimulation.

It should be noted that the role of ovarian imaging is much broader in the context of gynecology and oncology than presented here. In general, the first-line imaging role for any suspected ovarian mass should be transvaginal ultrasound. Ultrasound provides a superior evaluation and characterization of the ovaries and is less expensive than other modalities. However, there are scenarios where other modalities, such as CT or MRI, provide important information for the oncologist and gynecologist.

Fallopian tubes

The fallopian tubes serve as a hollow conduit to transport oocytes from the peritoneal cavity to the uterus. The tubes are typically 10–14 cm in length and divided into regions: interstitial, isthmic, ampullary, infundibulum and ending in fimbria. In reproductive medicine, imaging of the tubes is typically limited to evaluation of patency and distortion of normal anatomy, as in hydrosalpinges and salpingitis isthmica nodosum.

Evaluation of tubal patency is a routine step in the infertility evaluation. This is most easily performed with hysterosalpingography (HSG). HSG provides a series of fluoroscopic x-ray images to show the filling of the fallopian tubes and the passage of contrast material into the peritoneal cavity. Passage of contrast medium confirms patency of the tubes. Filling of the tube with contrast but without spillage indicates distal tubal disease. Filling of the uterus but without contrast fill of the fallopian tube indicates either proximal disease or tubal spasm. Premedication with antispasmodic agents prior to the procedure may reduce tubal spasm. HSG not only provides information on tubal patency, but can also assess the tubes for disease. Salpingitis isthmica nodosa (SIN) can appear as a honeycomb appearance of the contrast. Other abnormalities which have been detected by HSG include müllerian anomalies, uterine cancer, leiomyoma, DES exposure, adenomyosis, synechia, and tubal polyps [26].

As mentioned under uterine imaging, research has evaluated CT and MRI technology for combined uterine and tubal patency studies. The early data on these studies suggest it is effective for tubal imaging. However, routine use of this technology is limited by its cost.

Ultrasonographic evaluation of the fallopian tubes is often difficult in the absence of significant pathology. The exception to this is for hydrosalpinges. If the HSG shows a dilated tube, this could be secondary to distal obstruction with iatrogenic tubal contrast filling or due to hydrosalpinges. For patients who will undergo IVF, this distinction is important. On ultrasound, a hydrosalpinx will appear as a "sausage-shaped" hypoechoic area between the uterine cornua and the ovary. In a meta-analysis, Zeyneloglu et al. showed that patients with hydrosalpinges had 50% lower implantation rates and ongoing pregnancy rates than patients without hydrosalpinges [27]. For patients undergoing IVF, ultrasonography of the fallopian tubes to assess for hydrosalpinges is warranted.

Lower genital tract

The lower genital tract consists of the structures of the vulva and the lower portion of the vagina. The vulva contains the mons pubis, labia majorum and minorum, hymen, urethra, clitoris, vestibular bulbs, and Skene's and Bartholin's glands. The mons pubis is a fatty eminence overlying the symphysis pubis. The hymen is a thin membrane of squamous epithelium at the vaginal opening that is present in varying degrees in childhood. The clitoris is located at the superior aspect of the vestibule and is composed of vascular channels that function as erectile tissue. The urethra is also located in the superior vestibule, located inferior and internal to the clitoris. It is typically 3–5 cm in length and serves as a conduit of urine from the bladder to the outside of the body. Located adjacent to the distal urethra are the Skene's glands (para-urethral glands), which are the homologue to the male prostate. Bartholin's ducts open between the hymen and the labia minora and serve to drain the Bartholin's glands, which are located posterolateral to the vagina near the introitus.

The lower genital tract is separate from the remainder of the female reproductive tract embryologically. The clitoris develops from the genital tubercle, the labium from the genital folds, and the vestibule from the urogenital sinus. The urogenital sinus must meet with the müllerian ducts and undergo a process of fusion, elongation, and canalization. Whereas the gynecologist and oncologist may have numerous diseases of the lower genital tract to evaluate and treat, the majority of consultations in reproductive medicine involve improper fusion of the müllerian duct and urogenital sinus.

The most common clinical scenario involving lower genital tract imaging for the reproductive clinician entails the imperforate hymen. On examination, the clinician encounters a blocked vagina, anywhere from the level of the hymen up to the uterus. In most cases the location of the obstructing tissue and findings on physical examination often differentiate the imperforate hymen from the transverse vaginal septum, although addition imaging may be needed. If physical examination alone is insufficient, ultrasound can determine whether the uterus is present and evaluate for hematocolpos. Ultimately, MRI may be necessary in complex cases or those involving müllerian anomalies. CT scans can evaluate Skene's duct cysts and ureteral diverticula. In reproductive medicine, physical examination is typically adequate for lower urinary tract evaluation.

Pituitary

The pituitary gland is a roundish organ located at the base of the skull in the sella turcica. The pituitary is located inferior to the hypothalamus and the optic chiasm, which it may compress when it enlarges. The anterior pituitary secretes hormones in response to pituitary release hormones. The posterior pituitary consists of hypothalamic neurons which release antidiuretic hormone and oxytocin.

Pituitary imaging is mostly performed in reproductive medicine for the infertile patient with persistently elevated prolactin levels or with levels over 100 ng/ml. Although prolactin levels correlate with the size of pituitary adenomas, macroadenomas may present with only moderate elevations in prolactin [28]. MRI imaging appears to be superior to CT evaluation and has replaced the historical coned-down radiographic view for imaging of the sella turcica [29]. Microadenomas by definition are less than 10 mm in maximal dimension whereas macroadenomas are 10 mm or greater. Adenomas are identified as a lower-intensity T1-weighted signal on MRI [11]. Newer dynamic MRI studies are performed with IV contrast and show greater sensitivity in detecting microadenomas. In these studies the normal pituitary enhances, while microadenomas show only weak enhancement.

Peritoneum

Imaging is rarely performed in reproductive medicine specifically to evaluate for peritoneal disease. Laparoscopy is considered the gold standard for diagnosis of peritoneal processes such as endometriosis. CT has been shown to be effective in evaluation for peritoneal malignancy [30]. For evaluation of deep endometriosis, including the peritoneal surfaces, MRI has been shown to have high sensitivity and specificity [31]. The ability of these tests to detect very small areas of endometriosis and their broad clinical utility is uncertain at present.

Summary

Imaging techniques play a key role in the evaluation of reproductive diseases and an increasingly prominent role in the treatment of such diseases. The possible applications of newer technologies are promising. Three-dimensional dynamic magnetic resonance hysterosalpingography (3D dMR-HSG) and multislice computed tomography hysterosalpingography (MSCT-H) can offer evaluation of tubal patency with superior imaging of the uterine, tubal, and ovarian anatomy. Positron emission tomography (PET) and computed tomography (CT) scans can be overlayed to provide detailed anatomic information correlated with metabolic activity. Such testing shows increased activity in certain types of fibroids [32]. In addition, PET scans show variation in the uterus and the ovaries during different times of the menstrual cycle. What clinical relevance this has warrants investigation. The future applications of newer imaging modalities are numerous for reproductive imaging, though cost will continue to be a factor.

References

1. Rindfleisch W. Darstellung des Cavum uteri. *Klin Wochenschr* 1910; **4**: 780.

2. Tur-Kaspa I, Gal M, Hartman M, Hartman J, Hartman A. A prospective evaluation of uterine abnormalities by saline infusion sonohysterography in 1,009 women with infertility or abnormal uterine bleeding. *Fertil Steril* 2006; **86**: 1731–5.

3. Kelekci S, Kaya E, Alan E, Alan Y, Bilge U, Mollamahmutoglu L. Comparison of transvaginal sonography, saline infusion sonography, and office hysteroscopy in reproductive-aged women with or without abnormal uterine bleeding. *Fertil Steril* 2005; **84**: 682–6.

4. Perez-Medina T, Bajo-Arenas J, Salazar F, et al. Endometrial polyps and their implication in the pregnancy rates of patients undergoing intrauterine insemination: a prospective, randomized study. *Hum Reprod* 2005; **20**: 1632–5.

5. Lass A, Williams G, Abusheikha N, Brinsden P. The effect of endometrial polyps on outcomes of in vitro fertilization (IVF) cycles. *J Assist Reprod Genet* 1999; **16**: 410–15.

6. Unterweger M, Geyter CD, Fröhlich FM, Bongartz G, Wiesner W. Three-dimensional dynamic MR-hysterosalpingography; a new, low invasive, radiation-free and less painful radiological approach to female infertility. *Hum Reprod* 2002; **12**: 3138–41.

7. Carrascosa M, Baronio M, Capuñay C, López EM, Sueldo C, Papier S. Clinical use of 64-row multislice computed tomography hysterosalpingography in the evaluation of female factor infertility. *Fertil Steril* 2008; **90**: 1953–8.

8. Baronio JM, Carrascosa P, Ulla M, Papier S, Borghi M, Sueldo C. Virtual hysterosalpingography:A novel painless technique for the study of the female reproductive tract in infertile patients. *Fertil Steril* 2006; **86**: s51

9. Salim R, Lee C, Davies A, Jolaoso B, Ofuasia E, Jurkovic D. A comparative study of three-dimensional saline infusion sonohysterography and diagnostic hysteroscopy for the classification of submucous fibroids. *Hum Reprod* 2005; **20**: 253–7

10. Dueholm M, Lundorf E, Hansen ES, Ledertoug S, Olesen F. Accuracy of magnetic resonance imaging and transvaginal ultrasonography in the diagnosis, mapping, and measurement of uterine myomas. *Am J Obstet Gynecol* 2002; **186**: 409–15

11. Imaoka I, Wada A, Matsuo M, Yoshida M, Kitagaki H, Sugimura K. Imaging of disorders associated with female infertility: use in diagnosis, treatment, and management. *RadioGraphics* 2003; **23**: 1401–21

12. Stewart EA, Rabinovici J, Tempany CM, et al. Clinical outcomes of focused ultrasound surgery for the treatment of uterine fibroids. *Fertil Steril* 2006; **85**: 22–9.

13. Rabinovici J, Inbar Y, Eylon SC, Schiff E, Hananel A, Freundlich D. Pregnancy and live birth after focused ultrasound surgery for symptomatic focal adenomyosis: a case report. *Hum Reprod* 2006; **21**: 1255–9.

14. Hanstede MF, Tempany CM, Stewart EA. Focused ultrasound surgery of intramural leiomyomas may facilitate fertility: A case report. *Fertil Steril* 2007; **88**: 497.e5–7.

15. Kunz G, Beil D, Huppert P, Noe M, Kissler S, Leyendecker G. Adenomyosis in endometriosis – prevalence and impact on fertility. Evidence from magnetic resonance imaging. *Hum Reprod* 2005; **20**: 2309–16.

16. Ascher SM, Arnold LL, Patt RH, et al. Adenomyosis: prospective comparison of MR imaging and transvaginal sonography. *Radiology* 1994; **190**: 803–6.

17. Reinhold C. Pelvic MR imaging in infertility and recurrent pregnancy loss. *International Congress Series* 2004; **1266**: 401–8.

18. McWilliams GD, Frattarelli JL. Changes in measured endometrial thickness predict in vitro fertilization success. *Fertil Steril* 2007; **88**: 74–8.

19. Levi CS, Lyons EA, Lindsay DJ. Early diagnosis of non-viable pregnancy with transvaginal ultrasound. *Radiology*. **167**: 383–5.

20. Centers for Disease Control and Prevention, American Society for Reproductive Medicine, Society for Assisted Reproductive Technology. *2005 Assisted Reproductive Technology Success Rates: National Summary and Fertility Clinic Reports.* Atlanta GA: Centers for Disease Control and Prevention; 2007.

21. The Rotterdam ESHRE/ASRM-sponsored PCOS consensus workshop group. Revised 2003 consensus on diagnostic criteria and longterm health risks related to polycystic ovary syndrome (PCOS). *Hum Reprod* 2004; **19**: 41–7.

22. Frattarelli JL, Lauria-Costa DF, Miller BT, Bergh PA, Scott RT. Basal antral follicle number and meanovarian diameter predict cycle cancellation and ovarian responsiveness in assisted reproductive technology cycles. *Fertil Steril* 2000; **74**: 512–17.

23. Frattarelli JL, Levi AJ, Miller BT, Segars JH. A prospective assessment of the predictive value of basal antral follicles in in vitro fertilization cycles. *Fertil Steril* 2003; **80**: 350–5.

24. Hendriks DJ, Mol BJ, Bancsi LF, Velde DE, Broekmans FJ. Antral follicle count in the prediction of poor ovarian response and pregnancy after in vitro fertilization: a meta-analysis and comparison with basal follicle stimulating

hormone level. *Fertil Steril* 2005; **83**: 291–301.

25. Csokmay JM, Frattarelli JL. Basal ovarian cysts and clomiphene citrate ovulation induction cycles. *Obstet Gynecol* 2006; **107**: 1292–6.

26. Baramki TA. Hysterosalpingography. *Fertil Steril* 2005; **83**: 1595–606.

27. Zeyneloglu HB, Arici A, Olive DL. Adverse effects of hydrosalpinx on pregnancy rates after in vitro fertilization-embryo transfer. *Fertil Steril* 1998; **70**: 492–9.

28. Bayrak A, Saadat P, Mor E, Chong L, Paulson JP, Sokol RZ. Pituitary imaging is indicated for the evaluation of hyperprolactinemia. *Fertil Steril* 2005; **84**: 181–5.

29. Kulkarni MV, Lee KF, McArdle CB, Yeakley JW, Haar FL. 1.5-T MR imaging of pituitary microadenomas: technical considerations and CT correlation. *Am J Neuroradiol* 1987; **9**: 5–11.

30. Shaw MS, Healy JC, Reznek RH. Imaging the peritoneum for malignant processes. *Imaging*. 2000; **12**: 21–33.

31. Bazot M, Darai E, Hourani R, et al. Deep pelvic endometriosis: MR imaging for diagnosis and prediction of extension of disease. *Radiology* 2004; **232**: 379–89.

32. Blake MA, Singh A, Setty BN, et al. Pearls and pitfalls in interpretation of abdominal and pelvic PET-CT. *RadioGraphics* 2006; **26**: 1335–53.

Ultrasonography: physics and principles

Osama M. Azmy and Kareem El-Nahhas

Introduction

Ultrasound examination is now considered as part of almost every clinic setting (Figure 2.1). We will focus in this chapter on concise and simple understanding of the basics and principles of ultrasound, and how we produce an image from sound. Also, we should be aware of the possible risks that ultrasound energy might have whether on the woman or her developing fetus.

Ultrasound physics

Sonar (sound navigation and ranging) is the technique of sending sound waves and detecting the returning echoes to discover hidden objects. Sound is a vibration that travels through a medium as a wave. Sound waves consist of longitudinal alternating high-pressure pulses (*compression*) and low-pressure pulses (*rarefaction*) traveling through a medium (Figure 2.2).

Basic principles of sound

- The *frequency* is a measure of the number of occurrences of a repeating event per unit time, i.e., the number of compressions or rarefactions per second. The unit of frequency is hertz (Hz). For humans, hearing is limited to frequencies between about 20 Hz and 20 kHz. Ultrasound is a sound of a higher frequency (Figure 2.3) than that perceivable by normal human hearing. In the medical field, the ultrasound frequency used is from 1 MHz to 20 MHz, but imaging by ultrasound does not usually use frequencies higher than 10 MHz. Although higher frequencies give sharper images, they are fainter because tissues absorb higher-frequency energy more readily.

- The *wavelength* of sound is the distance between two successive compressions or two successive rarefactions (Figure 2.2). We should note that the frequency increases as the wavelength of sound decreases. The speed of propagation of ultrasound depends not only on its frequency but also on what medium it is passing through, since the medium through which the waves are traveling experiences cyclical variations in pressure. The denser the material, the faster the ultrasound waves travel. For

example, in air sound travels at 330 m/s, in water at 1480 m/s, in bone at about 3400 m/s, and in steel at 5000 m/s. Due to the high water content of tissues, the speed of sound in most tissues is very close to that in water. In fact, all ultrasound scanners are set up with the speed of sound in all tissues as 1540 m/s. Although this is not precisely true, it is a reasonable assumption. The wavelength becomes shorter as the frequency rises; for example, at frequency 3 MHz the wavelength is 0.51 mm, and it is only 0.15 mm at 10 MHz.

- Ultrasound *reflection* is similar to optical reflection. Ultrasound waves are reflected at the boundaries between different materials. Applying this to the human body, ultrasound waves reflect very well wherever different types of tissues meet each other, e.g., where soft tissues meet air or soft tissues meet bones. In a true reflection, the angle of incidence is equal to the angle of reflection (Figure 2.4). No matter how strong the reflecting surface is, it will not be displayed unless the angle of incidence is approximately 90°, otherwise the returning echo will miss the transducer and will not be displayed. When scanning the fetal head, for example, to measure the biparietal diameter, it is often noted that structures such as the cavum septum pellucidum and the lateral ventricles are best demonstrated clearly when insonated at 90°. The *characteristic acoustic impedance* is a property that is specific to an individual material and dependent upon the density of the material and the speed of sound in the material. The interface between two soft tissues has the same acoustic impedance on each side and would result in little reflection. This is of particular importance in practice where an interface between tissues and either gas or bone involves a considerable change in acoustic impedance and will create a strong echo. This is seen in the third-trimester scan when large calcified bones, e.g., ribs, can create misleading shadows behind them. Also, the concept of acoustic impedance explains why we use a coupling material between the transducer and the patient's skin. We need a material with an impedance value that is intermediate between that of the skin and the transducer; in practice we use gel but in principle, any material that

Ultrasonography in Reproductive Medicine and Infertility, ed. Botros R. M. B. Rizk. Published by CAMBRIDGE UNIVERSITY PRESS. © Cambridge University Press 2010.

displaces air from the transducer–skin interface would work, e.g., water.

- *Scattering* is a general physical process whereby sound waves are forced to deviate from a straight trajectory by one or more localized nonuniformities in the medium through which they pass. In an attempt to overcome the amplitude of sound

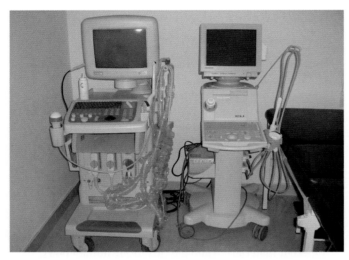

Figure 2.1. Commonly used medical ultrasound instruments in obstetric and/or gynecologic clinics.

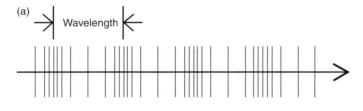

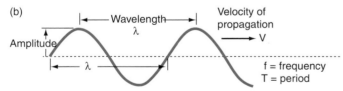

Fig. 2.2. (a) Sound waves are alternating compression and rarefaction of the medium. In the diagram, amplitude is represented by the density of the lines. (b) The relationship between wavelength and frequency. Note that the wavelength can be calculated if the speed of sound and the frequency are known from the equation: Wavelength = Speed of sound / Frequency.

scattering, the use of microbubble contrast media has been introduced in medical ultrasonography (*contrast-enhanced ultrasound*) to improve ultrasound signal backscatter.

- Sound waves can change their direction as they pass from one medium to another (Figure 2.4). This is called *refraction* and is accompanied by a change in speed and wavelength of the waves. It is most evident in situations where the wave passes through a medium with gradually varying properties. Additionally, ultrasound waves will bend when they face an obstacle in their path. This is called *diffraction* and has a strong influence on the shape of the beam generated by the transducer, which itself may act as an obstacle.

- *Absorption* is the direct conversion of the sound energy into heat and always occurs to some extent. It is generally undesirable but is inevitable. Higher frequencies are absorbed at a greater rate than lower frequencies.

- *Attenuation* is the decay of waves as they propagate through materials due to loss of energy, expressed as change in intensity; that is, when sound travels through a medium its intensity diminishes with distance. Further weakening results from scattering and absorption. When the ultrasound intensity becomes one-hundredth of the original value, the attenuation is −20 dB; if it is reduced to one-thousandth of the original value, the attenuation is −30 dB.

- *Focus*: We can reduce the width of the beam to a smaller dimension to produce better images if focusing technique is used. This can be carried in two basic ways: using lenses and using mirrors. The introduction of a lens has the effect of narrowing the beam at some selected depth, although it also causes extra divergence at other depths. The beam depth is inversely proportional to beam width, thus we need to compromise between beam width improvements at the focus point and beam width degradation elsewhere. This focusing technique is now achieved by electronic lenses and also by the curved front face of the transducer. Focusing is applied both on beam transmission and during detection of the echoes. The electronic lens can be set up to receive only those echoes originating from a defined region. However, whereas a transmitted beam consists of a single pulse traveling through the tissue, the received signal can consist of many echoes originating at a range of depths but separated in time. Therefore, a single transmitted pulse will normally result in the generation of many echoes. The focusing of these received echoes can be altered quickly (*dynamic focusing*) so that the focus is swept out simultaneously with the arrival of the echoes.

Fig. 2.3. The different frequency ranges of sound waves.

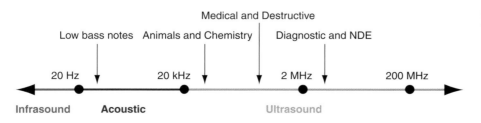

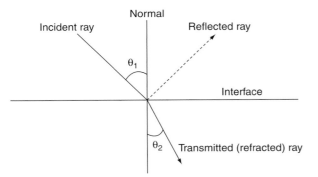

Fig. 2.4. Reflection, transmission, and refraction of sound waves.

From sound to image

The creation of an image from sound is achieved in three steps – producing a sound wave, receiving echoes, and interpreting those echoes.

Producing a sound wave

The transducer (*probe*) is a device that converts electrical signals into ultrasound waves at the desired frequency and vice versa (Figure 2.5). These sound waves bounce off body tissues and make echoes. The part of the transducer that converts electrical impulse to ultrasound and vice versa is known as the crystal or the active element. Transducers are made from materials that exhibit the property of piezoelectricity (a Greek word, *piezein*: to squeeze or press). Piezoelectricity is the ability of some materials to change their dimensions when an electric field is applied to them and conversely to develop electrical charges when they are deformed. Medical transducers are made from a synthetic ceramic material (lead zirconate titanate) that is fired in a kiln and therefore can be modeled into almost any shape. To establish an electrical connection, thin layers of silver are evaporated onto the surface to form electrodes. This device will expand and contract when a voltage is applied to it but will also create a voltage when subjected to a small pressure such as a returning echo might exert. Obviously the voltages generated when receiving echoes are normally much smaller than those applied to create the ultrasound wave in the first instance. The material on the face of the transducer is usually a rubbery coating, a form of impedance matching to enable the sound to be transmitted efficiently into the body. Thus, transducers in simple terms are metallic electrodes attached to a piezoelectric substance that converts electrical energy into acoustic energy when it is "switched on" and acoustic energy to electrical energy when it is "listening."

There are different types of transducers. All types have advantages and disadvantages and no single transducer can perform all functions. There are several classification of transducers. A *linear* transducer is a rectangular-shaped probe in which the elements are arranged in a line and involves a large number of parallel scan lines, whereas a *sector* (annular) transducer has the elements in the form of ring

shape and arranged concentrically. This results in a series of lines that all originate from a single location and travel outward in a pie-shaped wedge. Linear arrays are usually cheaper than sector scanners but have wider skin contact and therefore make it difficult to focus on some organs such as the heart. The linear arrays use a firing sequence of alternate groups of 3–4 elements. A *curved array* is similar to a linear array except that the image created is a sector type. A *linear phased array* applies voltage pulses to all elements as a group but with small time differences (phasing). The time difference is changed each time so that the sound pulses will be sent out in different directions. A phased array results in a sector image and has several advantages such as being smaller in size, the fact that the flat face allows better gel coupling, and the fact that the electronics create high frame rates compared with annular arrays. The main disadvantage is the poor superficial visualization because true phased arrays come to a point in the midline of the probe as the beam is made up of the whole group of elements. This can be overcome by exploiting the principles of phased and linear arrays to form a hybrid called *vector phased array*. Some transducers operate in a burst-excited mode that converts 1–2 cycles of alternating voltage bursts into alternating pressure, resulting in a sound pulse. It then receives echoes and converts them into voltage bursts. Others use a shock-excited mode. These create ultrasound pulses and also receive echoes and convert them into voltage bursts. The most common *mechanical* transducers are the oscillating probes and the rotating probes driven by a motor. These use a combination of single-element oscillation, multiple-element rotation, or a single element and set of acoustic mirrors to generate the sweeping beam for 2D mode. Mechanical probes are subject to wear but produce excellent images. On the other hand, *electrical probes* are not subject to wear but are generally more expensive.

Most transducers are only able to emit one frequency because the crystals have a certain inherent frequency. Accordingly, most ultrasonographers use multiple probes. Multifrequency probes do exist, however. These probes have multiple crystals with different frequencies and a specific frequency is selected by the user. They are convenient because they save time in not having to switch to different probes. Nevertheless, they do have slower frame rates and therefore are useful only for imaging static structures.

Receiving the echoes

The return of the sound wave to the transducer results in the same process that it took to send the sound wave, but in reverse. The return sound wave vibrates the transducer. The transducer turns the vibrations into electrical pulses that travel to the ultrasonic scanner where they are processed and transformed into a digital image.

Forming the image

The ultrasound scanner must determine two things from each received echo. First, how long did the echo take to be

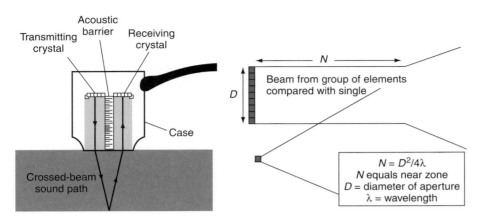

Fig. 2.5. A schematic representation of an ultrasound transducer and the difference in the beam shape between a single-element transducer and an array transducer.

received from the time the sound was transmitted? From this the focal length for the phased array is deduced, enabling a sharp image of that echo at that depth. Second, how strong was the echo? From these two answers the scanner determines which pixel in the image to light up and with what intensity and at what hue if frequency is processed. Furthermore, for the ultrasound scan to operate in *real time* – i.e., any real movement in tissue is instantly associated with a corresponding movement in the displayed image – it has to avoid judder such as can be seen on early cinema movies and the object being imaged must not move excessively between successive views. This can be maintained by a sufficiently high *frame rate*, which is the rate at which the image is updated or refreshed. To avoid judder, the image must be updated at a rate of approximately 25 times per second or higher. Scanners are also equipped with a facility often labeled *frame freeze* whereby the same image is written onto the screen about 25 times a second.

The returning echoes from tissues show a steady decline in amplitude with increasing depth due to attenuation. This is generally considered to be a nuisance and attempts are made to correct for it. The amount of amplification or gain given to the incoming signals is made to increase simultaneously with the arrival of echoes from the greater depth. This is called the *time gain compensation* (TGC) control and is now fitted to virtually all ultrasound scanners. Of course, the assumption that all echoes should be made equal is not really valid. The operator still needs to use the TGC control with care so as not to produce misleading images; for example, excessive TGC can turn a normally echo-poor area within a fluid-filled cyst into one that seems to have small echoes, thereby resembling a tumor.

The layout of the TGC controls varies from one machine to another. One of the most popular settings is a set of slider knobs. Normally each knob in the slider set controls the gain for a specific depth. It is the task of the operator to set each level for each patient and often it is necessary to adjust the TGC during the examination when moving from one anatomic region to another. TGC has also one important clinical application, to avoid *acoustic shadowing* and its opposite,

flaring or *enhancement*. Shadowing occurs when the desired organ to be examined is placed behind another organ that absorbs too much of the energy of the transmitted and received pulses. For example, we may see a break in the posterior uterine wall where it lies posterior to the fetal head. On the other hand, the posterior wall of an ovarian cyst may appear to be very bright because the path traveled by the pulse and its corresponding echoes is largely through cyst fluid, which absorbs very little of the beam energy. In addition, this can also be used to differentiate between some solid masses that are quite homogeneous and whose image can be devoid of internal echoes (i.e. *hypoechoic*). These can be confused with a cyst, which would also be expected to be hypoechoic. Nonetheless, the solid mass is much more likely to be absorptive than the cyst and hence the two can normally be distinguished by the presence or absence of flaring or shadowing posteriorly.

Modes of ultrasonography

Four different modes of ultrasound are used in medical imaging:

A-mode: This is the simplest type of ultrasound wherein a single-element transducer scans a line through the body with the echoes plotted on screen as a function of depth. It is therefore a one-dimensional view. Therapeutic ultrasound aimed at a specific tumor is A-mode, to allow for pinpoint accurate focus of the destructive wave energy.

B-mode: To produce a more useful two-dimensional (2D) scan, it is necessary to obtain a series of A-mode scans and assemble them in a convenient format. This is done either by moving the transducer using a suitable mechanical device or else by having more than one transducer. This second option is preferred in modern scanners and the transducer, which is hand-held by the operator, in fact contains a row (*array*) of many transducers (typically 100–200). In this way, a series of A-scans can be obtained in a closely packed regular format. The amplitude (height) of each echo is represented by the brightness of a spot at the position. This display mode, in which the x and y directions relate to real distance of organs and the use

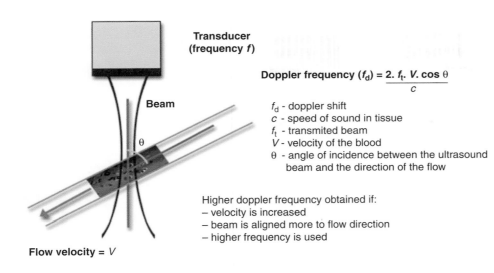

Fig. 2.6. Doppler frequency shift and the equation for calculating it.

Transducer
(frequency *f*)

Beam

θ

Flow velocity = *V*

Doppler frequency (f_d) = $\dfrac{2 \cdot f_t \cdot V \cdot \cos\theta}{c}$

f_d - doppler shift
c - speed of sound in tissue
f_t - transmited beam
V - velocity of the blood
θ - angle of incidence between the ultrasound
   beam and the direction of the flow

Higher doppler frequency obtained if:
– velocity is increased
– beam is aligned more to flow direction
– higher frequency is used

of gray scale to represent echo strength, is known as the B-mode scan.

M-mode: M-mode is a motion scan wherein a rapid sequence of B-mode images follow each other in sequence on the screen to enable physicians to see and measure a range of motion. This mode can be useful when imaging heart valves, because the movement of the valves will make distinct patterns.

Doppler mode: This mode produces an image of flow and is essentially obtained from measurements of movement. In ultrasound scanners, echoes from stationary tissue are the same from pulse to pulse. However, echoes from moving objects exhibit slight differences in the time for the signal to be returned to the receiver – the *Doppler effect*. In general, this refers to a change in the received frequency compared with the frequency emitted whenever there is relative motion between a sound source and the listener. These differences can be measured as a direct time difference or, more usually, in terms of a *frequency shift* from which the Doppler effect is obtained. This shift falls in the audible range of sound and is often presented audibly using stereo speakers to produce a very distinctive, although synthetic, pulsing sound. The Doppler frequency shift (Figure 2.6) depends on several factors:

1. *Blood velocity:* As velocity increases, so does the Doppler frequency.

2. *Ultrasound frequency:* Higher frequencies give increased Doppler frequency. However, this is a compromise between better sensitivity to flow or deeper penetration.

3. *The angle of insonation:* The Doppler frequency increases as the beam becomes more aligned to the direction of flow, i.e., as the angle between the beam and the direction of flow becomes smaller (Figure 2.7). Therefore, the maximum Doppler shift will occur at angles of 0° (*maximum positive Doppler shift*) and 180° (*maximum negative Doppler shift*) and at an angle of 90° there will be no Doppler shift as the cosine of 90° is 0.

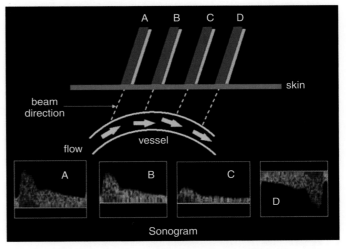

Fig. 2.7. Effect of the Doppler angle on the sonogram. A higher-frequency Doppler signal is obtained if the beam is aligned more in the direction of flow. In the diagram, beam A is more aligned than B and produces higher Doppler signals. The beam/flow angle in C is almost 90° and there is a very poor Doppler signal. The flow at D is away from the beam and there is a negative signal.

Types of Doppler ultrasound flow modes

The Doppler frequency shift information can be displayed graphically in various ways.

● **Color Doppler** (directional Doppler) uses a computer to convert the Doppler measurements into an array of colors. The transducer elements are switched rapidly between B-mode and color flow imaging to give an impression of a combined simultaneous image. Thus, color visualization is combined with a standard ultrasound picture of a blood vessel to show the speed and direction of blood flow (Figure 2.8). The assignment of color to frequency shifts is usually based on direction and magnitude: red for flow toward the ultrasound beam and blue for shifts away from it

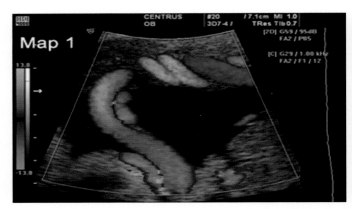

Fig. 2.8. Color Doppler (directional) showing the flow along the umbilical vein and arteries.

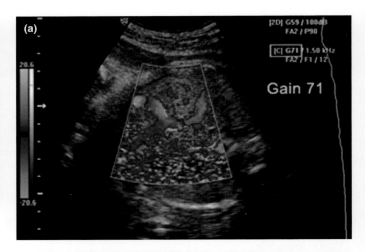

Fig. 2.10. Setting the color gain to minimize the signals (artifacts) from surrounding tissue: (a) color gain = 71; (b) decreasing the color gain to 35.

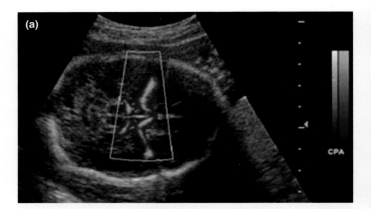

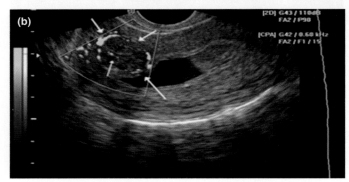

Fig. 2.9. Color power Doppler, showing its sensitivity to low flow. (a) Color power angiogram of the circle of Willis in the fetal head. (b) Color power angiography of a submucosal fibroid; note the small vessels inside the tumor.

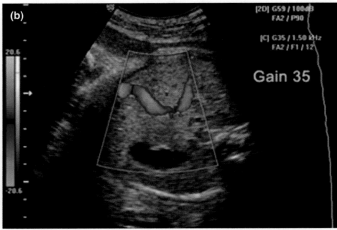

and different color hues or lighter saturation for higher frequency shifts. Color Doppler is very sensitive to low flow (Figure 2.9) and has the ability to render the directional information in different colors (*color flow maps*). However, it gives limited flow information and poor temporal resolution/flow dynamics as the frame rate can be low when scanning deep. The color Doppler image is dependent on the general Doppler factors, particularly the need for a good beam/flow angle. In practice, the experienced operator alters the scanning approach to obtain good insonation angles so as to get unambiguous flow images.

- Other factors that control the appearance of the color flow image include:
  1. *Power and gain:* Color flow uses higher-intensity power than B-mode. The values are set to obtain good signal for flow and to minimize the signals from surrounding tissue (Figure 2.10).
  2. *Frequency selection:* High frequencies give better sensitivity to low flow and have better spatial resolution. Nevertheless, low frequencies have better penetration and are less susceptible to aliasing at high velocities.
  3. *Velocity scale/pulse repetition frequency:* Low pulse repetition frequencies should be used to examine low velocities but aliasing may occur if high velocities are encountered (Figure 2.11).
  4. *Region of interest:* Because more pulses are needed to look at flow rather than for the B-mode image, reducing the width and maximum depth of the color flow area under investigation will usually improve frame rate and may allow a higher color scan line density with improved spatial resolution.

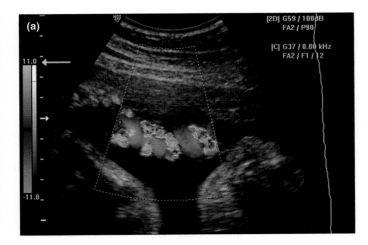

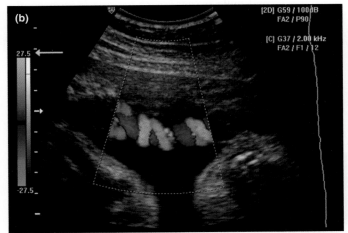

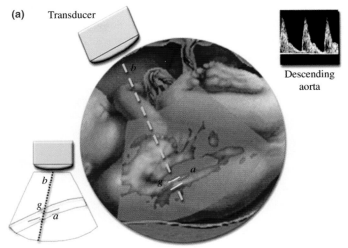

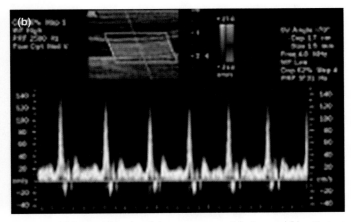

Fig. 2.11. Color flow imaging with effects of pulse repetition frequency or scale. (a) The pulse repetition frequency or scale is set low (yellow arrow). The color image shows ambiguity within the umbilical artery and vein and there is extraneous noise. (b) When the scale is set appropriately for the flow velocities, the color image shows the arteries and vein clearly and unambiguously.

Fig. 2.12. (a) Spectral Doppler of the common carotid artery and (b) setting up the sample volume in a sonogram of the descending aorta. With the angle correction the peak velocities can be measured, where *b* is the direction of the Doppler beam, *g* is the gate or sample volume, and *a* the angle of correction.

5. *Focus:* The focus should be at the level of the area of interest. This can make a significant difference to the appearance and accuracy of the image.

- **Power Doppler** (energy, amplitude flow, nondirectional Doppler) is a technique that is more sensitive in detecting blood flow than is color Doppler. It is able to obtain images that are difficult or impossible to obtain using standard color Doppler. It also provides greater detail of blood flow, especially in vessels that are located inside organs. However, it provides nondirectional information in some modes and has very poor temporal resolution and is susceptible to noise.

- **Spectral (pulsed) Doppler**, where instead of displaying the Doppler measurements visually they are displayed graphically (Figure 2.12). It is used to provide a measure of the changing velocity in the sample volume "gate." If an accurate angle correction is made, then absolute velocities can be measured. Spectral Doppler has the advantage of detailed analysis of distribution of flow and good temporal resolution and it can examine flow waveform and allows calculations of velocity and indices. Spectral Doppler images are affected by the same factors as color Doppler as well as the gate size; a large gate may include signals from adjacent vessels (Figure 2.13).

Since color flow imaging provides a limited amount of information over a large region, and spectral Doppler provides more detailed information about a small region, the two modes are complementary and, in practice, are used as such. Color flow imaging is used to identify vessels requiring examination, to identify the presence and direction of flow, to highlight gross circulation anomalies, and to provide beam/vessel angle correction for velocity measurements. Pulsed-wave Doppler is used to provide analysis of the flow at specific sites in the vessel under investigation. When using color flow imaging with pulsed-wave Doppler, the color flow/B-mode image is frozen while the pulsed wave Doppler is activated. Recently, some manufacturers have produced concurrent color flow imaging and pulsed-wave Doppler, sometimes referred to as *triplex scanning*. When these modes are used simultaneously, the performance of each is decreased. Because transducer elements are employed in three modes (B-mode, color flow, and pulsed-wave

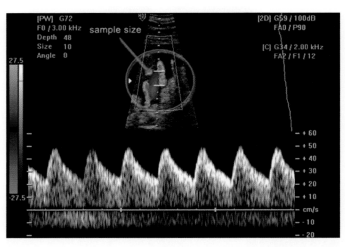

Fig. 2.13. Influence of gate size. The spectral Doppler gate insonates an artery and vein and the sonogram shows flow from both of these vessels. The calculation of mean velocity (arrow) is meaningless since velocities from one vessel subtract from those of the other.

Doppler), the frame rate is decreased, the color flow box is reduced in size, and the available scale is reduced, leading to increased susceptibility to aliasing.

When pulses are transmitted at a given sampling frequency (the *pulse repetition frequency* or the *scale*), the maximum Doppler frequency that can be measured unambiguously is half the scale. Therefore, if the blood velocity and beam/flow angle being measured combine to give a Doppler frequency value greater than half of the scale, ambiguity arises in the Doppler signal. This is *aliasing* and its bad effect can be corrected by reducing color gain or increasing the scale (Figure 2.14). The pulse repetition frequency is itself constrained by the range of the sample volume. The time interval between sampling pulses must be sufficient for a pulse to make the return journey from the transducer to the reflector and back. If a second pulse is sent before the first is received, the receiver cannot distinguish between the reflected signal from both pulses and ambiguity ensues. As the depth of investigation increases, the journey time of the pulse to and from the reflector is increased, reducing the pulse repetition frequency for unambiguous ranging. The result is that the maximum Doppler frequency measured decreases with depth. Therefore, low pulse repetition frequencies are employed to examine low velocities (e.g., venous flow) as the longer interval between

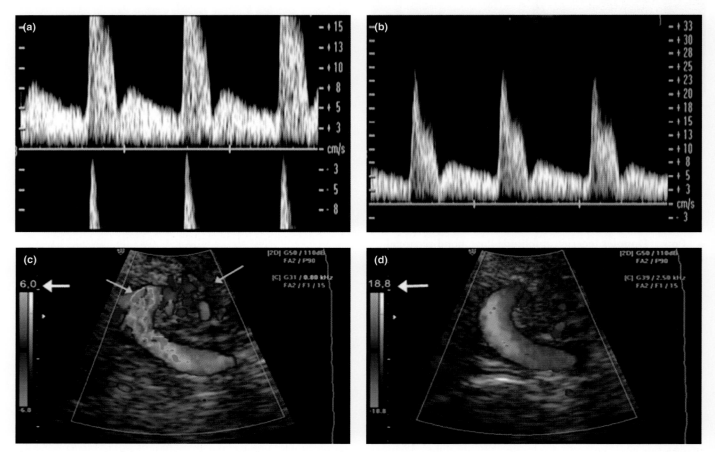

Fig. 2.14. An example of aliasing and its correction. (a) Abrupt termination of the systolic peak, with the truncated part of the peaks showing below the baseline. (b) The same case after correction by increasing the pulse repetition frequency and adjusting the baseline (downward). (c) Aliasing of the color flow (yellow arrows) is corrected by reducing the color gain and increasing the pulse repetition frequency (d).

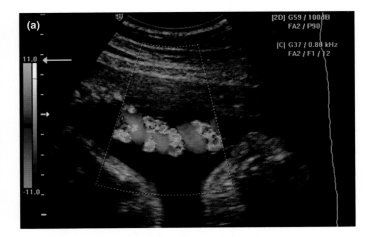

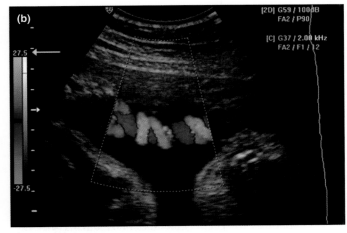

Fig. 2.15. The effects of pulse repetition frequency or scale on aliasing. (a) The pulse repetition frequency is set low (yellow arrow). The color image shows ambiguity within the umbilical artery and vein and there is extraneous noise. (b) The scale is set appropriately for the flow velocities and the color image shows the arteries and vein clearly and unambiguously.

pulses allows the scanner a better chance of identifying slow flow. Aliasing will occur if low scale is used and high velocities are encountered (Figure 2.15). Conversely, if a high scale is used, low velocities may not be identified.

Modes of Doppler waves

In the sonographic community, the terminology "Doppler" has been accepted to apply to both the continuous-wave and pulsed-wave systems despite the different mechanisms by which velocity is detected.

Continuous-wave Doppler (CW), as the name suggests, uses continuous transmission and reception of ultrasound by two separate elements within the transducer, e.g., for listening to fetal heart rate. Doppler signals are obtained from all vessels in the path of the beam until it becomes sufficiently attenuated due to depth. These machines are unable to determine the specific location or velocities and cannot be used to produce color flow images.

Pulsed-wave Doppler (PW) machines transmit pulses of ultrasound, and then switch to receive mode. As such, the

reflected pulse that they receive is not subject to a frequency shift, as the insonation is not continuous. However, the phase change in subsequent measurements can be used to obtain the frequency shift.

Blood flow measurements

- **Calculation of velocity**
  Theoretically, once the beam/flow angle is known, velocities can be calculated from the Doppler equation. Nonetheless, errors may still occur due to:
  (a) Use of multiple elements in array transducers.
  (b) Nonuniform insonation of the vessel lumen.
  (c) Insonation of more than one vessel.
  (d) Use of filters removing low-velocity components.
  (e) Use of high angles (>60°) may give rise to error because of the comparatively large changes in the cosine of the angle that occur with small changes of the angle.
  (f) The velocity vector may not be in the direction of the vessel axis.

  It is good practice to try to repeat velocity measurements, using a different beam approach, to gain a feel for the variability of measurements in a particular application.

- **Calculation of absolute flow**
  Total flow measurement using color or duplex Doppler ultrasound is fraught with difficulties, even under ideal conditions. Errors that may arise include:
  (a) Those due to inaccurate measurement of vessel cross-sectional area
  (b) Those originating in the derivation of velocity.

  These errors become particularly large when flow calculations are made in small vessels; errors in measurement of diameter are magnified when the diameter is used to derive cross-sectional area.

- **Flow waveform analysis**
  This has the advantage that derived indices are independent of the beam/flow angle. Furthermore, changes in flow waveform shape have been used to investigate both proximal disease (e.g., peripheral arterial circulation in adults) and distal changes (fetal circulation and uterine arteries). Many different indices have been used to describe the shape of flow waveforms. All are designed to describe the waveform in a quantitative way. In general, they are a compromise between simplicity and the amount of information obtained.

  The most commonly used indices available on most commercial scanners are:
  1. *Resistance index* (RI) (also called resistive index)
  2. *Systolic/diastolic ratio* (S/D) ratio, sometimes called the A/B ratio
  3. *Pulsatility index* (PI)

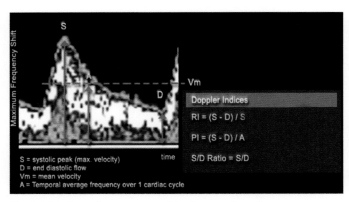

Fig. 2.16. Indices of measurement of the flow waveform shape.

These indices are all based on the maximum Doppler shift waveform and their calculation as described in Figure 2.16. Although PI takes slightly longer to calculate, it does give a broader range of values – for instance, in describing a range of waveform shapes when there is no end-diastolic flow. In addition to these indices, the flow waveform may be described or categorized by the presence or absence of a particular feature, e.g., absent end-diastolic flow in fetal compromise.

Safety issues

Despite its impressive safety record of ultrasound to date, the intensity (or acoustic output) level of ultrasound used to scan the fetus in utero has increased almost eightfold over the level that was allowed in the early 1990s. Therefore, the comfort obtained from the absence of any harm based on epidemiological evidence must be tempered by the fact that there are not enough studies appropriate and adequate for guiding current clinical practice.

On the basis of some concerns about the theoretical effects of ultrasound on the developing fetus, researchers have conducted epidemiological studies looking for associations between ultrasound exposure and various traits, particularly brain development (dyslexia, non-right-handedness, and delayed speech development), reduced birth weight, and childhood cancers. Meta-analyses of randomized controlled trials of adverse effects show only that there is a just-significant increased tendency to non-right-handedness in the offspring of women who have had scans; however, the complexity of the study makes the observation difficult to interpret [1]. Nevertheless, continual vigilance is necessary particularly in areas of concern such as the use of pulsed Doppler in the first trimester.

Ultrasound causes heating, referred to as *thermal and non-thermal effects*. The main areas of concern among nonthermal effects are cavitation and microstreaming, but effects due to movement of cells in liquids, electrical changes in cell membranes, and pressure changes also exist.

Thermal heating is a consequence of the absorption of the ultrasound wave by tissue. Absorption increases with increasing frequency, and the temperature rise caused by an ultrasound beam depends on many factors such as beam intensity and output power, focusing, beam size and depth, tissue absorption coefficient, tissue-specific heat and thermal conductivity, time, and blood supply. The Consensus Report on Potential Bioeffects of Diagnostic Ultrasound in 2007 [2] stated that "Due to the movement of the transducer and of the structures being imaged during clinical examination, the acoustic field remains fixed over a given structure or volume of tissue for brief periods of time, typically measured in seconds or fractions of a second. Under these conditions, the probability of local tissue or organ heating is small and unlikely to be of clinical significance."

Cavitation (bubble formation) is the growth, oscillation, and decay of small gas bubbles under the influence of an ultrasound wave. These bubbles often grow to some limiting size and continue to vibrate at the ultrasound frequency. The growth and collapse of these microbubbles focuses and transfers energy and produces extremely high localized pressures and temperatures that add further stress to cell boundaries. When bubbles expand and contract without growing to critical size, the activity is termed stable cavitation. Unstable cavitation does not occur in the therapeutic range in normal tissues except in air-filled cavities, most notably adult lung and intestine. Luckily, the fetal lung and intestine do not contain obvious air bubbles. Cavitation is limited by low-intensity and pulsed Doppler because there will be enough time for bubbles to regain their initial size during the "off" period.

Microstreaming when ultrasound passes through liquid causes a sort of stirring action termed acoustic streaming. As the acoustic pressure of the ultrasound increases, the flow of liquid speeds up. Cavitation sets up eddy currents in the fluid surrounding the vibrating bubbles and the eddy currents in turn exert a twisting and rotational motion on nearby cells. In the vicinity of vibrating gas bubbles, intracellular organelles are also subjected to rotational forces and stresses. This stirring action, in theory, could occur in fluid-filled parts of a patient's body, such as blood vessels, the bladder, or the amniotic sac. In experimental animals shearing can occur when streaming liquid comes near a solid object, and this can damage platelets and lead to abnormal blood clotting (thrombosis). It is not clear to what extent this effect occurs in humans exposed to diagnostic ultrasound.

Accordingly, the conclusion should always be that the diagnostic procedure should be performed only when there is a valid medical indication, with the lowest possible ultrasonic exposure setting to gain the necessary diagnostic information. This requires self-regulation on the part of the manufacturer and in part of the operator to keep the time limit as short and informative as possible.

References

1. Miller DL. Safety assurance in obstetrical ultrasound. *Semin Ultrasound CT MR*. 2008; **29**(2): 156–64.

2. Barnett SB, Duck F, Ziskin M. WFUMB symposium on safety of ultrasound in medicine: conclusions on recommendations on biological effects and safety of ultrasound contrast agents. *Ultrasound Med Biol* 2007; **33**(2): 233–4.

Suggested reading

Elvy M. Physics of medical ultrasound. http://www.qmseminars.co.nz/PDF/ElvyPhysicsMedicalUltrasound.pdf (Accessed May 10, 2008).

Kremkau FW. (2005). *Diagnostic Ultrasound Principles and Instruments*, 7th edn. Philadelphia, WB Saunders, 2005.

Deane C. Doppler ultrasound: Principles and practice. http://www.centrus.com.br/DiplomaFMF/SeriesFMF/doppler/capitulos-html/chapter_02.htm (Accessed April 20, 2008).

Evans T. Physics and instrumentation. In: Chudleigh T, Thilaganathan B, eds. *Obstetric Ultrasound: How, Why and When*. 3rd edn. Edinburgh, Churchill Livingstone, 2004; 1–15.

Chapter 3

Hysterosalpingography

Shawky Z. A. Badawy, Stuart J. Singer and Amr Etman

Introduction

The evaluation of the pelvic organs and pathology related to them has always been dependent on proper pelvic examination, rectal examination, and external palpation of the abdomen and pelvic areas. That there were marked limitations to such methods of evaluation was long realized by physicians. About a century ago various investigators developed technologies to visualize the pelvic organs. One of the earliest technologies was the introduction of air into the abdominal cavity using a needle, and there was discussion about what type of air medium should be introduced. Investigators started by using oxygen, but they realized that this gas takes many hours to be absorbed, thus subjecting the patient to unnecessary pain and discomfort after the procedure. They replaced the oxygen medium by carbon dioxide and found that within 15–20 minutes carbon dioxide is very easily absorbed into the circulation; patients therefore will not have any lasting discomfort and may go home comfortably after the procedure. The practice of introducing carbon dioxide into the abdominal cavity, producing pneumoperitoneum, developed in association with radiological science. After the production of pneumoperitoneum, radiography is used to visualize many organs in the abdominal cavity, including tumors and adhesions. Contraindications to the use of transabdominal pneumoperitoneum are, of course, the presence of large masses or the suspicion of massive adhesions; the technique is also contraindicated in patients who are suspected of having heart problems. This technique was useful for limited evaluation of the pelvic cavity and for outlining the pelvic organs.

Isodor Clinton Rubin introduced the technology of transcervical carbon dioxide insufflation for diagnosis of tubal pathology [1]. He used an apparatus that allowed him to monitor the flow of carbon dioxide as well as the pressure during the procedure. Carbon dioxide was introduced through the cervix into the uterus using a cannula with a rubber end that fitted onto the cervix and produced a seal with the external os. The carbon dioxide was then allowed to flow and Rubin noted that the pressure usually rose to 60–100 mmHg and then began to drop, indicating that carbon dioxide had easy access through the tubes into the peritoneal cavity and that at least one tube was patent. If the pressure continued to rise, reaching almost 200 mmHg without any drop, the patient started to suffer pain; this suggested that tubes were blocked and the procedure was then terminated. This was an elegant procedure to make a diagnosis of tubal factors in infertility. However, the limitations at that time involved whether one tube or both were patent, which could not be ascertained with this technique, depending on reading the intrauterine pressure with a special manometer. The procedure was supplemented by using a stethoscope to listen suprapubically to the sound of air passing through the tube if it was patent.

Limitations on the use of Rubin's insufflation test include acute or subacute pelvic infections and also the presence of cervical infection as diagnosed by purulent fluid discharging from the cervix.

The principle of transuterine insufflation appealed to other investigators, who introduced modification of the technique for producing pneumoperitoneum, which, associated with radiography of the pelvis, proved more useful in outlining pelvic pathology. Essentially, the patient was placed in the knee–chest position or Simm's position, the cannula was introduced into the cervix in that position, and transuterine insufflation was performed to produce pneumoperitoneum. Certainly if the tubes are open then pneumoperitoneum will be sufficient to show on the radiographs, thus outlining the uterus and ovaries and any pathology in the pelvis. Some uterine anomalies might even be diagnosed by this technology.

Clearly, transuterine insufflation was an important technology that laid the foundation for evaluation of the uterus, tubes, and pelvic organs and was an advance that preceded the use of dyes to outline the uterine cavity and the fallopian tube.

Hysterosalpingography

Hysterosalpingography is a technique introduced by Rubin used to visualize the uterine cavity and fallopian tubes. Many investigators have attempted to bypass this method in the evaluation of the infertile couple, going on to laparoscopic and hysteroscopic procedures instead. However, hysterosalpingography has withstood the test of time as a noninvasive procedure that is used without any anesthesia, and much of the

Ultrasonography in Reproductive Medicine and Infertility, ed. Botros R. M. B. Rizk. Published by Cambridge University Press. © Cambridge University Press 2010.

information obtained is extremely valuable in the future management of these patients.

The procedure is usually done in the proliferative phase of the cycle, preferably in the week following the end of the menstrual period. At this stage the endometrium is still on the thin side and does not interfere with any early pregnancy if the pneumoperitoneum is performed later in the cycle. The procedure is usually performed in the radiology suite with the patient placed on the radiology table in the lithotomy position and is usually done under completely aseptic conditions. The patient is draped with leggings as well as sterile towels on the front and on the back. The speculum is used to expose the cervix and the upper part of the vagina. The cervix and vagina are cleaned using an antiseptic lotion. The anterior lip of the cervix is then grasped using a tenaculum. The tip of the hysterosalpingography cannula is introduced through the cervical canal, producing a tight system. Usually the procedure is done with the help of fluoroscopic visualization via a monitor. In this way, the amount of radiation is minimized and at the same time this fluoroscopic technology allows the gynecologist, the radiologist, and the patient to view the procedure as it is being performed.

Two types of radiopaque solutions are used:

1. An oil-based solution, known as Lipoidol

2. A water-soluble solution

The advantages and disadvantages of these solutions will be discussed later in this chapter. The solution is usually warmed to body temperature before being used. The injection is usually done very slowly and gradually in order to visualize the various segments of the uterine cavity and to detect any pathology as the procedure progresses. The use of warm solution as well as gradual slow injection prevents spasm of the uterus and fallopian tubes. In addition, patients are instructed to take 600 mg of ibuprofen about two hours before the procedure; this leads to relaxation of the smooth muscle of the uterus by preventing prostaglandin release from the endometrium during the procedure. All these precautions minimize pain and discomfort during the procedure and allow patients to go home after the procedure in a very comfortable state.

Two types of device are used to deliver the radiopaque solution to the uterine cavity:

1. A thin, flexible catheter with a balloon at the end. This catheter is usually introduced through the cervical canal into the lower uterine segment and then the balloon is distended with about 1–2 ml of air. This keeps the radiopaque dye inside the uterine cavity during the injection until the procedure is completed. The disadvantage of the balloon is that it obliterates the view of the lower uterine segment and therefore any pathology in that segment will be missed. In order to visualize the lower uterine segment, at the end of the procedure the balloon is deflated and further radiographs are taken to visualize the lower uterine segment.

2. The rigid system, in which a hysterosalpingography cannula with a plastic tip and a rubber cone is used. The plastic tip is introduced into the cervical canal short of the lower uterine segment and the rubber cone is adjusted to fit on the external os, thus allowing a tight system. This system is preferable because it allows visualization of the whole uterine cavity.

Effects on fertility following the use of oil-based compared with water-soluble contrast medium

Hysterosalpingography carries with it a pregnancy rate within several months of the procedure provided that the tubes are patent and there are no other factors involved; the rate is about 30% within 3 months. There are several studies comparing the pregnancy rates following the use of oil-based contrast medium and water-soluble contrast medium. Several studies including retrospective as well as prospective randomized controlled studies have reported that there are more pregnancies following the use of oil-based contrast medium than with water-soluble medium [2]. However other investigators have also found that the use of oil-based contrast medium during hysterosalpingography reduced the time to conception compared with the use of water-soluble contrast medium [3].

There has been debate about the therapeutic value of hysterosalpingography in general and the use of the oil-based medium in particular [4,5,6]. Various investigators have suggested that hysterosalpingography flushes the fallopian tubes and therefore removes any mucous material that might have been clotted inside the tube leading to mechanical obstruction. The other explanation is the theory of immunomodulation as a result of the oil-based contrast medium. The investigators found that this oil-based medium will lead to a shift in the endometrial immune response toward the T-helper type II cells. These cells produce cytokines including interleukin-4, interleukin-5, and interleukin-10. These types of interleukins will certainly help the implantation and prevent the rejection of the embryo from the uterine endometrium. This is based on the fact that diminished secretion of these interleukins leads to recurrent miscarriages [3].

However, investigators also found that there are some side-effects associated with the use of the oil-based contrast medium for hysterosalpingography. These include intravasation of the medium into the blood vessels around the tube and the uterus, which will lead to embolization. Several investigators also found the development of granulomas in the fallopian tubes as well as in the pelvic cavity a month after the hysterosalpingography was done. These were discovered during laparoscopic evaluation of the pelvic cavity and during laparotomy procedures for correction of tubal pathology [7,8,9,10,11,12,13].

In another study to evaluate the effect of oil-based medium on the fallopian tube and the pregnancy rate, the investigators used an oil-based medium following the a water-soluble medium during selective catheterization of the fallopian tubes with obstruction at the isthmic portion. No significant benefit on the pregnancy rate was found with the use of this medium and the investigators concluded that the time to conception might be reduced [14].

Thus it appears from these various studies taken together that the use of oil-based contrast medium for hysterosalpingography might shorten the time to conception by a few months. However, it is associated with some complications that are undesirable for a test that is elective and should not carry any risks. Accordingly, the standard in our unit is the use of water-soluble contrast medium; this gives us the results immediately without any side-effects and patients are comfortable and go home on the same day after the completion of the procedure.

Uterine cavity and abnormalities

Hysterosalpingography allowed gynecologists and infertility specialists to study the uterine cavity, shape, and any abnormalities that could result from either congenital problems or acquired disease processes. The following represents a description supported by actual hysterosalpingograms from cases that we have evaluated in our Division of Reproductive Endocrinology and Infertility. The indications for hysterosalpingography in these cases included primary infertility, secondary infertility, patients with recurrent pregnancy losses, and some cases of amenorrhea following postpartum or postabortion uterine curettage.

Evaluation of a normal hysterosalpingogram starts with the visualization of the cervical canal. Normally it has serrated edges that represent the cervical glands. This will then end in the cervical uterine junction followed by visualization of the uterine cavity (Figures 3.1, 3.2). Normally the uterus, when it fills up with the radiopaque dye, shows a triangular appearance in the majority of cases. However, there are some variations to this picture. In some cases the fundus of the uterus may be convex; in other cases it may be concave. A concavity in the fundus of the uterus might lead to the suspicion of either a filling defect in the fundus or a congenital uterine anomaly. Usually with a filling defect that concavity is irregular. Concavity in the fundus less than 1 cm in depth, as measured from the center of a line drawn between the two cornua of the uterus, is termed arcuate uterus and is considered to be a normal variant of the uterine cavity (Figure 3.3).

In some cases, the uterus is either acutely anteflexed or acutely retroverted, and the picture of the fundus of the uterus will be superimposed on the cervix. This situation will not allow the gynecologist and radiologist a good view of the fundus as well as the cavity of the uterus. In such conditions, we suggest that the gynecologist pull down on the cervix with the tenaculum that is attached to the anterior lip of the cervix in order to straighten the uterus. This is of course made easy by direct visualization on the monitor during fluoroscopy. This technique has been very successful in visualization of the uterine cavity and the fundus and detection of any abnormalities in such situations.

Uterine anomalies

Hysterosalpingography has been extremely useful in diagnosing uterine anomalies. Uterine anomalies are the result of the failure of the normal development of the paramesonephric ducts or failure of fusion of the two paramesonephric ducts.

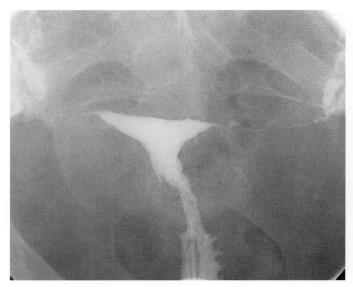

Figure 3.1. Cervical canal with serrated edges representing normal cervical glands.

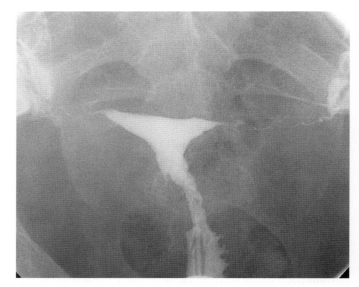

Figure 3.2. Normal triangular-shaped uterine cavity.

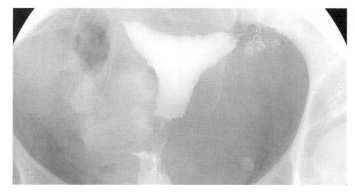

Figure 3.3. Arcuate uterus.

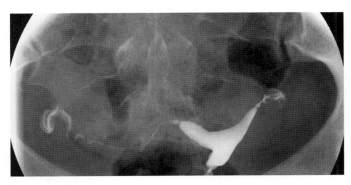

Figure 3.4. Uterine septum.

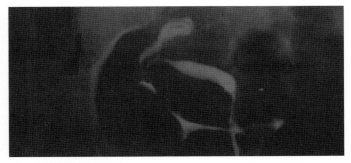

Figure 3.6. Unicornuate uterus.

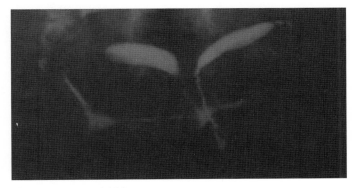

Figure 3.5. Uterus didelphys.

This can result in several anomalies including septate uterus, bicornuate uterus, uterus didelphys, unicornuate uterus, or absent uterus.

The hysterosalpingogram might not be very helpful in the differential diagnosis between a septum (Figure 3.4) and a bicornuate uterus. On the hysterosalpingogram, both types of uterine anomalies have two cavities, well outlined. Some investigators have tried to differentiate between a septum and a bicornuate uterus by measuring the angle of fusion at the lower ends of the two horns. If the angle of fusion is less than 90° then there is a septum, otherwise a bicornuate uterus. These types of angle measurements were used in the past before the introduction of the MRI visualization techniques. In these situations, MRI of the uterus will definitely lead to the correct diagnosis of a septate uterus where there is one uterine body with a septum or a bicornuate uterus where there are two uterine bodies. This is because of the ability of MRI to evaluate the soft tissue and the wall of the uterus very clearly. Therefore, nowadays once we find such anomalies in hysterosalpingography, it is supplemented with an MRI study as a noninvasive technique for the final diagnosis of the anomaly [15].

In cases of uterus didelphys there are two separate uterine cavities, two cervices, and two vaginas due to the presence of a longitudinal septum in the vagina (Figure 3.5). This represents failure of fusion of the two paramesonephric ducts. In order to study the uterine cavities and fallopian tubes in these cases, two sets of catheters are inserted, one in each cervix; following distension of the balloons, injection of the dye simultaneously through both catheters will outline the uterine cavities and the fallopian tubes. Each of these horns will have one fallopian tube. Again, MRI will be indicated to support the diagnosis.

The picture of the unicornuate uterus is usually very diagnostic (Figure 3.6) The cavity of the uterus, as revealed by the hysterosalpingogram, is banana-shaped and has only one fallopian tube, coming out of the cornu. The hysterosalpingogram cannot diagnose the presence of a functioning or nonfunctioning rudimentary horn that developed from the other paramesonephric duct. Again, in these circumstances an MRI will be very helpful in the final diagnosis.

The evaluation of uterine anomalies will help the reproductive endocrinologist and gynecologist to counsel patients about the effect of these anomalies on reproductive history. About 60% of patients with a uterine septum will have no problem with their reproductive career, but the rest of these patients will have problems related to recurrent miscarriages and/or premature deliveries. In these circumstances the uterine septum has to be removed. Historically this was done via laparotomy and various techniques including the Strassman procedure, the Jones procedure, and the Tompkins procedure. Following such procedures, these patients will be delivered by cesarean section. During the past several decades, hysteroscopic surgery became well advanced in our field and has allowed us to carry out various surgical procedures on the uterine cavity in an outpatient setup. The septum can be removed using hysteroscopic surgery with a YAG laser, or by the use of the resectoscope. The advantage of this procedure is that the patients may go home on the same day. Patients also will be delivered vaginally unless there is an obstetric indication [16,17].

Intrauterine adhesions or synechiae

Intrauterine adhesions form as a result of postpartum or post-abortion sharp curettage of the endometrial cavity [18]. The decidua of pregnancy is extremely vulnerable to trauma and infection. Sharp curettage in these cases will remove the decidua and injure the myometrium; the end result will be the formation of adhesions between the anterior and posterior walls of the uterus. The amount of adhesions formed will depend on the injury that was sustained by the endometrium. Most of these adhesions occur near the fundus of the uterus; however, some of them occur in the lower segment as well as near the junction of the cervix and uterus and some occur in the cervical canal itself.

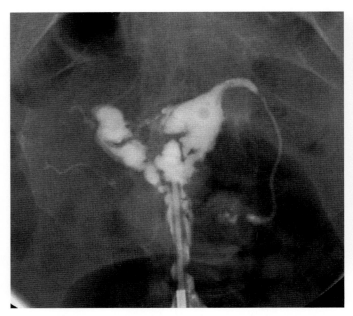

Figure 3.7. Intrauterine adhesions following postpartum curettage for bleeding and retained products of conception.

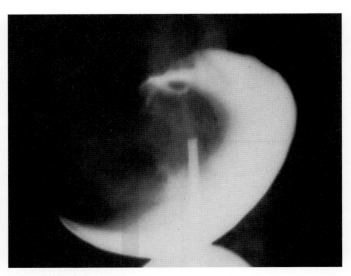

Figure 3.8. Submucous uterine myoma.

Hysterosalpingography has been helpful in the diagnosis of these cases. Of course if the cervical canal and the lower segment are completely obliterated with adhesions, the dye will not be able to penetrate into the uterine cavity and the procedure will fail. If the adhesions occupy the body of the uterus and the fundus of the uterus then the introduction of the dye into the uterine cavity will show these adhesions in the form of multiple linear filling defects, giving the cavity of the uterus a very irregular appearance. In some cases, the cavity of the uterus may be reduced to a very small cavity because the rest of the uterine cavity has been obliterated with adhesions (Figure 3.7).

At one point in the history of gynecology, intrauterine adhesions were common because of the frequent use of sharp curettage in patients with postpartum and postabortion uterine bleeding. More recently, with the use of the suction devices, the products of conception are removed without the use of any sharp curettage, thus avoiding trauma to the endometrium and uterine wall and consequently avoiding the formation of adhesions.

The patients usually have the typical history of sharp curettage because of postabortion and postpartum bleeding. Usually they complain of either oligomenorrhea, or hypomenorrhea and also infertility. Rarely, they may present with a picture of recurrent miscarriages.

The adhesions may be mild, in the form of strings extending across the uterine cavity, but some adhesions can be severe, fibrous, thick, and obliterating the major part of the uterine cavity. The effect on menstrual history depends on the severity of these adhesions [19,20,21]. These cases are treated using hysteroscopic lysis of the adhesions. Following the procedure, patients must be put on estrogen treatment for 6–8 weeks followed by progestogens for 10 days to produce withdrawal bleeding. The idea of estrogen treatment is to stimulate the remaining islands of the endometrium to grow and help heal the sites of injury. Patients also have to be counseled that these adhesions may recur, partially or totally. If pregnancy happens, there is a possibility of miscarriage or the development of placenta accreta, depending on the extent of the adhesions.

Hysterosalpingography in patients with irregular uterine bleeding

Irregular uterine bleeding is not an uncommon phenomenon during the reproductive years. Many of these cases are dysfunctional uterine bleeding that require endocrine evaluation as well as hematologic studies. They are usually treated conservatively using hormonal therapy and many of these cases are cured without any surgical intervention. Some of these cases are due to tumors of the uterine cavity [22,23,24]. Hysterosalpingography has been helpful in the evaluation of these tumors whether they are endometrial polyps or submucous myomas (Figure 3.8). Such cases are treated surgically using the resectoscope when the uterine function needs to be preserved for future pregnancies. The histopathological diagnosis is usually confirmatory and might sometimes reveal areas of malignant transformation, and this will allow for proper management. Many of these cases present because of infertility and the inclusion of hysterosalpingography as part of the work-up and management of these cases will certainly help these patients to achieve pregnancy.

Salpingography

Salpingography allows the gynecologist and infertility specialist to visualize the lumen of the fallopian tubes. Salpingography will identify a normal fallopian tube lumen or abnormalities related to iatrogenic factors such as tubal sterilization or pathology as a result of infection and various kinds of obstructive disease. The procedure is part of hysterosalpingography in which the radiopaque dye ascends into the uterine cavity and then enters the fallopian tubes and outlines the lining of these tubes.

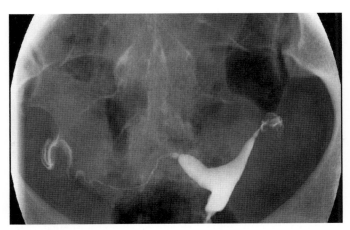

Figure 3.9. Hysterosalpingogram showing the triangular appearance of the interstitial segment of the fallopian tube.

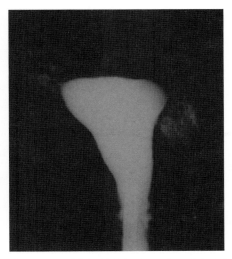

Figure 3.10. Salpingitis isthmica nodosa of the isthmic portion of the fallopian tube.

The fallopian tube is about 10–14 cm in length. It has several sections that vary in size. The intramural portion of the fallopian tube is located in the cornu of the uterus and it is the segment that connects the uterine cavity with the rest of the fallopian tube. This intramural portion of the tube is about 1–2 cm in length and its lumen is extremely narrow, about 0.2–0.4 mm.

The isthmic portion of the fallopian tube is the segment of the tube that connects the intramural portion with the ampulla. This segment is about 2–3 cm in length and its lumen is about 2 mm in diameter. The next segment of the fallopian tube is the ampulla and infundibulum which measures about 5–8 cm in length, and its diameter at the distal portion is about 5 mm. The infundibulum leads then to the fimbriated end of the fallopian tube. The fimbriae are small folds that spread out of the infundibulum of the tube, and their function is to embrace the surface of the ovary at the time of ovulation through a chemotactic action, thus allowing the oocyte to enter into the lumen of the fallopian tube.

The fallopian tube is lined with epithelial lining that has several types of cells including secretory cells, ciliated cells, and intercalary cells. In the region of the ampulla and infundibulum, the epithelial lining forms several folds known as rugae under normal conditions.

During hysterosalpingography and under normal conditions when the fallopian tube is healthy and open, the radiopaque dye travels through the tube starting from the interstitial portion, isthmus, ampulla and infundibulum and then, if the fimbriated end is open, the dye will spill out into the peritoneal cavity. All of this process can be visualized during fluoroscopy. Again, under normal conditions, the interstitial segment of the tube will be seen as a triangular cavity with its base toward the uterine cavity and its apex joining the isthmus of the tube (Figure 3.9). Sometimes one can see at the base of this triangle a small constriction that normally represents the junction between the tubal mucosa and the uterine mucosa. This is very clear to all physicians working in the field of reproductive endocrinology and infertility, as well as to radiologists who have the experience and have witnessed many instances of

hysterosalpingography. This phenomenon of the insterstitial portion of the tube must not be mistaken for pathological appearances of filling defects or spasm of the tube.

The isthmus is usually very thin and flows directly into the ampulla, which under normal conditions will exhibit the rugae suggesting that the mucous membrane lining of the tube is healthy. With the use of water-soluble opaque dyes, the spillage from the fimbriae can be seen immediately by fluoroscopy and under normal conditions the dye flows into the cul-de-sac freely without any loculations.

When we report on the results of hysterosalpingography, we must include description of the various segments of the fallopian tube and not miss any pathology localized to any segment of the tube.

Pathology of the isthmic portion of the fallopian tube

Various pathological conditions have been identified in the isthmic portion of the fallopian tube with the use of hysterosalpingography. One of these conditions is salpingitis isthmica nodosa (SIN: Figure 3.10). This is a proliferative process in which the endosalpinx proliferates into the muscle wall of the tube. The etiology is not known. Some investigators suggested that it is an inflammatory process, and others have suggested that it might be associated with intrauterine devices. The condition on a hysterosalpingogram will have the appearance of a honeycomb form. It is very characteristic but is sometimes missed in the diagnosis as a result of oversight. Salpingitis isthmica nodosa leads to constriction of the isthmic portion of the fallopian tube due to fibromuscular hyperplasia and is an important factor in infertility and also in tubal pregnancy.

Another condition that is diagnosed in the isthmus of the tube is isthmic obstruction, wherein the dye travels for only a very small distance in the isthmus of the tube and then comes to a standstill without visualization of the remaining portion of the fallopian tube (Figure 3.11). The etiology in this condition

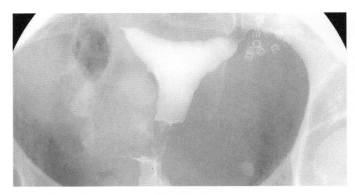

Figure 3.11. Isthmic occlusion of the fallopian tube.

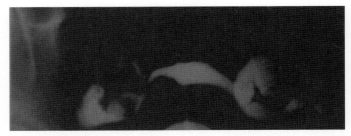

Figure 3.12. Hydrosalpinx.

may be related to pathological fibrosis as a result of chronic infection; in the majority of these cases it is due to spasm of the tube, especially if the patient is under stress or uncomfortable or when there is rapid injection of a large volume of the dye. The differentiation between pathological obstruction and spasm can be accomplished by tubal catheterization under sedation.

Pathology of distal part of fallopian tube

Another pathological entity identified by hysterosalpingography is hydrosalpinx. In this condition the distal end of the fallopian tube, that is the fimbriae, is either agglutinated together or completely obstructed as a result of chronic pelvic infection. Under such circumstances the secretions in the fallopian tube have no exit to the peritoneal cavity and the tube becomes distended and looks like a sack filled with fluid (Figure 3.12). This is a major factor in infertility. In addition to the obstruction of the distal end of the tube and therefore failure of the pick-up of the oocyte mechanically, the fluid inside this tube is toxic due to the presence of cytokines and prostaglandins and will lead to the demise of the early embryo [25].

Sometimes hysterosalpingography also can identify the presence of accessory ostia of the fallopian tube or rarely fistulas between the fallopian tube and other structures in the abdominal cavity.

The fallopian tube is an important anatomic structure that is essential for the normal process of fertilization and pregnancy, involving the pick-up of the oocyte by the fimbriae, the ciliary action of the lining cells, and contractility of the fallopian tube. The oocyte will be fertilized by the sperm in the ampullary portion of the tube. The early embryo then travels through the lumen of the tube into the uterine cavity where implantation will occur. If the fallopian tube is completely obstructed, these stages will not occur, leading to infertility. If the tube is partially obstructed, the early embryo might implant in the tube, leading to tubal pregnancy. Tubal disease is on the rise due to the increase in the rate of pelvic infections and sexually transmitted disease. Early diagnosis and aggressive treatment might prevent any residual effect. However, tubal disease is responsible for about 50% of the infertility factors in women.

Use of antibiotics prior to performing hysterosalpingography is indicated if the patient has a previous history of pelvic inflammatory disease. The test should not be done for 3–6 months after complete cure and until the white blood count and the sedimentation rate are normal. If there is no history of pelvic infection and the procedure is done and a hydrosalpinx is diagnosed, then the patient should be started immediately on antibiotics. The antibiotic of choice in these situations is doxycycline 100 mg twice a day for 5 to 7 days. This antibiotic has a wide range of coverage of bacteria including *Chlamydia*, which is a very serious offending microorganism.

Laparoscopic evaluation of the fallopian tubes is not a substitute for hysterosalpingography. Laparoscopy leads only to the diagnosis of peritubal and periovarian pathology; it does not give the infertility specialist any diagnosis of the condition of the lining and the lumen of the fallopian tubes. Hysterosalpingography therefore remains the primary diagnostic tool for the uterine cavity and the fallopian tube lumen [26].

Fallopian tube recanalization: an underutilized procedure for treatment of primary infertility

Infertility impacts 3.5 million couples in the USA. Fallopian tube disease is the single most common cause of infertility and women routinely undergo hysterosalpingography in the course of the infertility work-up to evaluate this factor. Physiological proximal fallopian tubal obstruction from spasm, mucus plugs, menstrual debris, and adhesion is responsible for infertility in 25–30% of women with fallopian tubal disease [27].

Fallopian tube recanalization (FTR) was first described in 1985 by Platia [28] and popularized in 1987 by Amy Thurmond MD, an Interventional Radiologist from Oregon Health Sciences University, Portland, Oregon [29,30]. The procedure was used to treat occluded cornual or interstitial obstruction of the fallopian tubes diagnosed by hysterosalpingography. The technique was so efficacious that in 1993 the Society of Reproductive Medicine (formerly the American Fertility Society) recommended in its Guidelines for Practice that fluoroscopically guided FTR is to be considered as the initial treatment of proximal fallopian tube obstruction [31]. It is critical to distinguish this population from those with coexisting distal tubal obstructions that require neosalpingostomy.

FTR is scheduled during the follicular phase of the menstrual cycle. The patient is pretreated with three days of 100 mg oral doxycycline twice a day and will take it for two days after the procedure. Typically, 50 μg of fentanyl and 1 mg of midazolam are given intravenously for analgesia and sedation.

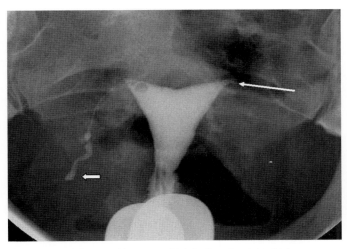

Figure 3.13. A 27-year-old woman with infertility after right distal salpingostomy for ectopic pregnancy. HSG shows distal right tubal obstruction seen during contrast (short arrow); left tubal cornual obstruction in remaining tube (long arrow).

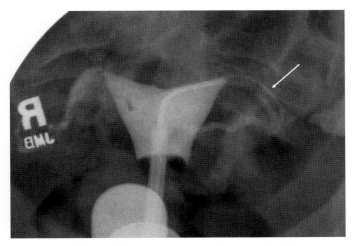

Figure 3.15. Selective left cornual contrast injection recanalized left tube (arrow).

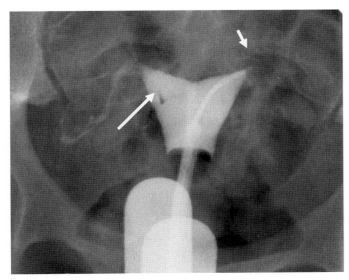

Figure 3.14. FTR one month later shows stable distal right tubal obstruction after contrast injection into the cervical cannula. 5F catheter tip in left cornua. Right uterine linear filling defect from adhesion.

Additional doses are generally needed during the procedure. In our practice, we have the referring gynecologist place and remove the cervical cannula using sterile technique, with the interventional radiologist doing the FTR. We feel that the patient is more comfortable with her gynecologist participating in the procedure. Paracervical block with lidocaine 1% precedes placement of the cervical cannula. Some practitioners use topical lidocaine spray on the cervix. A 14F double balloon cervical cannula (Mencini double balloon hysterosalpingography catheter, Cook Medical, Bloomington, Indiana) is placed into the uterine cavity using a cervical tenaculum and 3 ml of saline is injected into the intrauterine balloon. We usually do not inflate the external balloon since cervical distension is painful. The

malleable metal introducer can be shaped to facilitate cannula placement. After the intrauterine balloon is inflated, the interventional radiologist injects the uterine cavity with Omnipaque 300 (Iohexal injection, GE Healthcare, Princeton, New Jersey). Often, osteal tubal occlusions resolve through overcoming tubal spasm with the higher-pressure hysterosalpingography that can be tolerated after intravenous sedation and analgesia.

After the uterine cavity has opacified with nonionic contrast, a multipurpose 5.5F catheter (Fallopian tube catheterization set, Cook Medical) is placed through the uterine cannula and into the cornu under fluoroscopic control. An angled 0.035-inch hydrophilic guide wire (60 cm Roadrunner PC wire guide, Cook Medical) can help direct the catheter into the cornu. Hand injection of contrast into the cornu may overcome spasm and demonstrate tubal pathology such as salpingitis isthmica nodosa or hydrosalpinx. The proximal tube should be gently probed with the 0.035-inch Roadrunner guide wire to treat osteal and interstitial obstructions from menstrual debris, mucus plugs, and adhesions. If the guide wire meets resistance, it is removed and another contrast injection is made. Hydrodilation of the obstruction often will flush debris or dilate adhesions. If obstruction persists, the next step is to place a 3F microcatheter and 0.015-inch guide wire coaxially through the 5.5F catheter and probe the tubal obstruction (Fallopian tube catheterization set, Cook Medical). The microwire will either pass the obstruction or perforate the tube wall (Figures 3.13, 3.14, 3.15, 3.16). A hydrophilic microwire can be used through the microcatheter as a last resort.

Submucosal tubal perforation is confirmed when there is contained contrast extravasation or the parametrial veins are opacified. Transmural tubal perforation results in intraperitoneal spill of contrast. No additional tubal interrogation is made after tubal perforation and the other tube is addressed. Tubal perforation is an innocuous event since the patient has been pretreated with three days of oral doxycycline and will take it for two more days after the procedure. If the microwire passes the obstruction, the microcatheter is advanced through the obstruction and

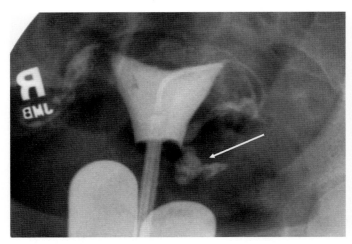

Figure 3.16. Additional contrast injection opacified distal left tube with peritubal adhesions and hydrosalpinx (arrow).

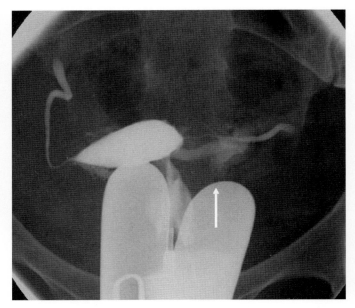

Figure 3.18. A 34-year-old woman who had reversal of tubal ligation after remarrying. She was not able to conceive after tubal reconstruction. Note bilateral ampullary tubal obstructions and venous extravasation during HSG (arrow).

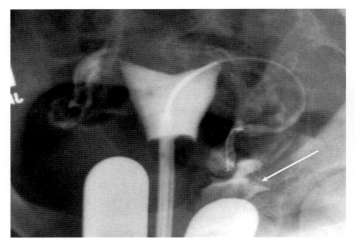

Figure 3.17. 3F microcatheter and 0.015-inch platinum-tipped guide wire placed across left ampullary tubal obstruction with intraperitoneal spill of contrast (arrow).

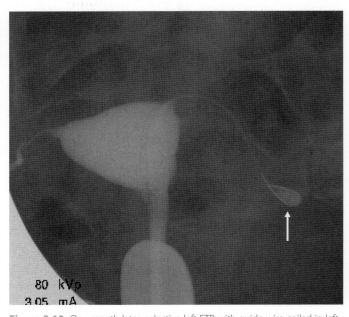

Figure 3.19. One month later; selective left FTR with guide wire coiled in left ampullary obstruction (arrow).

another hand injection of contrast is made. Distal tubal patency or obstruction is determined and then, if necessary, the contralateral fallopian tube obstruction is treated. A completion hysterosalpingogram is obtained to confirm postprocedure tubal patency (Figures 3.17, 3.18, 3.19, 3.20, 3.21, 3.22).

The radiation exposure with modern digital fluoroscopy is less than 1 rad (10 Gy), or the equivalent of a barium enema or an intravenous pyelogram (IVP) [32].

We review the results of the procedure with the patient and her partner. Most patients have pelvic pain, and cramps that can last up to 24 hours and respond to NSAIDs. Vaginal spotting can last up to three days. Normal activity including sexual intercourse can resume the next day. Patients are reminded both to complete the antibiotics and follow up with their gynecologist.

One-third of patients with recanalized fallopian tubes are radiographically normal with free peritoneal spill of contrast.

Another third have periampullary adhesions causing incomplete peritoneal spill. The remaining third of patients show residual tubal stenosis, SIN and/or hydrosalpinx [32]. Laparoscopic treatment of periampullary adhesions and hydrosalpinx with lysis of adhesions and neosalpingostomy is then indicated. We have recently placed guide wires through ampullary obstructions with peritoneal spill, but have not documented long-term patency or successful pregnancies (Figures 3.18–3.22).

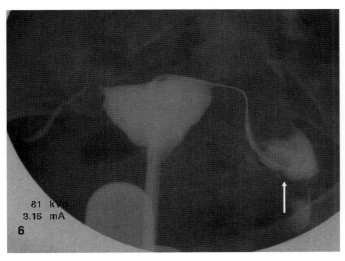

Figure 3.20. 3F microcatheter and 0.015-inch platinum-tipped guide wire placed through ampullary obstruction. Contrast contained within periampullary adhesions with some intraperitoneal spill (arrow).

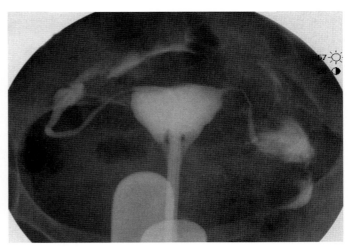

Figure 3.22. Completion HSG through cervical cannula shows bilateral intraperitoneal spill of contrast with periampullary adhesions. Outpatient transcervical balloon fimbrioplasty is planned in 3 months if the patient remains infertile.

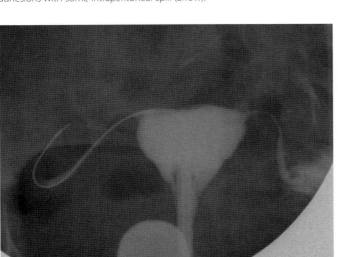

Figure 3.21. Right tubal ampullary obstruction probed with 3F microcatheter and platinum-tipped guide wire.

Meta-analysis of 1466 cases of FTR reported a success rate of 71–92% per treated proximal fallopian tube obstruction and 62–90% per patient [33]. FTR to treat occlusion after micro-surgical reanastomosis for tubal ligation has success rates from 44% [34] to 77% [35]. FTR for obstruction related to Salpingitis isthmica nodosa was successful in 77–82% of tubes but was technically more difficult [36,37]. In patients who had successful FTR and failed to become pregnant in 12 months, 38% of tubes had reoccluded. Repeat FTR is warranted in these cases rather than tubal microsurgery [38].

Other published pregnancy rates after FTR range from 9% [39] to 58% [40]. The lowest pregnancy rates are associated with more advanced tubal pathology and the highest pregnancy rates are associated with physiological obstructions. Microsurgical proximal tubal reanastomosis has a 30–50% pregnancy rate.

The ectopic pregnancy risk after FTR with residual tubal pathology is 3% [33]. The ectopic pregnancy risk after tubal reconstruction is 5–10% [41].

A recent series from Nagpur, India, of FTR performed at the time of diagnostic hysterosalpingography showed 31% 6-month, and 20% 1-month pregnancy rates in 200 infertile women who had FTR. There were no ectopic pregnancies. There was a 6% FTR failure rate and 3.5% incidence of hydrosalpinx. These results compare with a 30–50% 2-year pregnancy rate after tubal microsurgery and 10–15% pregnancy rate after IVF [42].

Since 1985, treatment of isolated proximal physiological fallopian tubal obstruction with guide wires and catheters has recanalized more than 80% of cases with a 30–50% 1-year intrauterine pregnancy rate. One-year tubal patency rates are greater than 50% even in women who do not conceive. The pregnancy rate falls to 30% with pathological tubal obstructions from salpingitis isthmica nodosa. The tubal pregnancy rate is 3% [1,4]. This population has traditionally been treated with in-vitro fertilization or tubal microsurgery [5].

FTR carries no general anesthetic risk, avoids laparoscopic surgery risks of uterine or ureteral injury, and has a one-hour recovery period. Patients can resume sexual relations the day after FTR, which is not the case with the 3–5 day recovery period after tubal reconstruction.

Fallopian tube recanalization is not recommended in patients with müllerian anomaly, corneal fibroids, or severe salpingitis isthmica nodosa. However, in the vast majority of infertility patients with tubal obstructions, FTR can diagnose and treat proximal tubal disease and spare patients unneeded hysteroscopy and tubal microsurgery. Bipolar (proximal and distal) tubal obstructions can be converted to unipolar distal obstructions, and appropriately treated with neosalpingostomy.

References

1. Rubin IC, ed. *Diagnostic Aids Offered by Transuterine and Transperitoneal Insufflation in Symptoms in Gynecology, Etiology and Interpretation with Notes on Diagnosis*. New York, Appleton, 1924; 253–92.

2. Yun AJ, Lee PY. Enhanced fertility after diagnostic hysterosalpingography using oil-based contrast agents may be attributable to immunomodulation. *Am J Radiol* 2004; **183**: 1725–7.

3. Steiner AZ, Meyer WR, Clark RL, Hartmann KE. Oil soluble contrast during hysterosalpingography in women with proven tubal patency. *Obstet Gynecol* 2003; **101**: 109–13.

4. Alper MM, Garner PR, Spence JEH, et al. Pregnancy rates after hysterosalpingography with oil and water soluble contrast media. *Obstet Gynecol* 1986; **68**: 6.

5. Decherney AH, Kort H, Barney JB, *et al*. Increased pregnancy rate with oil soluble hysterosalpingography dyes. *Fertil Steril* 1980; **33**: 407.

6. Schwabe MG, Shapiro SS, Haning RV Jr. Hysterosalpingography with oil contrast medium enhances fertility in patients with infertility of unknown etiology. *Fertil Steril* 1983; **40**: 604.

7. Aaron JB, Levine W. Endometrial oil granuloma following hysterosalpingography. *Am J Obstet Gynecol* 1954; **68** (6):1594–7.

8. Vang J. Complications of hysterosalpingography. *Acta Obstet Gynecol Scand* 1950; **29**: 383.

9. Bergman F, Gorton G, Norman O, Sjostets. Foreign body granulomas following hysterosalpingography with a contrast medium containing carboxymethyl cellulose. *Acata Radiol* 1955; **43**: 17.

10. Kantor HI, Kamholz JH, Smith A. Foreign body granulomas following the use of salpix: Report of a case simulating intrabdominal tuberculosis. *Obstet Gynecol* 1956; **7**: 171.

11. Karshmer N, Stein W. Oil embolism complicating hysterosalpingography. *J Med Soc New Jersey* 1951; **48**: 496.

12. Levinson JM. Pulmonary oil embolism following hysterosalpingography. *Fertil Steril* 1963; **14**: 21.

13. Williams ER. Venous intravasation during hysterosalpingography. *Br J Radiology* 1944; **17**: 13.

14. Pinto ABM, Hovsepian DM Wattanackumtornkul S, Pilgram TK. Pregnancy outcomes after fallopian tube recanalization: oil-based versus water soluble contrast agents. *J Vasc Interv Radiol* 2003; **14**: 69–74.

15. Letterie GS, Wilson J, Miyazawa K. Magnetic resonance imaging of Mullerian tract abnormalities. *Fertil Steril* 1988; **50**: 365.

16. Decherney AH, Russell JD, Graebe RA, et al. Hysteroscopic management of Mullerian fusion defects. *Fertil Steril* 1986; **45**: 726.

17. Fayez JA. Comparison between abdominal and hysteroscopic metroplasty. *Obstet Gynecol* 1986; **68**: 399.

18. Netter AP, Musset R, Lambert A, Salomon Y. Traumatic uterine synechiae: a common cause of menstrual insufficiency, sterility, and abortion. *Am J Obstet Gynecol* 1956; **71**: 368.

19. Buttram V, Turati G. Uterine synechiae: Variation in severity and some conditions which may be conducive to severe adhesions. *Int J Fertil* 1977; **22**: 98.

20. Jensen P, Stromme W. Amenorrhea after puerperal curettage. *Am J Obstet Gynecol* 1971; **113**: 150.

21. Jewelewicz R, Khalaf S, Neuwirth R, et al: Obstetric complications after treatment of intrauterine synechiae (Asherman's Syndrome). *Obstet Gynecol* 1976; **47**: 701.

22. Schenken JG, Margalioth EJ: Intrauterine adhesions: An update appraisal. *Fertil Steril* 1982; **37**, 593.

23. Norman O: Hysterography in cancer of corpus of the uterus. *Acta Radiol Suppl.* 1950: 79.

24. Foda MS, Yousseff AF, Shafeek MA, Kassem KA. Hysterography in diagnosis of abnormalities of the uterus. II. Acquired structural abnormalities. *Br J Radiol* 1962; **35**: 783.

25. Vandromme J, Chasse E, LeJeune B, VanRysselberg M, Delvigne A, LeRoy F. Hydrosalpinges in in-vitro fertilization. Unfavorable prognostic feature. *Hum Reprod* 1995; **10**: 576–9.

26. Hunt RB, Siegler AM. *Hysterosalpingography: Techniques and Interpretation*. Chicago, Yearbook Medical Publishers, 1990; 2–34.

27. Comb MC, Gomel. Cornual occlusion and its microsurgical reconstruction. *Clin Obstet Gynecol* 1980; **23**: 1229–41.

28. Platia MP, Krudy AF. Transvaginal fluoroscopic recanalization of a proximally occluded oviduct. *Fertil Steril* 1985; **44**: 704–6.

29. Thurmond AS, Rosch J, Patton PE, et al. Fluoroscopic transcervical fallopian tube catheterization for diagnosis and treatment of female infertility caused by tubal obstruction. *Radiographics* 1988; **4**: 621–40.

30. Thurmond AS, Novy M, Uchida BT, Rosch J. Fallopian tube obstuction: selective salpingography and recanalization. *Radiology* 1987; **174**: 571–2.

31. American Fertility Society. *Guideline for Tubal Disease*. Birmingham, Alabama, American Fertility Society (American Society for Reproductive Medicine), February 15, 1993.

32. Thurmond AS. Fallopian tube recanalization. *Semin Interv Radiol* 2000; **17**: 303–8.

33. Thurmond AS, Machan LS, Maubon AJ, et al. A review of selective salpingography and fallopian tube catheterization. *Radiographics* 2000; **20**: 1759–68.

34. Hayashi N, Kimoto T, Sakai T, et al. Fallopian tube disease: limited value of treatment with fallopian tube catheterization. *Radiology* 1994; **190**: 141–3.

35. Thurmond AS, Brandt KA, Gorrill MJ. Tubal obstruction after ligation reversal: results of catheter recanalization. *Radiology* 1999; **210**: 747–80.

36. Houston JG, Machan LS. Salpingitis isthmica nodosa: technical success and outcome of fluoroscopic transcervical fallopian tube recanalization. *Cardiovasc Interv Radiol* 1998; **21**: 31–5.

37. Thurmond AS, Burry K, Novy MJ. Salpingitis isthmica nodosa: results of transcervical fluoroscopic catheter recanalization. *Fertil Steril* 1995; **63**: 715–22.

38. Thurmond AS. Pregnancies after selective salpingography and tubal recanalization. *Radiology* 1994; **190**: 11–13.

39. Lang EK, Dunaway HE, Jr, Roniger WE. Selective osteal salpingography and transvaginal catheter

dilatation in the diagnosis and treatment of fallopian tube occlusion. *Am J Roentgonol* 1990; **154**: 735–40.

40. Thurmond AS, Rosch J. Nonsurgical fallopian tube recanalization for treatment of infertility. *Radiology* 1990; **174**: 371–4.

41. Zagoria RJ. Transcervical fallopian tube recanalization. *Appl Radiol* 1995; **24**: 34–9.

42. Dwivedi MK, Pal R, Jain M, et al. Efficacy of fallopian tube catheterization for treatment of infertility. *Indian J Radiol Imaging* 2005; **15**: 521–3.

Fertiloscopy

Antoine Watrelot

Introduction

The management of unexplained infertility is problematic, because in the absence of a clear diagnosis of the causes of infertility, treatment decisions are in effect therapeutic trials. The diagnosis of unexplained infertility is established classically when no pathology is found concerning the sperm value, ovulation, and the tubal patency. The problem is that the last is frequently only the conclusion of hysterosalpingography (HSG) or ultrasonography (US), which have both proven to be inaccurate [1]. Broadly, most patients with "unexplained" infertility are treated according to one or the other of two intervention strategies:

1. Offering some cycles (often 3–6) of stimulated or unstimulated intrauterine insemination (IUI) to see whether pregnancy occurs; if it does not, IVF is offered. In these cases, IUI has wasted both the patient's time and the payor's resources (the payor may be the patient/the patient's family or a third party payor, such as an insurer or a government).

2. Offering IVF immediately, because of the possibility that IUI will not work, with the risks of overtreating the patients, once again with a lack of cost-effectiveness.

A third alternative is abdominal laparoscopy. This is the currently accepted "gold standard" for establishing causes of infertility in the fallopian tubes and the peritoneal cavity surrounding the uterus [2,3]. However, laparoscopy is a nontrivial surgical procedure with significant risks. It is often performed without discovering any significant pathology, which, for the woman concerned, means being exposed to a surgical procedure that offers no benefit. Complications occur in about 3 out of every 1000 abdominal laparoscopies [4]. These complications include:

- Those related to general anesthesia
- Injury to blood vessels or organs that causes bleeding
- Damage to ducts or other structures that allow body fluids to leak out

The risks and trauma associated with laparoscopy, as well as the likelihood that the procedure will prove with hindsight to have been unnecessary (because the woman has no relevant disease), make doctors and patients understandably cautious about carrying out laparoscopy at an early stage. However, as noted, the resulting failure to diagnose the cause of the patient's "unexplained" infertility may mean that unnecessary treatment (for example, IVF which could have been avoided) or ineffective treatments (for example, intrauterine insemination for a woman with blocked fallopian tubes) are offered.

It was therefore of interest to find an alternative that was safe, minimally invasive, and reproducible to a relatively low cost: thus was developed the concept of fertiloscopy in 1998 after the pioneering work of Gordts on transvaginal hydrolaparoscopy (THL) (Figure 4.1) [5,6,7].

Fertiloscopy is the performance of a laparoscopy through the vagina using saline solution instead of CO_2 as working medium [8,9].

Important advantages are:

- It is safe, since no CO_2 or Trendelenburg position is required.

- Complication rate is low and no serious complication are anticipated.

- A perfect evaluation is possible of the genital tract, observed in a true physiological position without any need to manipulate the structures, which is not the case in laparoscopy.

- The procedure is minimally invasive and can be performed as an office procedure with local anesthesia or with general sedation in an ambulatory process.

Technique [10]

It is essential to carry out a careful vaginal examination prior to the procedure. This examination allows detection of pathology of the pouch of Douglas, such as nodules of the rectovaginal septum or fixed retroverted uterus. These situations are important contraindications for fertiloscopy because, when there is posterior endometriosis, the rectum is attracted close to the posterior vaginal vault and the risk of rectal injury is high when inserting the trocar. In case of a fixed retroverted uterus there is no space to penetrate the pouch of Douglas.

Ultrasonography in Reproductive Medicine and Infertility, ed. Botros R. M. B. Rizk. Published by Cambridge University Press. © Cambridge University Press 2010.

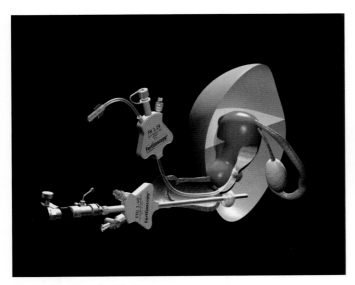

Fig 4.1. The principle of fertiloscopy.

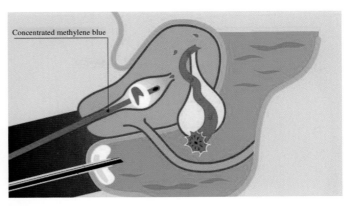

Fig. 4.2. The technique of fertiloscopy.

Strict local anesthesia can be used, or general sedation may be used. Strict local anesthesia is very useful in those countries where office surgical procedures are allowed. In the other cases, general sedation is normal; sometimes it is the choice of patients. The advantage of general sedation is the possibility to practice operative fertiloscopy at the same time when pathology is found. Strict local anesthesia is carried out by first inserting an anesthetic swab (Emla gel) for 10 minutes, and then a classical paracervical block is performed using lidocaine. General sedation is of the same kind as used for egg collection during IVF.

In all cases, fertiloscopy is performed as an ambulatory technique. There are five steps in the procedure: (1) hydropelviscopy (Figure 4.2); (2) dye test; (3) salpingoscopy; (4) microsalpingoscopy; (5) hysteroscopy.

1. Hydropelviscopy is performed by first inserting a Verres needle into the pouch of Douglas. This needle is inserted 1 cm below the cervix, and then saline solution is instilled through a perfusion line using no other pressure than gravity. When 150–200 ml has been instilled, the Verres needle is removed and replaced by the fertiloscope (FTO 1–40-Fertility Focus Ltd., UK). The sharp end of the fertiloscope allows a direct insertion without any incision. Also, the fertiloscope is fitted at its extremity with a balloon that prevents it being inadvertently pulled out of the peritoneal cavity (Figure 4.1). The optic is then introduced via the fertiloscope, and observation can start (it is important to use a 30° telescope of less than 4 mm outer diameter). On first use of fertiloscopy, the view is disconcerting to those accustomed to performing conventional laparoscopy because the view is inverted (Figure 4.1), but after a short learning period it becomes easy to see all the reproductive structures. It is important to have a systematic view of both ovaries, tubes (Figure 4.2), fossae ovaricae, posterior part of the uterus, uterosacral ligaments, and pelvic peritoneum.

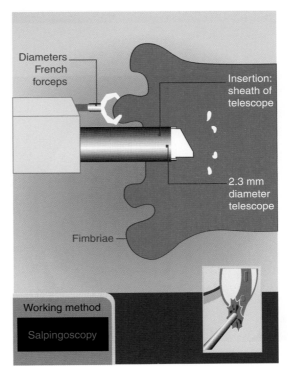

Fig 4.3. The technique of salpingoscopy.

2. When anatomy has been assessed, a dye test is performed through the uterine fertiloscope (FH 1–29-Fertility Focus Ltd., UK). Tubal patency is thus established.

3. Identification of tubal pathology such as intra-ampullary adhesions or flattened mucosal folds (see Figures 4.6, 4.7, 4.8) is important because in these cases the only valid therapeutic option is IVF. We therefore systematically perform salpingoscopy (Figure 4.3). It is straightforward to inspect the tubal ampulla using the same scope, so salpingoscopy may be practiced as a routine evaluation, which is not usually the case during laparoscopy where a second optic, a second cold light supply, and a separate irrigation are needed [11].

35

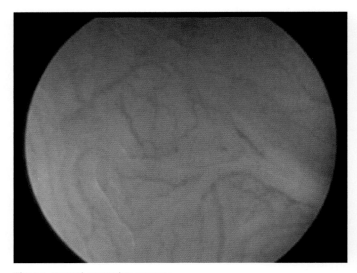

Fig 4.4. Normal microsalpingoscopy.

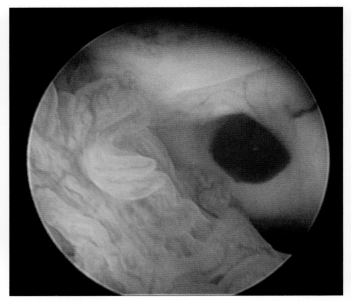

Fig 4.6. Minimal ovarian endometriosis.

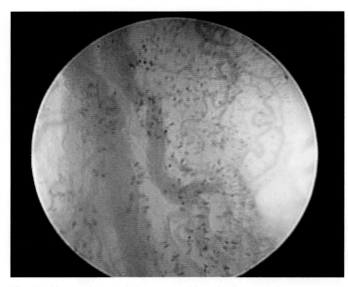

Fig 4.5. Abnormal microsalpingoscopy with nuclei dye stained.

4. Microsalpingoscopy is a further step. The concept was described by Marconi and Quintana [12] in1998, who clearly demonstrated that after the dye test, the more the nuclei are stained by the methylene blue dye, the more pathological the tube is (Figures 4.4, 4.5). Every dye-stained nucleus is a damaged cell (either inflammatory or in apoptosis). To perform microsalpingoscopy a special optic is used (Hamou II-K., Storz, Germany) that permits magnification up to 100 times, thus achieving real "in vivo" histology. Findings are classified as normal if none or few dye-stained nuclei are seen, or pathological when many nuclei are dye stained [13].

5. A standard hysteroscopy (through the same optic) is then performed in order to have a complete evaluation of the reproductive system.

At the end of the procedure, the scar is so small that it is not necessary to close the vaginal puncture site and we do not give any antibiotics.

Imaging

Introduction of a Verres needle and then of the fertiloscope in the pouch of Douglas sometimes raises fear of rectal injury. Even if it has been demonstrated that such an injury is avoidable and not of serious consequence, one may prefer to introduce the instrumentation with a visual control. The technique of ultrasound-guided entry has been proposed.

Operative fertiloscopy

In the beginning, fertiloscopy was purely diagnostic. But thanks to the operative channel provided on the fertiloscope, several forms of treatment have rapidly been developed and performed. We can now routinely practice adhesiolysis, treatment of minimal and sometimes mild endometriosis, and ovarian drilling [14].

In order for it to become generally accepted, it needed to be shown that operative fertiloscopy was as effective as the same procedure practiced during laparoscopy, and this requirement places some limitations on the procedures [15]. These are described below.

The operative channel is unique and small (5F, 1.5 mm diameter) and because of this only relatively limited adhesiolysis can be performed (especially when adhesions are found between the distal part of the tubes, ovaries, and fossa ovarica) (Figure 4.5). Similarly, endometriotic lesions can be treated only when minimal or moderate (Figures 4.3, 4.4).

Another requirement is to avoid any bleeding during operative fertiloscopy, since only a few drops of blood will obscure the field of vision. For this reason, very careful hemostasis is necessary and a bipolar probe should obviously be used to work in the liquid environment. Several such probes exist and we

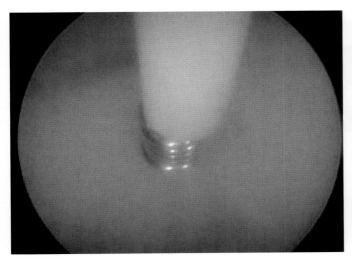

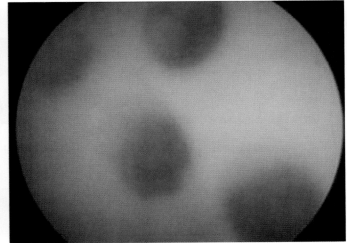

Fig 4.7. Ovarian drilling.

mostly use the disposable Versapoint (Gynecare, USA). For all these reasons, it is evident that operative fertiloscopy does not compete with operative laparoscopy: it is only an additional tool that may in some cases avoid unnecessary laparoscopy.

Justification of fertiloscopy

The fundamental question was to know at an early stage whether fertiloscopy was as accurate as laparoscopy, which was considered at that time the " gold standard" in infertility investigation.

To be able to answer this question, we designed a special study: the FLY study (acronym for fertiloscopy versus laparoscopy) [16]. This was a multicenter prospective randomized study in which first fertiloscopy and then laparoscopy were performed on the same infertile patient by two surgeons A and B randomized for the procedure. Every procedure was video recorded, the files being seen by two independent reviewers. This trial was approved by the French ethical committee under the Huriet law. Fourteen teaching hospitals centers were enrolled (12 in France, 1 in Belgium, and 1 in Tunisia), and 92 patients were studied.

Calculation of sensitivity and specificity was performed as well as concordance test using kappa score on the results from six sites (both ovaries, tubes, peritoneum, and ovaries), the total number of sites for analysis being 552 (92 × 6). The kappa score between sites varied from 0.75 to 0.91.

A correlation between two diagnostic tools is considered as excellent when the kappa score reaches 0.75 or more. Thus the conclusion of the FLY study was that "fertiloscopy should replace laparoscopy in infertile women with no obvious pathology."

Can fertiloscopy be used as a first-line infertility test?

For many years we have been looking for a simple, reproducible, safe, minimally invasive, and relatively cheap method to diagnose pelvic abnormalities in infertile patients. Many noninvasive tools such as hysterosalpingography (HSG) and hysterosonography (USG) or invasive as laparoscopy are available.

Their ability to assess the four important parameters to consider (i.e., tubal patency, tuboperitoneal environment, tubal mucosa, and uterine cavity) is variable. They are summarized in Figures 4.8, 4.9, 4.10, which demonstrate that fertiloscopy seems to be the most suitable exploration.

Strategy for fertiloscopy

According to the specific health system and the legislation concerning office procedure, two different strategies are available:

1. When office procedure is available and permitted, fertiloscopy may be practiced early in the infertile work-up (i.e., after one year of infertility). In this case fertiloscopy is performed under strict local anesthesia. If no abnormalities are detected then it is logical to practice expectant management up to two years of infertility since the chances of pregnancy per cycle are still 12% during the second year of infertility. After two years of infertility, the spontaneous pregnancy rate falls around 5% and it is then consistent to propose IUI. If pathology is detected, the patient is treated accordingly, which means further surgery in cases of endometriosis or pelvic adhesions or IVF if the tubes appear to be damaged beyond the possibility of surgical repair. This is often the case when tubal mucosa is involved.

2. When surgical office procedures are not available or not permitted, fertiloscopy is performed under general anesthesia in the operating room prior to beginning IUI or IVF (this means after 2 years of infertility except in patients aged over 38, when only one year of infertility is required, or over 40 years, when fertiloscopy is carried out directly). When fertiloscopy is normal, patients are referred for artificial reproductive technologies (ART) or treated according to the lesions encountered.

Advantages of local anesthesia are obvious; also it is a low-cost option. General anesthesia, on the other hand, allows for

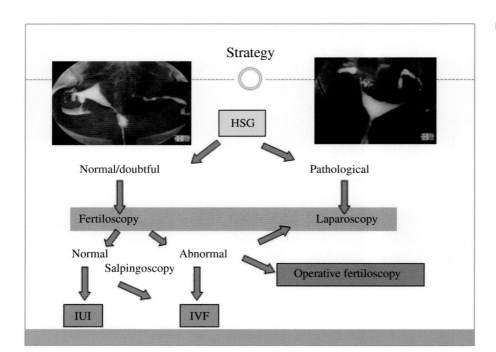

Fig 4.8. Strategy for fertiloscopy.

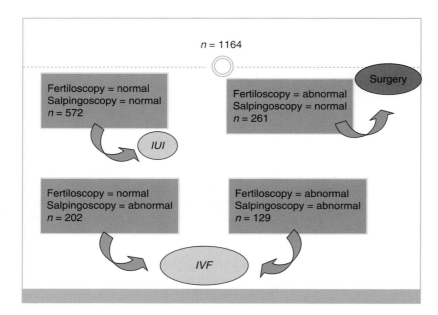

Fig 4.9. Results of fertiloscopy.

operative fertiloscopy or further laparoscopy when required at the same time. Indeed, the patient may choose between the two options, but the earlier the fertiloscopy is practiced the more likely it is that any pathology can be treated in order to obtain pregnancy in the shortest time.

Complications

Complications are rare if clinicians respect firstly the learning curve – which has been evaluated at 5 to 10 procedures according to the surgeon's skill – and secondly the contra-indications, which are pathology of the pouch of Douglas such as recto-

vaginal endometriosis or fixed retroverted uterus. These pathologies are detected by vaginal examination prior to the procedure. Any doubt should lead to cancellation of the fertiloscopy and to proposal of the necessary laparoscopy.

The only real complication is represented by rectal injury. However, such injury may be always treated conservatively with antibiotics without the need for further surgical intervention [17].

Case studies [18]

Between July 1997 and January 2008, 1589 patients presenting with infertility lasting more than one year were potentially

Scoring of diagnostic tools
0 = no value, 5 = very good value

Fig 4.10. Comparison of diagnostic tools

	Tubal patency	Uterine cavity	Tubo-peritoneal environment	Tubal mucosa	Total
HSG [1]	4	4	1	2	11
USG [2]	4	4	1	0	9
Laparoscopy [3]	5	0	5	1	11
Laparoscopy + hysteroscopy	5	5	5	1	16
Fertiloscopy [16]	5	5	5	5	20

enrolled for fertiloscopy. In all these patients, the sperm evaluation in the husband showed either a normal value or a value allowing the use of IUI. Also, every patient considered as normal or doubtful underwent HSG.

Out of 1589 candidate patients, ninety-one (5.7%) were excluded during the selection process due to abnormalities discovered during the preoperative clinical examination (as previously described, mainly endometriosis of the rectovaginal space or fixed retroverted uterus). These cases, being contraindicated for the technique, were referred to operative laparoscopy.

Thus, 1498 patients underwent fertiloscopy. Written consent was required for each patient. The mean age was 32 years (range 22–41); mean duration of infertility was 3.2 years (range 1–9). Primary infertility affected 1018 patients (68.0%).

Procedures

In 1490 patients (99.5%), fertiloscopy was performed as an ambulatory procedure; 288 patients (19.2%) were treated under strict local anesthesia; the remaining 1202 (80.8%) were treated under general sedation, which allowed operative fertiloscopy at the same time when necessary.

Findings of diagnostic fertiloscopy

Global results were as follows. Patients' macroscopic findings appeared to be normal in 1006 (67.1%) . We included in this category patients with subtle lesions such as paratubal cyst, nonconnective adhesions, very minimally endometriotic lesions, and minor tubal alterations such as sacculation or accessory tube.

Pathology was found in the other 492 (32.8%). Endometriosis was found in 112 patients (7.5%); in 79 (5.3%) cases the endometriosis was considered mild and in 33 cases

(2.2%) was severe. The frequency of endometriosis thus appears quite low. This is due firstly to the exclusion policy for patients with endometriosis of the rectovaginal septum and secondly to patients with minimal endometriosis being considered as having subtle lesions and classified as normal or having minimal impact on fertility. We should therefore add 72 cases of rectovaginal endometriosis and 139 cases of minimal endometriosis. Thus, 323 patients (21.6%) presented endometriosis at various stages or locations, which is consistent with findings in an infertile population.

Pelvic adhesions and tubal pathology were the second main pathologies, encountered in 380 patients (25.4%). We distinguished minimal adhesions with normal tubes in 114 patients (7.6%); 208 patients (13.9%) had mild adhesions associated with either a phimosis or hydrosalpinx, and 58 patients (3.9%) had a severe adhesion status associated with tubal lesions (phimosis, hydrosalpinx, or proximal tubal blockage). The group of patients with severe adhesions is rather small because very often lesions were seen on HSG and in these cases patients were directly referred to operative laparoscopy as mentioned above.

Initially fertiloscopy was exclusively diagnostic; then in 1999 we added the routine practice of microsalpingoscopy following the work of Marconi [12]. In the earlier period (prior to January 1999) 266 fertiloscopies were performed; 1232 have been performed since that time. We have shown that salpingoscopy and microsalpingoscopy are feasible routinely in a great number of cases. In our series it was possible to carry out both techniques in at least one tube in 1164 cases (94.3%).

From 1999 the results of microsalpingoscopy were taken into account, making it possible to distinguish four situations according to the tubal mucosa score (Figure 4.9): group 1, normal fertiloscopic findings and normal tubal mucosa; group 2, normal fertiloscopic findings but abnormal tubal mucosa;

group 3, abnormal fertiloscopic findings but with normal tubal mucosa; group 4, abnormal fertiloscopic findings and abnormal tubal mucosa. We had 572 patients in group 1, 202 in group 2, 261 in group 3, and 129 in group 4.

Patients of groups 2 and 4 (i.e., with abnormal tubal mucosa, were directly referred to IVF. Patients of group 1 were considered eligible for IUI, and patients of group 3 have had subsequent surgical treatment. Thus, 331 patients were referred for IVF (28.4%), 572 were referred for IUI (49.1%), and 261 were referred for surgery (22.4%).

Out of the 261 patients for whom surgery was decided, in 139 (53.3%) treatment was achieved through operative laparoscopy, 105 (40.2%) were treated by operative fertiloscopy, and only 17 (6.5%) were treated by microsurgical proximal anastomosis. When operative fertiloscopy was performed it involved distal ovarosalpingolysis in 78 cases and treatment of ovarian superficial lesions in 27 cases.

We were able to achieve a complete follow-up for only 6 months because of the varying geographic origins of the patients. Among the 572 patients referred for IUI, 118 (20.6%) became pregnant in the following 6 months and after 1–3 IUI attempts. Among the 331 patients referred for IVF, 121 (35.6%) became pregnant after 1 or 2 attempts. Among the 261 patients treated surgically, we obtained 92 (35.2%) pregnancies.

One hundred and five patients (40.2%) were treated through operative fertiloscopy and 29 pregnancies were achieved (27.6%). One hundred and thirty-nine patients (53.2%) had an operative laparoscopy and 53 pregnancies were obtained (38.1%). In the remaining 17 patients we performed a microsurgical anastomosis for proximal tubal obstruction and 10 pregnancies were obtained (58.8%). There was no significant difference between patients who had IVF and patients who underwent a surgical approach.

In all, 331 patients out of 1164 (28.4%) became pregnant in the following 6 months.

- As in all surgical procedures, complications may occur.
- We had three rectal injuries, all treated conservatively (i.e., antibiotics for 5 days without any further surgery).
- Only one infection (0.09%) occurred despite the fact that no antibiotics are routinely given.
- We also had two abnormal vaginal bleedings (0.17%); in such cases a stitch on the vaginal wall was required, which is not commonly the case.
- Lastly, we had 11 cases of false route (0.95%). That signifies that the fertiloscope was inserted between the peritoneum and the vaginal wall. This complication was the result of poor technique (essentially linked with a slow insertion of the needle in the pouch of Douglas instead of its insertion with a firm movement).
- There were no complications in patients who had operative fertiloscopy.

Conclusion

Our series demonstrates that fertiloscopy is useful for diagnosis of tubal diseases that are not openly visible after noninvasive exploration like HSG.

Results of the FLY study have shown that fertiloscopy is at least as accurate as laparoscopy and dye. However, fertiloscopy is less invasive and less risky than "lap-and-dye." Moreover, fertiloscopy allows a careful evaluation of the tubal mucosa. In this respect, fertiloscopy shows superiority in comparison with lap-and-dye. Indeed salpingoscopy allows us to explore only the distal part of the tube. The proximal portion is too narrow to be explored except by falloposcopy, which is still experimental because of the poor quality of imaging obtained. This disadvantage is counterbalanced by the fact that the distal part of the tube is not only the more common location of tubal lesions but is also the most important part of the tube where everything happens: oocyte retrieval and fertilization.

Microsalpingoscopy seems to have a good prognostic value but will require more studies before it is completely validated. Nevertheless, for the first time an "in-vivo histological" appreciation of the tubal mucosa is available

Therefore, patients who have been elected for tubal surgery have a pregnancy rate after 6 months that is not statistically different from the IVF group (35.2% and 35.6%, respectively). Tubal surgery remains a valid option after proper selection. Also, when tubal pathology is discovered we may in some circumstances propose treatment by operative fertiloscopy (in our series 105 patients [40.2%]).

Fertiloscopy also appears to be a relatively easy technique but it has to be learned by experience. In our experience we consider that the practice of 10 fertiloscopies is necessary for a "new" laparoscopic surgeon to be able to include fertiloscopy in his or her strategy.

At this stage we believe that fertiloscopy should be widely adopted as a precise minimally invasive tool as already demonstrated by several teams. Sharma et al. [3] considered fertiloscopy a safer method than laparoscopy and one that in addition allows salpingoscopy, Tanos et al. [19] performed 78 fertiloscopies and showed that the learning curve was short and the results were very accurate. More recently Nohuz et al. [20] performed fertiloscopy in 229 infertile women and discovered a pathology in 28.6% of cases. These results are similar to those observed in our study.

Fertiloscopy is an attractive alternative to lap-and-dye when tubal pathology is suspected. Accuracy of fertiloscopic findings has been demonstrated and allows a good selection for patients with tubal or peritubal pathology. When this is done, pregnancy rate after tubal surgery is the same as after IVF. A spontaneous pregnancy obtained after surgery has many advantages: it is cheaper, it is more physiological, and when the disease is treated several pregnancies can be achieved without further treatment.

References

1. Swart P, Mol BW, Van Beurden M, et al. The accuracy of hysterosalpingography in the diagnosis of tubal pathology: a meta-analysis. *Fertil Steril* 1995; **64**: 486–91.

2. Exacoustos C, Zupi E, Carusotti C, Lanzi G, Marconi D, Arduini D. Hysterosalpingo-contrast sonography compared with hysterosalpingography and laparoscopic dye pertubation to evaluate patency test. *J Am Assoc Gynecol Laparosc* 2003; **10**: 367–72.

3. Sharma A, Bhalla R, Donovan O. Endoscopy in ART an overview. *Gynecol Surg* 2004; **1(1)**: 3–10.

4. Chapron C, Querleu D, Bruhat MA, et al. Surgical complications of diagnostic and operative gynaecologic laparoscopy: a serie of 29,966 cases. *Hum Reprod* 1998; **13**: 867–72.

5. Odent M. Hydrocolpotomie et hydroculdoscopie. *Nouv Presse Med* 1973; **2**: 187.

6. Mintz M. Actualisation de la culdoscopie transvaginale en décubitus dorsal. Un nouvel endoscope à vision directe muni d'une aiguille à ponction incorporée dans l'axe. *Contra Fert Sex* 1987; **15**: 401–4.

7. Gordts S, Campo R, Rombauts L, Brosens I. Transvaginal hydrolaparoscopy as an outpatient procedure for infertility investigation. *Hum Reprod* 1998; **13**: 99–103.

8. Watrelot A, Gordts S, Andine JP, Brosens I. Une nouvelle approche diagnostique: La Fertiloscopie. *Endomag* 1997; **21**: 7–8.

9. Watrelot A, Dreyfus JM, Andine JP. Fertiloscopy; first results (120 cases report). *Fertil Steril* 1998; **70(Suppl)**: S-42.

10. Watrelot A, Dreyfus JM, Andine JP. Evaluation of the performance of fertiloscopy in 160 consecutive infertile patients with no obvious pathology. *Hum Reprod* 1999; **14**: 707–11.

11. Watrelot A, Dreyfus JM. Explorations intra-tubaires au cours de la fertiloscopie. *Reprod Hum Horm* 2000; **12**: 39–44.

12. Marconi G, Quintana R. Methylene blue dyeing of cellular nuclei during salpingoscopy, a new in vivo method to evaluate vitality of tubal epithelium. *Hum Reprod* 1998; **13**: 3414–17.

13. Watrelot A, Dreyfus JM, Cohen M. Systematic salpingoscopy and microsalpingoscopy during fertiloscopy. *J Am Assoc Gynecol Laparosc* 2002; **9**: 453–9.

14. Fernandez H, Alby JD. De la culdoscopie à la fertiloscopie opératoire. *Endomag* 1999; **21**: 5–6.

15. Chiesa-Montadou S, Rongieres C, Garbin O, Nisand I. A propos de deux complications au cours du drilling ovarien par fertiloscopie. *Gyn Obst Fertil* 2003; **31**: 844–6.

16. Watrelot A, Nisolle M, Hocke C, et al. Is laparoscopy still the gold standard in infertility assessment? A comparison of fertiloscopy versus laparoscopy in infertility. *Hum Reprod* 2003; **18**: 834–9.

17. Gordts S, Watrelot A, Campo R, Brosens I. Risk and outcome of bowel injury during transvaginal pelvic endoscopy. *Fertil Steril* 2001; **76**: 1238–41.

18. Watrelot A. Place of transvaginal fertiloscopy in the management of tubal factor disease. *RBMonline* 2007; **15(4)**: 389–95.

19. Tanos V, Bigatti G, et al. Transvaginal endoscopy: new technique evaluating female infertility in three Mediterranean countries' experiences. *Gynecol Surg*, 2005; **2(4)**: 241–3.

20. Nohuz E, Pouly JL, et al. Fertiloscopy: Clermont-Ferrand's experiment. *Gynécol Obst Fertil* 2006; **34**: 894–9.

Chapter 5

Sonohysterography

William W. Brown, III

Introduction

Saline infusion sonohysterography (SIS) is a minimally invasive office technique designed to maximize investigation of the female genital tract. Transvaginal sonography (TVS) is performed while sterile saline is simultaneously infused into the uterus to distend the endometrial cavity. The fluid contrast enhances ultrasound visualization by outlining intracavitary defects or growths. The result is a simple screening method for pelvic abnormalities with major advantages over other imaging modalities and without the invasive risks or expense of surgical evaluation.

Procedural method

Indications

Clinical applications for this diagnostic test include the following: abnormal uterine bleeding (AUB), infertility, recurrent pregnancy loss (RPL), postmenopausal bleeding, abnormal TVS finding, postoperative assessment, possible intrauterine adhesions, tamoxifen pretreatment evaluation, indistinct endometrium, and retained products of conception.

Contradictions

A very satisfying fact about this simple office procedure is that there are only two absolute contraindications: pregnancy or possible pregnancy, and active pelvic infection. If a history of chronic pelvic inflammatory disease is elicited, if painful dilated fallopian tubes are discovered during baseline TVS, if the pelvis is inexplicably tender on bimanual examination or with vaginal ultrasound probe palpation [1], or if a mucopurulent cervical discharge is noted on speculum examination, then SIS can be delayed and prophylactic antibiotic treatment offered. Active vaginal bleeding is only a relative contraindication to SIS, primarily because blood and clot can inhibit optimal imaging and confound interpretation.

Timing

Ideally, in a patient who is ovulating and menstruating regularly, this procedure should be performed sometime between cycle days 6 and 10; that is, after the end of the menstrual flow and prior to ovulation. This timing precludes the chance of interfering with a very early pregnancy, and the expected thin, symmetric follicular-phase endometrium will optimize the ability to visualize any uterine filling defects, if present (Figure 5.1). The more echodense luteal-phase endometrium, which thickens as the cycle advances and measures up to 14–16 mm immediately prior to menstruation, may obscure small intracavitary echogenic masses. Not only that, late secretory endometrium can look irregular and polypoid, thereby increasing the possibility of a false-positive diagnosis. As might be expected, careful timing for SIS is less of a consideration in those patients who are on hormonal contraception because pregnancy risk should be obviated and the suppressed endometrial growth enhances visualization. Lastly, although bleeding is not a contraindication, it is best to avoid this test when a patient is bleeding very heavily. Blood clots, especially, may hinder the validity of the results by masquerading as filling defects themselves and potentially obscuring true nearby lesions (Figure 5.2).

Practically speaking, however, it is not always possible to schedule this examination when it is best for both patient and physician. Menstrual histories are not always known or predictable, and ovulatory status can be uncertain. Pregnancy testing is always advised when appropriate in premenopausal women, but such testing can be falsely negative early in the luteal phase. Sexually active patients practicing unprotected intercourse can be given the option to return after their next menses or sign a written consent that acknowledges the potential risks of sonohysterography to an undiagnosed pregnancy.

Technique

Antibiotic treatment prior to sonohysterography is not routinely recommended; however, it is important to consider its use if the patient has already been noted to have certain particular gynecologic indications as described above. The American Heart Association 2007 guidelines for the prevention of infective endocarditis no longer consider any genitourinary procedures as high-risk and do not recommend routine use of prophylactic antibiotics, even in patients with the highest-risk cardiac conditions. Additionally, the need for any nonsteroidal

Ultrasonography in Reproductive Medicine and Infertility, ed. Botros R. M. B. Rizk. Published by Cambridge University Press. © Cambridge University Press 2010.

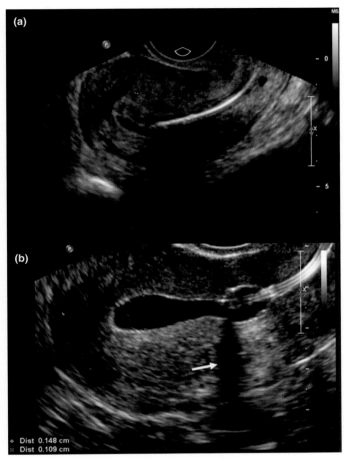

Figure 5.1. Saline infusion sonohysterography, sagittal view, normal empty uterine cavity. (a) SIS catheter advanced to the mid-body of the uterus. (b) Balloon catheter pulled back to the level of the internal cervical os. The thin, symmetric endometrium is easily seen and measured (calipers). A minute amount of air in the balloon filled with saline is responsible for the obvious linear shadow (arrow).

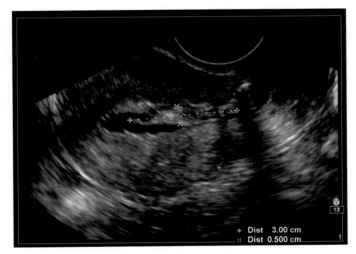

Figure 5.2. Longitudinal transvaginal SIS image of a blood clot (calipers). This echodense pseudo-mass can be confused with true pathology within the uterus and is characterized by shaggy and irregular borders, absence of vascular flow, free-floating position, and tendency to break apart when touched with an infusion catheter.

analgesia during the procedure is rare enough to warrant individualized treatment. In most practices, sonohysterography is immediately preceded by high-frequency TVS. Exact menstrual dating and latex allergy are documented first, and a negative pregnancy test is obtained, along with a signed informed consent, when appropriate. The purpose of the baseline ultrasound is to confirm all pelvic findings prior to the fluid enhancement study. Awareness of any extreme anterior or posterior uterine position can sometimes help facilitate placement of the infusion catheter, and the unexpected finding of painless hydrosalpinges is a reasonable indication for short-term postprocedure antibiotics, such as 200 mg doxycycline after the procedure and then 100 mg/day for a total of 5 days [2].

Upon completion of the baseline ultrasound, the vaginal probe is removed, set aside, and replaced with a speculum in the vagina to visualize the cervix. The cervix is cleansed thoroughly with a solution of either povidone iodine or chlorhexidine, depending upon the patient's allergy history. At this point, a catheter that has been pre-filled with sterile saline from an attached 10–12 ml syringe in order to avoid infusing air into the cavity and completely obscuring visualization, is inserted into the uterus. There are many catheter options available, such as intrauterine insemination catheters, 5F or 7F balloon hysterosalpingography (HSG) catheters, pediatric feeding tubes, small-gauge Foley catheters, in-vitro fertilization (IVF) embryo transfer catheters, and others. The choice of catheter is entirely up to the provider, and the selection depends upon cost, ease of insertion, ability to distend the uterus, and patient comfort. It is prudent, however, to have more than one catheter available for use during the procedure because it is unreasonable to expect one style to work best in all situations. If a balloon catheter is used, the balloon is now filled also with saline and pulled back with gentle traction to the level of the internal cervical os, so as to prevent egress of fluid during the saline infusion. Dessole et al. [3] compared six such catheters and found no statistical difference in their ability to correctly perform the SIS procedure.

After the catheter has been placed, the speculum is removed from around the catheter, while being careful not to dislodge it. The vaginal probe is inserted again into the vagina, and it is more comfortable for the patient if the examiner uses the fingers of a gloved free hand to open the labia and gently depress the perineum to facilitate insertion, especially if a larger three-dimensional ultrasound (3D) probe is used. Now imaging is carried out by recording multiple views of the uterine body and lower uterine segment in both sagittal and transverse planes while saline is being infused to physically separate the walls. The goal is to have a complete evaluation of the entire endometrial cavity, and this typically requires multiple static images in both planes. A typical study usually requires no more than 10–20 ml of saline infused, but the total amount is variable and patient-specific. If the additional technology is available, a 3D volume data set can be obtained in a matter of seconds, and this may both shorten the procedure time and improve specificity of the testing. Lastly, all instruments are removed from the uterus, cervix, and vagina and appropriate documentation of the study is completed. The patient should be informed that short-term spotting and pelvic cramping are not uncommon after this procedure.

Optimizing performance

The following suggestions are offered to help maximize the chance for procedural success and for troubleshooting, in advance, of some of the more common difficulties that can be encountered during SIS.

- *Sterile SIS tray.* The instruments – which should be part of a pre-set sterile tray, or wrapped separately and easily available – for use with each SIS procedure include: speculums of various sizes and widths, containers to hold the antiseptic bactericidal solution of choice and saline, a single-toothed tenaculum, cotton balls, ring forceps, small graduated cervical dilators, lubricating jelly, at least two options for intrauterine catheters – one containing a balloon tip, sterile saline, povidone iodine and Hibiclens, 10- or 12-ml infusion syringes, local anesthetic, and needles.

- *Speculum.* A single-hinged or open-sided speculum facilitates removal from the vagina around the catheter, especially if the attached syringe is a 20- or 30-ml size. If the only speculum available is the more typical double-hinged type, then, for the sake of patient comfort, do not attempt to open it at its base to allow pull-through of the catheter and syringe until it is completely outside of the introitus.

- *Uterine distension.* There will be occasions where inherent uterine pathology or laxity of the internal cervical os does not allow for adequate distention of the cavity, and a balloon catheter may help in this situation. The balloon should be filled with 1–2 ml saline (not air), which is usually quite adequate to allow it to be pulled back against the internal os under mild tension and act as a stopper to prevent retrograde leakage of fluid under pressure back out of the uterus and cervix. As noted above, a single rapid 3D sweep of insonation can also be beneficial when the uterus stays distended only briefly. The volume data set obtained in this manner can undergo postprocessing to create all the necessary images in any plane and does not require refilling of the syringe or the uterus.

- *Patient discomfort.* Mild cramping during or after this procedure does occasionally occur, so oral analgesic medication may be started immediately prior to the appointment or simply on an "as needed" basis. Significant procedural pain can potentially be averted by avoiding touching the uterine fundus with a firm catheter tip or by inflating a balloon catheter in the cervix rather than in the lower uterine segment prior to saline infusion [4]. It is always best to begin the infusion slowly and continue slowly while observing the patient's subjective reaction. Very rarely, even with only a minimal volume of saline instilled, a patient will suffer with extreme pain, cramping, nausea diaphoresis and faintness. Every office should be prepared to address such a vasovagal reaction.

- *Cervical stenosis.* Inability to adequately place a catheter is one of the main causes of procedural failure. Sometimes, all that is needed is a stronger, less-malleable catheter, such as the Shepard insemination catheter (Cook Medical, Bloomington, Indiana) that is equipped with a somewhat rigid inner cannula. Other catheters that have been proposed for this purpose include chorionic villus sampling catheters and the Echosight catheter (Cook Medical) [2]. It may be necessary to locate the cervical os or to serially dilate the endocervical canal and internal os with small disposable or metal dilators. This often requires use of a cervical tenaculum, which, otherwise, is almost never necessary for this procedure, in order to bring the uterus and cervix into an aligned, horizontal plane. Use of either spray or injectable local anesthesia on the cervical lip prior to tenaculum placement is patient-centered, as is also paracervical anesthetic block before any unusual or prolonged efforts to dilate the canal. Finally, although it is not an FDA-approved use, some physicians have also pretreated their patients with oral or vaginal misoprostol in an effort to successfully overcome severe cervical stenosis.

- *Sub-optimal visualization.* A large, fibroid uterus and a directly midplane uterus are two examples in which the imaging may actually be improved by performing transabdominal ultrasound with SIS, rather than TVS. Be sure, then, always to have an abdominal probe available for this express purpose, as well as to attempt imaging of adnexal structures which are not seen vaginally.

- *Lower uterine segment evaluation.* This area of the endometrial cavity also requires examination. If a balloon catheter is used, intracervical placement of the balloon allows full and complete visualization. Sometimes, however, a patulous or multiparous cervix simply will not hold the balloon, and the only location it will work is above the level of the internal cervical os. In this event, prior to termination of the procedure, the balloon should be deflated completely, and the lower uterine segment is imaged while the catheter is being withdrawn and final amounts of saline are infused simultaneously (Figure 5.3).

- *Endometrial sampling.* If endometrial sampling is necessary, SIS should be performed first so that disturbed or lifted endometrial mucosa does not confuse image interpretation. Common disposable biopsy samplers can be used for this purpose, or catheters that are specifically designed for the dual purpose of fluid infusion and endometrial biopsy are available, such as the Goldstein Sonobiopsy Catheter (Cook Medical).

Complications

SIS is a minor office procedure that is usually very well tolerated by the vast majority of women, although mild pelvic cramping and spotting are not uncommon side-effects. There are reports of occasional severe complications, and in a recent prospective study of 1153 patients [5] the stated incidence

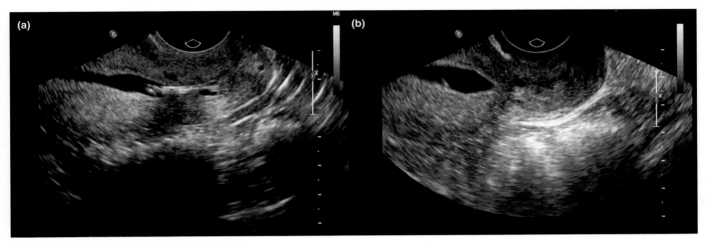

Figure 5.3. Optimal visualization of the lower uterine segment. (a) With the catheter tip at the level of the internal cervical os, instillation of fluid is begun as the catheter is completely withdrawn. (b) Distended lower uterine segment at the termination of the SIS procedure.

of peritonitis due to ascending pelvic infection was 0.95%. Patients, of course, should be apprised of this low-level risk and encouraged to call or return for evaluation in the event of postprocedural fever and progressive pelvic pain. In that same study, surprisingly, 8.8% of the participants experienced moderate or severe pain, vasovagal symptoms, or nausea or vomiting during the procedure; however, mostly intrauterine balloon catheters were used, and there is no mention of what other techniques, if any, were employed to prevent or reduce such reactions.

Failure of the procedure does also occur, unfortunately. de Kroon [6], in a meta-analysis of 24 studies and 2278 procedures, describes an overall failure rate of 7% – a figure that jumps to 13.5% in postmenopausal women, most likely due to cervical stenosis. A 5–7% range for procedural failure or incomplete investigation has also been reported by several other authors, with the larger fibroid uterus noted to be one of the other statistical predictors for a suboptimal result.

Finally, there remains the valid concern about fluid contrast hysterography and possible intraperitoneal spread of endometrial cancer. Two authors [7,8] have reported small prospective studies specifically designed to evaluate the risk of sonohysterography in patients with uterine cancer. The results differed substantially between the studies: the mean volume amount of saline instilled necessary to complete an adequate SIS examination varied from 8.5 to 33 ml, and the occurrence of malignant or suspicious cells recovered from tubal fluid spill ranged from 6% to 25%. What seems clear is that transtubal spill of fluid and endometrial cells into the peritoneal cavity does occur during SIS. Controversy still exists, however, regarding the prognostic significance of peritoneal washings positive for cancer cells, whether they be naturally occurring or artificially induced. Additionally, even if some dissemination of malignant cells into the pelvis does occur during a fluid contrast study and results in a small risk of upstaging early endometrial cancer, there currently is no definitive evidence that such an occurrence worsens long-

term prognosis [9]. More study is certainly needed in this area. In the meantime, since high fluid volumes and pressures during sonohysterography probably increase the rate of tubal spill, every effort should be made to avoid both during the procedure.

Diagnostic accuracy

The literature is now flush with multiple studies that document how very well SIS compares with other uterine imaging modalities in patients with AUB [10], infertility [11], and RPL [12]. Although sonohysterography provides an indirect look inside the uterus, its ability to accurately diagnose intracavitary filling defects, such as myomas and polyps and adhesions and even malformations, matches that of the "gold standard" hysteroscopy. Understandably, SIS adds more information than TVS alone; in addition, its performance is consistently much more sensitive and specific than that of hysterosalpingography, without exposing the patient to either ionizing radiation or contrast allergy. An improvement over hysteroscopy for the clinician, this procedure images far more in the female pelvis than simply the uterine cavity; yet, it is relatively simple to learn and perform, and it can easily be provided by those gynecology practices already offering TVS.

Specific imaging examples

Submucous myoma

Leiomyomas are hormone-dependent smooth-muscle tumors of the myometrium. Reported to be present in 20–40% of women during their reproductive years, they are the most common tumor found in females. Sonohysterography is an imaging technique with very high sensitivity for accurately diagnosing submucosal myomas, which penetrate variably into the endometrial cavity. The sonographic characteristics of these benign masses include broad-based heterogeneous echoes; isoechoic or hypoechoic appearance when compared with surrounding myometrium; an intracavitary component that is sometimes also clearly lined with endometrium (Figure 5.4); occasional poor sound transmission; distal shadowing when quite dense (Figure 5.5); hyperechoic foci if calcification is present; and a symmetrical and well-defined contour. Distortion of the endometrial cavity may or may not be associated with significant myometrial penetration, and the European Society of Hysteroscopy has developed a classification system to describe the relevant anatomy. A Type 0, or T:0, submucous fibroid has no intramural extension; T:1 has <50% extension, and T:2 has >50% intramural involvement [13]. This kind of classification allows authors around the world to speak in similar terms, and it also is a tool that can assist surgeons with preoperative planning. Hysteroscopic resection of T:0 and T:1 tumors can usually be accomplished completely (Figure 5.6), whereas T:2 myoma resection may require more than one procedure to complete, should be performed by only the most experienced hysteroscopists, and may be facilitated by the combined addition of either ultrasound or laparoscopic guidance.

Although the majority of women with myomas are asymptomatic, some patients with myomas may present with AUB in the form of pre- or postmenstrual spotting, heavy or prolonged periods, or intermenstrual spotting. The exact association between fibroids and AUB has not been clearly defined, but it has been theorized that excessive menorrhagia could be due to venous congestion in the myometrium and endometrium from the obstructive effect of myomas on uterine vasculature. Surgery can be an appropriate option to address the bleeding consequences of fibroids when conservative medical management fails, and complete hysteroscopic resection of submucous tumors has been shown by Corson and Brooks [14] to dramatically improve menorrhagia rates.

Many authors agree that leiomyomas alone are probably not a common cause of infertility [15], but the relationship of fibroids to reproductive outcome is not well characterized. Unfortunately, most of the studies that address this subject are fraught with a paucity of prospective, randomized, controlled trials and a lack of statistical power. Tumors that distort the endometrial cavity do appear to decrease fertility by 50–70% in the patients undergoing IVF due to failure of implantation, and their surgical correction can improve pregnancy rates to baseline [16]. So, given either infertility or RPL, surgery to remove submucosal myomas should be considered, but only after a thorough evaluation of all other causes and potential factors has been completed.

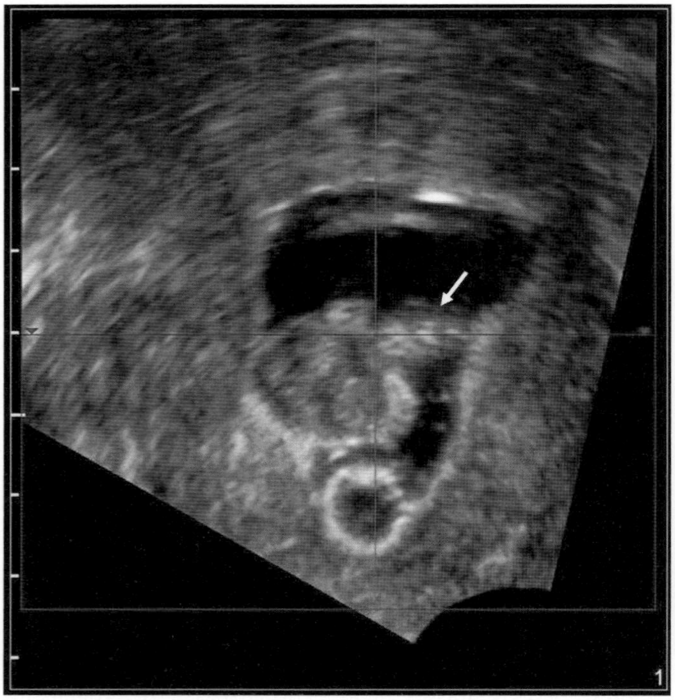

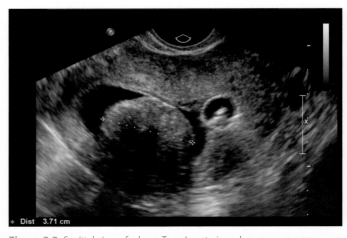

Figure 5.5. Sagittal view of a large Type I posterior submucous myoma (calipers) with minimal myometrial penetration. This solid, mostly spherical mass with mixed echoes and posterior acoustic shadowing has ultrasound characteristics that are typical for a fibroid, and it would be amenable to hysteroscopic resection.

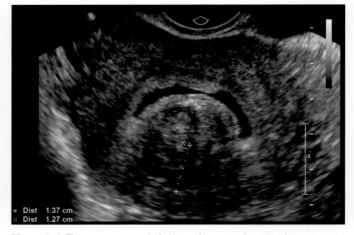

Figure 5.6. This uterus as seen in horizontal cross-section contains a submucous fibroid. Sonohysterography fluid contrast allows complete delineation of the posterior tumor, its depth of myometrial and endometrial extension (calipers), and its measured distance away from the exterior serosal surface.

Figure 5.4. Coronal view of the uterus filled with saline. A Type 0 submucous myoma is contained entirely within the cavity and arises from the right sidewall. The mass is incompletely lined by endometrium and blood clot (arrow).

Endometrial polyp

The most common filling defects identified by sonohysterography are polyps, which are growths of either mature or immature endometrium that are attached to a pedicle. Their sonographic characteristics are that they have a sessile or pedunculated base, usually an oval or fusiform shape, size varying from millimeters to centimeters, slightly greater echogenicity than myometrium, typically isoechoic with endometrium, and mostly homogeneous echoes though they may appear to have "microcysts" (Figure 5.7); they arise from the endometrium, do not distort the endo-myometrial junction, and often reveal a "feeder vessel" (Figure 5.8) on color Doppler evaluation. Patients with polyps may have no symptoms, may have fertility complaints, or may present with bleeding abnormalities similarly to women with fibroids. In fact, it is not necessarily uncommon to find that some women with AUB actually have coexisting submucous myomas and polyps (Figures 5.9, 5.10).

Endometrial polyps are usually surgically excised in symptomatic patients, although the exact association of polyps with AUB is not yet completely known. In a recent retrospective study of a mixed population of 300 women with polyps, 24.3% of whom were asymptomatic, the underlying rate of malignancy and complex hyperplasia with atypia was 1.6%. All of the cancer cases were in peri- or postmenopausal patients symptomatic with AUB [17]. Thus, the authors reaffirmed the need for symptomatic polyps to be removed. Although cancerous polyps have been found in asymptomatic women, there is currently no evidence-based standard that guides management decisions when the diagnosis of an endometrial polyp is completely incidental.

If there is a decisive relationship between infertility and the presence of polyps, that, too, needs further study. The mechanisms that regulate and impact implantation are mostly unexplained, but there is still concern that structural abnormalities in the uterine cavity may play a role in subfertility, implantation failure, and miscarriage. Reports about polyps, and whether or not their removal results in improved pregnancy rates, are conflicting [18,19]; however, it is still common clinical practice to screen the uterine cavity for abnormalities such as polyps in infertility patients, especially prior to IVF or after IVF failures, and SIS is an ideal way to accomplish this.

Postmenopausal women undergoing tamoxifen therapy are at increased risk for precancerous or cancerous change of the endometrium, but screening for these conditions in asymptomatic women using tamoxifen is not recommended. The presence of endometrial polyps in this group of patients prior to therapy, however, may increase the defined risk from this medication. Consequently, pretreatment sonohysterography to specifically investigate for polyps is a reasonable consideration.

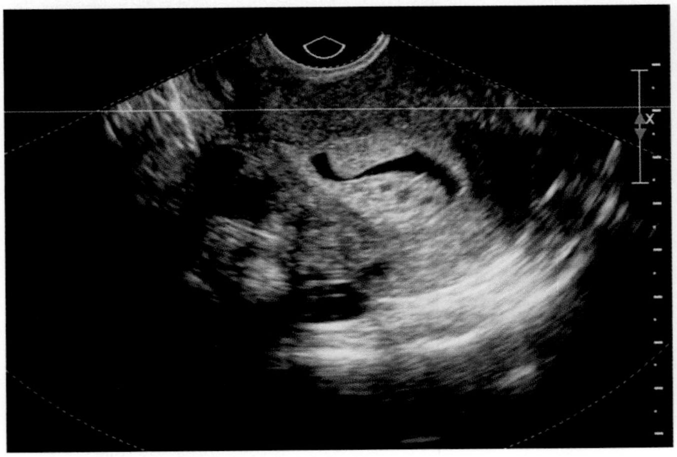

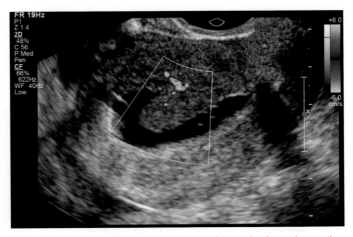

Figure 5.8. Color-flow image of an anterior endometrial polyp with a sessile base and a central "feeder vessel."

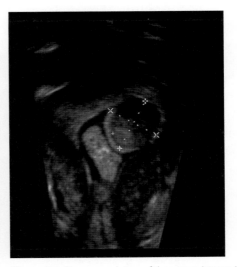

Figure 5.9. True coronal view of the uterus. Intracavitary fluid outlines two distinct masses: (1) a Type 0 submucous myoma (calipers) positioned near the left cornu and outlined with endometrium; (2) a central, brightly echogenic polyp.

Figure 5.7. Saline sonohysterography of a retroverted uterus with two polyps that are isoechoic with endometrium. The larger mass protruding from the anterior wall has a microcystic appearance.

Blood clot

It is necessary to appreciate fully the ultrasound characteristics of a blood clot due to its tendency to be confused with either adhesions or polyps when not free-floating. Most commonly, the surface contour of such a pseudo-filling defect is irregular. It is understandably avascular, may appear to move during active saline infusion, and is variably echodense depending upon its age (Figure 5.2). The diagnosis of a blood clot can sometimes be confirmed with the use of a firm catheter during SIS, which can be advanced into such an apparent mass and intentionally used to actively disrupt and scatter it.

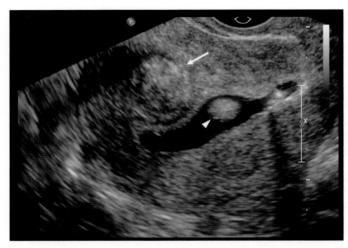

Figure 5.10. Combined findings of an anterior Type II submucous myoma (arrow), which is seen deviating the contour of the endometrial cavity, and an endometrial polyp (arrowhead).

Endometrial malignancy

A histological biopsy is required to make a firm diagnosis of either endometrial hyperplasia or cancer. When the disease is diffuse, endometrial sampling, even when performed in the office, is highly reliable. It is when the abnormality is found focally within the uterine cavity that false-negative results can and do occur. Clinical examples of where sonohysterography might be useful include histo-pathological results that denote inadequate sampling, such as "tissue insufficient for diagnosis" (Figure 5.11); a biopsy diagnosis that does not match the transvaginal ultrasound finding, such as "endometrial atrophy" in a postmenopausal woman whose endometrial stripe

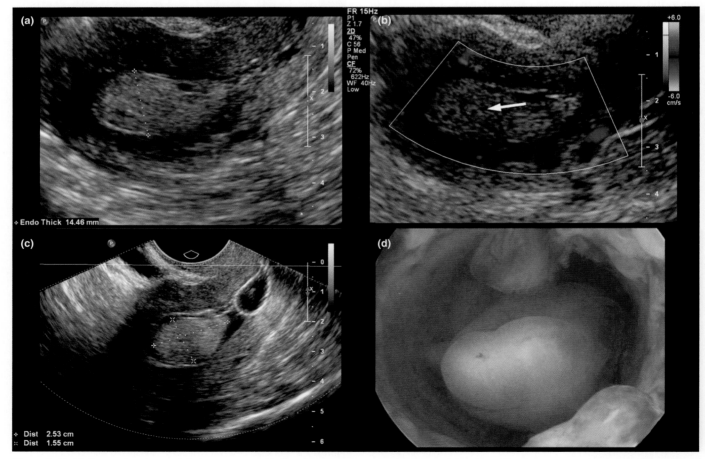

Figure 5.11. (a) Abnormal endometrial thickness measured (calipers) in a postmenopausal patient with bleeding. Office biopsy reported tissue insufficient for diagnosis. (b) Application of color-flow reveals a central "feeder vessel" (arrow). (c) Saline surrounds a homogeneously echodense filling defect (calipers), suggestive of polyp. The endometrium lining the cavity is very thin and symmetric, explaining the biopsy results. (d) Benign polyp confirmed on hysteroscopy.

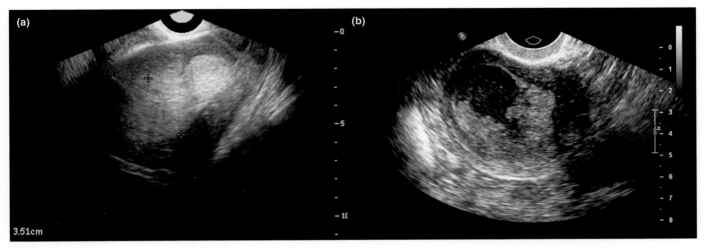

Figure 5.12. Two views of endometrial cancer. (a) Diffuse adenocarcinoma. Endometrium (calipers) is mostly homogeneous and very thick. (b) Focal carcinosarcoma appears irregular and echogenic. This is not an SIS image; rather, the fluid seen in this complex endometrial cavity is blood. Office biopsy can miss this diagnosis, especially given the thin, symmetric endometrium seen anteriorly.

is uncharacteristically thickened; or any patient with AUB whose endometrium on TVS is indistinct or not visible in its entirety, despite the biopsy results. Any focal findings on SIS deserve hysteroscopy and selective biopsy under direct visualization, and focal cancers tend to have irregular borders, may disrupt the endo-myometrial junction or reveal obvious myometrial invasion, and can be highly vascular (Figure 5.12). Finally of note is the fact that endometrial cancers may cause poor distensibility of the cavity during saline infusion [20].

Effects of tamoxifen

Most women undergoing adjuvant therapy for breast cancer with tamoxifen have no pathological endometrial changes. However, the estrogen-agonist effect of tamoxifen can be associated with endometrial polyps, hyperplasia, metaplasia, and cancer, so postmenopausal patients, especially, with any signs of bleeding, should be thoroughly evaluated. Unfortunately, the most common abnormal TVS finding in this situation is a nonspecific thickened endometrial stripe with scattered cystic changes (Figure 5.13). Because there are many diagnostic options, which include subepithelial stromal hypertrophy and subendometrial cysts, SIS can be used to help delineate true endometrial abnormalities when abnormal symptoms arise.

Intrauterine synechia

Intrauterine adhesions almost never occur de novo or spontaneously; rather, they are a recognized complication of uterine curettage necessitated by postpartum or postabortion retained products of conception or septic abortion. Patients with this condition may be entirely asymptomatic and present with unexplained infertility or RPL, or they may seek relief for menstrual complaints of amenorrhea, hypomenorrhea, or dysmenorrhea. An interrupted endometrial

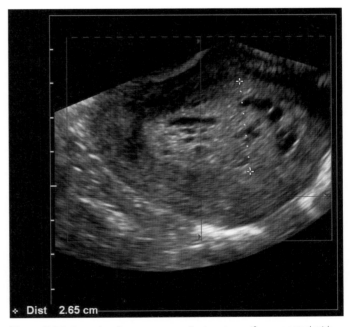

Figure 5.13. A previous breast cancer patient on tamoxifen presented with abnormal uterine bleeding. The thick endometrium (calipers) of this retroverted uterus on sagittal view appears heterogeneous and cystic. After endometrial sampling excluded hyperplasia and malignancy, sonohysterography revealed a large polyp whose final pathology was benign.

stripe seen on transvaginal ultrasound may suggest the possibility of synechia (Figure 5.14). SIS, however, is a simple and sensitive imaging method that can confirm the diagnosis, which manifests as thick, thin, firm, or undulating echogenic bridging bands extending from anterior to posterior uterine walls (Figure 5.15). The lateral walls and fundus of the uterus also may be involved, and true coronal plane views can help elucidate the extent of disease. Not surprisingly, distension of the cavity may be difficult and require increased injection pressures (Figure 5.16), or the most

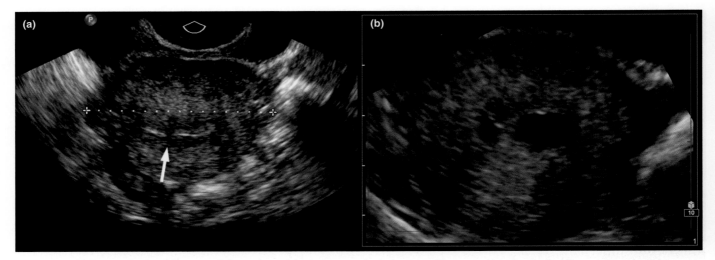

Figure 5.14. (a) Transverse view of the uterus. A thin endometrial stripe appears discontinuous and interrupted by a longitudinal linear structure (arrow) whose echodensity is similar to that of myometrium. (b) Sonohysterography confirms a thick adhesion to the right of midline bridging between anterior and posterior uterine walls.

severe cases of Asherman syndrome may result in a failed study altogether because adherent endometrial walls simply do not separate. Valle and Sciarra [21] showed many years ago that making the diagnosis of intrauterine adhesions is critical because hysteroscopic treatment can dramatically improve both menstrual disturbances and reproductive outcome in affected women.

Congenital uterine anomaly

In most studies to date, the prevalence of congenital uterine anomalies (CUA; also known as congenital uterine abnormalities) is similar in both infertile and fertile women at around 4–7%. In women with a diagnosis of RPL, however, the prevalence of this condition rises to nearly 17% [22]. Of the many known possible uterine malformations, complete or partial septate uterus is the most common major anomaly with a mean incidence of 35%, when present is associated with the poorest reproductive outcome, and is the most easily amenable to surgical treatment [23]. Uterine anomalies can result in impaired pregnancy outcomes, and obstetric complications are more frequent. The goal of hysteroscopic septum resection is to restore a normal uterine cavity, and successful treatment gives in near-normal pregnancy results with a term delivery rate of 75% and a live birth rate of 85% [24].

Sonohysterography is better able than HSG and TVS to differentiate a septate from a complete bicornuate uterus, and a precise diagnosis in this situation is of paramount importance to the gynecologic surgeon because the respective operations necessary to correct these two conditions are completely different from one another. The normal uterus has an endometrial cavity that is entirely empty and has a conelike appearance on sagittal view (Figure 5.1). The septate uterus has a convex, flat, or slightly indented fundal contour, while the cavity is divided

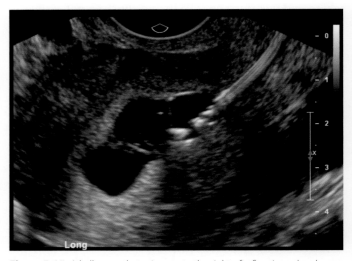

Figure 5.15. A balloon catheter is seen to the right of a fine, irregular, shaggy adhesion which stretches from the anterior to the posterior uterine wall.

either partially (subseptate) or completely (septate) by a midline longitudinal band of varying length and width with an echotexture similar to that of myometrium (Figure 5.17). The thickness of the septum and the relationship of the septum to the fundal myometrium are important data points when planning hysteroscopic metroplasty. Three-dimensional ultrasound technology, with the addition of its reconstructed coronal plane image, allows accurate measurement of dimensions and volume.

Additional studies

Although beyond the scope of this chapter, there are several other extrapolations of saline infusion ultrasound of the pelvis that deserve mention.

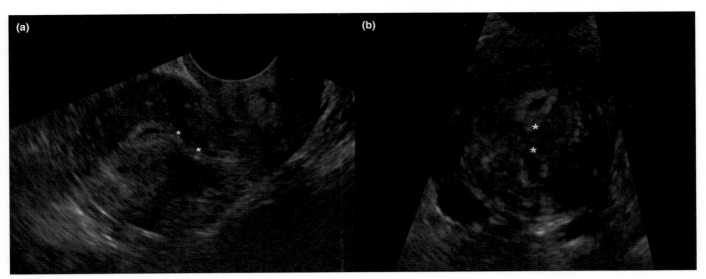

Figure 5.16. This patient presented with very light, short menses beginning after uterine curettage for spontaneous miscarriage. Both the sagittal view (a) and coronal view (b) show a thick adhesive band (calipers) that partially obliterates the uterine cavity.

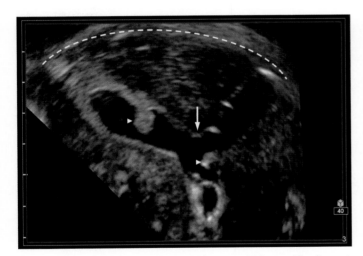

Figure 5.17. A subseptate uterus is seen in this coronal SIS image. The diagnosis is confirmed by visualizing a partial septum (arrow) in combination with a normal surface uterine contour (broken curved line). Endometrial polyps (arrowheads) are an incidental finding.

3D SIS

The ability to rapidly acquire and store a set of volume data about the entire uterus has some potential advantages: (1) the volume data can be evaluated in any plane desired, retrospectively, possibly reducing the usual amount of time necessary during two-dimensional SIS for uterine distension and multiple still images; (2) the true "C-plane," or coronal view, of the uterus maximizes the information about the endometrial cavity, the myometrium, and the fundal contour (Figure 5.18, and see Figures 5.16, 5.4, 5.9) to potentially improve diagnostic accuracy in the setting of CUA (Figure 5.17).

Sonosalpingography or hysterosalpingo-contrast sonography (HyCoSy)

This procedure uses a technique similar to SIS to evaluate tubal obstruction in infertility patients. Ultrasound-positive contrast media can distend the uterus and reveal the tubes, but an alternative is to use an agitated mixture of air and saline to observe for patency. Exacoustos et al. showed HyCoSy to be as effective as HSG in diagnosing tubal patency, and the detection rate for tubal obstruction was 80% [25].

Operative SIS

If there is a drawback to SIS alone, it is that, unlike office hysteroscopy, it does not allow guided biopsy at the time of diagnosis. There have been promising studies to evaluate the feasibility of using SIS guidance for both directed biopsy and polyp resection, but further randomized research is needed in this area.

Sonovaginography

Combining TVS with vaginal saline infusion may improve the ability to image structures surrounding the vagina, such as the rectovaginal septum for endometriosis.

Key points in clinical practice

1. SIS is a simple, minimally invasive, cost-effective imaging option that is applicable to many gynecologic conditions.

2. For evaluation of the endometrial cavity, the degree of accuracy for this office test approximates that of hysteroscopy and exceeds that of both HSG and TVS.

3. Sonohysterography is well tolerated by the patient, nearly risk-free, and can be learned easily by those physicians already experienced in transvaginal ultrasound.

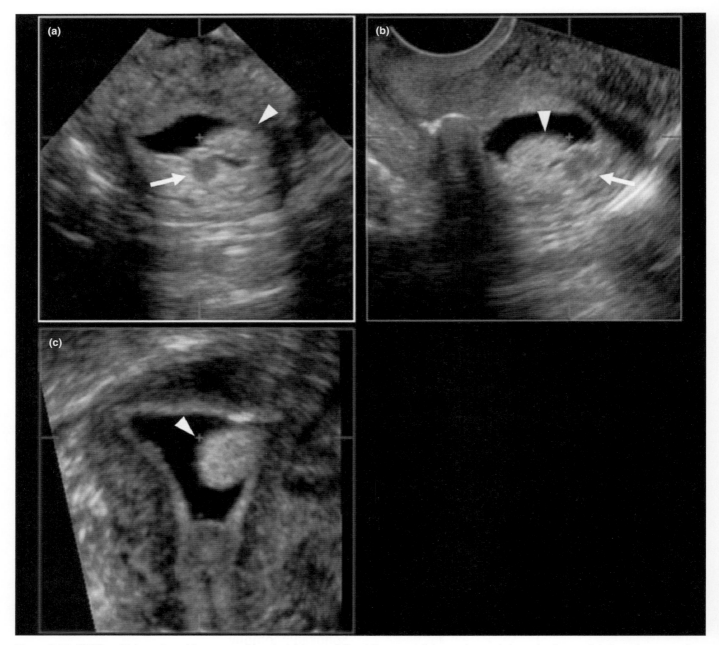

Figure 5.18. 3D SIS, multiplanar views: (a) transverse, (b) sagittal; (c) coronal. The ability to see all three orthogonal planes simultaneously helps to locate exactly the size and position of both a posterior submucous myoma (arrow) and a left lateral endometrial polyp (arrowhead).

References

1. Breitkopf D Goldstein SR, Seeds JW; ACOG Committee on Gynecologic Practice. ACOG technology assessment in obstetrics and gynecology. Number 3, September 2003. Saline infusion sonohysterography. *Obstet Gynecol* [Technology Assessment]. 2003; **102**: 659–62.

2. Lindheim SR, Sprague C, Winter TC 3rd. Hysterosalpingography and sonohysterography: lessons in technique. *AJR Am J Roentgenol.* 2006; **186**(1): 24–9.

3. Dessole S, Farina M, Capobianco G, Nardelli GB, Ambrosini G, Meloni GB. Determining the best catheter for sonohysterography. *Fertil Steril* 2001; **76**(3): 605–9.

4. Spieldoch RL, Winter TC, Schouweiler C, Ansay S, Evans MD, Lindheim SR. Optimal catheter placement during sonohysterography: a randomized controlled trial comparing cervical to uterine placement. *Obstet Gynecol* 2008; **111**(1): 15–21.

5. Dessole S, Farina M, Rubattu G, Cosmi E, Ambrosini G, Battista Nardelli G. Side effects and complications of sonohysterosalpingography. *Fertil Steril* 2003; **80**(3): 620–4.

6. de Kroon CD, de Bock GH, Dieben SW, Jansen FW. Saline contrast hysterosonography in abnormal uterine bleeding: a systematic review and

meta-analysis. *BJOG* 2003; **110**(10): 938–47.

7. Berry E, Lindheim SR, Connor JP, et al. Sonohysterography and endometrial cancer: incidence and functional viability of disseminated malignant cells. *Am J Obstet Gynecol* 2008; **199**(3): 240 e1–8.

8. Dessole S, Rubattu G, Farina M, et al. Risks and usefulness of sonohysterography in patients with endometrial carcinoma. *Am J Obstet Gynecol* 2006; **194**(2): 362–8.

9. Revel A, Tsafrir A, Anteby SO, Shushan A. Does hysteroscopy produce intraperitoneal spread of endometrial cancer cells? *Obstet Gynecol Surv* 2004; **59**(4): 280–4.

10. Jansen FW, de Kroon CD, van Dongen H, Grooters C, Louwe L, Trimbos-Kemper T. Diagnostic hysteroscopy and saline infusion sonography: prediction of intrauterine polyps and myomas. *J Minim Invasive Gynecol* 2006; **13**(4): 320–4.

11. Ragni G, Diaferia D, Vegetti W, Colombo M, Arnoldi M, Crosignani PG. Effectiveness of sonohysterography in infertile patient work-up: a comparison with transvaginal ultrasonography and hysteroscopy. *Gynecol Obstet Invest* 2005; **59**(4): 184–8.

12. Keltz MD, Olive DL, Kim AH, Arici A. Sonohysterography for screening in recurrent pregnancy loss. *Fertil Steril* 1997; **67**(4): 670–4.

13. Wamsteker K, Emanuel MH, de Kruif JH. Transcervical hysteroscopic resection of submucous fibroids for abnormal uterine bleeding: results regarding the degree of intramural extension. *Obstet Gynecol* 1993; **82**(5): 736–40.

14. Corson SL, Brooks PG. Resectoscopic myomectomy. *Fertil Steril* 1991; **55**(6): 1041–4.

15. Practice Committee of the American Society for Reproductive Medicine. Myomas and reproductive function. *Fertil Steril* 2006 Nov; **86**(5 Suppl 1): S194–9.

16. Pritts EA. Fibroids and infertility: a systematic review of the evidence. *Obstet Gynecol Surv* 2001; **56**(8): 483–91.

17. Shushan A, Revel A, Rojansky N. How often are endometrial polyps malignant? *Gynecol Obstet Invest* 2004; **58**(4): 212–15.

18. Perez-Medina T, Bajo-Arenas J, Salazar F, et al. Endometrial polyps and their implication in the pregnancy rates of patients undergoing intrauterine insemination: a prospective, randomized study. *Hum Reprod* 2005; **20**(6): 1632–5.

19. Lass A, Williams G, Abusheikha N, Brinsden P. The effect of endometrial polyps on outcomes of in vitro fertilization (IVF) cycles. *J Assist Reprod Genet* 1999; **16**(8): 410–15.

20. Laifer-Narin SL, Ragavendra N, Lu DS, Sayre J, Perrella RR, Grant EG. Transvaginal saline hysterosonography: characteristics distinguishing malignant and various benign conditions. *AJR Am J Roentgenol* 1999; **172**(6): 1513–20.

21. Valle RF, Sciarra JJ. Intrauterine adhesions: hysteroscopic diagnosis, classification, treatment, and reproductive outcome. *Am J Obstet Gynecol* 1988; **158**(6 Pt 1): 1459–70.

22. Saravelos SH, Cocksedge KA, Li TC. Prevalence and diagnosis of congenital uterine anomalies in women with reproductive failure: a critical appraisal. *Hum Reprod Update* 2008; **14**(5): 415–29.

23. March CM, Israel R. Hysteroscopic management of recurrent abortion caused by septate uterus. *Am J Obstet Gynecol* 1987; **156**(4): 834–42.

24. Grimbizis GF, Camus M, Tarlatzis BC, Bontis JN, Devroey P. Clinical implications of uterine malformations and hysteroscopic treatment results. *Hum Reprod Update* 2001; **7**(2): 161–74.

25. Exacoustos C, Zupi E, Carusotti C, Lanzi G, Marconi D, Arduini D. Hysterosalpingo-contrast sonography compared with hysterosalpingography and laparoscopic dye pertubation to evaluate tubal patency. *J Am Assoc Gynecol Laparosc* 2003; **10**(3): 367–72.

53

Diagnostic hysteroscopy

Tony Bazi and Tony G. Zreik

The history of hysteroscopy: light, optics, distension

It was in the first decade of the nineteenth century that a German-born physician by the name of Philipp Bozzini allegedly attempted to visualize the cavities of the living through a hollow tube, with the help of candlelight reflected by a mirror. At the time, his idea of "a magic lantern in the human body" was ridiculed.

The first reported successful direct visualization of the endometrial cavity was that of Pantaleoni in 1869, using a modified instrument previously invented by Desmoreaux for bladder visualization [1]. During the procedure, a "hemorrhagic uterine growth" was diagnosed and cauterized with silver nitrate, thus qualifying the procedure to be the first "operative hysteroscopy."

Maximilian Nitze (1848–1906) set the cornerstone for modern endoscopy by incorporating, within the viewing instrument, an optical lens system (such as in a microscope). This allowed a larger field of view, and the first of the "modern" cystoscopes was born in 1877, measuring 21-French.

In the following decades, several reported attempts at developing hysteroscopy met with technical obstacles. This was not the case with cystoscopy, which was evolving at a much faster pace. The reason lies in the inherent difference between the two organs to be visualized. The bladder is a storage organ of high compliance; distension and wall separation is a physiological phenomenon. The major challenge with hysteroscopy, on the other hand, was in transforming a small cavity with two apposing thick muscle layers into a space amenable to visual inspection. In addition, the tendency of the endometrium to bleed with the earlier inspection methods made satisfactory visualization too cumbersome. Another limitation was the light source, as the placement of incandescent bulbs in the vicinity of the inspected organ resulted in excessive heat dissipation.

The introduction of carbon dioxide (CO_2) as a distending medium [2], and the development of the "cold light system" are the two most important pillars upon which modern hysteroscopy was built.

In the cold light system, light is conducted from its source via bundles of fine glass fibers (hence the term fiberoptics), thus sparing the illuminated organ the effect of heat production. The first fiberoptic endoscope, a bronchoscope, was described in 1952 by Fourestiere et al. [1]. However, it did not use the "cold light system," as illumination was provided by miniature bulbs situated distally (next to the lens). Only the visual information was transmitted via a bundle of "coherent" fine glass fibers, i.e., fibers having exactly the same spatial arrangement at both ends of the cable. Thus, fiberoptic principles were applied in endoscopy for image transmission before their use in conducting light from a distant source [3].

Endoscopic visualization took a dramatic leap after the clinical application of the rod-lens system in the late 1960s, more than a decade after its conception by Harold Hopkins, a British physicist [3]. In the rod-lens system, fewer and narrower air–glass interfaces exist, thus reversing the roles of air and glass in conventional telescopes at the time. With air acting now as a lens through long glass rods, the system yields a brighter image, better resolution, and a wider viewing angle, all through a smaller-diameter telescope. In 1965, Karl Storz (1911–1996) licensed the idea of fiberoptic external cold light transmission coupled with the rod-lens optical system. This was the first prototype of the "rigid hysteroscope" known today.

Improvement in uterine distension, on the other hand, was facing a standstill, as the use of CO_2 was found to be associated with serious hazards, including acidosis, embolism, and death. It is very likely that such events were the result of uncontrolled infusion rates, a deviation from the original description by Rubin in 1925 [2]. This led to a relative pause in the implementation of hysteroscopy as a viable diagnostic procedure.

Distending the uterine cavity with a transparent rubber balloon inflated with air or saline was tried. While safe and mechanically sound, this method did not prove to be viable, as lesions could be easily missed, and the visual field could be compromised.

In 1970, Edstrom and Fernstrom reported on the use of 35% dextran solution as a distention medium in 30 women undergoing hysteroscopy. The view was described as clear enough to allow visualization of the "rhythmic contractions of the tubal ostia" [4].

By the early 1970s, there was a better understanding of the relationship between parameters of CO_2 insufflation and the

Ultrasonography in Reproductive Medicine and Infertility, ed. Botros R. M. B. Rizk. Published by Cambridge University Press. © Cambridge University Press 2010.

risk of adverse events. Lindelmann and Mohr, in a classic publication in 1976, showed that when keeping the intrauterine pressure between 40 and 80 mmHg, no complication was observed in more than 1200 hysteroscopies, including 450 transuterine tubal sterilizations [5]. Interestingly, this pressure range was almost identical to the one described by Rubin, using manometric control half a century earlier [2]. Technological advances allowing electronic monitoring of gas flow rate and intrauterine pressure led to the reintroduction and subsequent widespread use of CO_2 as a safe and effective distension medium.

The 1980s witnessed great technological improvements that benefited all fields of endoscopy. Specifically, the attachment of miniature chip cameras to transmit images to a screen allowed faster and more accurate procedures, and revolutionized the process of education.

During the 1990s, the development of fine bipolar operating instruments for use with saline as a distending medium improved the safety profile of the procedure, especially as related to fluid overload, and contributed to the increased adoption of the "see and treat" philosophy.

Distension media

Whether diagnostic or operative, hysteroscopy cannot be performed without distending the uterine cavity.

The ideal distension medium should

1. Be safe and nonallergenic
2. Have an optimal refractory index
3. Be readily absorbed by the human body, in case of intraperitoneal spill, without causing major hemodynamic changes
4. Be largely soluble in blood, so that no embolism would result from intravasation
5. Be readily cleared by the renal or respiratory system
6. Be available at a reasonable cost

The pressure required to separate the walls of a normal-sized uterine cavity (with saline) is less than 50 mmHg, while intraperitoneal spillage occurs between 70 and 110 mmHg, depending on the degree of tubal adhesive disease.

Hyskon®

Dextrans are polysaccharide polymers that have been in clinical use for decades for plasma expansion and thrombotic prophylaxis.

A solution containing 35% dextran 70 (molecular weight 70 000 kDa) was introduced in 1970 as a distending medium for hysteroscopy [4]. At a time when the choice of satisfactory distension media was limited, this solution was quickly adopted by gynecologists as it provided a clear view as a result of its excellent light conduction and its immiscibility with blood. Additional advantages include its nonconductive properties and electrolyte-free composition. Later marketed under the name Hyskon® (32% dextran 70 in 10% dextrose in water), it is introduced into the uterine cavity through the cannula of the hysteroscope under low pressure (~100 mmHg) until the uterus is sufficiently distended to permit adequate visualization. Usually less than 100 ml is sufficient for satisfactory diagnosis [4]. Due to its viscous nature, it sticks and crystallizes onto the equipment unless washed off with hot saline immediately after the procedure.

The main concern with Hyskon® was the emergence of safety issues following reports of pulmonary edema and disseminated intravascular coagulopathy (DIC) associated with its use, especially after long operative procedures [6]. Initially, this was believed to be partly due to its oncotic properties as a powerful plasma expander in case of intravasation (8.6 times its own volume). Fluid overload alone, however, may not explain the other serious events, such as hypoxia, hypotension, renal failure, and DIC. It is thus likely that Hyskon® may induce direct pulmonary toxicity with subsequent release of vasoactive mediators and activation of the coagulation cascade [6].

While the above complications, collectively referred to as the "Dextran syndrome" [6], have been related to the use of large amounts (>500 ml), anaphylaxis and anaphylactoid reactions may occur with much smaller volumes [7]. Although sensitization through previous exposure to sugar beets or some bacterial antigens may be responsible, there is no reliable way to identify the patient at risk [7]. The incidence of dextran 70-induced anaphylactoid reactions during its intravenous use for plasma expansion or thrombotic prophylaxis is about 1:2000. It is reasonable to assume that the incidence would be much less when used as a distension medium and in the absence of intravasation. Nevertheless, the possibility of occurrence of such a serious adverse event in a healthy woman undergoing an outpatient procedure is alarming. Fewer hysteroscopists are now using Hyskon®, which has been withdrawn from the market in some countries. It is the authors' opinion that there exist nowadays alternative satisfactory distension media that are safer than Hyskon®.

Low-viscosity electrolyte-free solutions

Use of 5% dextrose in water as a distending medium, while successful, was associated with hyponatremia and hyperglycemia, especially in long operative hysteroscopies [8].

Other sugar solutions, such as mannitol, sorbitol, or a combination of the two, as well as glycine in different concentrations (1.5% and 3.0%) have all been used in hysteroscopy, following extensive experience with their use in transurethral prostate procedures. As they are nonconductive, monopolar electrosurgery is judged to be safe, if needed. Dilutional hyponatremia, while possible with all three media (including mannitol, which theoretically by itself induces diuresis), is usually only encountered after prolonged operative procedures that involve endometrial injury [9]. Use of glycine has also been reported to temporarily affect vision in the postoperative period, secondary to its neurotransmitter inhibitory effect in the retina.

It is important to remember that, at least theoretically, any of these complications may be encountered in a strictly diagnostic hysteroscopy if the duration and infused volume exceed reasonable limits. It is therefore judicious to monitor infused volumes, at least manually, especially when supervising long procedures performed by trainees.

Currently, the two most commonly used distension media for diagnostic hysteroscopy are carbon dioxide (CO_2) and physiological saline. CO_2 is the only gas currently used for uterine distension. Use of air is precluded by embolism. Nitrous oxide (N_2O), when delivered through a laparoscopy insufflator (i.e., at much higher pressures than accepted) was found to increase the PCO_2 and possibly cause embolism as well. However, there is insufficient data about its use with modern insufflators with the recommended parameters for hysteroscopy.

Having a refractive index equivalent to that of air (1.00), CO_2 used as a distension medium provides a good-quality panoramic view of the uterine cavity. It suppresses combustion, is blood soluble, and is rapidly eliminated by the lungs. A potential limitation is the creation of gas bubbles when it is mixed with blood or mucus. This is especially the case when bleeding is unpreventable in case of dilation of the cervix. Experienced hysteroscopists have learned to overcome this transient problem, either by waiting for spontaneous clearing, or by flushing the bubbles with a readily available saline-filled syringe.

Safety concerns over the use of CO_2 originated from reports of potentially fatal gas embolism [10]. However, CO_2 is highly soluble in blood and is rapidly cleared by the lungs. It is therefore most likely that gas embolism is unrelated to the type of distension medium (CO_2), and actually represents venous entrapment of room air rather than CO_2 [10,11]. Not taking the distension medium into consideration, a 1991 survey recorded gas embolism in 0.02% of all hysteroscopies (diagnostic and operative) [12]. The incidence of subclinical emboli, suggested by a decrease in end-tidal CO_2, could be much higher [11]. Possible predisposing factors include steep Trendelenburg positioning, intrauterine bleeding, difficult cervical dilation (with possible creation of false myometrial tracks), and presence of air (instead of the distending medium) in the tubing system at the initiation of the procedure [10,11]. In fact, "deaerating" the supply tube, i.e., purging the tube with CO_2, was sufficient to eliminate subclinical embolism among 1261 consecutive diagnostic hysteroscopies [11].

It is safe to assume that, when modern insufflating devices are used, a strictly diagnostic hysteroscopy poses an unmeasurable risk of embolism. In addition, with an intrauterine pressure below 70 mmHg, and a flow rate not exceeding 60 ml per minute, the amount of CO_2 entering the peritoneal cavity during a diagnostic procedure is less than few hundred milliliters, allowing for rapid absorption and subsequent lung excretion without any risk of acidosis. Since CO_2 is used during laparoscopy at a much higher flow rate, at least 30 times that used for hysteroscopy, it is imperative to have the laparoscopy insufflators stored separately outside the hysteroscopy room, in order to avoid mistakes with potentially grave consequences.

Saline, having a refractory index of 1.37, offers the advantage of magnification of the area under examination. This characteristic, along with the inability of saline to "flatten" the endometrium, may lead to detection of subtle endometrial pathology (endometritis, adenomyosis) that would otherwise be missed with the use of CO_2 [13].

Arguably, saline flow during the introduction of the hysteroscope (up to 5.5 mm diameter) "opens up" the cervical canal, thus reducing the need for cervical dilation compared with CO_2 [13]. In addition, should bipolar operative instruments be needed during the same setting, no change of medium is necessary when saline is used. Finally, saline may be delivered without the need for calibrated electronic equipment, making it a cheap and safe distending medium.

A summary of randomized controlled trials evaluating saline versus CO_2 use in outpatient diagnostic hysteroscopy (with or without endometrial biopsy) is outlined in Table 6.1. It is important to note that the procedural steps (speculum, tenaculum, dilation) were not identical in these studies [13,14,15,16,17,18].

Although the discomfort associated with either medium is often described as "tolerable," there seems to be a trend, for various reasons, for more successfully completed examinations with saline use [13,14].

The shorter operative time with saline use is a result of two factors: (1) a more rapid expansion of the endometrial cavity, and (2) a quicker satisfactory diagnosis due to the absence of bubbles. The time saved, often in the order of few minutes, is especially important for the awake and anxious patient undergoing an outpatient procedure.

Preparing the cervix

Misoprostol, a synthetic prostaglandin E_1 analogue, is mainly used for the prevention of gastric ulcers due to its cytoprotective properties. Compared with placebo, use of misoprostol among premenopausal women before hysteroscopy was found to result in fewer cervical lacerations, most probably secondary to a reduced need for cervical dilation [19]. This benefit is counteracted by a higher incidence of cramping, elevated temperature, and uterine bleeding. The latter is particularly important as it may interfere with the diagnostic accuracy of the procedure. The route of administration and the exact dosage of misoprostol needed remain arbitrary.

Dinoprostone, a natural prostaglandin E_2 known for its use in labor induction, has also been used for cervical ripening prior to hysteroscopy. However, the lower cost of misoprostol and its stability at room temperature are clear advantages favoring its selection over other prostaglandins.

The use of Laminaria as cervical ripeners has been extensively cited in the obstetric literature. The complication rate is extremely low, and anaphylaxis has not been reported with the new synthetic version. Laminaria insertion three hours before diagnostic hysteroscopy with a 5 mm sheath was found to soften the cervix and facilitate the procedure.

Table 6.1. Randomized controlled trials evaluating saline vs. CO_2 use in outpatient diagnostic hysteroscopy

Study (Reference)	Patients (n)	Pain	Visibility	Time	Comments
Nagele et al., 1996 [14]	157	Worse with CO_2	Similar with both	Shorter with saline	
Pellicano et al., 2003 [15]	189 (all with infertility)	Worse with CO_2	Similar with both	Shorter with saline	Vaginoscopic approach
Brusco et al., 2003 [16]	74	Worse with CO_2	Similar with both	Shorter with saline	Vaginoscopic approach with saline; tenaculum use with CO_2
Litta et al., 2003 [17]	415	Worse with saline only in nulliparous; otherwise similar	Not studied	Shorter with saline	No cervical dilation in any. Pain always worse in nulliaprous
Shankar et al., 2004 [18]	300	Similar with both	Better with saline	Not studied	Mostly postmenopausal patients. Local anesthetic for tenaculum application
Paschopoulos et al., 2004 [13]	74	Similar with both	Saline better for detection of "subtle" endometrial lesions	Not studied	Vaginoscopic approach

Anesthesia/analgesia

Decades ago, a diagnostic hysteroscopy was mostly performed under general or regional anesthesia. With the introduction of smaller-caliber hysteroscopes, and with increasing experience and confidence of gynecologists, hysteroscopy gradually became an ambulatory office procedure. This allowed a faster recovery, better patient satisfaction, and cost control, while still yielding comparable findings to inpatient hysteroscopy [20].

Notwithstanding the anxiety associated with any office procedure, pain during diagnostic hysteroscopy results from any or all of the following:

(a) Application of the tenaculum to the cervix, when necessary

(b) Dilation of the cervix, when necessary

(c) Insertion of the hysteroscope

(d) Distension of the uterus, leading to visceral pain

(e) Inadvertent contact of a dilator or the hysteroscope with the endometrial surface, with subsequent muscle fiber stretching.

Conscious sedation

For years the term "conscious sedation" was vague, and use of different combinations of sedatives/analgesics during outpatient and inpatient procedures, by nonanesthesiologists, was lacking standard guidelines. In 2002, the American Society of Anesthesiologists (ASA) adopted the definitions of four levels of sedation–analgesia as follows [21]:

1. Minimal sedation (anxiolysis)

2. Moderate sedation/analgesia (conscious sedation)

3. Deep sedation/analgesia

4. General anesthesia

Moderate sedation/analgesia (conscious sedation) was defined as "a drug-induced depression of consciousness during which patients respond purposefully to verbal commands, either alone or accompanied by light tactile stimulation. No interventions are required to maintain a patent airway, and spontaneous ventilation is adequate. Cardiovascular function is usually maintained."

It is important to note that these levels represent a "continuum." Consequently, it is not possible to preoperatively identify the patient who may go into a deeper level of sedation than initially intended. Individuals administering moderate sedation/analgesia (conscious sedation) should therefore be able to rescue patients who enter a state of deep sedation/analgesia.

Recommendations and guidelines about use of conscious sedation may vary from one institution to another. It is imperative to abide by the institutional policies and the policies of the health care authorities, where applicable.

When no such policy exists, we find the guidelines detailed by the ASA to be a valuable reference. To maximize safety during conscious sedation, at least the following criteria should be met:

1. Monitoring of the patient is done before, during, and after the procedure, and is documented. This is done by a well-trained health care provider, possibly a nurse, who may not be involved with additional duties other than minor interruptible tasks and only after the patient's level of sedation–analgesia and vital signs have stabilized.

2. Pharmacologic antagonists and resuscitation medications should be immediately available. Appropriate equipment for establishing a patent airway, suctioning, and providing positive pressure ventilation with supplemental oxygen should be present and in good working order.

3. Education is provided to the patient and family, and discharge occurs only when specific written criteria are met, to minimize the risk of central nervous system or cardiorespiratory depression after discharge.

Local anesthetic injection

Despite the increasing adoption of hysteroscopy as an ambulatory procedure, protocols for local anesthesia and/or analgesia remain far from uniform. Notwithstanding the personal preferences of physicians, the pertinent literature allows for only limited conclusions regarding the ideal anesthetic/analgesic approach, when necessary, due to the following:

(a) Cultural differences are known to exist among patient populations regarding pain perception and tolerance.

(b) Parity and menopausal status, two factors affecting the cervical canal diameter, are not uniform in most data.

(c) The amount and concentration of the anesthetic/analgesic, the technique, the route, and the timing of administration as related to the actual procedure remain arbitrary.

(d) Comparison is not possible among procedures using instruments of different calibers, and different distending media at different intrauterine pressures.

(e) The extent and the duration of the operative component of hysteroscopy, when present, vary from one study to another.

Innervation of the upper vagina, the cervix, and the lower uterine segment is believed to pass through the plexuses of Frankenhauser, which are located posterolateral to the cervix, within the uterosacral folds. Paracervical block in this region is known to alleviate pain related to these organs. The uterine fundus, on the other hand, derives its innervation directly from the hypogastric plexus originating from T11–L1. It has been suggested that fibers from this plexus run deeply within the paracervical tissues. Except in women with endometriosis, the functional endometrial layer is totally devoid of nerve fibers, while the deeper portion of the basal layer may occasionally contain small unmyelinated nerve fibers.

In women of reproductive age, paracervical block does not seem to affect procedure-related pain with 5 mm hysteroscopes [22].

In addition, disadvantages related to paracervical block include injection pain and bleeding. The same is true about intracervical lidocaine injection, which was not found to be superior to saline. Interestingly, a sizable number of patients consider the injection itself to be as painful as the hysteroscopy [22]. Two points must be mentioned for an adequate evaluation of the data addressing anesthetic injections. First, there is continued controversy about what constitutes an "adequate paracervical block" with regard to sites, depth, and the number of injections. Second, a local anesthetic effect due to fluid tissue distension may not be ruled out when saline is used for placebo, as is the case in some of these studies.

Topical anesthesia

Topical anesthetics applied onto the cervix or within the cervical canal, in the form of gel, cream, or aerosol, may be of benefit prior to injection or application of a tenaculum. The effect of this method on procedure-related pain, however, has not been consistent in all studies [23]. While painless application and absence of bleeding represent obvious advantages, the cream form may affect visibility due to lens fogging.

Transcervical anesthesia

Transcervical intrauterine instillation of lidocaine before hysteroscopy, or mixing it with the saline distension medium during the procedure, has not yielded consistent results. Considering that the functional endometrial layer has no nerve endings, it is arguable that anesthetic effects and a possible decrease in the incidence of vasovagal reactions [22,23] are due to blockage of nerve endings at the level of the internal cervical os, or to absorption of the anesthetic into deeper layers.

No anesthesia

Decreasing the caliber of the hysteroscope is probably the most important modification clearly shown to reduce pain scores. The success of the 3.5 mm (outer sheath) hysteroscopy, without anesthesia, appears to be unrelated to the operator's experience or the patient's parity [24]. This is largely due to the easier introduction of the scope without the need for cervical dilatation.

In the last few years, hysteroscopes with outer dimensions down to 2 mm have been introduced to the market. This has definitely allowed for more procedures to be performed without anesthesia or analgesia.

Vaginoscopic approach

This approach, also called "no touch technique," was pioneered by Bettocchi and Selvaggi in the 1990s [25]. As no speculum is used, the pressure generated by the distension medium (usually saline) suffices for the expansion of the vagina and subsequent introduction of the telescope. The latter is then "negotiated," under direct video monitoring, through the cervical canal without the application of a tenaculum. This technique, described exclusively with rigid scopes, allows satisfactory diagnostic hysteroscopy, in addition to targeted endometrial biopsies and removal of polyps, without the need for analgesia or anesthesia.

Rigid or flexible hysteroscopy?

A "rigid hysteroscope" is rigid by virtue of its glass rod optical system. In a "flexible hysteroscope," fiberoptic bundles (flexible) transmit the image to the eyepiece or the camera. In both systems, however, light is separately transmitted from its source via a flexible fiberoptic cable. Either system may be used with CO_2 or saline as a distending medium.

Several decades ago, rigid scopes were almost exclusively used in hysteroscopy, due to the superior quality image delivered by the glass rod system. Since then, substantial technological improvements in flexible scopes have led to much improved image size, resolution, and brightness, especially after replacement of image fiber bundles with video chips. By the early 1990s, the flexible instrument had been quickly adopted for office hysteroscopy. Enthusiasts cited an easier entry into the cervical canal, without the need for dilation or tenaculum placement [26]. This was, however, at a time when most available rigid hysteroscopes were substantially larger than the 3.6 mm flexible model. At present, small diameter is no longer

Table 6.2. Advantages and disadvantages of flexible hysteroscopy compared with rigid hysteroscopy

Advantages	Disadvantages
Usually smoother entry in the cervical canal.	Entry could be difficult in the stenotic cervical canal.
Less likelihood of creation of "false canals" and uterine perforations, due to the non traumatic distal tip.	Equipment is more expensive.
Better visualization in the irregularly shaped uterus.	More problematic care and maintenance; probably shorter lifespan.
Less painful.	Limited operative accessories.
Lower incidence of vasovagal reactions.	Longer learning curve

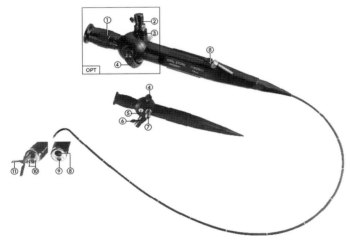

Figure 6.1. A flexible hysteroscope. (Courtesy Karl Storz.) 1, Focusing ring; 2, suction valve insert; 3, valve nozzle; 4, up/down control; 5, valve for pressure compensation and leakage tester connection; 6, suction outlet; 7, light inlet piece; 8, instrument channel; 9, objective lens; 10, light outlet; 11, instrument in instrument channel.

a virtue exclusive to flexible hysteroscopes; and the choice of one system over the other, in nonoperative interventions, remains a personal preference.

Most flexible hysteroscopes (Figure 6.1) come with a 0° viewing angle, compared with 0°, 5°,12°, or 30° angles found in the rigid version. An angulation control lever-mounted on the handle and manipulated by the operator's thumb allows for steering the end of the distal tip up to 160° in each direction. This permits easy visual access to the cornual areas, a feature especially important in irregularly shaped uteri.

A summary of some of the variables that may influence the operator's choice is depicted in Table 6.2.

Performing the procedure: instruments and techniques

Expectations of the duration of the procedure and related pain should be discussed with the patient. Assurance should be given, in case of no anesthesia, that the procedure will be stopped at any time, on her command. If a video monitor is available, she is given the choice to observe the findings and ask questions. Acceptability of outpatient hysteroscopy without anesthesia, while multifactorial, is believed to be improved by adequate preparation, by communication, and by allowing the patient to view the monitoring screen as a distraction from pain.

Hysteroscopy is best performed during the proliferative phase, when the endometrium is thin, vascularity is minimal, and the risk of early pregnancy is minimal.

The operator and the assistants should be familiar with the equipment. Web-based training and telesurgery are not substitutes for preceptorship. Instruments should be assembled and ready to use prior to the patient's positioning. The light source, however, is turned on exactly at the beginning, and turned off immediately at the completion of the procedure, in order to avoid inadvertent burns, especially with paper drapes. Currently used light sources include halogen or xenon. The lowest intensity necessary for satisfactory viewing should be used. With the technologically advanced cameras, high light intensity is no longer crucial for image transmission.

Preferably after emptying her bladder, the patient may change clothes in a private environment, and position herself in the lithotomy position, with legs on stirrups, and buttocks well supported on the table. Trendelenburg position, uncomfortable for most, is not necessary, especially with the availability of the video monitor. A digital pelvic examination determines the axis of the uterus (anteverted or retroverted). Although the speculum type depends on the operator's preference, the smallest size judged to be satisfactory should be used. The vagina and cervix are cleansed with an antiseptic solution.

Should local or paracervical anesthesia be used, the diluted form is preferable as it results in less burning sensation than with the concentrated form. Especially for short procedures, use of epinephrine with local anesthetics is better avoided, in order to prevent unpleasant epinephrine-related systemic effects. In case of paracervical block, a few minutes should be allowed for the anesthetic to act. It is the authors' experience that starting the injection during a patient's cough greatly reduces the discomfort associated with the initial needle penetration.

Many authorities advise against sounding the uterus prior to hysteroscopy. Sounding is the leading cause of the rare perforations that may occur. In addition, it may provoke, on contact with the fundus, a painful stimulus in the awake patient. Information about uterine dimensions can be easily obtained by ultrasound.

It is imperative to purge the tubing with the distension medium prior to starting the procedure.

In case of CO_2 use, pressure and flow parameters are adjusted as described in previous paragraphs. With saline, one may choose between calibrated equipment and infusion by gravity. When using the latter, a 3-liter saline bag set at 1.5 m above the hysteroscope level, and connected via large-bore urological tubing (not a standard intravenous tube), would result in a mean intrauterine pressure of 105 mmHg.

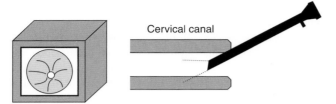

Figure 6.2. Wrong view on the screen, corresponding to wrong alignment of the instrument with the cervical canal. (Adapted on [27].)

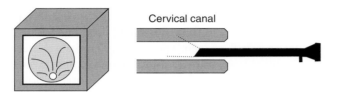

Figure 6.3. Correct view on the screen, corresponding to correct alignment of the instrument with the cervical canal. (Adapted from [27].)

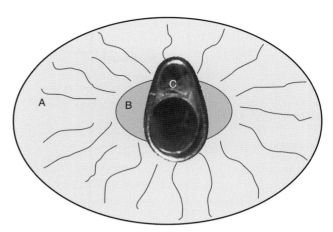

Figure 6.4. Perspective view of the internal cervical os and the hysteroscope profiles in a traditional introduction: A, cervix; B, internal cervical os; C, hysteroscope profile. (Based on [27].)

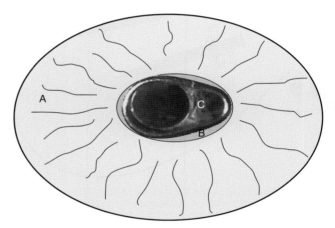

Figure 6.5. Perspective view of the internal cervical os and hysteroscope profiles after 90° rotation :A, cervix; B, internal cervical os; C, hysteroscope profile. (Based on [27].)

The hysteroscope is negotiated through the cervical canal under direct viewing (or video monitoring). At this point, it is especially important to interpret the image as a function of the viewing angle of the telescope. If using a 0° telescope, the cervical canal should appear in the center of the screen. On the other hand, when using a 30° telescope, a cervical canal appearing in the lower half of the screen would indicate a correct anatomical position. If the image is in the center of the screen (with a 30° telescope), the tip of the scope would be pushing against the endocervical mucosa, thus stretching stroma and muscle fibers and causing related pain (Figures 6.2, 6.3) [27].

An oval hysteroscope, instead of the traditional round one, was reported to better conform to the shape of the oval internal cervical os. The passage is therefore facilitated by rotating the scope on the endocamera by 90° to align the longitudinal axis of the scope with the transverse axis of the internal cervical os (Figures 6.4, 6.5) [27].

Visualization of the tubal ostia confirms an intrauterine location. The appearance of crisscrossing muscle fibers, with unusual resistance, signifies a "false canal," while sudden loss of intrauterine pressure alerts to perforation.

Once successfully inside the cavity, inspection of the uterine walls is performed, with the help of the focusing knob, as needed. If bubbles are encountered with CO_2 use, the insufflation pressure may be lowered, or the bubbles "flushed" with warm saline readily available in a 50 ml syringe. Magnification and brightness are both inversely proportional to the distance from the viewed object. One should avoid touching the mucosa with the tip of the instrument as this may cause unnecessary discomfort and bothersome oozing. If an intervention such as a biopsy or a lesion excision is necessary, it should be delayed till the end of the procedure, i.e., after the diagnostic part is satisfactorily completed. Such interventions are probably more convenient with the 12° rather than the 30° telescope, as the former allows easier visualization of the tip of the operative instrument.

As the rigid telescope has a panoramic view of 60–90°, rotating the scope around the camera offers visual coverage of all uterine aspects, thus avoiding the uncomfortable jittering of the hysteroscope from side to side and from up to down. With the flexible hysteroscope, deflecting the distal tip in all directions, using the operator's thumb on the special angulation control lever, achieves the same results. For comparative scale purposes, a tubal ostium is about 1.0–1.5 mm. Consequently, once both ostia are visualized, and the maneuvers described above are performed, no significant lesion is likely to be missed.

After the completion of the procedure, instruments are removed, and the patient is allowed to assume the sitting position, but only with help as vasovagal reactions may occur at this stage.

Documentation of findings without delay is obviously imperative. Still pictures and video recordings, when available, are of great value in the patient's record.

The patient is discharged with instructions to avoid intercourse for a week. She may resume her regular activities the following day. While light bleeding per vagina is expected for a few days, she is instructed to report fever, persistent pain, or heavy bleeding. Mild shoulder tip pain secondary to diaphragmatic irritation following CO_2 use is not uncommon. Over-the-counter analgesics are usually sufficient in case of discomfort.

Instrument care

- While in storage, light cables and flexible scopes should not be bent excessively or laid at the bottom of other stored items. It does not take excessive mishandling to damage expensive fiberoptic equipment.

- Regular autoclaving may not be used for most telescopes and plastic accessories (including the plastic nipples).

- While glutaraldehyde may be used for most instruments, one has to adhere strictly to the manufacturer's recommendations.

Applications

Discussion of the numerous applications for operative hysteroscopy is beyond the scope of this chapter. The following is an overview of the use of office hysteroscopy in the setting of a reproductive endocrinology and infertility unit.

Should hysteroscopy be a part of the basic infertility workup?

Historically hysterosalpingography (HSG), providing a clear picture of the uterus and fallopian tubes (including patency), has been commonly used as part of the basic infertility workup. With the advent of office hysteroscopy, more reproductive endocrinologists have replaced HSG with this outpatient procedure. However, a prospective randomized study concluded that office hysteroscopy and HSG were comparable in evaluating the uterine cavity in infertile women [28].

The latest World Health Organization report continues to recommend HSG for the study of the uterine cavity in the standard evaluation of infertile women. Until 1997 most reproductive endocrinologists were routinely ordering HSG as the initial screening test for the evaluation of the uterine cavity [29].

However, in view of the improved safety profile, recent endoscopic technological advances, and minimal time requirement, hysteroscopy has been advocated as a routine procedure in all infertile women undergoing diagnostic laparoscopy, as well as in the evaluation of female infertility in populations where the risk of prior pelvic infections is considerable [30].

Routine office hysteroscopy in the investigation of infertile couples before assisted reproduction

A significant percentage of infertile women have intracavitary lesions that may impair the success of fertility treatments [31,32]. The most common abnormalities found are endometrial polyps, small uterine septa, small uterine fibroids, endometritis, and adhesions [32,33,34].

These simple-to-treat pathologies may affect endometrial receptivity and implantation. Lower pregnancy rates have been reported following in-vitro fertilization (IVF) in patients with such uterine cavity abnormalities [33], while their correction has been associated with improved pregnancy rates [32,34].

In a retrospective study of 145 patients who systematically underwent office hysteroscopy before the first stimulation cycle, Feghali et al. noted pathological abnormalities in 45% of hysteroscopies. The treatment of these pathologies improved the pregnancy rates to equal those encountered in patients with normal cavities [34].

In a prospective study of 300 patients who underwent hysteroscopy before the first IVF cycle, Doldi et al. [32] noted unsuspected intrauterine abnormalities in 40% of their patients. Women who underwent hysteroscopy prior to IVF had a significantly higher pregnancy rate than those who did not, suggesting that hysteroscopy should be routinely performed prior to the first IVF cycle.

The reportedly poor agreement (43%) between hysteroscopy and HSG [35] is likely due to the limited accuracy of the latter in the diagnosis of intrauterine adhesions and endometritis [30]. In addition, hysteroscopy may allow the physician to diagnose small abnormalities not evident on HSG.

In 1992 Bonilla-Musoles et al. [36] introduced saline infusion hysterosonography (SIS) for the evaluation of the uterine cavity. Since then various studies have suggested the superiority of SIS over traditional transvaginal sonography in the evaluation of submucous/intramural myomas, and for endometrial evaluation in patients with abnormal uterine bleeding. More recently, its use has been described in the work-up of infertile women. A prospective, investigator-blinded study compared traditional hysteroscopy in the operating room setting with the three outpatient procedures commonly used in the evaluation of the uterine cavity: HSG, SIS, and office hysteroscopy. No significant advantage regarding the diagnostic accuracy was found for any of the three outpatient procedures, or any combination of two [28].

Recurrent IVF treatment failure

Commonly referred to as mechanical infertility, failure of conception despite the repeated transfer of apparently good-quality embryos is a significant clinical problem in IVF practice.

Endometrial abnormalities were detected in 18–45% of women with at least three previous unexplained IVF failures [37,38], and the treatment of these abnormalities was demonstrated to improve the pregnancy rates [38].

In a prospective observational study of patients with at least two failed IVF cycles despite the transfer of good-quality embryos, Oliveira et al. found hysteroscopic abnormalities of the uterine cavity, such as polyps, adhesions, or endometritis, in 45% of the patients. In only half of these patients were the abnormalities suspected on transvaginal ultrasound prior to hysteroscopy, while none were seen on HSG performed within the previous year. Following hysteroscopic treatment, 52% conceived on repeat IVF cycles [38].

In conclusion, evaluation of the uterine cavity in infertile women should be performed in the most sensitive and accurate way possible. Hysteroscopy is of value in patients undergoing IVF, especially in those with recurrent IVF failures. Furthermore, technological advances in hysteroscopic equipment and instrumentation have allowed the office-based hysteroscopy to become the gold standard for uterine cavity evaluation.

Complications

At present, most complications of diagnostic hysteroscopy are considered minor, and consequently may be underreported in retrospective reviews.

In a prospective multicenter study of 13 600 hysteroscopies in the Netherlands in 1997, complications occurred in 0.13% of diagnostic procedures (all were uterine perforations) and 0.95% of operative procedures, and there was no mortality [39].

An *unsuccessful hysteroscopy* could be the most common procedure-related complication. It has been reported in 5% of combined cases performed by operators of different levels of expertise [40]. An unsuccessful hysteroscopy may be secondary to difficulty negotiating the cervical canal, intolerable pain in an outpatient setting, the occurrence of vasovagal syndrome, or unsatisfactory visualization.

Bleeding from a *cervical laceration* may be managed by tamponade, application of silver nitrate, or sutures.

Half of the *uterine perforations* are entry related [12,39]. Although there is no consensus on whether to proceed with diagnostic hysteroscopy following uterine perforation [39], it is probably prudent to abandon the procedure and observe the patient for signs of bleeding, especially if the perforation is suspected to be on the lateral aspect of the uterus. Ultrasound assessment may be of value in this situation.

Vasovagal syndrome may be secondary to anxiety or pain, or arguably to pressure on "carotid sensors," presumably present in the cervix, such as known to occur during intrauterine device insertion. In this particular setting, the classical "near faintness" symptom, due to bradycardia and hypotension, usually responds to leg elevation or Trendelenburg position, and subsides in few minutes. It is reportedly more common with CO_2 than with saline distension, and with the use of a rigid rather than a flexible hysteroscope. The incidence of vasovagal syndrome may be decreased by the use of local anesthesia [22].

Except for the rare association of Hyskon® with anaphylactoid reactions, the risk of *distension media-related complications* is negligible in diagnostic hysteroscopy. Purging the tubing system with the distension medium, abiding by the recommended CO_2 insufflation parameters, and monitoring of the infused fluid volume should be standard practice.

Endometritis may complicate operative hysteroscopy in fewer than 1% of the cases. The incidence is expected to be much lower with strictly diagnostic procedures. Most gynecologists do not prescribe prophylactic antibiotics, especially in

view of the lack of evidence for efficacy. An exception continues to apply for the patient with moderate/high risk for infective endocarditis, such as one with prosthetic heart valves.

Pregnancy and genital tract infections are obvious contraindications to hysteroscopy. It is wise to obtain a pregnancy test on the day of the procedure. It is also prudent to postpone the procedure in the presence of prodromal symptoms in a patient with a history of genital herpes.

References

1. Lau WY, Leow CK, Li AK. History of endoscopic and laparoscopic surgery. *World J Surg* 1997; **21**: 444–53.

2. I. C. Rubin. Uterine endoscopy, endometroscopy with the aid of uterine insufflation. *Am J Obstet Gynaecol* 1925; **10**: 313–27.

3. Linder TE, Simmen D, Stool SE. Revolutionary inventions in the 20th century. The history of endoscopy. *Arch Otolaryngol Head Neck Surg* 1997; **123**: 1161–3.

4. Edstrom K, Fernstrom I. The diagnostic possibilities of a modified hysteroscopic technique, *Acta Obstet Gynaecol Scand* 1970; **49**: 327–30.

5. Lindelmann HJ, Mohr J. CO_2 hysteroscopy: diagnosis and treatment. *Am J Obstet Gynecol* 1976; **124**: 129–33.

6. Ellingson TL, Aboulafia DM. Dextran syndrome. Acute hypotension, noncardiogenic pulmonary edema, anemia, and coagulopathy following hysteroscopic surgery using 32% dextran 70. *Chest* 1997; **111**: 513–18.

7. Ahmed N, Falcone T, Tulandi T, Houle G. Anaphylactic reaction because of intrauterine 32% dextran-70 instillation. *Fertil Steril* 1991; **55**: 1014–16.

8. Moghadami-Tabrizi N, Mohammad K, Dabirashrafi H, Zandimejad K. The hyperglycemia and hyponatremia response of patients during operative hysteroscopy with 5% dextrose in water (D5W).

J Am Assoc Gynecol Laparosc 1994; **1**: S23.

9. Phillips DR, Milim SJ, Nathanson HG, Phillips RE, Haselkorn JS. Preventing hyponatremic encephalopathy: comparison of serum sodium and osmolality during operative hysteroscopy with 5.0% mannitol and 1.5% glycine distention media. *J Am Assoc Gynecol Laparosc* 1997; **4**: 567–76.

10. Corson SL, Brooks PG, Soderstrom RM. Gynecologic endoscopic gas embolism. *Fertil Steril* 1996; **65**: 529–33.

11. Brandner P, Neis KJ, Ehmer C. The etiology, frequency, and prevention of gas embolism during CO_2 hysteroscopy. *J Am Assoc Gynecol Laparosc* 1999; **6**: 421–8.

12. Hulka JF, Peterson HB, Phillips JM, Surrey MW. Operative hysteroscopy. American Association of Gynecologic Laparoscopists 1991 membership survey. *J Reprod Med* 1993; **38**: 572–3.

13. Paschopoulos M, Kaponis A, Makrydimas G, et al. Selecting distending medium for out-patient hysteroscopy. Does it really matter? *Hum Reprod* 2004; **19**: 2619–25.

14. Nagele F, Bournas N, O'Connor H, Broadbent M, Richardson R, Magos A. Comparison of carbon dioxide and normal saline for uterine distension in outpatient hysteroscopy. *Fertil Steril* 1996; **65**: 305–9.

15. Pellicano M, Guida M, Zullo F, Lavitola G, Cirillo D, Nappi C. Carbon dioxide versus normal saline as a uterine distension medium for diagnostic vaginoscopic hysteroscopy in infertile patients: a prospective, randomized, multicenter study. *Fertil Steril* 2003; **79**: 418–21.

16. Brusco GF, Arena S, Angelini A. Use of carbon dioxide versus normal saline for diagnostic hysteroscopy. *Fertil Steril* 2003; **79**: 993–7.

17. Litta P, Bonora M, Pozzan C, et al. Carbon dioxide versus normal saline in outpatient hysteroscopy. *Hum Reprod* 2003; **18**: 2446–9.

18. Shankar M, Davidson A, Taub N, Habiba M. Randomised comparison of distension media for outpatient hysteroscopy. *BJOG* 2004; **111**: 57–62.

19. Crane JM, Healey S. Use of misoprostol before hysteroscopy: a systematic review. *J Obstet Gynaecol Can* 2006; **28**: 373–9.

20. Tahir MM, Bigrigg MA, Browning JJ, Brookes ST, Smith PA. A randomised controlled trial comparing transvaginal ultrasound, outpatient hysteroscopy and endometrial biopsy with inpatient hysteroscopy and curettage. *Br J Obstet Gynaecol* 1999; **106**: 1259–64.

21. American Society of Anesthesiologists. Task Force on Sedation and Analgesia by Non-Anesthesiologists: Practice guidelines for sedation and analgesia by non-anesthesiologists. *Anesthesiology* 2002; **96**: 1004–17.

22. Readman E, Maher PJ. Pain relief and outpatient hysteroscopy: a literature review. *J Am Assoc Gynecol Laparosc* 2004; **11**: 315–19

23. Hassan L, Gannon MJ. Anaesthesia and analgesia for ambulatory hysteroscopic surgery. *Best Pract Res Clin Obstet Gynaecol* 2005; **19**: 681–91.

24. Campo R, Molinas CR, Rombauts L, et al. Prospective multicentre randomized controlled trial to evaluate factors influencing the success rate of office diagnostic hysteroscopy. *Hum Reprod* 2005; **20**: 258–63.

25. Bettocchi S, Nappi L, Ceci O, Selvaggi L. Office hysteroscopy. *Obstet Gynecol Clin North Am* 2004; **31**: 641–54.

26. Bradley LD, Widrich T. State-of-the-art flexible hysteroscopy for office gynecologic evaluation. *J Am Assoc Gynecol Laparosc* 1995; **2**: 263–7.

27. Bettocchi S, Nappi L, Ceci O, Selvaggi L. What does 'diagnostic hysteroscopy' mean today? The role of the new techniques. *Curr Opin Obstet Gynecol* 2003; **15**: 303–8.

28. Brown SE, Coddington CC, Schnorr J, et al. Evaluation of outpatient hysteroscopy, saline infusion hysterosonography, and hysterosalpingography in infertile women: a prospective, randomized study. *Fertil Steril* 2000; **74**: 1029–34.

29. Glatstein IZ, Harlow BL, Hornstein MD. Practice patterns among reproductive endocrinologists: the infertility evaluation. *Fertil Steril* 1997; **67**: 443–51.

30. Shokeir TA, Shalan HM, El-Shafei MM. Combined diagnostic approach of laparoscopy and hysteroscopy in the evaluation of female infertility: Results of 612 patients. *J.Obstet Gynaecol Res* 2004; **30**: 9–14.

31. Hinckley MD, Milki AA. 1000 office-based hysteroscopies prior to in vitro fertilization: feasibility and findings. *JSLS* 2004; **8**: 103–7.

32. Doldi N, Persico P, Di Sebastiano F, et al. Pathologic findings in hysteroscopy before in vitro fertilization-embryo transfer (IVF-ET). *Gynecol Endocrinol* 2005; **21**: 235–7.

33. Shamma FN, Lee G, Gutmann JN, Lavy G. The role of office hysteroscopy in in vitro fertilization. *Fertil Steril* 1992; **58**: 1237–9.

34. Feghali J, Bakar J, Mayenga JM, et al. Systematic hysteroscopy prior to in vitro fertilization. *Gynecol Obstet Fertil* 2003; **31**: 127–31.

35. Cicinelli E, Matteo M, Causio F, Schonauer LM, Pinto V, Galantino P. Tolerability of the mini-pan-endoscopic approach (transvaginal hydrolaparoscopy and minihysteroscopy) versus hydrosalpingography in an outpatient infertility investigation. *Fertil Steril* 2001; **76**: 1048–51.

36. Bonilla-Musoles F, Simon C, Serra V, Sampaio M, Pellicer A. An assessment of hysterosalpingosonography (HSSG) as a diagnostic tool for uterine cavity defects and tubal patency. *J Clin Ultrasound* 1992; **20**: 175–81.

37. Kirsop R, Porter R, Torode H, Smith D, Saunders D. The role of hysteroscopy in patients having failed IVF/GIFT transfer cycles. *Aust NZ J Obstet Gynecol* 1991; **341**: 263–4.

38. Oliveira FG, Abdelmassih VG, Diamond MP, Dozortsev D, Nagy ZP, Abdelmassih R. Uterine cavity findings and hysteroscopic interventions in patient undergoing in vitro fertilization-embryo transfer who repeatedly cannot conceive. *Fertil Steril* 2003; **80**: 1371–5.

39. Jansen FW, Vredevoogd CB, van Ulzen K, Hermans J, Trimbos JB, Trimbos-Kemper TC. Complications of hysteroscopy: a prospective, multicenter study. *Obstet Gynecol* 2000; **96**: 266–70.

40. Di Spiezio Sardo A, Taylor A, Tsirkas P, Mastrogamvrakis G, Sharma M, Magos A. Hysteroscopy: a technique for all? Analysis of 5,000 outpatient hysteroscopies. *Fertil Steril* 2008; **89**: 438–42.

Ethics of ultrasonography

Osama M. Azmy and Kareem El-Nahhas

Ethics is the branch of science that deals with human morality – right and wrong behavior or virtues and vices. The prime question that ethics addresses is "What ought our behavior to be?" In medicine, ethics has been embodied in the venerable Hippocratic Oath and aphorisms that have provided a guide over the centuries to how physicians should deal with their patients. Over centuries, medical ethics has been influenced by traditions, attitudes, cultural and religious beliefs, and social obligations. Indeed, issues of civil and women's rights added to concepts of individual autonomy and outlined principal lines that should be considered within the context of ethics.

Because the implementation of innovative medical technologies can raise unprecedented ethical, legal and social dilemmas, ethics is nowadays an emerging subdiscipline in ultrasound practice as several clinical situations can only be identified and addressed by ethical appreciation. This is particularly so in the area of antenatal screening, which is dominated by the language of risk and probabilities. By their definitions, obstetrics and gynecology are the branches of medicine that touch most closely maternity and the privacy of the family. Among all civilizations and cultures, dealing with women has its own particular form and codes. In some ancient cultures, women are gods in temples and their lives are taboos surrounded with secrets.

Ethics has two main principles: beneficence and autonomy of the patient; in other words, the best interests of the patient and her or his right to choose.

The principle of beneficence

The physician should serve the best interests of the patient. This can be considered from different perspectives; one is the doctor's perspective whereby, based on scientific knowledge, shared clinical experience, and rigorous clinical judgment, the doctor can identify and serve what is best for his or her patient [1]. The other perspective acknowledges that the health-related interests of patients are a function of the competencies of medicine as a social institution rather than a function of the personal or subjective outlook of the physician [2].

The principle of autonomy

The principle of autonomy recognizes that it is the voluntary decision of the patient to authorize or refuse clinical management based on adequate and complete disclosure by the physician about the patient's condition and management with the understanding of this information by the patient [3]. This is the basis of the concept of informed consent.

In the area of obstetric ultrasound, these rights are complete and integral, but they may conflict with one another [4] because, on the one hand, the mother and child are independent beings and are incommensurable bearers of these rights. But at the same time the pregnant woman and her unborn child are interconnected in such a way that what benefits one may harm the other.

There are obviously beneficence-based and autonomy-based obligations to the pregnant woman during ultrasound examination. Although the unborn child does not possess any legal rights, in terms of autonomy or beneficence, it is expected that each mother will by nature look after the best interests of her unborn child [5].

Women's autonomy

Indeed, ultrasound examination is considered by women a safe procedure that causes no physical damage. They consider it "intervention" only when the transducer is introduced through an orifice such as the vagina. Although concerns have been raised about pregnant women viewing ultrasound scans as benign, many of the women reported having thought carefully through their own moral beliefs and values prior to screening [6]. Furthermore, the American College of Obstetricians and Gynecologists has endorsed the "Prudent Use" statement from the American Institute of Ultrasound in Medicine based on ethical purposes discouraging the use of obstetric ultrasonography for nonmedical reasons, e.g., solely to create keepsake photographs or videos [7]. Thus, ultrasound examination requires the woman's consent as this examination collects information about her physical condition. When the examination is indicated and is done solely for the health of the woman, consent is easily secured. Generally this indication exists if the

Ultrasonography in Reproductive Medicine and Infertility, ed. Botros R. M. B. Rizk. Published by Cambridge University Press. © Cambridge University Press 2010.

examination is expected to produce a result that has therapeutic implications (even if it is the absence of a condition [8] that would have therapeutic implications, i.e., no treatment is required). One study [9] has emphasized that women's understanding of ultrasound does not meet the requirements of informed choice. This cross-sectional study evaluated women's understanding of prenatal ultrasound and was conducted to evaluate how information is provided, women's perceived value of the information received, and their understanding of ultrasound in relation to the principles of informed choice. One hundred and thirteen women completed a questionnaire prior to their 18-week ultrasound scan. Fifty-five percent stated they received no information from their care provider. Only 31.9% considered health care providers as a "very helpful" source of information. Yet 69.0% stated that their care provider gave them information that facilitated their understanding. Specifically, 46.0% did not view ultrasound as a screen for anomalies; some were uncertain about the safety (18.6%), diagnostic capabilities (26.5%), and limitations of testing (37.2%).

If the woman refuses the ultrasound examination, her wish must be respected. The woman has the right to refuse without giving any reason for her refusal. In this situation, the physician has to counsel the patient of the possible consequences and hazards that may affect her upon this refusal. If the patient refuses the ultrasound examination due to the fears of its harmful effects, the physician must clarify the facts to the patient, support her, and illuminate her fears. During obstetric ultrasound scanning and in occasional circumstances where the unborn child may suffer from a condition that needs a treatment and this treatment threatens the mother's life, there must not be any obligation upon her to tolerate this treatment [10]. All fetal treatment necessitates accessing the fetus through the pregnant woman's body, and nonsurgical treatments have long been a part of pregnancy care. However, recent developments in this area, including the increasing routinization of sophisticated antenatal ultrasound screening and the introduction of treatments including fetal surgery, may mark a shift in this specialty. There are apparent effects of the orientation of fetal medicine on prevalent conceptualizations of the maternal–fetal relationship, and some of the consequences of this. It is argued that new forms of uncertainty, including complex risk and diagnostic information, and uncertain prognostic predictions set within the rhetoric of nondirective counseling and women's choice, are leading to unprecedented ethical issues within this area [11]. More widespread debate about such potential dilemmas needs to take place before, rather than following, their introduction. In other words, the pregnant woman has the right to accept or refuse this treatment even if the treatment would be life-saving for the unborn child. No such treatment is conceivable that does not act on the child by going "through the mother" in some way, inevitably invading the physical integrity of the pregnant woman. So any treatment for the child requires consent from the mother and the pregnant woman is not held responsible for the consequences of not treating her unborn child [12].

The unborn child's autonomy

Special situations are unique to obstetric ultrasound scanning, where the physician is dealing with two living individuals at the same time and where treating one may inevitably produce harmful or untoward effects on the other.

The autonomy of the unborn child is an area of debate. The silence that surrounded rigorous ethical debate served to highlight where discussion lay – namely, with the justifications offered for the unborn child added to the dilemma of autonomy. In the authors' view and that of others [13], the fetus is a human being that has all the appropriate rights from the date of conception. However, because we lack a method of communicating with and understanding the unborn's needs, and he or she does not have the opportunity to express their own decisions, we cannot uphold that right. Furthermore, the development of 4D ultrasound technology has revolutionized fetal imagery by offering direct visual access to realistic images of the fetus in utero. These images, which claim to show a responsive being capable of complex behavior, have renewed debate about the personhood of the fetus [14]. The application of this statement should not contradict with the woman's right to choose. Others believe that the fetus has autonomy only if viable and not as such in the pre-vital state, and that only the woman can confer such status on it [15]. Concerning the health aspects of the unborn child, the responsibility may be on the mother, the father, and/or the physician. However, this responsibility and authority must be subordinate to the mother's right of self-determination over her own body, because anything done to the unborn child has to "go through" the mother. Thus, only the mother can represent her unborn child when prenatal treatment is required. The woman is free to act or not to act according to her own values and beliefs. The responsibility of the managing physician to the fetus in all cases should be balanced against the obligations to the pregnant woman. Also, one should not ignore that the ethical problems surrounding prenatal screening are intensified in low-income settings [16], which points to the need for research that takes into account the wider social context that structures ethical dilemmas.

Key points in clinical practice

- Always maintain professionalism. The patient must be addressed by her preferred name. Never make remarks relating to bodily appearance such as tattoos, piercing, or suntan.

- Be careful and explain to the patient what you are going to do in the examination and provide ample information to the patient about the purpose of the procedure.

- Contain and respect the patient's autonomy and the right to refuse the procedure and do not begin it until she gives her consent.

- During examination, always maintain the patient's dignity. The patient should not be left undressed for long. Use a gown or a sheet to cover her body during examination. Make sure that the examination room is secured from unexpected intrusion.

- Ensure the patient's privacy, by providing comfortable and pleasant conditions and adapt a comfort place in which the patient can change in privacy.

- Always obtain a chaperone. This chaperone is a source of support, guidance, and help for the patient.

- Give your patient your mind and your full attention. Let her feel that the time of examination belongs exclusively to her and respond to the patient's questions and concerns. This attitude will pay healthy dividends for both of you.

- Maintain confidentiality of the acquired patient information, and discuss the findings on the screen with your patient.

Conclusion

Ethics as a subdiscipline of ultrasound examination and intervention has significant clinical implications. Failure to consider these clinical implications of the ethical principles of beneficence and women's autonomy is regarded as unacceptable and unprofessional. Ultrasound societies should include training in ethics, the use and misuse of ultrasound, and good technique and understanding of implications for clinical care to improve sensitivity. It is argued that innovative health technologies may be changing the roles of both women and health practitioners, and raising new issues, including ethical, legal, and social dilemmas.

References

1. Cooper TR, Caplan WD, Garcia-Prats JA, Brody BA. The interrelationship of ethical issues in the transition from old paradigms to new technologies. *J Clin Ethics* 1996; **7**(3): 243–50.

2. Gorincour G, Tassy S, LeCoz P. The moving face of the fetus-the changing face of medicine. *Ultrasound Obstet Gynecol* 2006; **28**(7): 979–80.

3. Boyle RJ, de Crespigny L, Savulescu J. An ethical approach to giving couples information about their fetus. *Hum Reprod* 2003; **18**(11): 2253–6.

4. Chervenak FA, McCullough LB. Scientifically and ethically responsible innovation and research in ultrasound in obstetrics and gynecology. *Ultrasound Obstet Gynecol* 2006; **28**(1): 1–4.

5. Strauss RP. Beyond easy answers: Prenatal diagnosis and counseling during pregnancy. *Cleft Palate Craniofac J* 2002; **39**(2): 164–8.

6. Kongnyuy EJ, van den Broek N. The use of ultrasonography in obstetrics in developing countries. *Trop Doct* 2007; **37** (2): 70–2.

7. ACOG Committee Opinion. Non-medical use of obstetric ultrasonography. *Obstet Gynecol* 2004; **104**(2): 423–4.

8. Chervenak FA, McCullough LB. Ethics in fetal medicine. *Baillieres Best Pract Res Clin Obstet Gynaecol* 1999; **13**(4): 491–502.

9. Williams C. Dilemmas in fetal medicine: premature application of technology or responding to women's choice? *Sociol Health Illn* 2006; **28**(1): 1–20.

10. Kohut RJ, Dewey D, Love EJ. Women's knowledge of prenatal ultrasound and informed choice. *J Genet Couns* 2002; **11**(4): 265–76.

11. McFadyen A, Gledhill J, Whitlow B, Economides D. First trimester ultrasound screening. Carries ethical and psychological implications. *BMJ* 1998; **317**(7160): 694–5.

12. Gagen WJ, Bishop JP. Ethics, justification and the prevention of spina bifida. *J Med Ethics* 2007; **33**(9): 501–7.

13. Savell K. Life and death before birth: 4D ultrasound and the shifting frontiers of the abortion debate. *J Law Med* 2007; **15**(1): 103–16.

14. Greenland P, Lloyd-Jones D. Critical lessons from the ENHANCE trial. *JAMA* 2008; **299**(8): 953–5.

15. Barnett SB. Live scanning at ultrasound scientific conferences and the need for prudent policy. *Ultrasound Med Biol* 2003; **29**(8): 1071–6.

16. Gammeltoft T, Nguyen HT. Fetal conditions and fatal decisions: ethical dilemmas in ultrasound screening in Vietnam. *Soc Sci Med* 2007; **64**(11): 2248–59.

8

3D Ultrasonography and infertility

Jose M. Puente and Juan A. Garcia-Velasco

Introduction

Imaging in gynecology, and specifically gynecologic imaging as it pertains to reproduction, refers almost exclusively to ultrasound imaging. In recent years, we have witnessed tremendous advances in ultrasound (US) techniques such as 2D, 3D, and 4D B-mode US. Reproductive medicine has also greatly benefited from advances in pulsed, color, and power Doppler.

Three-dimensional US is a valuable new tool for the reproductive field. The ability to acquire and store ultrasonographic volumes provides several advantages over preexisting techniques. First, we can load the volume in a computer for later analysis: thus, the images can be evaluated after patient consultation and can easily be sent to a colleague for further analysis if necessary. Second, 3D US is a great tool for teaching. The ability to recreate a volume allows visualization of images in the three orthogonal space sections and also allows generation of any section in which the desired organ can be visualized perfectly; this is something that can be difficult to achieve using 2D US.

Three-dimensional US also has some unique capabilities that significantly enhance diagnosis. For example, it is quite difficult to obtain a coronal section using 2D US but very simple using 3D US. This greatly facilitates accurate diagnosis and characterization of uterine abnormalities, especially the difficult differential diagnosis of a septate uterus versus a bicornuate uterus. Through tomographic US imaging (TUI), a series of extremely useful tomographic images are obtained which can be used, for example, to visualize a uterine leiomyoma protruding toward the endometrial cavity (Figure 8.1). The inverted mode of 3D US facilitates evaluation of antral follicles (Figure 8.2). Organ volume can be calculated using the software provided with the ultrasound equipment; the most widely used is "virtual organ computer-aided analysis" or VOCAL. This imaging program calculates organ volume from the areas of the three orthogonal sections, allowing very precise calculation of ovarian and endometrial volumes (Figure 8.3).

Combining power Doppler and 3D US allows the study of tissue vascularization. First, the organ volume is obtained using power Doppler. Subsequently, indexes such as the vascularization index (VI), the flow index (FI), and the vascularization-flow index (VFI) are obtained by comparing the number and intensity of the colored voxels (similar to pixels in 2D US) with the gray voxels. This technology has proved useful in the development of endometrial receptivity markers and oocyte quality/quantity predictors based on endometrial/ovarian vascularization status. Although results so far have been mixed, new studies will help further refine this method There are some drawbacks to 3D US. The equipment can pose technical difficulties – since the techniques involved are complex and there is a very wide spectrum of possible applications, there is a longer learning curve for users. In addition, different commercial machines and software lack compatibility, complicating or even preventing data interchange and multicenter studies. Finally, delayed image-processing means that 3D US involves extra work and thus extra time. There is tremendous potential for the use of 3D US in two scenarios: for use in basic research and in clinical studies, and for wider use in all reproductive medicine units, so that clinicians who currently routinely use 2D US can benefit from the advantages of this newer technology.

Estimating the ovarian reserve with 3D US

Antral follicle count in both ovaries, preferentially performed during the menstrual cycle or in the early follicular phase, is currently considered the gold standard for estimating the ovarian reserve. Follicle count can be evaluated by either 2D US or 3D US [1], since both modalities have shown good inter- and intra-observer correlation. The antral follicle count results using 2D and 3D US are generally very similar, although 3D US is superior for estimates in ovaries with a very high antral follicle population. Some US machines display "inversion mode," which provides an inverted image, similar to the image in a photographic negative. Using the inversion mode, visualization of the ovarian parenchyma is suppressed and follicles, which appear white, can be counted more easily. Image or volume rotation, either manually or automatically using cine-loop, facilitates this process. Inversion mode can be used to diagnose low responders and is easy to implement.

Currently, the greatest disadvantage of 3D US is the amount of time required to perform it. It has been estimated that an expert professional needs 20–30 minutes [2], and another additional 5–10 minutes are required if vascular flow is analyzed. This reduces the chances of real-time decision-making and the

Ultrasonography in Reproductive Medicine and Infertility, ed. Botros R. M. B. Rizk. Published by Cambridge University Press. © Cambridge University Press 2010.

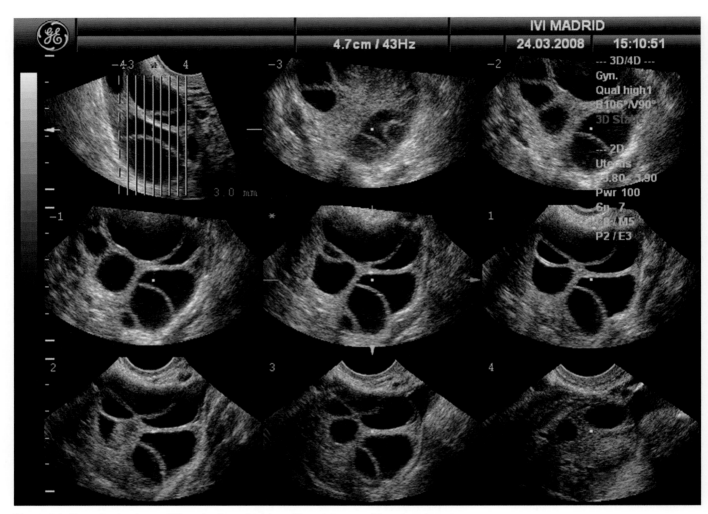

Figure 8.1. Hyperstimulated ovary. TUI mode allows obtaining millimetric images of the selected structure.

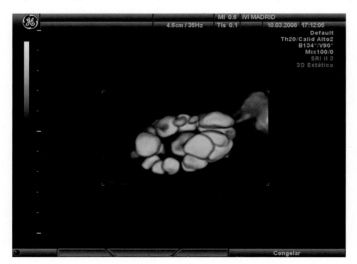

Figure 8.2. Antral follicle count by inversion mode.

possibility of discussing the findings with the patient. To address this, new software has been developed that can automatically calculate follicle diameter and volume. The operator simply captures the ovarian volume, and the software immediately calculates the volume and mean follicle diameter. This method reduces human error due to measuring only two sections, and also saves time and enables immediate discussion with patients about changes in medication. This software may improve follicle measurements, although studies are needed before its widespread use is implemented (Figure 8.4).

Three-dimensional US is an excellent technique for calculating ovarian volume very precisely. Using the VOCAL program and observing the ovary with rotating angles between 9° and 15°, the ovarian volume can easily be estimated with a sagittal section. Low ovarian reserve and poor response to controlled ovarian hyperstimulation in assisted reproductive technology (ART) is associated with ovarian volumes <3 ml, whereas polycystic ovaries are associated with volumes >6.6 ml. Similarly, evaluation of ovarian volume on the day of hCG administration discriminates between women who have moderate versus severe OHSS (271 ± 87 vs. 157.30 ± 54 ml) [3].

Evaluating ovarian stroma flow with 3D US

It is possible that poor ovarian vascularization impairs access of gonadotropin to the ovarian follicles, hampering follicular

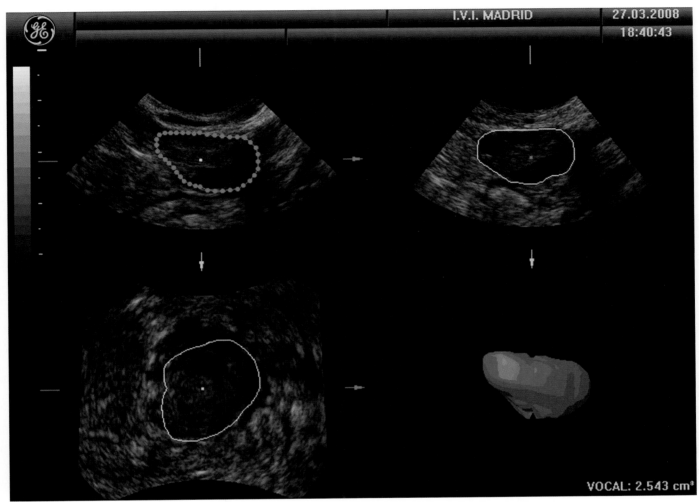

Figure 8.3. Ovarian volume calculation through VOCAL software (virtual organ computer-aided analysis) in a patient with low ovarian reserve. Total ovarian volume is 2.5 ml.

growth and development. Power Doppler US, in combination with 3D US and VOCAL, is a very good approach for investigating the global ovarian vascular network and its correlation with ovarian response in ART. An ovarian vascular "map" is easily obtained from a sagittal section of the ovary. It is crucial to avoid patient or US probe movements, as well as interposition of the bowel, while capturing the volume. Once captured, vascular flow indexes can be analyzed at a later stage using software. It should be noted that not all groups report similar results [2,3,4]. While some report good correlation between ovarian vascular flow, the number of eggs retrieved, and better pregnancy rates [5], others have not found such a correlation. This is most likely due to the very low reduction in ovarian vascular flow with aging. This decline may not appear until later, and so may not be useful in early detection of low responders. Thus, we conclude that investigating ovarian stroma vascular flow is not an independent tool for estimating the ovarian response in ART, as it does not provide additional information to the already known antral follicle count and ovarian volume evaluation by 2D US [6,7].

Three-dimensional power Doppler has also been used to predict oocyte and embryo quality, a key step for successful ART. The rationale behind this is that adequate follicular vascularization on the day of hCG administration is related to adequate intrafollicular oxygen concentration, which may facilitate oocyte development and maturation. Low oxygen concentration has been correlated with oocyte cytoplasmic defects and embryo abnormalities. However, currently there is not enough evidence to extrapolate data from 3D power Doppler to embryo development and pregnancy rates.

Evaluating uterine pathology and müllerian anomalies using 3D US

Three-dimensional US has become a key tool for diagnosing uterine malformations. It has revolutionized this field as it is noninvasive, reproducible, relatively inexpensive, and well tolerated compared with techniques such as laparoscopy/hysteroscopy, MRI, or hysterosalpingography (HSG). Three-dimensional US is very reliable, since a coronal section can be obtained, and a septate uterus can now be distinguished from a

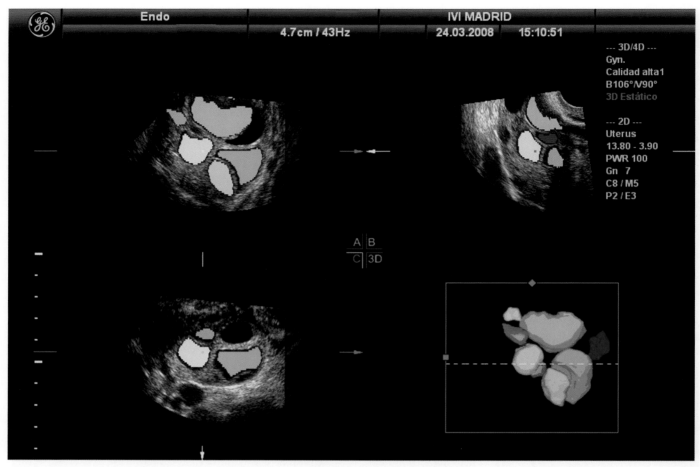

Figure 8.4. SonoAVC software permits both follicular diameter and volume calculation (automated volume calculation). The operator just needs to capture ovarian volume and the application analyzes and determines diameter as well as volume of the sonolucent areas found.

bicornuate uterus without the need of a laparoscopy. In case of a septate uterus, 3D US is more accurate than HSG when estimating the depth of the septum. Multiplanar navigation allows complete evaluation of the septum and the distance from the septum to the fundus. If we incorporate 3D power Doppler, vascularization of the septum can also be determined. The accuracy of diagnosing septate uteri using 3D US is almost 98% [7].The main sources of error are uterine leiomyomas, synechiae, or other distorting processes within the cavity.

Diagnosing benign uterine pathologies: endometrial polyps and leiomyomas

Leiomyomas and endometrial polyps are the most frequent benign uterine pathologies, and both can interfere with the reproductive process. Three-dimensional US can be used to precisely establish the size, vascularization and location of myomas and can determine their relation to the endometrial cavity. At our institution, we recommend removing myomas that distort the endometrial cavity, so 3D US is a valuable tool when surgery is being discussed. Similarly, 3D US provides a more reliable postsurgical evaluation of the uterine cavity than 2D US, avoiding the need for a postsurgery diagnostic hysteroscopy.

The extraordinary capacity of the multiplanar mode to study the whole endometrium simplifies identification of polyps, which can hamper embryo implantation if they are larger than 10 mm. The introduction of fluid into the uterine cavity (for 3D hysterosonography) improves diagnostic accuracy and is also very useful when evaluating intrauterine synechiae. The TUI mode provides tomographic sections of the uterus, permitting global evaluation of the uterus.

Analyzing the endometrium

The human endometrium undergoes intense angiogenesis during the menstrual cycle, and angiogenesis is a key process for successful embryo implantation and development. Power Doppler combined with 3D US is a noninvasive way to study the layers of the whole endometrium using perfusion analysis. Raine-Fenning et al. [8] investigated changes in endometrial and subendometrial flow in 27 healthy, fertile volunteers with regular menstrual periods. They performed 3D power Doppler on alternate days, starting on cycle D3 until ovulation, and then every 4 days afterward until initiation of menses. With the use of VOCAL, the vascular indexes were calculated for each time point. For the subendometrial vascular index, an arbitrary limit of 5 mm was established, and the inner third of the endometrium and the area irrigated by radial arteries. They found that both endometrial and subendometrial vascular flow increased to a maximum 3 days prior to ovulation, then decreased until postovulatory D5, and finally began a gradual increase during the rest of the luteal phase. The proliferative phase increment was related to estradiol levels and its vasodilating effects, while the luteal phase increase was related to serum progesterone. Interestingly, the flow indexes continued to increase during menstruation regardless of a drastic drop in progesterone levels; this might be explained by the high endometrial vascular density due to progressive compaction of the spiral arteries. The reduction in the postovulatory vascular indexes is explained by vasodilation of the subepithelial capillary plexus, which induces the required stromal edema to allow embryo implantation.

Jokubkiene et al. [9] conducted a similar study, finding that the lowest vascularization index occurred 2 days after ovulation and progressively increased during the luteal phase. Thus, 3D US is a reliable technique for investigating cyclic, physiological changes in endometrial vascularization, showing that there are maximum values 2–3 days prior to ovulation, decreasing to minimal values 2–5 days postovulation, and increasing thereafter. Vascular flow is delicately orchestrated in order to provide human embryos a favorable microenvironment for implantation, although the amount of oxygen the embryo needs from the endometrium during the implantation process is still controversial. Some authors believe that a drop in vascularization would induce a relative hypoxia that could facilitate embryo implantation. However, the increase in vascularization observed during the days in which implantation takes place does not support this hypothesis. More studies are needed to definitively establish the role of endometrial/subendometrial vascular oscillations in embryo implantation.

The endometrium in infertile women

Evaluation of the endometrium is very important in studying infertile women. Three-dimensional US facilitates noninvasive evaluation of the human endometrium and identifies some organic problems that can negatively influence the implantation process [10,11]. Specifically, endometrial volume determination and evaluation of endometrial angiogenesis using vascularization indexes can easily and accurately be performed using 3D US.

Endometrial neoangiogenesis may differ in natural cycles versus stimulated cycles, such as in IVF. The vascularization indexes are different in fertile women than in patients with unexplained infertility; the latter show a dramatic decrease in both endometrial and subendometrial vascularization indexes that are unrelated to both estradiol or progesterone levels and to endometrial thickness and volume. This suggests that vascular dysfunction may compromise embryo implantation [12]. Similarly, vascular changes that take place during natural menstrual cycles have been compared with those that occur in stimulated cycles. Ng et al. [13] compared vascular changes in natural and stimulated cycles in the same patient and found a

35% decrease in endometrial and subendometrial vascularization in stimulated cycles.

Endometrial studies in women undergoing ART

Only 30% of embryos transferred into the uterine cavity after ART successfully implant. In many cases, this may be due to the embryo, but in other cases, endometrial receptivity may also be impaired. Prognostic endometrial receptivity markers are still needed to identify patients with a good, fair, or poor prognosis. Patients with a good prognosis might benefit from single embryo transfer, whereas patients with a poor prognosis may be advised to have the embryo frozen, and transferred at a later stage in a natural cycle.

Throughout the years, multiple variables relating cycle outcome with endometrial thickness and pattern have been identified based on 2D US assessment of endometrial perfusion at the uterine, arcuate, radial, and spiral arteries. Endometrial/subendometrial mapping with color Doppler and power Doppler has also been used [14,15]. Some have reported a positive correlation between endometrial thickness, volume and/or texture and IVF cycle outcome [16,17,18]; others have not observed this positive correlation [19,20,21]. Two reports concluded that pregnancy cannot result if the endometrial volume is less than 1–2 ml [16,22].

Initially, pulsed Doppler studies of uterine arteries appeared extremely promising in terms of determining a cut-off value for predicting pregnancy, but subsequent studies failed to confirm this link. This may be due to the lack of correlation between the uterine artery pulsatility index and endometrial vascularization. A positive correlation between the subendometrial blood flow morphology in the spiral arteries and IVF cycle results was also reported [23], although not all studies supported this conclusion [24].

Three-dimensional US allows prompt, integrated evaluation of all known receptivity markers by measuring endometrial thickness, texture, pattern, volume, and global perfusion. Endometrial/subendometrial perfusion provides a more direct estimate of endometrial receptivity. It has been evaluated in different phases of the stimulated ART cycle: on the day of hCG administration [6,22,25,26], the day of egg retrieval [27], and the day of embryo transfer [16,23]. Some investigators focused only on endometrial vascularization [6], expecting a close correlation of the implantation process with the tissue in which the embryo implants. Others also investigated the relationship of subendometrial vascularization to implantation [7], speculating that a more favorable environment with better subendometrial perfusion would positively influence implantation.

There is no generally accepted consensus about the area that should be studied for adequate assessment of subendometrial vascularization. While some groups consider 1 mm outside the endometrium adequate [27], others postulate that a 5 mm [8] or 10 mm margin [26] should be used. The choice of a smaller margin (i.e., 1 mm) is based on the fact that cyclic changes in vascularization occur in that region in response to sex steroid

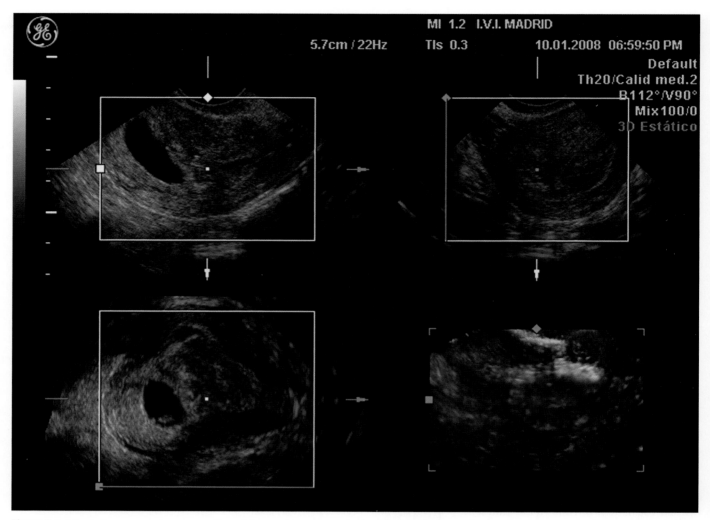

Figure 8.5. Intrauterine vs. cornual pregnancy. On certain occasions, an excessive lateralization of the gestational sac toward the uterine horn may confuse the operator and prompt a wrong diagnosis of corneal pregnancy. The image in the coronal section (bottom left) enables the visualization of the adequate placement of the gestational sacs in close contact with the uterine cavity

secretion throughout the cycle. A wider margin may inadvertently include leiomyomas, which could interfere with the accuracy of the indexes. Not unexpectedly, the results of these studies have been highly variable. Some authors found a direct relationship between pregnancy rates and subendometrial vascularization (VI, FI, VFI) on the day of hCG administration [25,28] or on the day of embryo transfer [2], whereas others found no correlation with the day of hCG [27], or even found the opposite (a higher pregnancy rate when endometrial/subendometrial flow was absent). Although no differences were found in patients with a good prognosis, cycle outcome seemed improved in patients with poor embryo quality but with better endometrial vascularization (VI, FI, VFI). This was true for in-vitro fertilization [6,28] as well as for cryopreserved embryo transfers [29].

Endometrial/subendometrial vascularization may also serve as a prognostic marker of ongoing pregnancy, as lower perfusion correlates with miscarriages [30]. None of the other study parameters – endometrial thickness, volume, or texture – had any predictive value in terms of pregnancy evolution. This finding may be helpful in order to appropriately counsel patients with a high chance of miscarriage and also as a guideline for implementing early preventive measures.

In summary, there is currently no reliable ultrasonographic predictor of endometrial receptivity for patients undergoing ART [31], except for predicting which patients will have little chance of achieving a pregnancy. Study of the global endometrial perfusion with 3D power Doppler US appears very promising. However, further comparative studies are needed to establish cut-off values in order for practitioners to counsel patients about their prognosis regarding endometrial receptivity. Studies performed during the embryo transfer procedure as well as during the window of implantation are needed to fully understand the vascular modifications that take place in the endometrium during this time. This information might help improve these processes as well as help doctors make informed decisions about how many embryos to transfer.

Early pregnancy

There are multiple advantages to using 3D US to diagnose complications in early pregnancy. In reproductive medicine, it is crucial to exclude ectopic pregnancy as early as possible. 3D US is a more accurate technique for evaluating the relationship between the gestational sac and uterine septum and for differentiating between a cornual pregnancy and a displaced intracavitary pregnancy (Figure 8.5). Similarly, 3D US is of great help in evaluating the risk of miscarriage, as it can accurately estimate the presence as well as the volume of subchorionic hematomas. Decreased gestational sac volume has been correlated with a higher frequency of chromosomal abnormalities, and lower placental volume has been associated with preeclampsia. Evaluation of vascular indexes by 3D power Doppler can provide information about spiral artery remodeling associated with the placentation process, allowing early intervention in cases of inadequate tissue remodeling.

In summary, 3D US has significantly improved diagnostic accuracy, not only for evaluating infertility but also for ART and follow-up of early pregnancy. In the coming years, 3D US will become even more useful both for performing common, simple procedures and for furthering advanced, clinically oriented research.

References

1. Scheffer GJ, Broekmans FJ, Bancsi LF, Habbema DJF, Looman CWN, te Velde ER. Quantitative transvaginal two- and three dimensional sonography of the ovaries: reproducibility of antral follicle counts. *Ultrasound Obstet Gynecol* 2002; **20**: 270–5.

2. Kupesic S, Kurjak A, Bjelos D, Vujisic S. Three-dimensional ultrasonographic ovarian measurements and *in vitro* fertilization outcome are related to age. *Fertil Steril* 2003; **79**: 190–7.

3. Oyesanya OA, Parsons JH, Collins WP, Campbell S. Total ovarian volume before human chorionic gonadotropin administration for ovulation induction may predict the hyperstimulation syndrome. *Hum Reprod* 1995; **10**: 3211–12.

4. Ng E, Chan C, Yeung W, Ho P. Effect of pituitary downregulation on antral follicle count, ovarian volume and stromal blood flow measured by three-dimensional ultrasound with power Doppler prior to ovarian stimulation. *Hum Reprod* 2004; **19**: 2811–15.

5. Pan H, Wu M, Cheng Y, Wu L, Chang F. Quantification of ovarian stromal Doppler signals in poor responders undergoing in vitro fertilization with three-dimensional power Doppler ultrasonography. *Am J Obstet Gynecol* 2004; **190**: 338–44.

6. Merce LT, Barco MJ, Bau S Troyano JM. Prediction of ovarian response and IVF/ICSI outcome by three-dimensional ultrasonography and power Doppler angiography. *Eur J Obstetr Gynecol Reprod Biol* 2007; **132**: 93–100.

7. Kupesic S. Three-dimensional ultrasound in reproductive medicine. *Ultrasound Rev Obstetr Gynecol* 2005; **5**: 304–15.

8. Raine-Fenning NJ, Campbell BK, Kendall NR, Clewes JS, Johnson IR. Quantifying the changes in endometrial vascularity throughout the normal menstrual cycle with three-dimensional power Doppler angiography. *Hum Reprod* 2004; **19**: 330–8.

9. Jokubkiene L, Sladkevicius P, Rovas L, Valentin L. Assessment of changes in endometrial and subendometrial volume and vascularity during the normal menstrual cycle using three-dimensional power Doppler ultrasound. *Ultrasound Obstet Gynecol* 2006; **27**: 672–9.

10. Nargund G. Time for an ultrasound revolution in reproductive medicine. *Ultrasound Obstet Gynecol* 2002; **20**: 107–11.

11. Lindhard A, Ravn V, Bentin-Ley U, et al. Ultrasound characteristics and histological dating of the endometrium in a natural cycle in infertile women compared with fertile controls. *Fertil Steril* 2006; **86**: 1344–55.

12. Raine-Fenning NJ, Campbell BK, Kendall NR, Clewes JS, Johnson IR. Endometrial and subendometrial perfusion are impaired in women with unexplained subfertility. *Hum Reprod* 2004; **19**: 2605–14.

13. Ng EH, Chan CC, Tang OS, Yeung WS, Ho PC. Comparison of endometrial and subendometrial blood flow measured by three-dimensional power Doppler ultrasound between stimulated and natural cycles in the same patients. *Hum Reprod* 2004; **19**: 2385–90.

14. Zaidi J, Campbell S, Pittrof R, Tan SL. Endometrial thickness, morphology, vascular penetration and velocimetry in predicting implantation in an in vitro fertilization program. *Ultrasound Obstet Gynecol* 1995; **6**: 191–8.

15. Pierson RA. Imaging the endometrium: are there predictors of uterine receptivity? *J Obstet Gynaecol Can* 2003; **25**: 360–8.

16. Raga F, Bonilla-Musoles F, Casan EM, Klein O, Bonilla F: Assessment of endometrial volume by three-dimensional ultrasoundprior to embryo transfer: clues to endometrial receptivity. *Hum Reprod* 1999; **14**: 2851–4.

17. Richter KS, Bugge KR, Bromer JG, Levy MJ. Relationship between endometrial thickness and embryo implantation, based on 1,294 cycles of in vitro fertilization with transfer of two blastocyst-stage embryos *Fertil Steril* 2007; **87**: 53–9.

18. Zhang X, Chen CH, Confino E, Barnes R, Milad M, Kazer RR. Increased endometrial thickness is associated with improved treatment outcome for selected patients undergoing in vitro fertilization-embryo transfer. *Fertil Steril* 2005; **83**: 336–40.

19. Puerto B, Creus M, Carmona F, Civico S, Vanrell JA, Balasch J. Ultrasonography as a predictor of embryo implantation after in vitro fertilization: a controlled study. *Fertil Steril* 2003; **79**: 1015–22.

20. Garcia-Velasco JA, Isaza V, Caligara C, Pellicer A, Remohi J, Simon C. Factors that determine discordant outcome from shared oocytes. *Fertil Steril* 2003; **80**: 54–60.

21. Soares S, Troncoso C, Bosch E, et al. Age and uterine receptiveness: predicting the outcome of oocyte donation cycles. *J Clin Endocrinol Metab* 2005; **90**(7): 4399–404.

22. Yaman C, Ebner T, Sommergruber M, Polz W, Tews G. Role of

three-dimensional ultrasonographic measurement of endometrium volume as a predictor of pregnancy outcome in an IVF-ET program: a preliminary study. *Fertil Steril* 2000; **74**: 797–801.

23. Kupesic S, Bekavac I, Bjelos D, Kurjak A. Assessment of endometrial receptivity by transvaginal color Doppler and three-dimensional power Doppler ultrasonography in patients undergoing in vitro fertilization procedures. *J Ultrasound Med* 2001; **20**: 125–34.

24. Schild RL, Holthaus S, d'Alquen J, et al. Quantitative assessment of subendometrial blood flow by three-dimensional-

ultrasound is an important predictive factor of implantation in an in-vitro fertilization programme. *Hum Reprod* 2000; **15**: 89–94.

25. Wu HM, Chiang CH, Huang HY, Chao AS, Wang HS, Soong YK. Detection of the subendometrial vascularization flow index by three-dimensional ultrasound may be useful for predicting the pregnancy rate for patients undergoing in vitro fertilization-embryo transfer. *Fertil Steril* 2003; **79**: 507–11.

26. Jarvela IY, Sladkevicius P, Kelly S, Ojha K, Campbell S, Nargund G. Evaluation of endometrial receptivity during in-vitro fertilization using three-dimensional power Doppler

ultrasound. *Ultrasound Obstet Gynecol* 2005; **26**: 765–76.

27. Ng Eh, Chan CC, Tang OS, Yeung WS, Ho PC: The role of endometrial and subendometrial blood flows measured by three-dimensional power Doppler ultrasound in the prediction of pregnancy during IVF treatment. *Hum Reprod* 2006; **21**: 164–70.

28. Mercé LT, Barco MJ, Bau S, Troyano J. Are endometrial parameters by three-dimensional ultrasound and power Doppler angiography related to in vitro fertilization/embryo transfer outcome?. *Fertil Steril* 2008; **89**: 111–17.

29. Ng EH, Chan CC, Tang OS, Yeung WS, Ho PC. The role

of endometrial and subendometrial vascularity measured by three-dimensional power Doppler ultrasound in the prediction of pregnancy during frozen-thawed embryo transfer cycles. *Hum Reprod* 2006; **21**: 1612–17.

30. Ng EH, Chan CC, Tang OS, Yeung WS, Chung H. Endometrial and subendometrial vascularity is higher in pregnant patients with livebirth following ART than in those who suffer a miscarriage *Hum Reprod* 2007; **22**: 1134–41.

31. Alcázar JL. Three-dimensional ultrasound assessment of endometrial receptivity: a review. *Reprod Biol Endocrinol* 2006; **4**: 56.

Ultrasonography and diagnosis of polycystic ovary syndrome

Manubai Nagamani and Rebecca Chilvers

Introduction

Polycystic ovary syndrome (PCOS) is the most common endocrine disorder, affecting 5%–10% of women of reproductive age [1]. Although the association of polycystic ovaries and amenorrhea was first described by Stein and Leventhal in 1935, the definition of PCOS is still not well established [2]. Hallmark signs and symptoms include hyperandrogenism, anovulation, and oligomenorrhea, but the phenotypic expression of the syndrome is quite variable. Even though hyperinsulinemia and other metabolic factors have been associated with the pathophysiology of PCOS, ovarian dysfunction is central to the diagnosis of PCOS. Since patients with PCOS are at risk for significant reproductive and metabolic consequences, establishment of criteria for accurate diagnosis of PCOS becomes imperative [3]. Advances in ultrasound technology provide an accurate view of the internal structure of the ovary. We will analyze the published data to investigate what ultrasound parameters of ovarian morphology are useful for diagnosing PCOS and highlight the role of ultrasound in the diagnosis and management of PCOS.

Diagnostic criteria for PCOS

NIH criteria

In April 1990 the NIH convened a conference to determine the diagnostic criteria of PCOS. The experts summarized the syndrome into the following criteria in order of importance: (1) hyperandrogenism, (2) oligo-ovulation, and (3) exclusion of disorders, such as Cushing syndrome, hyperprolactinemia, and congenital adrenal hyperplasia that can present in a similar fashion (Table 9.1) [4]. These criteria comprise the most commonly used definition of PCOS used today in the USA [5]. A fourth criterion, polycystic ovary (PCO) on ultrasound, was not included in the diagnostic criteria since it was considered controversial. Even though the prevalence of PCOs is increased severalfold in women with PCOS, PCOs have also been observed in patients without any endocrine abnormalities [6]. There is also difficulty in predicting the degree of the disorder from the ultrasound features. Neither the polycystic morphology nor the volume of the ovaries identifies the distinctive metabolic or reproductive abnormalities in women with PCOS [7].

Rotterdam criteria

In 2003 a joint meeting of the European Society of Human Reproduction and Embryology (ESHRE) and the American Society of Reproductive Medicine (ASRM) was held in Rotterdam. At this PCOS Consensus Workshop, in addition to hyperandrogenism and anovulation, ultrasound evidence of PCO was also included as a criterion for the diagnosis of PCOS [8] (Table 9.1). A diagnosis of PCOS is to be made when at least two of three elements are present: chronic anovulation, clinical or biochemical hyperandrogenism, and clearly defined PCOs on ultrasound [8]. It also specified that there be exclusion of other androgenic and anovulatory disorders prior to the diagnosis of PCOS. These new diagnostic criteria resulted in diagnosis of PCOS in patients who were previously excluded by the 1990 NIH criteria, such as anovulatory normoandrogenic women and ovulatory hyperandrogenic women with PCOs on ultrasound scan. The Rotterdam definition increases the phenotypic heterogeneity of the disorder, and some investigators have criticized it on the grounds that the additional phenotypes included in the definition by the Rotterdam consensus have few supportive data and could decrease the efficiency of research such as finding a genetic abnormality common to PCOS women [5].

Even though there is not a global consensus on its diagnostic value, ultrasound is frequently used as a morphologic indicator of polycystic ovaries and is thus supportive of the diagnosis of PCOS. Technical recommendations for ultrasound assessment of PCO recommended by the Rotterdam consensus are shown in Table 9.2 [8].

In 2006 the Androgen Excess Society met and discussed the rationale of the use of ultrasound imaging as part of the diagnostic criteria for PCOS [6]. Review of the literature revealed that polycystic ovaries are detected by transvaginal ultrasound in only approximately 75% of women with a clinical diagnosis of PCOS, and they highlighted that 25% of women with PCOS do not have characteristic findings on ultrasound. The task force also recognized that the false-positive rate is relatively

Ultrasonography in Reproductive Medicine and Infertility, ed. Botros R. M. B. Rizk. Published by Cambridge University Press. © Cambridge University Press 2010.

Table 9.1. Diagnostic criteria of polycystic ovary syndrome

1990 NIH Criteria (both 1 and 2)
1 Chronic anovulation
2 Clinical/or biochemical signs of hyperandrogenism and exclusion of other causes

Revised 2003 Rotterdam Criteria (2 out of 3)
1 Oligo-ovulation or anovulation
2 Clinical/or biochemical signs of hyperandrogenism
3 Polycystic ovaries and exclusion of other causes

Table 9.2. Technical recommendations for ultrasound assessment of PCO from the 2003 Rotterdam PCOS consensus [8]

State-of-the-art equipment operated by appropriately trained personnel.

Whenever possible, the transvaginal approach should be used.

Regularly menstruating women should be scanned in the early follicular phase (cycle days 3–5). Oligo-/amenorrheic women should be scanned either at random or between days 3 and 5 after a progestin-induced withdrawal bleeding.

Calculation of ovarian volume is performed using the simplified formula for a prolate ellipsoid (0.5 × length × width × thickness).

Follicle number should be estimated both in longitudinal and antero-posterior cross-sections of the ovaries. The size of follicles <10 mm should be expressed as the mean of the diameters measured on the two sections.

high, as evidenced by the high rate of polycystic ovaries in the general population. The task force noted that the diagnosis of polycystic ovaries requires strict criteria and should not be assigned solely on the basis of a polycystic or multicystic appearance of the ovary. They indicated that the diagnostic sonographic features of PCOS should be follicle number and ovarian volume [6]. The diagnosis of polycystic ovaries has recently been reviewed [9]. The most commonly used criteria today are those proposed by Jonard and colleagues [10] and reaffirmed in the Rotterdam 2003 consensus, which indicate that diagnosis of polycystic ovaries can be established when at least one ovary demonstrates an ovarian volume of greater than 10 cm³ (10 ml) and/or 12 or more follicles measuring 2–9 mm in diameter [8]. In the task force's assessment, women with oligoamenorrhea and polycystic-appearing ovaries on ultrasonography, but no evidence of hyperandrogenism, do not have PCOS.

Ultrasound assessment of polycystic ovary

Before the availability of ultrasound, PCOs were assessed by direct visualization of the ovaries during laparotomy and histological evaluation of a wedge biopsy of the ovaries [2]. The advent of ultrasound has allowed less invasive means of accurately viewing the ovaries (Figure 9.1a, b). Currently, ultrasound is the most widely used noninvasive means of evaluating ovarian morphology in women with suspected PCOS. Although the most commonly used diagnostic sonographic features of PCOS are follicle number and ovarian volume, there is no complete consensus regarding the best criteria for ultrasound diagnosis. The role of stromal echogeneity, stromal volume, and ovarian and uterine blood flow in the diagnosis of PCOS is still being debated. In this chapter we will address optimal ultrasound techniques, different ultrasound criteria for PCOs diagnosis, and the possible role of three-dimensional (3D) and Doppler techniques in the diagnosis of PCOS.

Ultrasound techniques

Transabdominal ultrasound

The first definition of PCO in 1985 was established using transabdominal sonography [11]. Transabdominal ultrasound has been largely superseded by transvaginal scanning because of

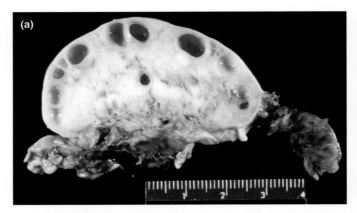

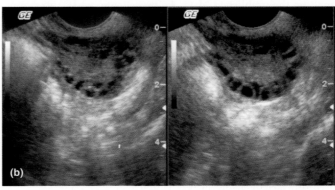

Figure 9.1. (a) Cut surface of a typical PCO with antral follicles arranged peripherally around a dense core of stroma, which is increased. (b) Sagittal ultrasound images of the ovaries in a patient with PCOS obtained with a 6.5-MHz transvaginal transducer. Small follicles less than 9 mm are arranged around increased ovarian stroma.

greater resolution and, in many cases, patient preference. Since the need for a full bladder is avoided, it saves time and is more convenient for the patient. The transabdominal route is, of course, required in adolescent girls and virginal women who decline a transvaginal scan. A transabdominal scan offers a whole view of the pelvic cavity, and so may be useful if the transvaginal scan fails to visualize displaced ovaries. Although a full bladder is required for visualization of the ovaries, one should be cautious that an overfilled bladder can compress the ovaries, yielding a falsely increased length. This emphasizes the need for assessing the ovarian size by measuring the area or the volume. Transvaginal ultrasound is a more sensitive method than the transabdominal scan for the detection of polycystic ovaries. For example, polycystic ovaries were not detected in 30% of women with PCOS when a 3.5 MHz transabdominal transducer was used, and a 7.5 MHz transvaginal probe was found to be more reliable [12].

Transvaginal ultrasound

Much of the interest in ultrasound came from the advent of endovaginal probes in the later 1980s, which have allowed for more accurate assessment of the ovaries. Two-dimensional ultrasonography remains the standard for those who image PCOs, and the current consensus from the Rotterdam meeting rests on this technique [8]. Transvaginal ultrasound provides a more accurate view of the internal and external morphologic features of the ovary than the abdominal ultrasound, especially in obese patients. It is recommended to use a high-frequency probe (>6 MHz) for transvaginal examination of the ovaries. It has a better spatial resolution but less examination depth, which is acceptable because the ovaries are usually in the cul-de-sac of the pelvis and close to the transducer.

Three-dimensional ultrasound

Three-dimensional ultrasound is a relatively new imaging modality that has the potential to improve the sensitivity and specificity of ultrasound in the diagnosis of PCOS. Three-dimensional ultrasound facilitates the quantitative assessment of follicle count, measurement of total ovarian and stromal echogenicity, and assessment of volume and blood flow in a way that has not been possible with 2D ultrasound. Three-dimensional ultrasound not only permits improved spatial awareness and volumetric and quantitative vascular assessment, but also provides a more objective tool to examine stromal echogenicity through the assessment of the mean grayness of the ovary [13]. The mean echogenicity of the gray voxels represents the mean tissue density or echogenicity in the region of interest and provides a new measure that can be objectively quantified. Aside from the disadvantage of needing more expensive equipment and further training in ultrasonography to use the technology, 3D ultrasonography has been shown to allow for easier assessment of follicular and stromal volume. It permits improved volumetric calculation and quantitative assessment of the vascularity within a defined volume of tissue [14]. However, the criteria for the diagnosis of PCO by 3D ultrasonography need to be defined and tested prospectively alongside 2D ultrasound parameters before it can be used in routine clinical care. There have been no well-designed studies to compare 2D and 3D ultrasound techniques in the assessment of PCOs.

Timing of the ultrasound examination

The Rotterdam criteria for ultrasound assessment specify that a baseline ultrasound scan of the pelvis should be performed in the early follicular phase (days 1–3) when the ovaries are relatively quiescent. If the patient does not have regular menses, then the ultrasound may be performed at a random time or after progestin withdrawal bleeding [8]. Additionally, time of day should be recorded if Doppler studies of ovarian blood flow or uterine blood flow are performed, since diurnal variation has been observed [15]. It is recommended that if a dominant follicle or corpus luteum is observed during the baseline scan, the scan be repeated in the early follicular phase of the patient's next menstrual cycle. The uterine dimensions should also be recorded during the baseline scan with measurement of endometrial thickness, since women with PCOS are at increased risk for endometrial cancer. More details of the various ultrasound parameters that can be measured in PCOS patients are discussed below.

Ultrasound criteria for diagnosis of PCOS

Antral follicle count

The ESHRE/ASRM consensus included PCO on ultrasound as a criterion for diagnosis of PCOS. The Rotterdam criteria for the diagnosis of PCOs include the presence of 12 or more follicles in each ovary measuring 2–9 mm in diameter and/or increased ovarian volume (>10 ml). Even though the Rotterdam criteria do not mention distribution of follicles in the ovary, typical PCO has follicles measuring 2–9 mm arranged peripherally around a dense core of stroma or scattered throughout the increased ovarian stroma (Figure 9.1b). Each ovary should be scanned from the inner to outer margins in order to count the total number of follicles/cysts. The evaluation of the follicular distribution was omitted from the definition of PCO. The presence of a single PCO is sufficient to meet the ovarian morphology criterion for diagnosis of PCOS. The PCO should be differentiated from the multifollicular ovary (MFO), which is defined as 6 or more follicles 4–10 mm in size with normal stroma (Figure 9.2). The most frequent causes of MFOs are a normal early follicular phase, puberty, hypothalamic

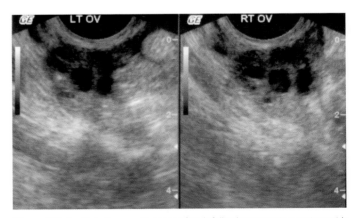

Figure 9.2. Sagittal ultrasound images of multifollicular ovaries in a patient with hypothalamic amenorrhea. The ovary contains follicles 4–10 mm in size, with normal stroma.

amenorrhea, and hyperprolactinemia, which can also be seen in conjunction with hypothyroidism [16].

Antral follicle count (AFC), which includes follicles measuring 2–9 mm by the Rotterdam criteria, is one of the most important ultrasound features of PCOS. In a comprehensive comparison of PCOS subjects and controls with 3D ultrasonography, women with PCOS had significantly higher AFCs (9–35 follicles, with a median of 16.3) than the controls (1–10 follicles, with a median of 5.5) [14]. Ovaries should be scanned in the longitudinal plane for determination of follicle count. The orthogonal plane should be used to estimate the size and distribution of follicles. The mean diameter of each follicle should be based on two orthogonal measurements [8]. Using a 7 MHz 3D transvaginal probe in 214 PCOS patients and 112 controls, the threshold of 12 follicles between 2 and 9 mm in at least one ovary was found to be most diagnostic for PCOS, thus supporting the Rotterdam consensus. Also of interest, the follicle number per ovary of follicles within the 6–9 mm range was found to be significantly and negatively related to body mass index (BMI) and fasting serum insulin level [10]. An excess of 2–5 mm follicles seen at ultrasonography has been associated with the follicular arrest in PCOS [17].

Total ovarian volume

Ovaries of PCOS patients are often enlarged and tend to be more spherical than ovoid. Ovarian volume is used as a surrogate for stromal hypertrophy. The Rotterdam criterion for diagnosis of PCO is an ovarian volume of >10 ml. Jonard criticized the Rotterdam consensus threshold of 10 cm³ for being "reached without appropriate studies such as receiver operator characteristics (ROC) curve analysis," and he validated his own threshold for ovarian volume as indicative of PCOS [18]. He compared 154 patients who met NIH criteria for PCOS with 57 controls and showed that the threshold of 7 cm³ offered the best compromise between sensitivity (67.5%) and specificity (91.2%) compared with the sensitivity of 45% and specificity of 98.3% of the 10 cm³ threshold [18]. The most commonly used formula to calculate ovarian volume is the prolate ellipsoid: length × width × height or thickness × 0.5. The use of 3D ultrasound makes calculation of ovarian volume easier. Ovarian area can be used as a surrogate for ovarian volume in difficult cases.

Stromal area and ovarian area

Stromal hypertrophy is a specific feature in ovarian androgenic dysfunction. The most severe form of stromal hypertrophy is referred to as hyperthecosis [19]. These women have long-standing hirsutism, have testosterone levels in tumor range (>6.94 nmol/l [200 ng/dl]), and have noncystic ovarian enlargement (Figure 9.3a). Histological examination reveals large nests of steroidogenically active luteinized thecal cells in the ovarian stroma (Figure 9.3b), which explains the high testosterone levels observed in these women. Ultrasound examination shows bilateral enlarged, solid-appearing ovaries with no antral follicles (Figure 9.3c). In these women, the whole ovary is replaced by ovarian stroma. Although an increase in stromal volume represents one of the most specific features of PCO, assessment of stromal volume is not practical in routine clinical practice, and therefore ovarian volume has been used as a good surrogate. Both qualitative and quantitative stromal evaluation had previously been viewed as merely subjective and were therefore excluded from the consensus definition of PCO [8].

Dewailly et al. proposed the presence of ovarian hypertrophy (an ovarian area >5.5 cm² unilaterally or bilaterally) as a morphological indicator of PCOS [20]. The stromal area is measured by "outlining with the caliper the peripheral profile of the stroma, identified by a central area slightly hyperechoic with respect to the other ovarian area." The ovarian area is calculated by outlining with the caliper the external limits of the ovary in the maximum plane section. The average of the parameters for both ovaries is used to determine mean ovarian area and stromal area and then calculate the stromal area to ovarian area ratio (S/A ratio) [21]. These investigators also were able to verify the feasibility of the determination of the S/A ratio in routine clinical use and confirmed its value for predicting hyperandrogenism in PCOS. In fact, the S/A ratio had the strongest correlation with serum androgens when compared with total ovarian area, stromal area, ovarian volume, and AFC. The androgens that showed significant correlation were testosterone and androstenedione, whereas DHEAS (dehydroepiandrosterone sulfate) did not show a significant relation. There was also a significant correlation of the S/A ratio to insulin AUC [21]. This group of investigators was able to define cut-off values for ultrasonographic parameters, with 0.34 as the S/A ratio at or above which PCOS was diagnosed at 100% sensitivity and 100% specificity [22]. Belosi et al. also observed that the S/A ratio showed the most significant correlation with the androgen levels and insulin secretion in PCOS patients [23].

Stromal echogenicity

Data from the literature indicate that increased ovarian stroma is an important marker for the presence of PCOS. An increase in the echogenicity of the stroma corresponds to histological findings of prominent theca and fibrotic thickening of the albuginea described by Stein and Leventhal [2]. Several investigators have shown increased stromal echogenicity in patients with PCOS compared with controls [23]. However, these studies were subjective until Buckett et al. described a method to calculate mean echogenicity of a given area [24]. Using 2D transvaginal ultrasound and newly advanced software, the brightness, or echogenicity, of the ovarian stroma was determined objectively and showed that the mean stromal echogenicity was similar between PCOs and normal ovaries. The total echogenicity of PCOs was shown to be significantly less than the total echogenicity of control ovaries, and this can be explained by the presence of the many hypoechoic cysts in PCOs. They observed that the stromal index (stromal echogenicity/total ovarian echogenicity) was significantly higher in PCOS than in control ovaries. They concluded that the subjective appearance of brighter stroma in PCOS patients in previous studies was due to the difference

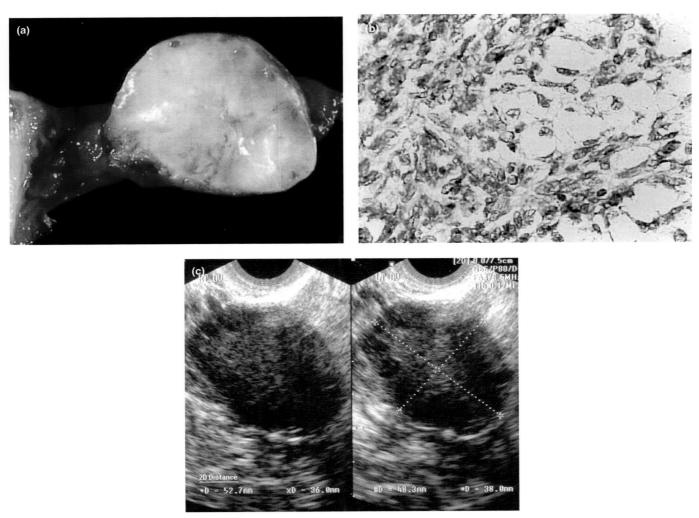

Figure 9.3. (a) Cut surface of an ovary with severe hyperthecosis showing abundant ovarian stroma that is completely replacing the ovary. (b) Diagnosis confirmed by histological examination – large nests of luteinized thecal cells in the ovarian stroma. (c) Sagittal ultrasound images of hyperthecotic ovaries. Note the complete lack of antral follicles and stroma replacing the ovary.

between the echogenicity of the stroma and total ovarian echogenicity and not due to a difference between the stroma of PCO and normal ovaries. Studies with 3D ultrasound also failed to show any difference in the stromal echogenicity between polycystic and normal ovaries [14]. Therefore, ultrasonic measurement of ovarian stromal echogenicity in the routine ultrasound assessment is not warranted.

Vascularity

Doppler analysis of stromal vascularity was not included in the Rotterdam criteria since the results are controversial. Stromal blood flow was shown to be most elevated in lean, hirsute women as compared with obese, normoandrogenic women [25]. This finding suggests that ovarian stroma plays an important role in the development of hyperandrogenism. It also may explain why patients with PCOS are hyperresponsive to gonadotropins and thus prone to developing ovarian hyperstimulation syndrome (OHSS). Three-dimensional ultrasonography is especially useful in the quantitative assessment of the vascularity within a defined

volume of tissue [14]. Interestingly, Jarvela et al. did not find any difference in the vascularization of polycystic ovarian stroma compared with normal ovarian stroma [13]. Several investigators have looked at uterine artery blood flow, which can be assessed by transvaginal Doppler ultrasound, but so far there have been conflicting results. Ozkan et al. observed that the ovarian artery pulsatility index (PI) and resistance index were significantly reduced in patients with PCOS. Increased uterine arterial resistance to blood flow may be a cause for poor endometrial receptivity of embryos, with a resultant decrease in fertility in these patients [25].

Key points in clinical practice

The role of ultrasonography in the diagnosis of PCOS is quite controversial and it was therefore excluded from the NIH criteria in 1990. However, it was included in the revised Rotterdam criteria in 2003, which indicate that diagnosis of PCO can be established when at least one ovary demonstrates an ovarian volume of greater than $10 \, cm^3$ (10 ml) and/or 12 or more follicles measuring 2–9 mm in diameter. The NIH criteria are more widely used in the USA, while the Rotterdam criteria are used mainly in Europe. It is to be hoped that the use of ultrasonography in PCOS patients will be more clearly defined as our technology in the area of ultrasound improves and our understanding of the pathophysiology focuses our attention on the more pertinent ultrasonographic features. From the literature, the S/A ratio has the strongest correlation with serum androgens when compared with total ovarian area, stromal area, ovarian volume, and AFC. It appears that the S/A ratio holds most promise for being adopted into routine clinical practice and use as an adjunctive marker in the diagnosis of PCOS whenever ultrasonography is used. Regardless of what methods are adopted as diagnostic tools, there is clearly a need for standardized definitions of PCOS to validly improve the comparability of data between studies, which is essential for furthering efficient research of PCOS. Three-dimensional (3D) ultrasound is a relatively new imaging modality that has the potential to improve the sensitivity and specificity of ultrasound in the diagnosis of PCOS.

References

1. Carmina E, Lobo RA. Polycystic ovary syndrome (PCOS): arguably the most common endocrinopathy is associated with significant morbidity in women. *J Clin Endocrinol Metab* 1999; **84**: 1897–9.

2. Stein IF, Leventhal ML. Amenorrhea associated with polycystic ovaries. *Am J Obstet Gynecol* 1935; **29**: 181–91.

3. Azziz R, Marin C, Hoq L, Badamgarav E, Song P. Health care-related economic burden of the polycystic ovary syndrome during the reproductive life span. *J Clin Endocrinol Metab* 2005; **90**: 4650–8.

4. Zawadski JK, Dunaif A. Diagnostic criteria for polycystic ovary syndrome: toward a rational approach. In: Dunaif A, Givens JR, Haseltine FP, Merriam GR, eds., *Polycystic Ovary Syndrome.* Boston, MA: Blackwell Scientific, 1992, pp. 377–84.

5. Azziz, R. Controversy in clinical endocrinology: diagnosis of polycystic ovary syndrome: the Rotterdam criteria are premature. *J Clin Endocrinol Metab* 2006; **91**: 781–5.

6. Azziz R, Carmina E, Dewailly D, et al. Position statement: criteria for defining polycystic ovary syndrome as a predominantly hyperandrogenic syndrome: an Androgen Excess Society guideline. *J Clin Endocrinol Metab* 2006; **91**: 4237–45.

7. Legro R, Chiu P, Kunselman AR, Bentley CM, Dodson WC, Duanif A. Polycystic ovaries are common in women with hyperandrogenic chronic anovulation but do not predict metabolic or reproductive phenotype. *J Clin Endocrinol Metab* 2005; **90**: 2571–9.

8. The Rotterdam ESHRE/ ASRM-sponsored PCOS consensus workshop group. Revised 2003 consensus on diagnostic criteria and long-term heath risks related to polycystic ovary syndrome (PCOS). *Hum Reprod* 2004; **19**: 41–7.

9. Balen A, Laven JSE, Tan SL, Dewailly D. Ultrasound assessment of the polycystic ovary: international census definitions. *Hum Reprod* 2003; **9**: 505–14.

10. Jonard S, Robert Y, Cortet-Rudelli C, Pigny P, Decanter C, Dewailly D. Ultrasound examination of polycystic ovaries: is it worth counting the follicles? *Hum Reprod* 2003; **18**: 598–603.

11. Adams J, Polson DW, Franks S. Prevalence of polycystic ovaries in women with anovulation and idiopathic hirsutism. *Br Med J.* 1986; **293**: 355–9.

12. Fox R, Corrigan E, Thomas PA, Hull MG. The diagnosis of polycystic ovaries in women with oligo-amenorrhoea: predictive power of endocrine tests. *Clin Endocrinol (Oxf)* 1991; **34**: 127–31.

13. Jarvela IY, Mason HD, Sladkevicius R, et al. Characterization of normal and polycystic ovaries using three-dimensional power doppler ultrasonography. *J Assist Reprod Genet* 2002; **19**: 582–90.

14. Lam PM, Johnson IR, Raine-Fenning NJ. Three-dimensional ultrasound features of the polycystic ovary and the effect of different phenotypic expressions on these parameters. *Hum Reprod* 2007; **22**: 3116–23.

15. Zaidi J, Tan SL, Pitroff R, Campbell S, Collins W. Blood flow changes in the intra-ovarian arteries during the peri-ovulatory period–relationship to the time of day. *Ultrasound Obstet Gynecol* 1996; **7**: 135–40.

16. Brown MA, Chang RJ. Polycystic ovary syndrome: clinical and imaging features. *Ultrasound Q* 2007; **23**: 233–8.

17. Dewailly D, Catteau-Jonard S, Reyss AC, Maunoury-Lefebvre C, Poncelet E, Pigny P. The excess in 2–5 mm follicles seen at ovarian ultrasonography is tightly associated to the follicular arrest of the polycystic ovary syndrome. *Hum Reprod* 2007; **22**: 1562–6.

18. Jonard S, Robert Y, Dewailly D. Revisiting the ovarian volume as a diagnostic criterion for polycystic ovaries. *Hum Reprod* 2005; **20**: 2893–8.

19. Nagamani M. Polycystic ovary syndrome variants: Hyperthecosis. In: Adashi EY, Rock JA, Rosenwaks Z, eds. *Reproductive Endocrinology, Surgery and Technology.* Philadelphia, PA: Lippincott-Raven, 1996; 1258–69.

20. Dewailly D, Robert Y, Helin Y, et al. Ovarian stromal hypertrophy in hyperandrogenic women. *Clin Endocrinol (Oxf)* 1994; **41**: 557–62.

21. Fulghesu AM, Ciampelli M, Belosi C, Apa R, Pavone V, Lanzone A. A new ultrasound criterion for the diagnosis of polycystic ovary syndrome: the ovarian stroma/total area ratio. *Fertil Steril* 2001; **76**: 326–31.

22. Fulghesu AM, Angioni S, Frau E, et al. Ultrasound in polycystic ovary syndrome–the measuring of ovarian stroma and relationship with circulating androgens: results of a multicentric study. *Hum Reprod* 2007; **22**: 2501–8.

23. Belosi C, Selvaggi L, Apa R, et al. Is the PCOS diagnosis solved by ESHRE/ASRM 2003 consensus or could it include ultrasound examination of the ovarian stroma? *Hum Reprod* 2006; **21**: 3108–15.

24. Buckett WM, Bouzayen R, Watkin KL, Tulandi T, Tan SL. Ovarian stromal echogenicity in women with normal and polycystic ovaries. *Hum Reprod* 1999; **14**: 618–21.

25. Ozkan S, Vural B, Caliskan E, Bodur H, Turkoz E, Vural F. Color doppler sonographic analysis of uterine and ovarian artery blood flow in women with PCOS. *J Clin Ultrasound* 2007; **35**: 305–13.

Chapter 10

Ultrasonography and the treatment of infertility in polycystic ovary syndrome

Carolyn J. Alexander

Introduction

Ultrasonography has evolved into a highly developed technology with high resolution capable of measuring structures within an accuracy of millimeters. Among fertility patients with polycystic ovary syndrome (PCOS), controlled ovarian hyperstimulation (COH) poses exquisite challenges and must be performed with vigilance in order to prevent ovarian hyperstimulation syndrome (OHSS) and higher-order multiple pregnancy. Defined by Stein and Leventhal [1] in 1935, PCOS is now considered to be one of the most prevalent endocrine disorders in young women, affecting 6–10% of women of child-bearing age [2] and accounting for 70% of anovulatory subfertility [3]. The application of real-time ultrasonography to ovarian follicular monitoring has advanced the understanding of follicular dynamics and its regulation. In 1988, Polson et al. [4] reported that 23% of 158 regularly menstruating women had polycystic ovaries on ultrasound; meanwhile, in another study, 83% of 173 with hirsutism had polycystic-appearing ovaries [5]. The overarching goal of this chapter is to highlight the role of ultrasound in the management of PCOS during ovulation induction for insemination as well as for in-vitro fertilization.

Historical perspective

In 1966, von Micsky et al. noted the possibility of using ultrasound to outline normal ovaries [6]. Among the first to identify ovarian follicles were Kratochwil et al. [7], using abdominal ultrasound. An abdominal ultrasound image of a single ovarian follicle is shown in Figure 10.1. In 1980, Hill et al. [8] reported the assessment of human follicular development by ultrasound for infertility patients using a 3.5 MHz transducer. Since 1986, pelvic ultrasonography has been used to identify polycystic ovaries [9]. Transvaginal (TV) ultrasonography has increased our appreciation of the physiological changes in the ovary and endometrium that occur during controlled ovarian hyperstimulation, especially in women with PCOS.

Briefly, the Rotterdam Consensus Workshop on PCOS in 2003 changed diagnostic guidelines by adding the ultrasonographic criteria of a mean of 12 follicles per ovary (FNPO) of both ovaries or ovarian volume of 10 ml (calculated using the formula $0.5 \times$ length $\times$ width $\times$ thickness) to hyperandrogenism

and oligo-ovulation; Two of the three criteria must be present to diagnose PCOS [10]. It was suggested that follicle distribution and an increase in stromal echogenicity and volume be eliminated as diagnostic criteria [11]. Women with PCOS have abnormal follicular development, including low follicular fluid estradiol concentrations and high levels of follicular fluid androgens [12]. Pelvic ultrasonography is indicated in patients with high serum androgen levels associated with a possible ovarian androgen-secreting tumor. The following findings are of concern: size >5 cm, solid masses, complex cysts, septations that are persistent over 4–6 weeks. Furthermore, women with nonovarian causes of hirsutism, such as congenital adrenal hyperplasia and adrenal tumors, may have polycystic-appearing ovaries.

Figure 10.2 demonstrates polycystic-appearing ovaries in a patient undergoing laparoscopy. This image reveals many antral follicles that can be seen protruding on the ovarian stroma in these enlarged ovaries. The transvaginal probe can identify ovarian follicles and cysts as small as 3–5 mm in diameter and thecal cell hyperplasia as shown in Figure 10.3. Historically, the monitoring of follicular growth revolved around total urinary estrogens [13] and by 1974, plasma 17β-estradiol levels were used [14]. Ultrasound examinations for follicle size and endometrial thickness have become standard of care during ovulation induction cycles with gonadotropins.

Ultrasound evaluation of the endometrium in women with PCOS

During COH in patients with PCOS, the endometrial thickness is typically thick because the response to gonadotropins increases the estradiol levels. When patients are seen at the initial visit, it is important to establish the endometrial thickness. Transvaginal ultrasonography is a noninvasive means of distinguishing women with PCOS with a concerning endometrial thickness of greater than 15–20 mm. In women with long-standing amenorrhea >6 months with a thickened endometrial complex, an endometrial biopsy may also be indicated to exclude endometrial hyperplasia (Figure 10.4), which is common in PCOS due to unopposed estrogenic activity. A thicker lining is evaluated further by office biopsy, hysteroscopy with

Ultrasonography in Reproductive Medicine and Infertility, ed. Botros R. M. B. Rizk. Published by Cambridge University Press. © Cambridge University Press 2010.

directed biopsy, or D&C. Endometrial adenocarcinoma becomes increasingly more frequent relative to benign disease as the endometrial thickness approaches 20 mm, especially in older patients. In one study with older patients, 20 mm was the mean endometrial thickness in 759 women with endometrial

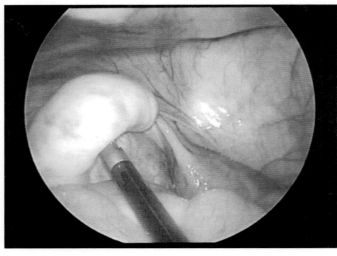

Figure 10.1. Abdominal ultrasound image of a single ovarian follicle.

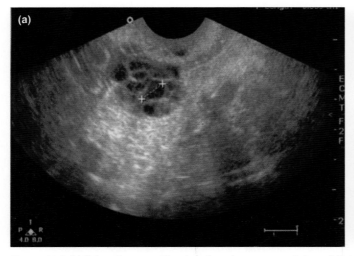

Figure 10.2. Laparoscopic image of a polycystic ovary.

cancer [15]. It is essential to keep in mind the risk of endometrial hyperplasia with and without atypia in women with PCOS before proceeding to COH.

Three-dimensional ultrasound: use in women with PCOS

Three-dimensional (3D) ultrasound technologies are beneficial in some applications of obstetrics and gynecology and may aid in the evaluation of abnormal ovaries. Figure 10.5 is a 3D image of a polycystic ovary diagnosed based on >12 antral follicles on 2D ultrasound. A review of the literature reveals a limited number of studies discussing the use of 3D US during COH in women specifically with PCOS. Although the diagnostic criteria of PCOS do not include 3D imaging, Allemand et al. [16] performed a study establishing the diagnostic threshold for 3D ultrasonography of PCOS. A threshold of 20 mean FNPO using 3D transvaginal ultrasound may be appropriate to minimize false-positive diagnoses of PCO. An advantage of 3D ultrasonography is that ovarian volumes of images can be analyzed with the patient off the examination table. The time required to review the volumes of images depended on the complexity of the ovary. Reconstruction of the volume images, storage capacities, and viewing of all three orthogonal planes are challenges of this technology.

The evaluation of vascular flow to the ovary and flow pattern has been performed using 3D power Doppler technology, which is less angle-dependent than 2D US. The total vascularized volume of the ovary can be expressed in volume units and quantification of vascularization using histogram software. Frequency-based color Doppler analyzes the frequency shift of blood velocity, whereas power Doppler uses the amplitude component of the signals received to present the number of blood cells moving. The vascularization index (VI) measures the ratio of color voxels to all the voxels in the region of interest (ROI). It represents the density of vessels in the tissue and is expressed as percentage (%). The total vascularized volume in the ovary (in ml) was obtained by multiplying VI by the volume of the ovary. The flow index (FI) is the mean value of the color

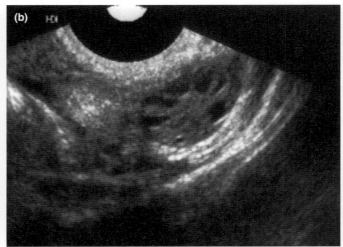

Figure 10.3. (a) Polycystic ovary with string-of-pearls appearance 3–5 mm follicles. (b) Thickened ovarian stroma in a patient with PCOS.

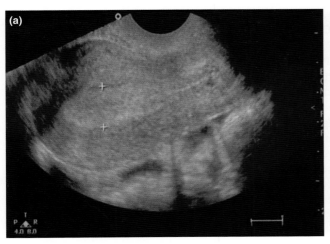

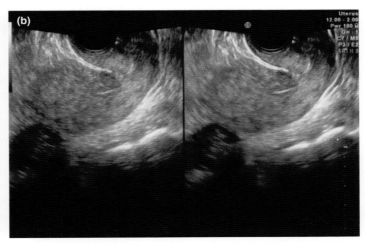

Figure 10.4(a, b). Images of a thickened endometrial stripe in PCOS patient with 8 months of amenorrhea.

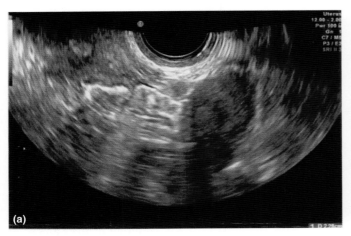

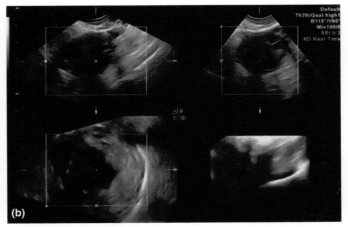

Figure 10.5(a, b). 3D ultrasound imaging of polycystic ovaries.

voxels, representing the average intensity of flow. The vascularization flow index (VFI), the mean color value in all the voxels in the ROI, is a feature of both vascularization and flow.

A previous study reported that after ovarian FSH stimulation, polycystic ovaries were larger and had higher VI, FI, and VFI values than the normal ovaries [17]. After the hCG trigger injection, there were no other differences than the larger volume in PCOs, which was observed prior to stimulation. These differences may have implications for angiogenesis and altered blood supply in polycystic ovaries. Recent advances in 3D ultrasound have the potential of improving our understanding of follicular development, ovulation, and uterine receptivity.

Follicular monitoring during COH using transvaginal ultrasound

The administration of gonadotropins for both insemination cycles as well as in-vitro fertilization cycles relies upon the use

of serial real-time ultrasound examinations. In 1961, urinary human menopausal gonadotropins (hMG), in which the ratio of LH to FSH bioactivity is 1:1, became available for ovulation induction. Recombinant human FSH became available in 1996 with a subcutaneous administration. Synchronous growth of small (4–5 mm) antral follicles, followed by the selection and growth of one dominant follicle that achieves the largest diameter and suppresses the growth of the subordinate follicles, can be followed via ultrasound.

There are many choices for infertile patients with PCOS, such as clomiphene citrate, possibly aromatase inhibitors, or gonadotropins for ovulation induction, in-vitro fertilization and embryo transfer, ultrasound-guided immature follicle puncture, and in-vitro maturation and fertilization of oocytes from unstimulated cycles. Individualized treatment according to the medical treatment conditions is the ideal. In patients with PCOS, a low-dose, step-up protocol with FSH allows a gradual stimulation, ideally with fewer than 5 follicles. Figures 10.6, 10.7, 10.8

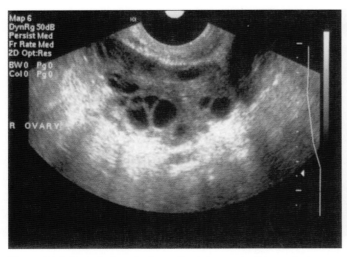

Figure 10.6. Controlled ovarian hyperstimulation on day 3 in a patient with PCOS.

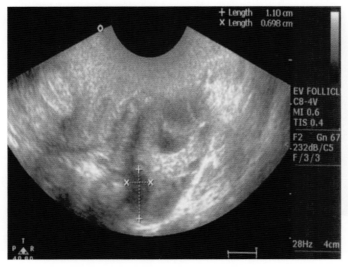

Figure 10.7. Controlled ovarian hyperstimulation on day 7 in a patient with PCOS.

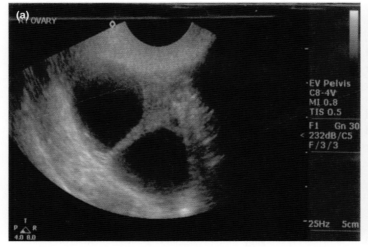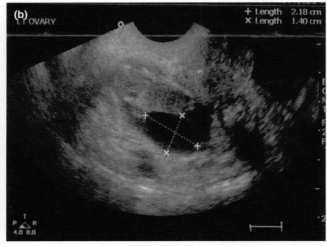

Figure 10.8(a, b). Controlled ovarian hyperstimulation on day 9 in a patient with PCOS.

reveal a series of 2D US images of a 32-year-old G0 with PCOS undergoing COH with a subcutaneous dose of FSH 37.5 increased to 75 IU/day on day 7; she was triggered with hCG on day 11 and subsequently conceived with artificial insemination (total motile sperm 121 million). In general, the dose is increased only if no response is documented on ultrasonography and serum estradiol monitoring. Ideally, increments of 37.5 IU are then given at weekly intervals up to a maximum of 225 IU/day for insemination cycles. The endometrial stripe typically is trilaminar, as shown in Figure 10.9. The temptation to stimulate a patient with PCOS with a higher dose of FSH must be weighed against the risk of stimulating >5 follicles and cancellation as a consequence in order to prevent the complication of multiple pregnancy. The images in Figures 10.10 and 10.11 reveal patients with PCOS after stimulation with starting doses of FSH 150 IU and FSH 225 IU; both recruited >5 follicles and were cancelled.

For in-vitro fertilization cycles, if a patient has undergone a previous cycle, the dose is titrated on the basis of her response to previous stimulation. If a patient with PCOS also has another indication to proceed to IVF, the starting dose is dependent on the patient's age, antral follicle count, and day 3 FSH. Minimal evidence is available on the optimal interval for increasing the dose in PCOS patients. When the ovarian follicles are mature (17–18 mm), human chorionic gonadotropin (hCG), both urinary and recombinant, may be used to trigger ovulation. A dose of 250 μg of recombinant hCG appears to be equivalent to the standard doses of urinary hCG (5000–10 000 units).

Serial follicular monitoring utilizing ultrasound is a reliable technique when undergoing COH, especially in patients with PCOS, who have a higher likelihood of developing OHSS (Figure 10.12). On counting of the number of follicles and measurement of their sizes, PCOS patients may need to be cancelled in order to prevent severe OHSS [18]. In Chapter 36 Rizk et al. discuss OHSS in detail. Rizk and Aboulghan [19] suggest that certain individuals may benefit

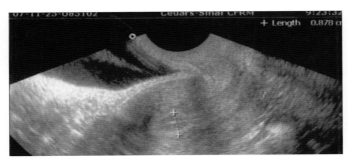

Figure 10.9. Ultrasound imaging of a trilaminar endometrial stripe on day 7 of controlled ovarian hyperstimulation.

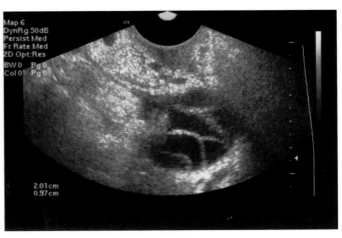

Figure 10.11. Image of a patient undergoing controlled ovarian hyperstimulation with FSH 225 IU on day 7 of stimulation.

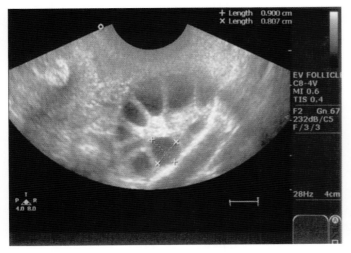

Figure 10.10. Image of a patient undergoing controlled ovarian hyperstimulation with FSH 150 IU on day 5 of stimulation.

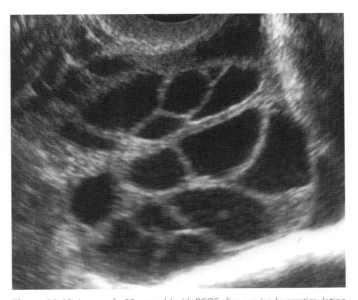

Figure 10.12. Image of a 39-year-old with PCOS after ovarian hyperstimulation with FSH 225 IU and human menopausal gonadotropin 150 IU for 6 days

from measurement of serial serum estradiol levels, which in conjunction with ultrasound may assist in close follicular monitoring and timing of the hCG trigger [19,20,21]. Furthermore, real-time ultrasound examinations provide an excellent means of following follicular development, and in the case of gonadotropin with insemination may detect >4 dominant follicles with subsequent cancellation to prevent multiple pregnancies. Universal follicle tracking proved to be time consuming and required significant resources.

Conclusions

To summarize, the advent of ultrasound has provided a diagnostic tool with clinical efficacy that is essential in evaluating and managing fertility treatment in women with PCOS. In clinical practice, TV ultrasound monitoring during COH is performed to improve safety and precise monitoring of ovarian response to gonadotropin stimulation. PCOS patients have an increased number of preantral follicles; hence, close monitoring for OHSS is essential. Three-dimensional ultrasound is a relatively new imaging modality that may improve the sensitivity and specificity of ultrasound.

Key points in clinical practice

- Ultrasound monitoring for follicular development in women with PCOS undergoing controlled ovarian hyperstimulation is a useful tool, with the goal of prevention of ovarian hyperstimulation syndrome and multiple pregnancy.
- Low-dose gonadotropin stimulation in women with PCOS for ovulation induction is the ideal.
- Development of >4 follicles in women undergoing insemination may warrant cycle cancellation.
- Recent advances in 3D ultrasound have the potential to better our understanding of follicular development, ovulation, and uterine receptivity.

References

1. Stein I, Leventhal M. Amenorrhea associated with bilateral polycystic ovaries. *Am J Obstet Gynecol* 1935; **29**: 181–91.

2. Azziz R, Woods K, Reyna R. The prevalence and features of PCOS in an unselected population. *J Clin Endocrinol Metab* 2004; **89**: 2745–9.

3. Hamilton-Fairley D, Taylor A. ABC of subfertility: anovulation. *BMJ* 2003; **327**: 5469.

4. Polson DW, Adams J, Wadsworth J, Franks S. Polycystic ovaries – a common finding in normal women. *Lancet* 1988; **1**(8590): 870–2.

5. Adams J, Polson DW, Franks S. Prevalence of polycystic ovaries in women with anovulation and idiopathic hirsutism. *Br Med J (Clin Res Ed)* 1986; **293**(6543): 355–9.

6. von Micsky LI. Cited by: Kratochwil A, Urban G, Friedrich F. Ultrasonic tomography of the ovaries. *Ann Chir Gynaecol Fenn* 1972; **61**: 211–14.

7. Kratochwil A, Jentzsch K, Brezina K. Ultraschallanatomie des weiblichen Beckens und ihre klinische Bedeuntung. *Arch Gynaecol* 1973; **214**: 273–5.

8. Hill L, Breckle R, Coulam C. Asssessment of human follicular development by ultrasound. *Mayo Clin Proc* 1982; **57**: 176–80.

9. Adams, J, Polson, DW, Franks, S. Prevalence of polycystic ovaries in women with anovulation and idiopathic hirsutism. *Br Med J* 1986; **293**: 355.

10. Rotterdam ESHRE/ASRM-Sponsored PCOS Consensus Workshop Group. Revised 2003 consensus on diagnostic criteria and long-term health risks related to polycystic ovary syndrome. *Fertil Steril* 2004; **81**: 19–25.

11. Welt, CK, Arason, G, Gudmundsson, JA, et al. Defining constant versus variable phenotypic features of women with polycystic ovary syndrome using different ethnic groups and populations. *J Clin Endocrinol Metab* 2006; **91**: 4361.

12. Mason HD, Willis DS, Beard RW, Winston RM, Margara R, Franks S. Estradiol production by granulosa cells of normal and polycystic ovaries: relationship to menstrual cycle history and concentrations of gonadotropins and sex steroids in follicular fluid. *J Clin Endocrinol Metab* 1994; **79**(5): 1355–60.

13. Brown JB, Beischer NA. Current status of estrogen assay in gynecology and obstetrics. *Obstet Gynecol* 1972; **27**: 205–35.

14. Black WP, Coutt JR, Dodson KS, Rao LG S. An assessment of urinary and plasma steroid estimations for monitoring treatment of anovulation with gonadotropins. *Br J Obstet Gynecol* 1974; **81**: 667–75.

15. Karlsson B, Granberg S, Wikland M, et al. Transvaginal ultrasonography of the endometrium in women with postmenopausal bleeding – a Nordic multicenter study. *Am J Obstet Gynecol* 1995; **172**: 1488.

16. Allemand MC, Tummon IS, Phy JL, Foong SC, Dumesic DA, Session DR. Diagnosis of polycystic ovaries by three-dimensional transvaginal ultrasound. *Fertil Steril* 2006; **85**(1): 214–19.

17. Järvelä IY, Sladkevicius P, Kelly S, Ojha K, Campbell S, Nargund G. Comparison of follicular vascularization in normal versus polycystic ovaries during in vitro fertilization as measured using 3-dimensional power Doppler ultrasonography. *Fertil Steril* 2004; **82**(5) 1358–63.

18. Blankstein J, Shalev J, et al. Ovarian hyperstimulation syndrome: prediction by number and size of preovulatory ovarian follicles. *Fertil Steril* 1987; **47**: 597–602.

19. Rizk B, Aboulghar M. Modern management of ovarian hyperstimulation syndrome. *Hum Reprod* 1991; **6**: 1082–7.

20. Rizk B, Aboulghar M. Classification, pathophysiology and management of ovarian hyperstimulation syndrome. In: Brinsden PR, ed. *A Textbook of In Vitro Fertilization and Assisted Reproduction: The Bourn Hall Guide to Clinical and Laboratory Practice.* 2nd edn. New York, Parthenon Publishing Group, 1991; pp. 131–55.

21. Rizk B, Aboulghar M. Ovarian hyperstimulation syndrome. In: Rizk B ed. *Ovarian Hyperstimulation Syndrome. Epidemiology, Pathophysiology, Prevention and Management.* Cambridge University Press, 2010; pp. 118–24.

Ultrasonography of uterine fibroids

Angela Clough and Yakoub Khalaf

Introduction

A fibroid or leiomyoma is a benign smooth-muscle growth of the uterus that can occur as a single lesion, though it more often presents as multiple lesions. Fibroids are found in 20–40% of women, generally from age 30 onwards, with a steady increase in incidence with age [1]. Ultrasound is a noninvasive, well tolerated, and relatively inexpensive way to accurately measure and locate fibroids within the uterus/pelvis. Assessment of fibroid size and location can be helpful for surgical planning or for monitoring fibroid changes over time, whether they are managed conservatively, medically or surgically.

This chapter sets out to examine the role of ultrasound in evaluating fibroids, by looking first at the etiology and classification of fibroids, then at fibroid diagnosis, prognosis, and treatment.

Etiology and classification

The fibroid mass originates from neoplastic smooth-muscle cells that undergo multiple division. It can vary in size from just several millimeters to that of a huge pelvic mass that can extend into the abdominal cavity. Fibroids are responsive to estrogen and progesterone and, therefore, are not present before puberty and tend to shrink after menopause. The prevalence of fibroids in women of African descent is significantly higher, and lesions are often larger and more numerous [2]. The predisposition to having fibroids can be hereditary.

The fibroid mass is usually round in shape, well circumscribed, and separated from the adjacent myometrium by a pseudocapsule of connective tissue. The fibroid tissue has a whirl-like or trabecular formation owing to the way smooth muscle interlaces concentric bands of connective tissue. The fibroid has a characteristic peripheral blood supply located in the pseudocapsule, which feeds smaller centripetal vessels supplying the center. If the fibroid grows rapidly, or to a significant size, then the blood supply to the center can become insufficient, and ischemic necrosis may occur. Fibroids can increase rapidly in size during pregnancy, resulting in an acute painful condition called "red degeneration" in which there is extensive necrosis involving the whole fibroid mass. Fibroids in the nonpregnant uterus can undergo a more chronic reduction of blood supply, which can result in hyaline, cystic, fatty, and myxomatous degeneration.

Fatty changes within a fibroid can later result in fibrous replacement or calcification, with the latter commonly seen in lesions of postmenopausal women.

Location of fibroids

Fibroids can develop in any part of the uterine or cervical muscle and can be confined to the muscle wall (intramural fibroids), can form under the endometrial lining (submucosal fibroids) or under the serosal covering of the uterus (subserosal fibroids) (Figures 11.1 and 11.2). However, not all fibroids fall clearly into these three groups and they often have a shared location; for example, an intramural fibroid may partially intrude into the endometrial cavity, or a subserosal fibroid may have a significant intramural component (see Table 11.2). Occasionally, a fibroid may grow separately from the muscle wall from which it arises, connected only by a pedicle that conveys blood vessels to the mass. These fibroids can either pedunculate into the uterine or cervical cavity (fibroid polyp) or outward into the pelvic cavity (pedunculated or exophytic fibroid). Rarely, these fibroids can develop within the broad or round ligaments. Cervical fibroids are relatively uncommon (1–3%) though they can be problematic, with a higher incidence of infection and bladder symptoms, and may give rise to dystocia in labor.

Classification of fibroids impinging on the uterine cavity

When fibroids originate from the uterine wall, but impinge on the cavity, it is useful to describe the degree of cavity distortion using the Wamsteker and de Blok classification [3].

Fibroids are classified as type 0 if they pedunculate 100% into the cavity; as type I if they arise from the myometrium but more than 50% of their mass is within the cavity; and as type II if they again arise from the myometrium but have the greater part of their mass within the myometrium, i.e., less than 50% in the cavity. (See Table 11.1. and Figure 11.6.)

Ultrasonography in Reproductive Medicine and Infertility, ed. Botros R. M. B. Rizk. Published by Cambridge University Press. © Cambridge University Press 2010.

Table 11.1. Classification of fibroids impinging on the uterine cavity

Classification of fibroids impinging on the uterine cavity
0: pedunculated into the uterine cavity
I: extend >50% into the uterine cavity
II: extend <50% into the uterine cavity

Table 11.2. Classification of intramural and subserosal fibroids

Classification of intramural and subserosal fibroids
0: pedunculated subserosal fibroid
I: involvement of <50% of the outer uterine wall
II: involvement of >50% of the myometrial wall
III: fibroids that extend from the mucosa to the serosa

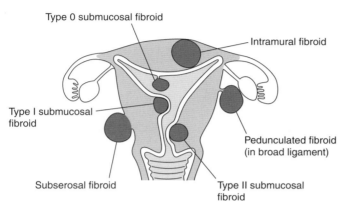

Figure 11.1. Schematic diagram of varying fibroid locations in the uterus.

This assessment is often difficult to make on a 2D scan alone and saline infusion sonohysterography is usually required (described in the next section). An accurate diagnosis is essential to help decide on presurgical treatment and the mode of surgery, and will help in giving an accurate prognosis to the patient [3]. A similar classification system has been proposed for intramural and subserosal fibroids to denote the degree of involvement in the myometrial wall (see Table 11.2) [4]. This classification may have a place in studies looking specifically at the precise effect of intramural fibroids on fertility and pregnancy.

Diagnosis

Ultrasound instrumentation and technique

The conventional way to image fibroids is by two-dimensional (2D) scanning. Other imaging options are available for more problematic fibroids, and these will be covered at the end of this section.

For good visualization of fibroids, particularly of the outline, the best imaging technique is the transvaginal scan (TVS). With a transvaginal approach, the probe is in closer proximity to the uterus and a higher frequency can be employed, thus providing better tissue definition. A TVS is performed with an empty bladder using a curvilinear, multifrequency, endocavity transducer with a typical central frequency of 6.5 MHz. Fibroids can be highly attenuating of the ultrasound beam due to their dense and mixed tissue make-up, and this may result in poor through-transmission and shadowing (see Figure 11.3). Because of this, it is sometimes necessary to select a lower frequency to allow for better penetration of the fibroid in order to view its posterior aspect. If a uterus is significantly enlarged by fibroids, TVS may fail to demonstrate the whole uterus and a transabdominal scan

(TAS) is required. TAS is performed using a multihertz curvilinear abdominal transducer with a central frequency of 3.5 MHz. This approach provides a greater field of view to give adequate demonstration of an enlarged uterus. The transabdominal transducer can also provide lower frequencies for better penetration. TAS generally requires a full bladder for good visualization of the pelvic organs, but this is seldom required in cases where the uterus is grossly enlarged by fibroids. This is because the loops of bowel that usually obscure the pelvic organs are displaced by the enlarged uterus.

In addition to changing the ultrasound frequency, harmonic selection and higher power settings may also serve to improve an ultrasound view of the fibroid uterus.

Ultrasound appearance of fibroids

A fibroid outline is usually well visualized by TVS, even in the very small lesion, because of the pseudocapsule. The mixed tissue make-up of the fibroid produces a heterogeneous echo pattern on an ultrasound scan and can be highly attenuating of the ultrasound beam in some lesions. It is important to recognize that the fibroid has a definite outline because a heterogeneous myometrium with ill-defined margins may represent adenomyosis (see differential diagnoses). Fibroids are commonly hypoechoic compared with the adjacent myometrium, but they can also be isoechoic or even hyperechoic, in comparison, particularly if they undergo fatty or fibrous changes. Cystic degeneration is seen on ultrasound as a central anechoic area that may sometimes contain internal echoes and fluid/fluid levels [5]. Fibrous replacement within the fibroid tissue can be recognized on ultrasound as an overall increase in reflectivity. Calcification can also occur, and is denoted by the presence of echogenic foci or a bright outer rim, which often produce posterior acoustic shadowing on an ultrasound image (see Figure 11.3).

Differential diagnoses

Adenomyosis

Adenomyosis is a common differential diagnosis and is sometimes misdiagnosed as fibroids or "fibroid change." As with fibroids, adenomyosis is a common condition (20–40% in hysterectomy specimens) and presents with similar symptoms of menorrhagia and dysmenorrhea. Careful examination by ultrasound will identify a more diffuse heterogeneous echo pattern, with an absence of discrete encapsulated masses, even when the adenomyosis is present in a localized collection or "adenomyoma." An ultrasonic diagnosis of adenomyosis is further strengthened by the detection of small cystic areas within the

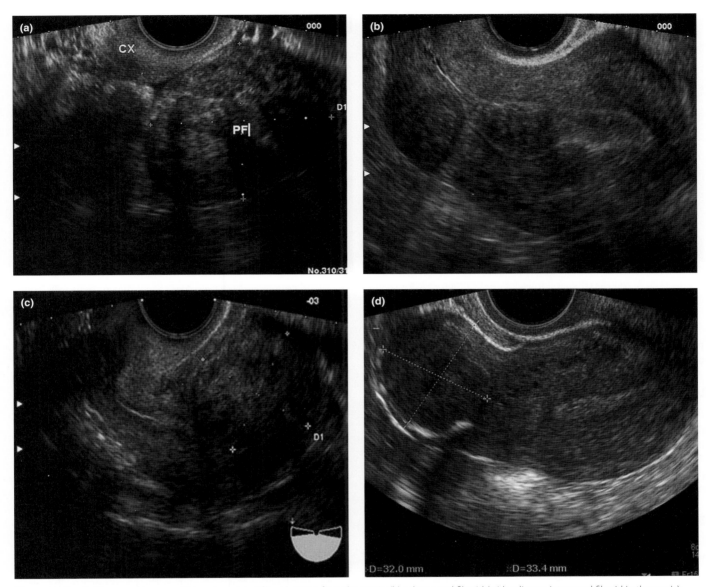

Figure 11.2a–d. Ultrasound images of (a) pedunculated fibroid arising from the cervix; (b) submucosal fibroid (with adjacent intramural fibroid in the cervix); (c) intramural fibroid (with indeterminate intrusion on the cavity); and (d) subserosal fibroid.

myometrium, a bulky myometrium, and irregularity of the endometrial/myometrial outline (see Figure 11.4a). Of note, studies show that in 35–55% of women, fibroids and adenomyosis coexist [6].

Diffuse leiomyomatosis

Diffuse leiomyomatosis is a rare condition in which there is diffuse and uniform involvement of the entire myometrium by multiple fibroids (see Figure 11.4b).

Endometrial polyps

A differential diagnosis for a submucosal fibroid is an endometrial polyp. Polyps are common cavity lesions that originate from endometrial rather than myometrial tissue. The ultrasound appearance of the polyp is typically more hyperechoic than that

of a fibroid polyp and has a classic "tongue" shape, rather than the rounder form of a fibroid (see Figure 11.4c,d) Because the polyp is echogenic it is more easily identified within the proliferative phase of the cycle, whereas a small submucosal fibroid would be more easily seen in the secretory phase. Color Doppler (as mentioned later) is a useful tool for distinguishing between a polyp and a submucosal fibroid.

Ovarian mass

A pedunculated fibroid can be easily mistaken for an ovarian mass, particularly an ovarian fibroma (see Figure 11.2a). Ultrasound confirmation of a pedunculated fibroid can be made if both ovaries are identified separately from the fibroid. If the fibroid is of a significant size, or located in the broad or round ligament, it may not be possible to separate it from the

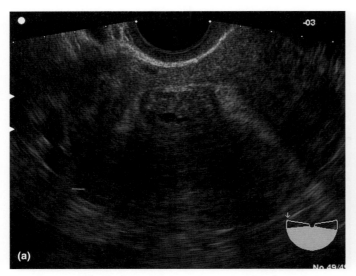 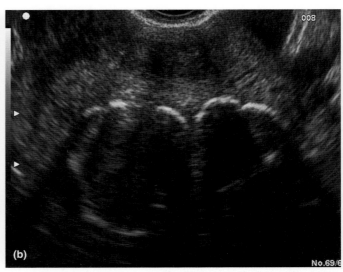

Figure 11.3. (a) A longitudinal section and transverse section view of a submucosal fibroid that has a small central cystic lesion. (b) Posterior wall intramural fibroids with calcified outlines; note how the strong posterior acoustic shadowing obscures the posterior uterine outline.

ovary. In this case, it is important to use color Doppler to positively identify a pedicle connecting the fibroid mass to the uterus (see Figure 11.7).

Leiomyosarcoma

A leiomyosarcoma is a rare smooth-muscle neoplasm that can give the ultrasonic appearance of a large fibroid. Typically presenting in a woman in her mid-fifties, the warning signs are rapid growth, abnormal bleeding, pain, and occasionally pyrexia. A definitive diagnosis is only determined from a microscopic specimen.

Disseminated peritoneal leiomyomatosis

Disseminated peritoneal leiomyomatosis is a rare condition in which multiple small benign smooth-muscle lesions diffusely stud the peritoneal and omental surfaces. Although their distribution suggests a metastatic process, the lesions are generally benign.

Other pelvic masses

Other pelvic masses that may be confused with pedunculated fibroids include bowel masses, pelvic kidneys, lymph nodes. Braxton Hicks contractions can also mimic a fibroid in the pregnant uterus.

Ultrasound reporting

A useful way to record fibroids identified by ultrasound is to state their size, type, and location. The fibroid may be measured in three dimensions, though two may suffice as the lesions are invariably round in shape. The location is noted in two planes, first in the transverse plane, i.e., anterior, posterior, or right/left lateral wall; then in the longitudinal plane, i.e., cervical, uterine body, or fundus. Multiple fibroids may be listed, for example, "A 30 × 31 × 36 mm intramural fibroid was identified in the right lateral fundal wall". If the fibroid is pedunculated, then mention

of the uterine origin and location in the pelvic cavity is required. Electronic ultrasound-reporting packages usually allow for categorization of the fibroids into size, type, and uterine location and some will even produce a computer-generated schematic diagram of the fibroid positions in the uterus.

Other diagnostic options

3D scanning

2D scanning is limited to demonstrating a fibroid in the transverse and longitudinal planes. 3D scanning can show the fibroid in the coronal plane, and this is particularly useful when assessing a fibroid that is within, or impinging on, the cavity. If there is good image contrast between the fibroid and endometrial lining, then clear visualization of the fibroid may be obtained. Optimum contrast is most likely to be obtained during the secretory phase of the cycle, when the endometrium becomes hyperechoic (see Figure 11.5).

Saline infusion sonohysterography

Saline infusion sonohysterography (SIS) has become a vital tool in the assessment of cavity distortion caused by fibroids [7]. This test involves introducing a small amount of saline into the uterine cavity via a uterine cannula. By distending the cavity with saline, it is usually possible to view clearly both the separated cavity surfaces for significant cavity wall distortion or irregularity, and the "potential cavity" for space-occupying lesions. If a fibroid impinges on the cavity then assessment is made of what percentage of the lesion projects into the cavity, and its degree of extension into the myometrium. It can then be categorized as a Type 0, I, or II (as previously described) to help plan the mode of surgical treatment.

3D scanning can be performed in conjunction with SIS to provide the additional coronal plane for further diagnostic accuracy.

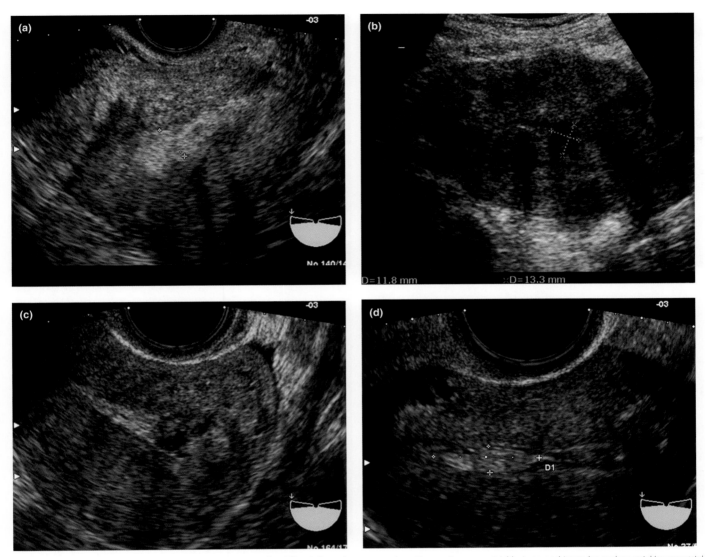

Figure 11.4. (a) Typical appearance of adenomyosis; note the diffusely irregular myometrium, tiny cystic myometrial lesions, and irregular endometrial/myometrial interface. (b) Transabdominal view of an enlarged uterus with multiple small fibroids throughout the myometrium suggestive of diffuse leiomyomatosis. (c) Small submucosal fibroid; note the round outline and hypoechogenic appearance. (d) Endometrial polyp – in contrast with the fibroid the polyp is "tongue-shaped" and hyperechogenic.

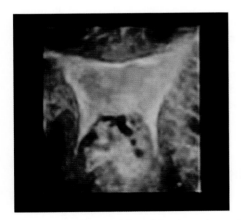

Figure 11.5. 3D coronal view of the uterus demonstrating a large submucosal fibroid centrally located in the body of the uterine cavity.

Hystero-contrast sonography (HyCoSy)

If a fibroid is situated close to the ostia, a HyCoSy test may help to clarify whether the fibroid is causing an ostial obstruction, as indicated by an absence of cornual exit of contrast. Echovist (the contrast used for HyCoSy) also provides a "positive" contrast for clearly outlining submucosal fibroids, as demonstrated in Figure 11.6.

Use of color/power Doppler

Color or power Doppler can be a useful in the assessment of the fibroid blood supply. It is particularly useful in identifying the pedicle connecting a pedunculated fibroid to the uterus when there is uncertainty about the etiology of a fibroid lying within the pelvis (Figure 11.7) [8]. It can also be used to help distinguish between an endometrial polyp and submucosal fibroid. The polyp vessels typically have a central feeder vessel branching

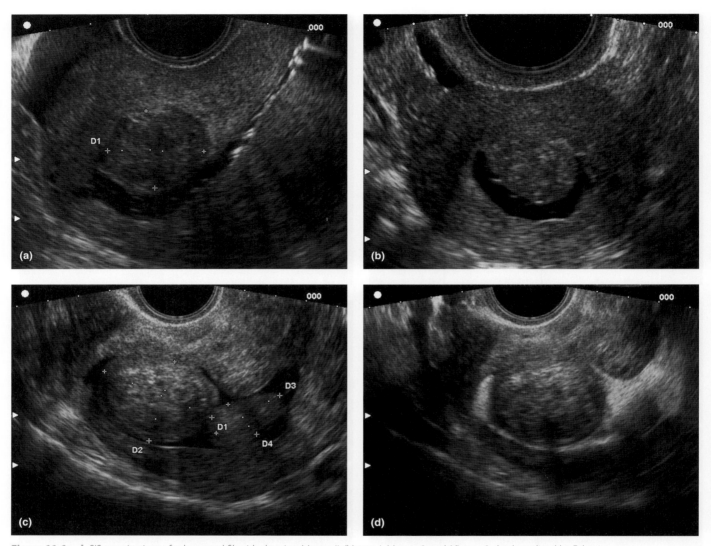

Figure 11.6a–d. SIS examinations of submucosal fibroids showing (a) type II, (b) type I, (c) type 0, and (d) type 0 clearly outlined by Echovist.

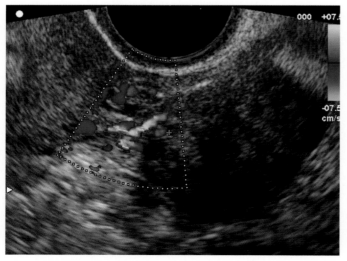

Figure 11.7. Color Doppler identifies the pedicle between a pedunculated fibroid (right) and the uterus.

into smaller vessels, whereas the blood vessels to the fibroid are identified at its periphery [8]. Color Doppler has also been used for treatment planning and post-treatment follow-up for radiologic treatment of fibroids, such as uterine artery embolization.

Magnetic resonance imaging

Magnetic resonance imaging (MRI) is a valuable alternative imaging technique providing good soft-tissue contrast and tissue specificity. The cost and availability of MRI can be restrictive, however, and it is therefore usually reserved for complicated cases.

Prognosis

Gynecological, obstetric, and postpartum complications

The most common gynecological symptoms of fibroids are menorrhagia and dysmenorrhea and, when significantly enlarged, they can also cause compression of adjacent pelvic structures. This "mass effect" may result in bladder or rectal frequency and occasionally hydronephrosis. It should be noted, however, that fibroids are usually asymptomatic, and can often be an incidental finding on an ultrasound scan.

In pregnancy, pain is the most common complication caused by fibroids, and can be severe enough to require hospitalization. Fibroid pain is problematic as it can precipitate preterm delivery, which has been reported as the most frequent cause of neonatal morbidity. The exact mechanism that causes such acute pain is unknown, but it is often accompanied by the ultrasonic finding of a central anechoic lesion within the fibroid, which suggests acute degeneration known as "red degeneration." However, this finding is not conclusive as these appearances can also be present in asymptomatic fibroids [9,10]. Pedunculated fibroids are at increased risk of torsion during pregnancy due to the increasing uterine size.

Cesarean rates have been shown to be higher when fibroids are present, and this is generally due to malpresentation [11,12].

There is also a higher incidence of postpartum hemorrhage and this is most likely due to an associated decrease in uterine contractility when fibroids are present [9,12]. Placental abruption is a much less common complication, but has been mildly associated with fibroids, particularly when submucosal or retroplacental in position [9]. Previously there has been some concern that fibroids are associated with small-for-dates babies, premature rupture of membranes, and retained placenta. However, a number of studies have shown that there is no significant link between fibroids and any of these obstetric complications [9,12].

Fertility

The relationship of fibroids to fertility is of great interest to those working in reproductive medicine, but there are still many uncertainties about their true impact. It is helpful to first look generally at how they might affect fertility, and then specifically at the impact of fibroids on IVF outcome.

Implantation

Many studies have set out to show the extent of the impact of fibroids on implantation. The precise effect and mechanisms have yet to be proven by randomized controlled trials (RCT). The mechanisms that have been postulated to affect implantation include mechanical disturbance (as in the case of a submucosal fibroid); reduced uterine contractility; altered uterine/endometrial perfusion; abnormal endocrine patterns; and chronic endometrial inflammation [13].

An intramural fibroid that is situated near the cornua may potentially cause a physical obstruction of the ostia, thus affecting sperm and gamete transfer [13].

Implantation and cavity-distorting fibroids

Fibroids that significantly distort the cavity, as in the case of a submucosal (type 0), or an intramural fibroid with extension into the cavity (types I and II), can cause a significant adverse effect on implantation [14]. A systematic review has shown that submucosal fibroids may decrease the implantation rates from 11.5% to 3% [15]. Studies of women who have undergone hysteroscopic resection of submucosal fibroids have shown a significant improvement in pregnancy rates, which were comparable to rates within the control groups [16,17]. The strength of evidence showing an adverse impact of submucosal fibroids on fertility, means that their removal has become both an accepted and a recommended practice to improve the chances of pregnancy [15,16].

Intramural fibroids and implantation

The precise effects of intramural fibroids on implantation are much less certain, and RCTs are required to understand their true impact on fertility. Studies to date have given conflicting results, with some studies showing an adverse impact of fibroids on implantation and pregnancy rates (particularly with larger fibroids) [18,19,20,21], while other studies show no impact [22,23]. Some studies have looked at fertility rates following myomectomy and have shown an encouraging increase in implantation rates [24,25]. The disparity of these findings makes it difficult not only to understand the impact of intramural fibroids but also to establish the best treatment options, particularly for infertile women.

Studies indicate that subserosal and pedunculated fibroids have no adverse impact on implantation rates [21].

Miscarriage

Most studies that have examined the relationship between fibroids and miscarriage rates have looked predominantly at intramural fibroids, with few data available on impact of submucosal fibroids [15]. Review of several studies shows an increase in the miscarriage rate from 8% to 15% when intramural fibroids are present [15]. The presence of multiple fibroids has also been shown to be a significant predictor of spontaneous loss [11]. An adverse impact of fibroids on pregnancy loss is supported by a review of reports on miscarriage rates following myomectomy for symptomatic fibroids, which identified a decrease from 41% to 19% [26].

IVF outcome

The literature suggests that the percentage of women whose infertility is caused solely by fibroids is very low (1–2.4%) [27]. One study indicated that fertility is decreased by fibroids and identified that 43% of women with fibroids, presenting in labor, had at least a two-year history of infertility [28]. Recent prospective studies looking at how fibroids affect IVF patients have also shown that IVF outcome is reduced in the fibroid group [19,20].

As mentioned previously, the removal of submucosal fibroids is a generally recognized practice for improving fertility. However, the value of removing intramural fibroids, particularly when there is no deformation of the cavity, is more uncertain. Furthermore, there is conflicting evidence on the impact of fibroid size, number, and extent of symptoms [14].

Studies so far have shown that spontaneous conception following myomectomy increases significantly (50–60%) [28], and that the rates of first- and second-trimester miscarriage are reduced [25,26].

There is general consensus in the literature that fibroids affect fertility, but what remains to be established is whether the surgical removal of fibroids prior to IVF will significantly improve the outcome and at the same time outweigh the risks of surgery.

Unfortunately, as yet, no RCTs have been conducted to test the value of performing a myomectomy, and the methodological limitations of existing studies make it difficult to draw clear guidelines for the management of fibroids in the IVF patient.

With no conclusive evidence, a case for surgical treatment prior to IVF could be considered on an individual basis, taking into account the presence of fibroid symptoms and reproductive history, including any previous failed IVF attempts.

Treatment

Medical treatment

Gonadotropin-releasing hormone analogue therapy

Gonadotropin-releasing hormone analogues (Gn-RHa) are used as a short-term therapy for women with symptomatic fibroids. However, as a hormone therapy that alters estrogen and progesterone production, it is not compatible with reproduction and therefore has no useful therapeutic effect for the subfertile woman. These analogues can, however, be used in this group of women as a pre-operative treatment prior to a myomectomy to help shrink fibroids, restore hemoglobin levels, and possibly reduce operative blood loss. Ultrasound has been shown to be useful as a predictor and gauge of response for Gn-RH therapy [29].

Surgical treatment

Hysteroscopic myomectomy

Hysteroscopic myomectomy is the treatment of choice for the removal of submucosal fibroids. This method often requires a repeat procedure, and risks include intrauterine adhesions and uterine perforation.

Laparoscopic myomectomy

The laparoscopic myomectomy procedure is less invasive than abdominal myomectomy, with a reduced risk of pelvic adhesions. The procedure is restricted to fibroids of a certain size. Risks include a higher incidence of fibroid recurrence and of uterine rupture in a subsequent pregnancy.

Abdominal myomectomy

Abdominal myomectomy is required when there are large or multiple fibroids and when entry into the cavity is expected. There is a greater risk of bleeding and adhesion formation than with previous methods. There is also increased risk of hysterectomy, particularly in cases of recurrence.

Radiologic treatment

Uterine artery embolization

Uterine artery embolization is performed under radiologic control and involves advancing a catheter into the uterine artery via the femoral artery. Once it is in the uterine artery, the arterial branches supplying the fibroid are identified, and injected with an embolic agent (small synthetic particles). Fibroid shrinkage occurs within 2–3 months and heavy bleeding is usually decreased in the cycle following treatment.

Some studies have indicated an improvement in fertility rates post treatment, with one study showing that all types of fibroid treated have the potential to improve future fertility [30]. Despite these initial findings, this treatment option is not currently recommended for women wishing to preserve fertility until there is more evidence on its impact on fertility [31]. Ultrasound has a role in pre- and post-treatment assessment for this treatment, and can identify treatment complications with accuracy [32].

Myolysis

Myolysis is ablation of a fibroid mass by use of radiofrequency (RF) electricity, cryoprobes or focused ultrasound. The most recent treatment involves the use of focused ultrasound under the guidance of MRI – or magnetic resonance imaging-guided focused ultrasound (MRIgFUS). It has been shown to be a safe and effective treatment for non-obese patients with symptomatic fibroids [33]. There is, however, a risk of uterine rupture in a subsequent pregnancy and it is therefore not currently recommended for the woman wishing to preserve her fertility.

Key points in clinical practice

- Fibroids occur in 20–40% of women, with a higher incidence in women of African descent.
- 2D ultrasound provides a low-cost, effective assessment of fibroids.
- Fibroids may be located within the uterine cavity, in the myometrium, or under the serosal layer or may pedunculate into the pelvic cavity.
- Fibroids are clearly visualized on ultrasound, appearing round in shape and heterogeneous in reflectivity. They may undergo cystic, fibrotic, and calcified changes, all of which are readily identified on 2D ultrasound.
- Differential diagnoses for fibroids include adenomyosis, ovarian masses, leiomyosarcoma, endometrial polyps, some pelvic masses such as pelvic kidney, lymph nodes, and bowel lesions.
- Other ultrasound techniques such as SIS, color Doppler, HyCoSy, and 3D scanning can offer valuable additional information
- Fibroids are generally asymptomatic. If symptoms are present they include menorrhagia, dysmenorrhea, and a bulk effect.

- Obstetric complications for fibroids include pain, pre-term delivery, postpartum hemorrhage, and higher cesarean rates.
- Submucosal fibroids have a significant impact on implantation and their removal can improve fertility.
- The impact of intramural fibroids on implantation is less certain and surgical removal should be considered on an individual basis.
- The chance of early miscarriage is increased when fibroids are submucosal in origin and to a lesser extent when they are intramural.
- Medical therapy in subfertile women is restricted to pre-operative treatment. Radiologic treatments are not currently recommended. Therefore surgical removal is the main treatment for fibroids.

References

1. Practice Committee of the ASRM. Myomas and reproductive function. *Fertil Steril* 2004; **82**: S111–16.

2. Marshall LM, Spiegelman D, Barbieri RL, et al. Variation in the incidence of uterine leiomyoma among premenopausal women by age and race. *Obstet Gynecol* 1997; **90**: 967–73.

3. Wamsteker K, de Blok S. Resection of intrauterine fibroids In: Lewis BV, Magos AL, eds. *Endometrial Ablation*. Edinburgh, UK: Churchill Livingstone, 1993.

4. Cohen L, Valle R. Role of vaginal sonography and hysterosonography in the endoscopic treatment of uterine myomas. *Fertil Steril* 2000; **73**: 197–204.

5. Reddy N, Jain KA, Gerscovich EO. A degenerating cystic uterine fibroid mimicking an endometrioma on sonography. *J Ultrasound Med* 2003; **22**(9), 973–6.

6. Ferenczy A. Pathophysiology of adenomyosis. *Hum Reprod Update* 1998; **4**(4): 312–22.

7. Sylvestre C, Child TJ, Tulandi T, Tan SL. A prospective study to evaluate the efficacy of two- and three-dimensional sonohysterography in women with intrauterine lesions. *Fertil Steril* 2003; **79**(5): 1222–5.

8. Bhatt S. Doppler imaging of the uterus and adnexae. *Ultrasound Clin* 2006; **1**(1): 201–21.

9. Exacoustos C, Rosati P. Ultrasound diagnosis of uterine myomas and complications in pregnancy. *Obstet Gynecol* 1993; **82**: 97–101

10. Katz VL, Dotters DJ, Droegemueller W. Complications of uterine leiomyomas in pregnancy. *Obstet Gynecol* 1989; **73**: 593–6.

11. Benson CB, Chow JS, Chang-Lee W, Hill JA, Doubilet PM. Outcome of pregnancies in women with uterine leiomyomas identified by sonography in the first trimester. *J Clin Ultrasound* 2001; **29**: 261–4.

12. Qidwai IG, Caughey AB, Jacoby AF. Obstetric outcomes in women with sonographically identified uterine leiomyomata. *Obstet Gynecol* 2006; **107**: 376–82.

13. Farhi J, Ashkenazi J, Feldberg D, Dicker D, Orvieto R, Ben Rafael Z. The effects of uterine leiomyomata on in-vitro fertilization treatment. *Hum Reprod* 1995; **10**: 2576–8.

14. Pritts EA. Fibroids and infertility: a systematic review. *Obstet Gynecol Surv* 2001; **56**: 483–91.

15. Klatsky P, Tran D, Caughey A, Fujimoto V. Fibroids and reproductive outcomes: a systematic literature review from conception to delivery. *Am J Obstet Gynecol* 2008: **198**(4): 357–66.

16. Shokeir TA. Hysteroscopic management in submucous fibroids to improve fertility. *Arch Gynecol Obstet* 2005; **273**(1) 50–4.

17. Narayan R, Rajat, Goswamy K. Treatment of submucous fibroids, and outcome of assisted conception. *J Am Assoc Gynecol Laparosc* 1994; **1**: 307–11.

18. Stovall DW, Parrish SB, Van Voorhis BJ, Hahn SJ, Sparks AET, Syrop CH. Uterine leiomyomas reduce the efficacy of reproduction cycles. *Hum Reprod* 1998; **13**: 192–7.

19. Hart R, Khalaf Y, Yeong CT, Seed P, Taylor A, Braude P. A prospective controlled study of the effect of intramural uterine fibroids on the outcome of assisted conception. *Hum Reprod* 2001; **16**: 2411–17.

20. Check JH, Choe JK, Lee G, Dietterich C. The effect on IVF outcome of small intramural fibroids not compressing the uterine cavity as determined by a prospective matched control study. *Hum Reprod* 2002; **17**: 1244–8.

21. Elder-Geva T, Meagher S, Healy DL, Maclachlan V, Breheny S, Wood C. Effect of intramural, subserosal, and submucosal uterine fibroids on the outcome of assisted reproductive technology treatment *Fertil Steril* 1998; **70**: 687–91.

22. Rinehart J. Myomas and infertility: small intramural myomas do not reduce pregnancy rate in vitro fertilization. Presented at the 53rd Annual meeting of the American Society for Reproductive medicine, Cincinnati, Ohio, 1997; 18–22.

23. Yarali H, Bukulmez O. The effect of intramural and subserous uterine fibroids on implantation and clinical pregnancy rates in patients having intracytoplasmic sperm injection. *Arch Gynecol Obstet* 2002; **266**: 30–3.

24. Surrey ES, Lietz AK, Schoolcraft WB. Impact of intramural leiomyomata in patients with a normal endometrial cavity on in vitro fertilization-embryo transfer cycle outcome. *Fertil Steril* 2001; **75**: 405–10.

25. Bulletti C, De Zeigler D, Setti P, Cicinelli E, Polli V, Stefanetti M. Myomas, pregnancy outcome and in vitro fertilization. *Ann NY Acad Sci* 2004; **1034**; 84–92.

26. Buttram VCJr, Reiter RC. Uterine leiomyomata: etiology, symptomology, and management. *Fertil Steril* 1981; **36**: 433–45.

27. Donnez J, Jadoul P. What are the implications of myomas on fertility? – A need for a debate? *Hum Reprod* 2002; **17**(6): 1424–30.

28. Hasan F, Arumugam K, Sivanesaratnam V. Uterine leiomyomata in pregnancy. *Int J Gynaecol Obstet* 1990 **34**, 45–58.

29. Kanelopoulos N, Dendrinos S, Oikonomou A, Panagopoulos P, Markussis V. Doppler-ultrasound as a predictor of uterine fibroid response to GnRH therapy. *Int J Gynaecol Obstet*. 2003 Jul; **82**(1): 41–7.

30. Walker WJ, Bratby MJ Magnetic resonance imaging (MRI) analysis of fibroid location in women achieving

pregnancy after uterine artery embolization *Cardiovasc Intervent Radiol* 2007; **30**(5): 876–81.

31. ACOG Committee Opinion. Uterine artery embolization. *Obstet Gynecol* 2004; **103**(2): 403–4.

32. Ghai S, Rajan DK, Benjamin MS, Asch MR, Ghai S. Uterine artery embolization for leiomyomas: pre- and postprocedural evaluation with US. *Radiographics* 2005 Sep-Oct; **25**(5): 1159–72; discussion 1173–6.

33. Mikami K, Murakami T, Okada A, Osuga K, Tomoda K, Nakamura H. Magnetic resonance imaging-guided focused ultrasound ablation of uterine fibroids: early clinical experience. *Radiat Med* 2008; **26**(4): 198–205.

Chapter 12

Ultrasonography of the endometrium

Richard Palmer Dickey

Introduction

Recognition of a relationship between endometrial characteristics visualized by ultrasound (US) and ability to become pregnant in assisted reproductive technology (ART), ovulation induction, and even spontaneous cycles is one of the important advances in infertility treatment during the last 20 years. Ultrasound measurement of the endometrium is now an indispensable part of ovulation induction monitoring and assisted reproductive technologies. It also has a role in evaluation of unexplained infertility. Before ultrasound, the condition of the endometrium could be evaluated only by progesterone challenge to induce withdrawal bleeding or by invasive procedures, biopsy, curettage, and hysteroscopy. This chapter will describe the use of ultrasound in the evaluation of infertility and monitoring of ovulation induction for timed intercourse or artificial insemination, as well as for ART.

Endometrial evaluation

Endometrial pattern

Evaluation of the endometrium in infertility was initially focused on its appearance or pattern and only later was the importance of endometrial thickness fully appreciated. Smith et al. are credited with being the first to use the appearance and thickness of the endometrium to decide when to administer human chorionic gonadotropin (hCG) to initiate ovulation [1]. They classified endometrial patterns as: (1) type A, a multilayered "triple-line" endometrium consisting of a prominent outer and central hyperechogenic line and inner hypoechogenic or black regions (Figure 12.1); (2) type B, an intermediate isoechogenic pattern, with the same reflectivity as the surrounding myometrium and a nonprominent or absent central echogenic line (Figure 12.2); and (3) type C, an entirely homogeneous endometrium without a central echogenic line (Figure 12.3). Subsequently, Gonen et al., in a report that was widely cited, reversed the ABC order [2]. The ABC classification is infrequently used in current literature. When endometrial pattern is reported, it is usually described as "triple-line" or "homogeneous," the two most common endometrial patterns. A third term, "post ovulation", may be used to describe the bright hyperechogenic pattern seen normally in the mid luteal phase (Figure 12.4).

Endometrial thickness

Endometrial thickness is customarily measured from outside to outside in an anterior–posterior view at the widest point; if measured inside to outside, the difference can be as much as 2 mm (Figure 12.5). The difference in how thickness is measured can explain some of the difference in values critical for successful implantation reported in the literature. Endometrial thickness measured by transvaginal US correlates well with histological endometrial maturation according to Hofmann et al. [3]. However, others found no relationship between endometrial thickness and histological dating of endometrial tissue obtained by biopsy[4,5].

Endometrial waves

Endometrial wavelike activity is often seen on ultrasound throughout spontaneous cycles and during ovulation induction with human menopausal gonadotropin (hMG) or follicle-stimulating hormone (FSH) [6]. The highest rate of activity is seen during the periovulatory period when opposing waves from the fundus to the cervix and from the cervix to the fundus occur in 30–40% of spontaneous cycles at a rate of 3–4 waves per minute [6]. Endometrial wavelike activity was found in 100% of hMG cycles at the time of ovulation. No waves from the fundus to the cervix occurred during the mid-luteal phase of hMG cycles. The clinical importance of endometrial waves is undetermined. No relationship between the presence or absence of endometrial waves and the outcome of ovulation induction (OI) or in-vitro fertilization (IVF) has been reported.

Endometrial changes during spontaneous cycles

In spontaneous cycles, endometrial thickness increases from a mean of 4.6 mm during menstruation, 9–13 days before the luteinizing hormone (LH) surge, to 12.4 mm on the day of the LH surge [7]. Although the increase in thickness is generally constant, averaging less than 1 mm per day, thickness may

Ultrasonography in Reproductive Medicine and Infertility, ed. Botros R. M. B. Rizk. Published by Cambridge University Press. © Cambridge University Press 2010.

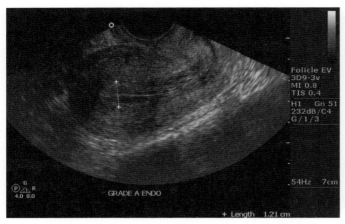

Figure 12.1. Triple-line pattern (Smith et al. [1] type A; Gonan et al. [2] type C); follicular phase day 12. The endometrial pattern is multilayered triple-line with a clearly demarked center line and with the echogenicity of the outer lines less than half that of the myometrium. The triple-line pattern may be found from approximately day 6 before the LH surge until 2–5 days after the LH surge, when the triple-line pattern becomes obscured by the increasingly hyperechogenic pattern of the postovulation luteal phase endometrium. Implantation does not occur, or is reduced, if the endometrium lacks a triple-line pattern on the day of hCG administration in ovulation induction cycles for IVF. With permission from reference [26].

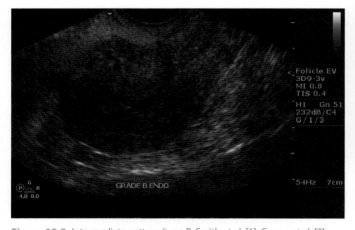

Figure 12.2. Intermediate pattern (type B, Smith et al. [1], Gonan et al. [2]; follicular phase days 6–8. The endometrial pattern is at an intermediate stage with a thin central line and echogenicity similar to that of the myometrium. With permission from reference [26].

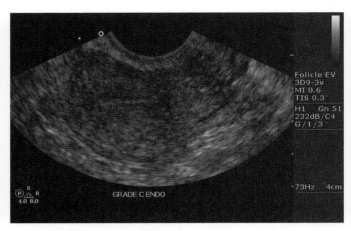

Figure 12.3. Homogeneous pattern (Smith et al. [1] type C; Gonan et al. [2] type A); follicular phase day 3. The endometrial pattern is entirely homogeneous and hyperechogenic without a central echogenic line; the endometrial thickness is typically less than 6 mm. With permission from reference [26].

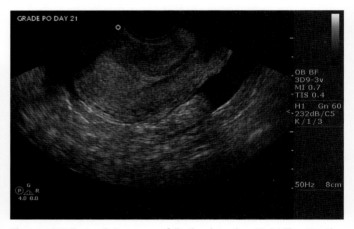

Figure 12.4. Postovulation pattern; follicular phase days 18–24. The normal endometrial pattern at this time is homogeneous and hypoechogenic; endometrial thickness is typically 9 mm or greater. With permission from reference [26].

increase by as much as 2 mm a day in the late proliferative phase. Endometrial thickness normally decreases by 0.5 mm on the day of LH surge, before beginning to increase again by an additional 2 mm during the luteal phase [8]. The endometrial pattern develops a triple-line appearance from day 6 before the LH surge until 7 days after the LH surge, when the triple-line pattern becomes obscured by the increasingly hyperechogenic pattern of the endometrium [9].

Uterine pathology may affect results of endometrial ultrasound scans. Sher et al. discovered uterine pathology (leiomyomas, severe uterine synechiae, diethyl stilbestrol DES anomalies,

adenomyosis) in 93.8% of patients with homogeneous endometrial patterns, compared with 30% of patients with triple-line pattern and endometrial thickness <9 mm and 5.8% of patients with triple-line pattern and thickness >9 mm [10].

Endometrial changes during ovulation induction

When clomiphene citrate (CC) is used for ovulation induction, endometrial thickness is often decreased compared with spontaneous cycles during and immediately following the days CC is taken, because of its antiestrogen effect [7] (Figure 12.6). During the late proliferative phase, endometrial thickness increases at a faster rate in CC cycles than in spontaneous cycles as it escapes from the antiestrogen, and the effect of increased estrogen due to multiple follicle growth becomes manifest. During ovulation

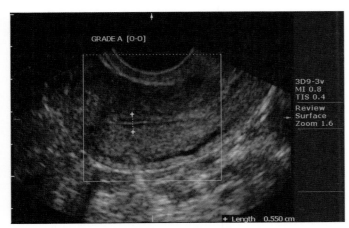

Figure 12.5. Endometrial measurement. Thickness measured in an anterior–posterior view at the widest point from outside to outside in an anterior-posterior view at the widest point (O–O). The pattern is triple-line. With permission from reference [26].

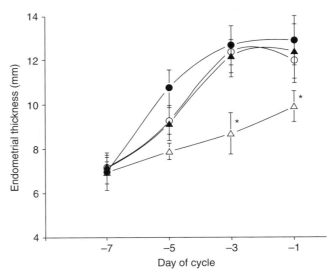

Figure 12.7. Distribution of mean (± SEM) of endometrial thickness at four points in the cycle. O, Controls; ●, human menopausal gonadotropin (hMG); △, clomiphene; ▲, clomiphene + ethinyl estradiol. *$P < 0.01$ compared with the control cycle result at the same phase of the cycle. From Yagel et al. (1992) [11]. Reproduced with permission of the authors and the publisher, the American Society for Reproductive Medicine (The American Fertility Society).

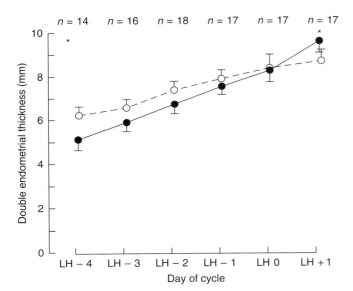

Figure 12.6. Double endometrial thickness (mm) in spontaneous (O) and clomiphene citrate (●) cycles (mean + SEM). LH 0 = day of onset of luteinizing hormone surge. *$P < 0.05$. From Randall and Templeton (1991) [7]. Reproduced with permission of the authors and the publisher, the American Society for Reproductive Medicine (The American Fertility Society).

induction with hMG and FSH, without CC, endometrial thickness is greater than in spontaneous cycles (Figure 12.7) [11].

During stimulation cycles for IVF, an average increase in length of the endometrial cavity by 3.8 mm and length of the cervical canal by 1.9 mm correlated with increase in endometrial thickness [12].

Critical ultrasound values for ovulation induction

Endometrial pattern

A triple-line pattern on the day of hCG administration has been reported by some authors to be necessary for implantation in controlled ovarian hyperstimulation (COH) cycles, where hMG or FSH is administered,. However, Dickey et al. found no difference in initial pregnancy rate between a triple-line pattern (10.9%) and intermediate pattern (10.2%) in CC and COH cycles for ovulation induction before intrauterine insemination, but noted a difference in continuing pregnancy rates of 9.4% for the triple-line pattern and 7.3% for the intermediate pattern [13].

Endometrial thickness

Decreased endometrial thickness is linked to failure to conceive and biochemical pregnancy in CC, hMG, and spontaneous cycles [13,14,15]. In a study of endometrial thickness on the day of hCG administration for timed intrauterine insemination (IUI), optimal pregnancy and birth (continuing pregnancy) rates occurred only when endometrial thickness was 9 mm or greater on the day of hCG administration (Table 12.1). More importantly, no pregnancies occurred when endometrial thickness was less than 6 mm in spontaneous, CC, or hMG IUI cycles [13,14].

The type of drug used for ovulation induction was significantly related to endometrial thickness on the day of hCG administration [13] (Table 12.2) Endometrial thickness was >9 mm in 59.2% of HMG cycles, compared with 47.2% of clomiphene cycles and 34.8% of spontaneous cycles. Endometrial thickness was <6 mm in 9.1% of CC cycles, but was also <6 mm in 8.7% of spontaneous cycles for donor insemination. By contrast, endometrial thickness on the day of hCG was less than 6 mm in only 2.0% of hMG cycles. The antiendometrial effect of CC was clearly apparent when CC and hMG (hMG+CC) were used in the same cycle.

Table 12.1. Endometrial thickness vs. outcome in ovulation induction intrauterine insemination cycles

Thickness (mm)	% of total cycles	Pregnancy/outcome			
		Pregnancy rate (%)	Biological pregnancy (%)	Clinical abortion (%)	Term (%)
<6	9.1	0	0	0%	0
6–8	43.6	8.1	21.9	15.6	62.5
≥9	47.2	14.0	0	12.2	87.8

Adapted from Dickey et al. [13]. Reproduced with permission of the publisher.

Table 12.2. Endometrial thickness according to ovulation regimen: percent cycles; figures in parentheses are number of cycles

Regimen	No. cycles	<6 mm	6–8 mm	>9 mm
None	23	8.7% (2)	56.5% (12)	34.8% (8)
CC	197	9.1% (18)	43.6% (86)	47.2% (93)
hMG	49	2.0% (1)	38.8% (19)	59.2% (29)
hMG+CC	205	11.2% (23)	55.6% (114)	33.2% (68)

CC, clomiphene; hMG human menopausal gonadotropin.
Adapted from Dickey et al. [13]. Reproduced with permission of the publisher.

Critical ultrasound values for IVF cycles

Endometrial pattern

The importance of endometrial pattern and thickness to successful outcome in IVF and gamete intrafallopian transfer (GIFT) was first described by Smith et al. [1]. They found that implantation did not occur, or occurred less often, if the endometrium lacked a triple-line pattern on the day of, or one day before, ovum retrieval in IVF cycles. This finding was latter confirmed by others [2,15]. A triple-line endometrial pattern on the day of hCG administration in IVF cycles is related to serum estradiol level, the number of mature oocytes, and the number of top-quality embryos and is unrelated to serum progesterone levels [15].

Endometrial thickness

Pregnancy does not occur in IVF cycles, presumably because of failure of embryos to implant, if the endometrium is too thin on the day of hCG administration according to the majority of studies. However, other studies have reported no relationship between thickness and pregnancy in IVF cycles. Many of the studies that failed to find a relationship between thickness and outcome compared mean thickness in conception and non-conception cycles, while most studies that found a relationship reported critical or "cut-off" values below which no pregnancies occurred. In most studies, the critical thickness value is reported as 6 mm, but the range is from 4 mm [16] to 7 mm [17]. One reason for these differences is that endometrial thickness can change, either increasing or decreasing, between the day hCG is administered and the day implantation is presumed to occur, a difference of 8–9 days. Importantly, in all studies of

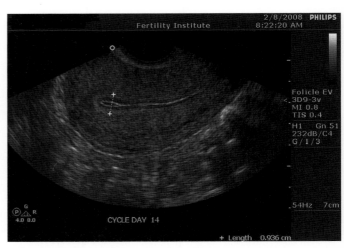

Figure 12.8. Fluid within the endometrial cavity. Gonadotropin cycle. Endometrial cavity with 3 mm of fluid. Fluid in the endometrial cavity on the day of embryo transfer in IVF or 6 days after ovulation is incompatible with implantation. With permission from reference [26].

oocyte donation, endometrial thickness on the day of embryo transfer has been found to be critical for implantation.

As is true for OI and IUI, optimal ART pregnancy and birth rates occur when endometrial thickness on the day of hCG administration is equal to or greater than 9 mm [10,15] or 10 mm [18,19]. Endometrium that is too thick, 14 mm or greater on the day of hCG administration, may reduce the chance of a clinical pregnancy [15,20]. Increased susceptibility to injury at the time of embryo transfer has been proposed as the reason for decreased clinical pregnancies by Dickey et al., who found that biochemical pregnancies were more frequent in IVF cycles when endometrial thickness was less than 9 mm or greater than 13 mm [15]. No relationship between endometrial thickness on the day of hCG and biochemical pregnancy was observed in IVF cycles in another study [21]. An excessively thick endometrium may have its origins in the previous cycle. It is common practice not to start ovulation induction in ART and IUI cycles following menstruation when endometrial thickness is greater than 6 mm.

Other ultrasound findings

Implantation rarely occurs when endometrial fluid is present on ultrasound on the day of embryo transfer, even when the fluid is aspirated (Figure 12.8) [22]. Endometrial polyps less than 2 cm do not decrease pregnancy rates, but there is a trend toward increased pregnancy loss (Figures 12.9, 12.10) [23].

Preclinical miscarriage (biochemical pregnancy)

Preclinical miscarriage, also referred to as biochemical pregnancy, in which quantitative hCG levels initially indicate pregnancy but decrease before a gestational sac can be seen on ultrasound, and clinical miscarriage of embryos with karyotype may be the result of inadequate endometrial development. Because there are no products of conception (POC) for chromosome analysis in biochemical pregnancy, the reason for failure

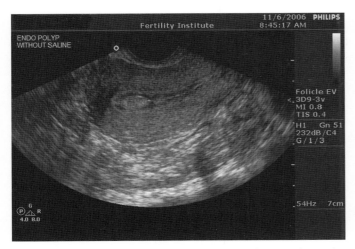

Figure 12.9. Endometrial irregularity, which could be either an endometrial polyp or submucosal fibroid. From reference [26].

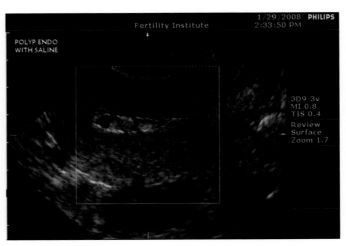

Figure 12.10. The same patient as in Figure 12.9 scanned using sonohysterography. The endometrial polyp is sharply outlined on the sonohysterography scan and clearly distinguished from a submucosal fibroid. From reference [26].

cannot be determined. However, because the karyotype of the POC is normal in 52% of spontaneous miscarriages it is sensible to hypothesize that inadequate endometrial development is responsible for a proportion of early pregnancy loss [24]. In a study of the relationship of endometrial thickness and pattern to pregnancy outcome following ovulation induction cycles for IUI, 21.9% of pregnancies were biochemical pregnancies if endometrial thickness was 6–8 mm at the time of hCG administration, compared with none when the thickness was 9 mm or greater [14] (Table 12.1). The incidence of clinical abortion after a gestational sac had been seen on ultrasound was 15.6% when endometrial thickness was 6–8 mm, compared with 12.2% when the thickness was 9 mm or greater. In the same study, biochemical pregnancies were significantly related to endometrial thickness and pattern, and were unrelated to maternal age or number of previous spontaneous abortions. By contrast, clinical abortions were significantly related to maternal age and previous abortion, and were unrelated to endometrial thickness or pattern.

Clinical management

For optimal pregnancy and birth results, endometrial thickness should be 9 mm or greater at the time of spontaneous LH surge or when hCG is administered in OI cycles for timed intercourse or IUI and when hCG is administered in IVF cycles. When endometrial thickness is less than 9 mm but 6 mm or greater, or there is fluid in the endometrial cavity, three treatment options are available.

Administration of hCG can be delayed to allow thickness to increase and fluid to disappear. Delay in administering hCG is particularly useful in CC cycles, because during the late proliferative phase endometrial thickness increases at a faster rate as it escapes from the antiestrogen effect of clomiphene than in spontaneous cycles [7] (Figure 12.6). If delay is not possible because a spontaneous LH surge is starting or because estrogen levels are rising too rapidly, there are still two treatment options.

The OI or IVF cycle can be allowed to proceed and estrogen can be given in the expectation that endometrial thickness will increase by the time implantation occurs or embryos are transferred.

The OI or IVF cycle can be cancelled and a different regimen of follicle recruitment can be used in a later cycle; or in the case of IVF, hCG can still be administered and all embryos cryopreserved for transfer at a later time. When the endometrium is too thin in a CC cycle, endometrial thickness may be improved in subsequent cycles by starting CC earlier, on menstrual day 3 instead of 5 [13], because the antiestrogen effect of CC lasts no more than 3–4 days after the last dose: (1) by giving a lower dose of CC; (2) by giving estrogen along with CC [11] (Figure 12.7); or (3) by switching to tamoxifen, an antiestrogenic structurally similar to CC that has less antiestrogen effect on the endometrium and cervical mucus. When tamoxifen is used in place of CC, a dose of 20–25 mg is approximately as effective as 50 mg of CC in ovulation induction. When the endometrium is too thin in an hMG or FSH cycle, the dose of gonadotropin can be increased in a subsequent cycle in the expectation, not always realized, that estrogen levels will be higher and result in a better endometrial pattern and thickness.

A potential disadvantage of estrogen administration in nongonadotropin cycles is that high doses may suppress natural FSH secretion or block a spontaneous LH surge. Therefore, estrogen should not be started until after hCG is given or an LH surge has occurred. When oral estrogen is given before an LH surge or hCG, low doses should be taken 2–4 times daily, instead of a single large dose once a day, to minimize serum levels. An alternative method of administrating estrogen in clomiphene cycles is to start with four times a day and step down one tablet a day. The rationale for this approach is that it takes approximately 3 days to induce endometrial changes in response to estrogen. An alternative to oral estrogen is administration by injection, skin patches, or vaginally; the type of estrogen is not important. In the author's clinic a 2 mg micronized estradiol oral tablet ordinarily prescribed for hormonal replacement in menopause symptoms is self-administered vaginally twice daily. There have been several reports of successful use of drugs other than estrogen to correct a thin endometrium or adverse pattern, but with the exception of low-dose aspirin none has been verified in a prospective randomized study. Low-dose aspirin (81 mg daily) increased the incidence of triple-line pattern and pregnancy rates without significantly increasing endometrial thickness [25].

References

1. Smith B, Porter R, Ahuja K, Craft I. Ultrasonic assessment of endometrial changes in stimulated cycles in an in vitro fertilization and embryo transfer program. *J IVF-ET* 1984; **1**: 233–8.

2. Gonen Y, Casper RF, Jacobson W, Blankier J. Endometrial thickness and growth during ovarian stimulation: a possible predictor of implantation in in vitro fertilization. *Fertil Steril* 1989; **52**: 446–50.

3. Hofmann GE, Thie J, Scott RT, Navot D. Endometrial thickness is predictive of histologic endometrial maturation in women undergoing hormone replacement for ovum donation. *Fertil Steril* 1996; **66**: 380–3.

4. Sterzik K, Abt M, Grab D, Schneider V Strehler E. Predicting the histologic dating of an endometrial biopsy specimen with the use of Doppler ultrasonography and hormone measurements in patients undergoing spontaneous ovulatory cycles. *Fertil Steril* 2000; **73**: 94–8.

5. Rogers PAW, Polson D, Murphy CR, Hosie M, Susil B, Leoni M. Correlation of endometrial histology, morphometry, and ultrasound appearance after different stimulation protocols for in vitro fertilization. *Fertil Steril* 1991; **55**: 583–7.

6. Ijland MM, Evers JLH, Dunselman GAJ, van Katwijk C, Lo CR, Hoogland HJ. Endometrial wavelike movements during the menstrual cycle. *Fertil Steril* 1996; **65**: 746–9.

7. Randall JM, Templeton A. Transvaginal sonographic assessment of follicular and endometrial growth in spontaneous and clomiphene citrate cycles. *Fertil Steril* 1991; **56**: 208–12.

8. Randall JM, Fisk MM, McTavish A, Templeton AA. Transvaginal ultrasonic assessment of endometrial growth in spontaneous and hyperstimulated menstrual cycles. *Br J Obstet Gynaecol* 1989; **96**: 954–9.

9. Bakos O, Lundkvist O, Bergh T. Transvaginal sonographic evaluation of endometrial growth and texture in spontaneous ovulatory cycles–a descriptive study. *Hum Reprod* 1993; **8**: 799–806.

10. Sher G, Herbert C, Maassarani G, Jacobs MH. Assessment of the late proliferative phase endometrium by ultrasonography in patients undergoing in-vitro fertilization and embryo transfer. *Hum Reprod* 1991; **6**: 232–7.

11. Yagel S, Ben-Chetrit A, Anteby E, et al. The effect of ethinyl estradiol on endometrial thickness and uterine volume during ovulation induction by clomiphene citrate. *Fertil Steril* 1992; **57**: 33–6.

12. Strohmer H, Obruca A, Radner KM, Feichtinger W. Relationship of the individual uterine size and the endometrial thickness in stimulated cycles. *Fertil Steril* 1994; **61**: 972–5.

13. Dickey RP, Olar TT, Taylor SN, Curole DN, Matulich EM. Relationship of endometrial thickness and pattern to fecundity in ovulation induction cycles: effect of clomiphene citrate alone and with human menopausal gonadotropin. *Fertil Steril* 1993; **59**: 756–60.

14. Dickey RP, Olar TT, Taylor SN, Curole DN, Harrigill K. Relationship of biochemical pregnancy to preovulatory endometrial thickness and pattern in patients undergoing ovulation induction. *Hum Reprod* 1993; **8**: 327–30.

15. Dickey RP, Olar TT, Curole DN, Taylor SN, Rye PH. Endometrial pattern and thickness associated with pregnancy outcome after assisted reproduction technologies. *Hum Reprod* 1992; **7**: 418–21.

16. Sundstrom P. Establishment of a successful pregnancy following in-vitro fertilization with an endometrial thickness of no more than 4 mm. *Hum Reprod* 1998; **13**: 1550–2.

17. Shoham Z, De Carlo C, Patel A, Conway GS, Jacobs HS. Is it possible to run a successful ovulation induction program based solely on ultrasound monitoring? The importance of endometrial measurements. *Fertil Steril* 1991; **56**: 836–41.

18. Check JH, Nowroozi K, Choe J, Lurie D, Dietterich C. The effect of endometrial thickness and echo pattern on in vitro fertilization outcome in donor oocyte-embryo transfer cycle. *Fertil Steril* 1993; **59**: 72–5.

19. Isaacs JD, Wells CS, Williams DB, Odem RR, Gast MJ, Strickler RC. Endometrial thickness is a valid monitoring parameter in cycles of ovulation induction with menotropins alone. *Fertil Steril* 1996; **65**: 262–6.

20. Weissman A, Gotlieb L, Casper RF. The detrimental effect of increased endometrial thickness on implantation and pregnancy rates and outcome in an in vitro fertilization program. *Fertil Steril* 1999; **71**, 147–9.

21. Krampl E, Feichtinger W Endometrial thickness and echo patterns. *Hum Reprod* 1993; **8**: 1339.

22. Mansour RT, Aboulghar MA, Serour GI, Riad R. Fluid accumulation of the uterine cavity before transfer: a possible hindrance for implantation. *J IVF-ET* 1991; **8**: 157–9.

23. Lass A, Williams G, Abusheikha N, Brinsden P. The effect of endometrial polyps on outcomes of in vitro fertilization cycles. *J Assist Reprod Genet* 1999; **16**: 410–15.

24. Boué J, Boué A, Lazar P. Retrospective and prospective epidemiological studies of 1500 karyotyped spontaneous human abortions. *Teratology* 1973; **12**: 11–26.

25. Hsieh YY, Tsal HD, Chang CC, Lo HY, Chen CL. Low-dose aspirin for infertile women with thin endometrium receiving intrauterine insemination: a prospective randomized study. *J Assist Reprod Genet* 2000; **17**: 174–7.

26. Dickey RP, Brinsden PR, and Pyrzak R, eds., *Manual of Intrauterine Insemination and Ovulation Induction.* Cambridge: Cambridge University Press, 2010.

Chapter 13

Ultrasonography of the cervix

Mona Aboulghar and Botros Rizk

Introduction

Ultrasound is an essential diagnostic tool in gynecologic and obstetric practice and is of special importance for management of infertile patients. With the advancement of ultrasound technology and ultrasound machines and the introduction of three-dimensional (3D) technology as well, detailed examination of the uterine cervix and anatomy and accurate measurements have become possible [1]. This has broadened the uses of sonographic examination in infertile patients as well as in pregnancy, mainly due to the importance of examination of the uterine cervix for prediction of preterm labor [2].

Morphology of the uterine cervix [3]

The cervix is the cylindrical portion of the uterus which enters the vagina and lies at right angles to it. It measures 2–4 cm in length. The point of junction to the uterus is called the isthmus. Branches of the uterine arteries are situated lateral to the cervix and can be seen by color Doppler by transvaginal ultrasound.

By transvaginal ultrasound the cervix is seen in the sagittal plane as a cylindrical, moderately echogenic structure with a central canal (Figure 13.1). The internal os is better identified during pregnancy. The cervical mucus is more prominent during pregnancy, facilitating the recognition of the cervical canal (Figure 13.2). The cervical gland area is an area surrounding the cervical canal that is either hypo- or hyperechoic; its absence has been related to preterm labor [4,5,6].

Route of ultrasound evaluation of the cervix

The transvaginal route (TVS) is the preferred route for examining the cervix, whether in the nonpregnant or pregnant state. Rizk et al. (1990) demonstrated that the transvaginal route is superior to the transabdominal route, as confirmed by other investigators [7,8,9,10].

It avoids limitations of the transabdominal route, which include difficulties due to maternal habitus and the need for a full bladder [11]. In addition, the cervical length as measured may be falsely increased by the transabdominal route [12].

Transperineal route

Comparison of the transvaginal and transperineal routes for assessment of the cervix (in pregnancy) found good agreement and very similar measurements of cervical length for both routes [13,14,15,16], in all but one study [17].

The need to evaluate the possibility of the transperineal (translabial) route arose because some authors argued against transvaginal ultrasound in some conditions, as in patients with threatened preterm labor, in patients with rupture of membranes (ROM) for fear of chorioamnionitis, and the risk of bleeding in patients with placenta previa; however, it has been shown that these are not true clinical risks [18,19]. In our practice we have not found this to be a contraindication for transvaginal ultrasonography; in patients with ROM a sterile sheath is used.

Technique of transvaginal ultrasound

The patient should be examined in the supine position with hips abducted and with an empty bladder. A high-frequency probe, a 3.5–8.0 MHz transvaginal transducer covered with a condom, is inserted midway between introitus and cervix. In pregnancy, the entire length of the cervical canal should be measured, from the internal os (demarcated by the junction with the amniotic membrane) and to external os.

Benign gynecologic conditions seen by US in the nonpregnant state include nabothian cysts, cervical polyps, fibroids, and müllerian anomalies [20].

Nabothian cysts

Nabothian cysts represent a reparative upward growth of squamous epithelium, causing obstruction of the ducts of the endocervical glands. Retention of mucus within these glands results in nabothian cysts. The are very common and can be single or multiple; by ultrasound they appear as anechoic cysts within cervical tissue [3] (Figures 13.3, 13.4).

Cervical polyps

Cervical polyps are common findings, and in most cases difficult to distinguish from cervical mucus. A large polyp can be seen

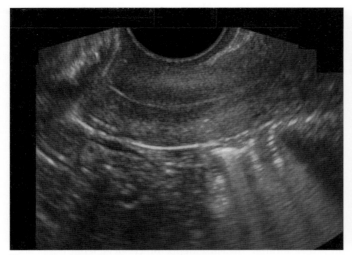

Figure 13.1. Normal cervix – nonpregnant state.

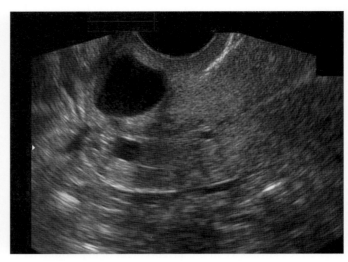

Figure 13.4. Nabothian cyst (large).

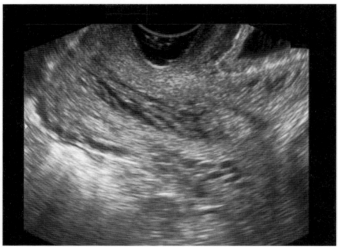

Figure 13.2. Cervix in pregnancy.

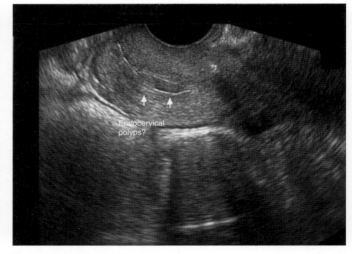

Figure 13.5. Endocervical polyps.

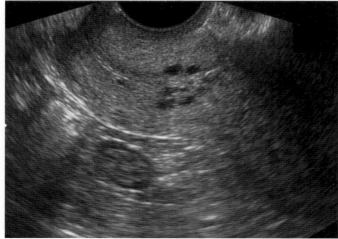

Figure 13.3. Nabothian cysts (small).

as an echogenic mass in the cervical canal, and this could be made easier by saline infusion (sonohysterography).

Evaluation of the cervical anatomy is important during investigation of infertility, as surgical procedures might be needed (polypectomy) before embarking on treatments such as intra-uterine insemination (IUI) and in-vitro fertilization (IVF) (Figure 13.5), and difficulties might be encountered during catheter introduction [21]. It is our routine practice to have an ultrasound image of the cervical canal and uterus, measuring cervical length and uterine body length, to assist during embryo transfer.

Cervical fibroids

Most commonly fibroids arise from the uterine body, extending into the cervical canal, i.e., pedunculated fibroids; or rarely they arise primarily from the cervix. In both instances sonohysterography enhances visualization of the fibroid, and its exact origin [22,23] (Figures 13.6 and 13.7).

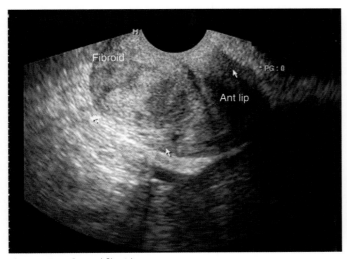

Figure 13.6. Cervical fibroid.

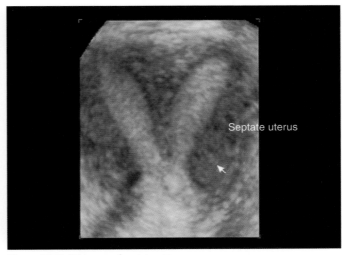

Figure 13.9. 3D image of septate uterus.

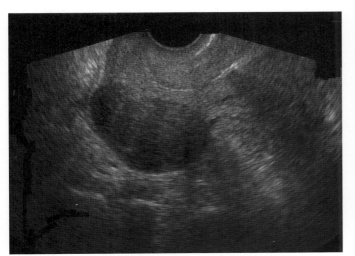

Figure 13.7. Müllerian anomaly; 3D image of cervical fibroid.

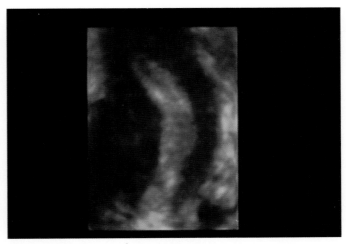

Figure 13.10. 3D image of unicornuate uterus.

Müllerian anomalies

The prevalence of müllerian anomalies is reported in various studies to range from 1% to 26% of infertile females [24]. Two-dimensional (2D) ultrasound is a good screening test with high sensitivity for detection of müllerian uterine anomalies [25,26]. However, 2D US has a limited ability to distinguish different types of uterine abnormalities and is operator dependent [26,27,28]. Consequently, 3D US is now used extensively, with advantages due its ability to demonstrate the coronal view of the uterus and cervix. It can therefore differentiate different müllerian anomalies with good reported sensitivity and specificity [29,30]. This is of course important in infertile patients with asymmetrical division, vaginal septa, or uterine horns, especially if IVF is to be performed with embryo transfer to be done in the correct body (Figures 13.7, 13.8, 13.9, 13.10).

Assessment of cervical length in this specific group of patients is of importance due to their higher incidence of preterm labor; it was found that a short cervical length on transvaginal ultrasonography in women with uterine anomalies had a

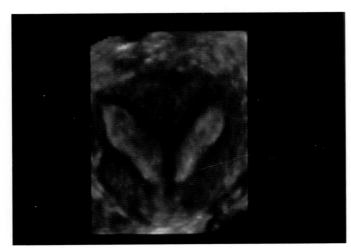

Figure 13.8. 3D image of complete septate uterus.

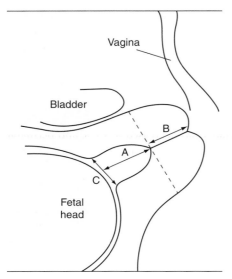

Figure 13.11. Cervical funneling.

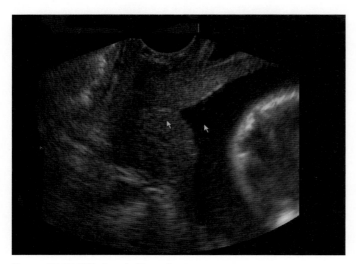

Figure 13.12. TVS of cervical funneling in pregnancy.

13-fold risk for preterm birth. Of all müllerian anomalies unicornuate uterus had the highest rate of cervical shortening and preterm delivery [31].

Ultrasound examination of the cervix in pregnancy

It is well documented in the literature that pregnancy following assisted reproductive technologies (ART) has a higher risk of adverse outcomes. A meta-analysis comparing IVF with spontaneous conceptions showed that IVF singleton pregnancies had significantly higher odds of perinatal mortality (odds ratio [OR] 2.2; 95% confidence interval [CI] 1.6 to 3.0); preterm delivery (OR 2.0; 95% CI 1.7–2.2); low birth weight (OR 1.8; 95% CI 1.4–2.2); very low birth weight (OR 2.7; 95% CI 2.3–3.1); and small-for-gestational-age births (OR 1.6; 95% CI 1.3–2.0) [32,33,34].

Similarly, IVF/ICSI (intracytoplasmic sperm injection) twins had a 10-fold increased age- and parity-adjusted risk of delivery before 37 completed weeks (OR 9.9; 95% CI 8.7–11.3) and a 7.4-fold increased risk of delivery before 32 completed weeks (OR 7.4, 95% CI 5.6–9.8) compared with singletons. Correspondingly, ORs of birth weight <2500 g and birth weight <1500 g in twins were 11.8 (95% CI 10.3–13.6) and 5.4 (95% CI 4.1–7.0), respectively [33,34].

Even spontaneous pregnancies of untreated but infertile women are reported to have a higher risk for obstetric complications and perinatal mortality than spontaneous pregnancies in fertile women [34].

Prediction of preterm labor is important in IVF patients. However, a recently published study (by our group) showed that mid-trimester cervical length measurement was not a predictor of preterm labor, as the majority of cases that delivered preterm still had long cervices (>28 mm) [35].

Cervical assessment at midtrimester

Sonographic assessment of cervical length is better than digital examination in screening for preterm delivery, in a low-risk population as well as in high-risk patients [36,37,38,39,40]. Shortened cervical length in comparison with a high Bishop score was found to have 12-fold higher positive likelihood ratio for preterm delivery in a low-risk population (37.4; 95% CI 8.2–170.7 versus 3.2; 95% CI 1.1–9.2) [36].

Cervical length measurement by ultrasound proved to be the most important predictor of preterm labor. The relative risk of preterm delivery increased as the length of the cervix decreased [41].

Cervical funneling

Funneling is described as dilatation of the internal os so that the cervical canal changes in shape, with bulging of the bag of membranes through the dilated cervix into the cervical canal. The funnel has a width and a length and usually the residual cervical length is measured as well (Figures 13.11, 13.12 and 13.13). Care must be taken as funneling can be falsely ascribed when the bladder is overdistended, during contractions, or with undue vaginal pressure of the probe on the cervix. It is always advised to keep the vaginal probe midway between the introitus and the cervix and also to wait for 3–5 minutes before assessing cervical length and morphology, as it might change [42,43]. Most studies have found funneling to be of significance in predicting preterm labor in addition to a short cervical length [44,45,46]. However To and co-authors found cervical length to be of more significance [47].

The finding of a dynamic cervix occurs more frequently in patients at risk for preterm labor; in these cases it is important to measure the residual cervical length [42,48,49].

The measurement of cervical length was also shown to be of benefit in patients presenting with threatened preterm labor. Sonographic measurement of cervical length helps to avoid overdiagnosis of preterm labor in women with preterm contractions and to distinguish between true and false labor. A cut-off of 15 mm was reported in two studies to be the best for prediction of delivery within 7 days from admission and ultrasound evaluation of the cervix. Logistic regression analysis demonstrated that the only significant contributor in the prediction of delivery within 7 days was cervical length <15 mm (OR 101; 95% CI 12–800; $P < 0.0001$) [50,51].

Timing of ultrasound examination of the cervix during pregnancy: when to perform the cervical ultrasound assessment?

Early ultrasound assessment of the cervix (between 11 and 14 weeks) was not found to be a reliable screening method in prediction of spontaneous preterm delivery [52]. Comparing early assessment at 11–14 weeks with midtrimester assessment at 22–24 weeks showed that cervical length at 11–14 weeks was not significantly different between the groups that delivered at term and preterm. However, at the 22–24-week evaluation, cervical length was significantly shorter in the group that had preterm delivery than in that with term delivery ($P = 0.0001$). This confirms that there is a spontaneous shortening in the pregnant cervix from the first to the second trimester of pregnancy, and thus this is the best timing for screening of the cervix [53].

Ultrasound-guided embryo transfer: transabdominal ultrasound-guided ET and importance of uterocervical angle

Ultrasound-guided embryo transfer [ET] has been introduced and studied by several authors, many of whom found an increase in pregnancy rates [54,55], while others found it to be equivalent to clinical touch transfers [56]. However, two recent meta-analyses done by our group [57] found higher rates of live birth, ongoing pregnancy, clinical pregnancy, and implantation and easier transfers with the ultrasound-guided technique [58].

The advantage of transabdominal ultrasound-guided transfer with a full bladder is mainly attributed to straightening of the uterocervical angle, facilitating entry of the catheter into the uterine cavity. However, it has the disadvantages of patient discomfort, and the fact that obesity and retroversion of the uterus might cause inadequate visualization of the endometrial cavity. A study done to compare the empty bladder with the full bladder at the time of transabdominal ultrasound-guided ET showed comparable results for all three groups of full bladder and empty bladder (both guided transabdominally) or clinical touch ET [59].

Another study examined the effect of molding the ET catheter to the uterocervical angle (measured by transabdominal ultrasound). Molding the ET catheter according to the uterocervical angle significantly increased clinical pregnancy (OR 1.57; 95% CI 1.08–2.27) and implantation rates (OR 1.47; 95% CI 1.10–1.96) compared with the "clinical touch" method. It also significantly reduced difficult transfers (OR 0.25; 95% CI 0.16–0.40) and bleeding during transfers (OR 0.71; 95% CI 0.50–0.99). Patients with large angles (>60 degrees) had

significantly lower pregnancy rates compared with those with no angle [OR 0.36; 95% CI 0.16–0.52] [60]. This confirms the need for assessment of the cervix as regards angle, length, and body length with ultrasound before ET [21].

Placenta previa

The incidence of placenta previa is 1:200, and increases with parity. Maternal mortality has decreased to <1%, and perinatal mortality to 5%, with modern treatment. It is essential, therefore, to diagnose placenta previa during pregnancy and to determine its type and the need for cesarean section according to the relation of the placenta to the internal os. The incidence of placenta previa is reported to be higher in pregnancies following ART. A 6-fold increased risk of placenta previa was found compared with naturally conceived pregnancies [61].

Ultrasound should be the main tool used to diagnose placenta previa and for follow-up as well. Diagnosis of placenta previa in the second trimester of pregnancy showed, with ultrasound follow-up, that approximately 85% of cases ended up with a normally situated placenta [62].

Comparing the routes of ultrasound for confirmation of placenta previa and determination of its exact relation to the internal cervical os, transvaginal ultrasound appears to be a superior method to transabdominal [63,64,65,66,67,68]; it is also a safe route that does not show an increased risk of vaginal bleeding [19,66,67] (Figure 13.14).

The importance of transvaginal ultrasound lies in its ability to determine the exact distance of the placental edge from the internal os, which will determine the mode of delivery. Studies suggest that a distance of ≥2 cm from the internal cervical os to the placental edge indicates safe vaginal delivery [69,70,71]. Management differs for placentas lying at a distance of 1–2 cm, but the probability of cesarean section is very high, reaching 40% in one of the studies [70], while in another study all patients underwent cesarean section [69,71].

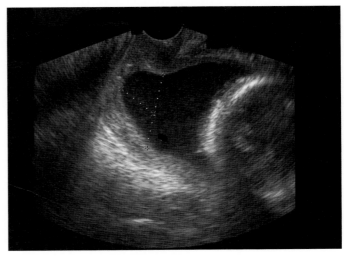

Figure 13.13. Marked cervical funneling.

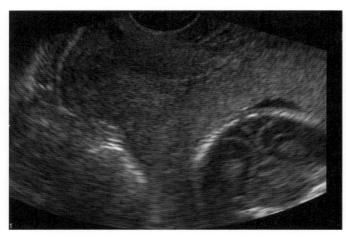

Figure 13.14. Placentia Previa.

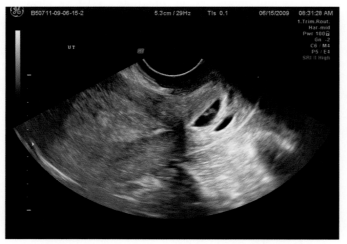

Figure 13.15. Cervical twin pregnancy; sagittal view from the fundus to the cervix.

Vasa previa

Vasa previa is defined as fetal vessels coursing within the membranes between the presenting part and cervix. The incidence is 1:1200 to 1:5000 pregnancies [72,73,74]. In anatomical variants the vessels over the cervix can lead from the placenta to a velamentous cord insertion, or connect the main bulk of the placenta to a succenturiate lobe.

Vasa previa carries a high fetal morbidity and mortality, since fetal vessels within the membranes are unprotected by Wharton's jelly; they are prone to compression during labor and may tear when the membranes rupture, resulting in fetal exsanguination.

The classic presentation is rupture of membranes followed by painless, dark vaginal bleeding associated with profound fetal distress or fetal demise. Vasa previa can cause abnormal intrapartum fetal heart rate patterns, including sinusoidal tracings [74] and severe variable decelerations [75]. Clinically the diagnosis is occasionally made on the basis of the palpation of fetal vessels within the (intact) membranes at the time of vaginal examination, and can also be made by amnioscopy [76].

It is now more often diagnosed by ultrasound, either abdominally or transvaginally and in some instances a combination of both [77,78]. In addition, color and power Doppler studies are essential in confirming vasa previa [79].

It has been recommended to attempt to visualize the cord insertion in the placenta and to perform a sweep across the lower uterine segment to look for velamentous vessels; and if a low-lying succenturiate lobe is seen, to examine the region over the cervix using color Doppler. Serial sonograms should be done and, in case of confirmed vasa previa, maternal rest and close monitoring are advised, with delivery by cesarean section after confirmation of fetal lung maturity.

In an evaluation of the outcomes and predictors of neonatal survival in pregnancies complicated by vasa previa, comparing outcomes in prenatally diagnosed cases of vasa previa with those not diagnosed prenatally, it was found that the only significant predictors of neonatal survival were prenatal diagnosis of vasa previa ($P < 0.001$) and gestational age at delivery ($P = 0.01$). The overall perinatal mortality reported was high (36%), and this was reduced in cases diagnosed prenatally and when cesarean section was done early in cases of rupture of membranes, labor, or significant bleeding [80].

Some reports indicate that there could be increased incidence of vasa previa in pregnancies following IVF due to a suggested higher incidence of velamentous and marginal insertions of the umbilical cord [81]. Disturbed orientation of the blastocyst at implantation, a contributing factor to vasa previa, is probably related to the IVF-ET procedure [82].

Cervical pregnancy

Cervical pregnancy is a rare ectopic pregnancy defined as implantation of the gestational sac in the endocervix (Figure 13.15). Several publications have suggested that ART may be associated with an increased risk of ectopic pregnancy [83,84,85,86].

Ultrasound is the main diagnostic tool (see Chapter 33). It is reported to have improved pretreatment diagnosis, up to 81.8%. Obligatory sonographic criteria of cervical pregnancy include endocervical localization of the gestational sac and trophoblastic invasion [87] (Figure 13.16). Doppler is also a very important tool for confirming viability; up to 60% of cervical ectopic pregnancies are viable [87].

Because of its difficult diagnosis, cervical pregnancy should be differentiated from the cervical stage of spontaneous abortion, nabothian cyst, and cervical choriocarcinoma The risk of cervical pregnancy is mainly severe hemorrhage necessitating hysterectomy in many situations; this usually occurs in nulliparous or low-parity women, adding to the dilemma of management.

Management of cervical pregnancy is mainly conservative: giving methotrexate systemically and in some cases curettage, curettage and Foley catheter tamponade, cervical cerclage, ligation of the descending branches of uterine arteries, or ligation of hypogastric arteries. Intra-amniotic injection of

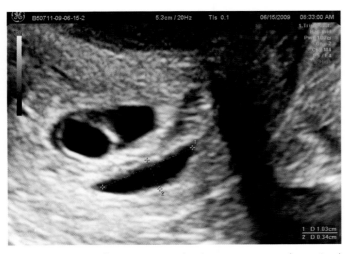

Figure 13.16. Cervical twin pregnancy showing an empty second gestational sac and a yolk sac in the first gestational sac

methotrexate (or potassium chloride) has also been described with success [88,89,90,91,92,93,94,95) and with excellent recovery.

Key points in clinical practice

- Advances in ultrasound technology, especially 3D, have allowed good imaging of the uterine cervix in both nonpregnant and pregnant states. The cervix is seen well by transvaginal ultrasound, especially during pregnancy, when cervical mucus renders the cervical canal prominent and demarcates the internal os well when measurement of cervical length is necessary.

- Ultrasound examination of the cervix is best done by transvaginal ultrasound, rather than by the transabdominal route. The transperineal route is also an option in cases of bleeding or premature rupture of membranes, but transvaginal ultrasound is not contraindicated in these situations.

- Benign gynecologic findings seen by ultrasound include nabothian cysts, cervical polyps, cervical fibroids, and müllerian anomalies. In the last case, 3D imaging provides higher sensitivity and specificity. Müllerian anomalies should be diagnosed before IVF trials, so that problems will not be faced during embryo transfer. An image of the cervical canal and uterine body and measurements of the length of each are very helpful in the clinical touch technique of embryo transfer.

- Cervical length at mid trimester is the best predictor for preterm labor. The relative risk of preterm labor increases with decrease in cervical length. This is of special importance in pregnancies following ART, as this group of patients is known to have a higher incidence of adverse perinatal outcomes; preterm labor is one of the risks. Cervical funneling and dynamic cervix are both predictors of preterm labor, and in both cases the residual cervical length is of importance.

- Transabdominal ultrasound-guided embryo transfer in IVF increases pregnancy rates; the advantage comes from straightening of the uterocervical angle. Molding of the ET catheter to fit the uterocervical angle increases pregnancy rates as well.

- Placenta previa occurs six times more frequently in pregnancies following ART.

- Mortality and morbidity due to placenta previa have decreased with modern management. An essential part of this has been ultrasound diagnosis, especially by transvaginal ultrasonography, which is superior to abdominal. It confirms the diagnosis of placenta previa and gives accurate measurements of distance from placental edge to internal cervical os. This will determine the mode of delivery, so that a placenta >2 cm from the cervical os allows safe vaginal delivery.

- Incidence of vasa previa is reported to be higher in pregnancies following ART.

- Vasa previa is diagnosed by transvaginal or transabdominal ultrasound, and with Doppler flow studies. The main significant predictor of neonatal survival is prenatal diagnosis of vasa previa. Delivery before ROM decreases perinatal mortality. Cervical pregnancy, defined as implantation in the endocervix, has a higher risk in ART pregnancies. The diagnosis is essentially by ultrasound and the management is conservative: methotrexate systemically or transvaginally, ultrasound-guided. Conservative management aims at reducing the risks of hemorrhage and the need for hysterectomy.

References

1. Sladkevicius P, Campbell S. Advanced ultrasound examination in the management of subfertility. *Curr Opin Obstet Gynecol* 2000; **12**(3): 221–5.

2. Kagan K, To M, Tsoi E, et al. Preterm birth: the value of sonographic measurement of cervical length. *BJOG* 2006; **113**(s3): 5–56.

3. Di Saia PJ. Disorders of uterine cervix. In: Scott JR, DiSaia P, Hammond CB, et al., eds. *Danforth's Obstetrics and Gynecology*, 7th ed. Philadephia, PA: JB Lippincott, 1994.

4. Sekyia T, Yoshimatsu K, et al. Detection rate of the cervical gland area during pregnancy by transvaginal sonography in the assessment of cervical maturation. *Ultrasound Obstet Gynecol* 1998; **12**: 328.

5. Yoshimatsu K, Sekiya T, Ishihara K, Fukami T, Otabe T, Araki T. Detection of the cervical gland area in threatened preterm labor using transvaginal sonography in the assessment of cervical maturation and the outcome of pregnancy. *Gynecol Obstet Invest* 2002; **53**(3): 149–56.

6. Pires CR, Moron AF, Mattar R, et al. Cervical gland area as an ultrasonographic marker for preterm delivery. *Int J Gynaecol Obstet* 2006; **93**(3): 214–19.

7. Rizk B, Steer C, Tan SL, Mason BA. Vaginal versus abdominal ultrasound guided

oocyte retrieval in IVF. *Br J Radiol* 1990; **63**: 638.

8. Steer C, Rizk B Tan SL, Mason BA. Vaginal versus abdominal ultrasound for obtaining uterine artery Doppler flow velocity waveforms. *Br J Radiol* 1990; **63**: 398–9.

9. Steer C, Rizk B Tan SL, Mason BA, Campbell S. Vaginal colour Doppler assessment of uterine artery impedance in subfertile population. *Br J Radiol* 1990; **63**: 638.

10. Qureshi IA, Ullah H, Akram MH, et al. Transvaginal versus transabdominal sonography in the evaluation of pelvic pathology. *J Coll Physicians Surg Pak* 2004; **14**(7): 390–3.

11. To MS, Skentou C, Cicero S, et al. Cervical assessment at the routine 23-weeks' scan: problems with transabdominal sonography. *Ultrasound Obstet Gynecol* 2000; **15**(4): 292–6.

12. Andersen HF. Transvaginal and transabdominal ultrasonography of the uterine cervix during pregnancy. *J Clin Ultrasound* 1991; **19**(2): 77–83.

13. Raungrongmorakot K, Tanmoun N, Ruangvutilert P, et al. Correlation of uterine cervical length measurement from transabdominal, transperineal and transvaginal ultrasonography. *J Med Assoc Thai* 2004; **87**(3): 326–32.

14. Cicero S, Skentou C, Souka A, To MS, Nicolaides KH. Cervical length at 22–24 weeks of gestation: comparison of transvaginal and transperineal-translabial ultrasonography. *Ultrasound Obstet Gynecol* 2001; **17**(4): 335–40.

15. Kurtzman JT, Goldsmith LJ, Gall SA, Spinnato JA.

16. Ozdemir I, Demirci F, Yucel O. Transperineal versus transvaginal ultrasonographic evaluation of the cervix at each trimester in normal pregnant women. *Aust N Z J Obstet Gynaecol* 2005; **45**(3): 191–4.

17. Carr DB, Smith K, Parsons L, et al. Ultrasonography for cervical length measurement: agreement between transvaginal and translabial techniques. *Obstet Gynecol* 2000; **96**(4): 554–8.

18. Carlan SJ, Richmond LB, O'Brien WF. Randomized trial of endovaginal ultrasound in preterm premature rupture of membranes. *Obstet Gynecol* 1997; **89** (3): 458–61.

19. Timor-Tritsch IR, Yunis RA. Confirming the safety of transvaginal sonography in patients suspected of placenta previa. *Obstet Gynecol*, 1993; **81**: 742.

20. Bajo J, Moreno-Calvo FJ, Uguet-de-Resayre C, et al. Contribution of transvaginal sonography to the evaluation of benign cervical conditions. *J Clin Ultrasound* 1999; **27**(2): 61–4.

21. Mansour R. T, Aboulghar MA. Optimizing the embryo transfer technique. *Hum Reprod* 2002; **17**(5): 1149–53.

22. Wongsawaeng W. Transvaginal ultrasonography, sonohysterography and hysteroscopy for intrauterine pathology in patients with abnormal uterine bleeding. *J Med Assoc Thai* 2005; **88**(Suppl. 3): S77–81.

23. Leone FP, Lanzani C, Ferrazzi E. Use of strict sonohysterographic methods for preoperative assessment

of submucous myomas. *Fertil Steril* 2003; **79**(4): 998–1002.

24. Grimbizis GF, Camus M, Tarlatzis BC, et al. Clinical implication of uterine malformations and hysteroscopic treatment results. *Hum Reprod Update* 2001; **7**(2) 161–74.

25. Valdes C, Malini S, Malikanak LR. Ultrasound evaluation of female genital tract anomalies: a review of 64 cases. *Am J Obstet Gynecol* 1984; **47**: 89–93.

26. Nicolini U, Bellotti M, Bonazzi B, et al. Can ultrasound be used to screen uterine malformations? *Fertil Steril* 1987; **47**: 89–93

27. Reuter KL, Daly DC, Cohen SM. Septate versus bicornuate uteri: errors in imaging diagnosis. *Radiology* 1989; **172**: 749–52.

28. Randoph JF Jr, Ying YK, Maier DB, et al. Comparison of real time ultrasonography, hysterosalpingopraphy, and laparoscopy/hysteroscopy in the evaluation of uterine abnormalities and tubal patency. *Fertil Steril* 1986; **5**: 828–32.

29. Raga F, Bonilla-Musoles F, Blanes J, et al. Congenital mullerian anomalies: diagnostic accuracy of three-dimensional ultrasound. *Fertil Steril* 1996; **65**: 523–8.

30. Wu MH, Hsu CC Huang KE. Detection of congenital mullerian duct anomalies using three-dimensional ultrasound. *J Clin Ultrasound* 1997; **25**: 487–92.

31. Airoldi J, Berghella V, Sehdev H, et al. Transvaginal ultrasonography of the cervix to predict preterm birth in women with uterine anomalies. *Obstet Gynecol* 2005; **106**(3): 553–6.

32. Jackson RA, Gibson KA, Wu YW, et al. Perinatal outcomes in singletons following in vitro

fertilization: a meta-analysis. *Obstet Gynecol* 2004; **103**(3): 551–63.

33. Pinborg A, Loft A, Nyboe Andersen A. Neonatal outcome in a Danish national cohort of 8602 children born after in vitro fertilization or intracytoplasmic sperm injection: the role of twin pregnancy. *Acta Obstet Gynecol Scand* 2004; **83**(11): 1071–8.

34. Allen VM, Wilson RD, Cheung A. Pregnancy outcomes after assisted reproductive technology. *J Obstet Gynaecol Can* 2006; **28**(3): 220–50.

35. Aboulghar MM, Aboulghar MA, Mourad L, Serour GI. Ultrasound cervical measurement and prediction of spontaneous preterm birth in ICSI pregnancies: a prospective controlled study. *Reprod Biomed Online* February 2009; **18**(2): 296–300.

36. Matijevic R, Grgic O, Vasilj O. Is sonographic assessment of cervical length better than digital examination in screening for preterm delivery in a low-risk population? *Acta Obstet Gynecol Scand* 2006; **85**(11): 1342–7.

37. Guzman ER, Walters C, Ananth CV, et al. A comparison of sonographic cervical parameters in predicting spontaneous preterm birth in high-risk singleton gestations. *Ultrasound Obstet Gynecol* 2001; **18**(3): 204–10.

38. Heath VC, Southall TR, Souka AP, Elisseou A, Nicolaides KH. Cervical length at 23 weeks of gestation: prediction of spontaneous preterm delivery. *Ultrasound Obstet Gynecol* 1998; **12**(5): 312–17.

39. Leung TN, Pang MW, Leung TY, Poon CF, Wong SM, Lau TK. Cervical length at 18–22 weeks of gestation

for prediction of spontaneous preterm delivery in Hong Kong Chinese women. *Ultrasound Obstet Gynecol* 2005; **26**(7): 713–17.

40. Cook CM, Ellwood DA. The cervix as a predictor of preterm delivery in 'at-risk' women. *Ultrasound Obstet Gynecol* 2000; **15**(2): 109–13.

41. Iams JD, Goldenberg RL, Meis PJ, et al. The length of the cervix and the risk of spontaneous premature delivery. National Institute of Child Health and Human Development Maternal Fetal Medicine Unit Network. *N Engl J Med* 1996; **334**(9): 567–72.

42. Kikuchi A, Kozuma S, Marumo G, et al. Local dynamic changes of the cervix associated with incompetent cervix before and after Shirodkar's operation. *J Clin Ultrasound* 1998; **26**: 371.

43. Parulekar SG, Kiwi R. Dynamic incompetent cervix uteri: sonographic observations. *J Ultrasound Med* 1988; **7**(9): 481–5.

44. Rust OA, Atlas RO, Kimmel S, et al. Does the presence of a funnel increase the risk of adverse perinatal outcome in a patient with a short cervix? *Am J Obstet Gynecol* 2005; **192**(4): 1060–6.

45. Vayssiere C, Favre R, Audibert F, et al. Cervical length and funneling at 22 and 27 weeks to predict spontaneous birth before 32 weeks in twin pregnancies: a French prospective multicenter study. *Am J Obstet Gynecol* 2002; **187**(6): 1596–604.

46. Berghella V, Kuhlman K, Weiner S, et al. Cervical funneling: sonographic criteria predictive of preterm delivery. *Ultrasound Obstet Gynecol* 1997; **10**(3): 161–6.

47. To MS, Skentou C, Liao AW, et al. Cervical length and funneling at 23 weeks of gestation in the prediction of spontaneous early preterm delivery. *Ultrasound Obstet Gynecol* 2001; **18**(3): 200–3.

48. Bergelin I, Valentin L. Cervical changes in twin pregnancies observed by transvaginal ultrasound during the latter half of pregnancy: a longitudinal, observational study. *Ultrasound Obstet Gynecol* 2003; **21**(6): 556–63.

49. Bergelin I, Valentin L. Normal cervical changes in parous women during the second half of pregnancy – a prospective, longitudinal ultrasound study. *Acta Obstet Gynecol Scand.* 2002; **81**(1): 31–8.

50. Tsoi E, Akmal S, Rane S, et al. Ultrasound assessment of cervical length in threatened preterm labor. *Ultrasound Obstet Gynecol* 2003; **21**(6): 552–5.

51. Fuchs IB, Henrich W, Osthues K, Dudenhausen JW. Sonographic cervical length in singleton pregnancies with intact membranes presenting with threatened preterm labor. *Ultrasound Obstet Gynecol* 2004; **24**(5): 554–7.

52. Conoscenti G, Meir YJ, D'Ottavio G, et al. Does cervical length at 13–15 weeks' gestation predict preterm delivery in an unselected population? *Ultrasound Obstet Gynecol* 2003; **21**(2): 128–34.

53. Carvalho MH, Bittar RE, Brizot ML, et al. Cervical length at 11–14 weeks' and 22–24 weeks' gestation evaluated by transvaginal sonography, and gestational age at delivery. *Ultrasound Obstet Gynecol* 2003; **21**(2): 135–9.

54. Coroleu B, Carreras O, Veiga A, et al. Embryo transfer under ultrasound guidance improves pregnancy rates after in-vitro fertilization.

Hum Reprod 2000; **15**(3): 616–20.

55. Matorras R, Urquijo E, Mendoza R, et al. Ultrasound-guided embryo transfer improves pregnancy rates and increases the frequency of easy transfers. *Hum Reprod* 2002; **17**(7): 1762–6.

56. Flisser E, Grifo JA, Krey LC. Transabdominal ultrasound-assisted embryo transfer and pregnancy outcome. *Fertil Steril* 2006; **85**(2): 353–7.

57. Abousetta A, Mansour RT, El Inany H, et al. Among women undergoing embryo transfer is the probability of pregnancy and live birth improved with ultrasound guided over clinical touch alone? A systematic review of meta-analysis of prospective randomized trials. *Fertil Steril* 2007; **88**(2): 333–41

58. Brown JA, Buckingham K, Abou-setta A, et al. Ultrasound versus clinical touch for catheter guidance during embryo transfer in women (Review). Cochrane Library 2007; issue 1.

59. Lorusso F, Depalo R, Bettocchi S, et al. Outcome of in vitro fertilization after transabdominal ultrasound-assisted embryo transfer with a full or empty bladder. *Fertil Steril* 2005; **84**(4): 1046–8.

60. Sallam HN, Agameya AF, Rahman AF, et al. Ultrasound measurement of the uterocervical angle before embryo transfer: a prospective controlled study. *Hum Reprod* 2002; **17**(7): 1767–72.

61. Romundstad LB, Romundstad PR, Sunde A, et al. Increased risk of placenta previa in pregnancies following IVF/ICSI; a comparison of ART and non-ART pregnancies in the same mother. *Hum Reprod* 2006; **21**(9): 2353–8.

62. Chama CM, Wanonyi IK, Usman JD. From low-lying implantation to placenta praevia: a longitudinal ultrasonic assessment. *J Obstet Gynaecol* 2004; **24**(5): 516–18.

63. Smith RS, Lauria MR, Comstock CH, et al. Transvaginal ultrasonography for all placentas that appear to be low-lying or over the internal cervical os. *Ultrasound Obstet Gynecol* 1997; **9**(1): 22–4.

64. Ghorab S. Third-trimester transvaginal ultrasonography in placenta previa: does the shape of the lower placental edge predict clinical outcome? *Ultrasound Obstet Gynecol* 2001; **18**(2): 103–8.

65. Heer IM, Muller-Egloff S, Strauss A. Placenta praevia – comparison of four sonographic modalities. *Ultraschall Med* 2006; **27**(4): 355–9.

66. Tan NH, Abu M, Woo JL, Tahir HM. The role of transvaginal sonography in the diagnosis of placenta praevia. *Aust N Z J Obstet Gynaecol* 1995; **35**(1): 42–5.

67. Sunna E, Ziadeh S. Transvaginal and transabdominal ultrasound for the diagnosis of placenta praevia. *J Obstet Gynecol* 1999; **19**(2): 152–4.

68. Chen JM, Zhou QC, Wang RR. Value of transvaginal sonography in diagnosis of placenta previa. *Hunan Yi Ke Da Xue Xue Bao* 2001; **26**(3): 289–90.

69. Bhide A, Prefumo F, Moore J, et al. Placental edge to internal os distance in the late third trimester and mode of delivery in placenta praevia. *BJOG.* 2003; **110**(9): 860–4.

70. Dawson WB, Dumas MD, Romano WM, et al: Translabial ultrasonography

and placenta praevia: does measurement of the os-placenta distance predict outcome? *J Ultrasound Med* 1996; **15**: 441.

71. Opeheimer LW, Farine D, Ritchie JW, et al. What is a low lying placenta. *Am J Obstet Gynecol* 1991; **165**: 1036.

72. Fung TY, Lau TK. Poor perinatal outcome associated with vasa previa: Is it preventable? A report of three cases and review of literature. *Ultrasound Obstet Gynecol* 1998; **12**(6): 430–3

73. Nomiyama M, Toyota Y, Kawano H. Antenatal diagnosis of velamentous umbilical cord insertion and vasa previa with color Doppler imaging. *Ultrasound Obstet Gynecol* 1998; **12**: 426–9

74. Pent D. Vasa previa. *Am J Obstet Gynecol* 1979; **134**: 151–5.

75. Antoine C, Youn BK, Silverman F, et al. Sinusoidal fetal heart rate pattern with vasa previa in twin pregnancy. *J Reprod Med* 1982; **27**: 295–300

76. Codero DR, Helgott AW, Landy HJ, et al. Non hemorrhagic manifestation of vasa previa. A clinicopathologic case. *Obstet Gynecol* 1993; **82**: 689–701.

77. Young M, Yu N, Barham K. The role of light and sound technologies in the detection of vasa previa. *Reprod Fertil dev* 1991; **3**: 439–51

78. Catanzarite V, Maida C, Thomas W, et al. Prenatal sonographic diagnosis of vasa previa: ultrasound findings and obstetric outcome in ten cases. *Ultrasound Obstet Gynecol* 2001; **18**(2): 109–15.

79. Baschat AA. Ante and intrapartum diagnosis of vasa praevia in singleton pregnancies by colour coded Doppler sonography. *Eur J Obstet Gynecol Reprod Biol* 1998; **79**(1): 19–25.

80. Oyelese Y, Catanzarite V, Prefumo F, et al. Vasa previa: the impact of prenatal diagnosis on outcomes. *Obstet Gynecol* 2004; **103** (5 Pt 1): 937–42.

81. Burton G, Saunders DM. Vasa praevia: another cause for concern in in vitro fertilization pregnancies. *Aust N Z J Obstet Gynaecol* 1988; **28**(3): 180–1.

82. Englert Y, Imbert MC, Van Rosendael E, et al. Morphological anomalies in the placentae of IVF pregnancies: preliminary report of a multicentric study. *Hum Reprod* 1987; **2**(2): 155–7.

83. Pyrgiotis E, Sultan KM, Neal GS, Liu HC, Grifo JA, Rosenwaks Z. Ectopic pregnancies after in vitro fertilization and embryo transfer. *J Assist Reprod Genet* 1994; **11**(2): 79–84.

84. Ginsburg ES, Frates MC, Rein MS, et al. Early diagnosis and treatment of cervical pregnancy in an in vitro fertilization program. *Fertil Steril* 1994; **61**(5): 966–9.

85. Rizk B, Brindsen PR. Embryo migration responsible for ectopic pregnancies. *Am J Obstet Gyneciol* 1990; **163**(4): 1639.

86. Aboulghar M, Rizk B. Ultrasonography of the cervix. In: Rizk B, ed. *Ultrasonography in Reproductive Medicine and Infertility*, chapter 16. Cambridge: Cambridge University Press, 2008; 143–151.

87. Ushakov FB, Elchalal U, Aceman PJ, et al. Cervical pregnancy: past and future. *Obstet Gynecol Surv* 1997; **52**(1): 45–59.

88. Kim TJ, Seong SJ, Lee KJ, et al. Clinical outcomes of patients treated for cervical pregnancy with or without methotrexate. *J Korean Med Sci* 2004; **19**(6): 848–52.

89. Doekhie BM, Schats R, Hompes PG. Cervical pregnancy treated with local methotrexate. *Eur J Obstet Gynecol Reprod Biol* 2005; **122**(1): 128–30.

90. Sherer DM, Lysikiewicz A, Abulafia O. Viable cervical pregnancy managed with systemic Methotrexate, uterine artery embolization, and local tamponade with inflated Foley catheter balloon. *Am J Perinatol* 2003; **20**(5): 263–7.

91. Mitra AG, Harris-Owens M. Conservative medical management of advanced cervical ectopic pregnancies. *Obstet Gynecol Surv* 2000; **55**(6): 385–9.

92. Pascual MA, Ruiz J, Tresserra F, et al. Cervical ectopic twin pregnancy: diagnosis and conservative treatment: case report. *Hum Reprod* 2001; **16**(3): 584–6.

93. Hassiakos D, Bakas P, Creatsas G. Cervical pregnancy treated with transvaginal ultrasound-guided intra-amniotic instillation of methotrexate. *Arch Gynecol Obstet* 2005; **271**(1): 69–72

94. Yildizhan B. Diagnosis and treatment of early cervical pregnancy: a case report and literature review. *Clin Exp Obstet Gynecol* 2005; **32** (4): 254–6.

95. Kirk E, Condous G, Haider Z, Syed A, Ojha K, Bourne T. The conservative management of cervical ectopic pregnancies. *Ultrasound Obstet Gynecol* 2006; **27**(4): 430–7.

Color Doppler imaging of ovulation induction

Osama M. Azmy and Alaa El-Ebrashy

There is a definite urge to search for a noninvasive procedure that will improve precision of the knowledge of oocyte maturity, the predictability of the number and quality of the oocytes, and assessment of the most appropriate timing of the administration of human chorionic gonadotropin in cases of assisted conception. Understanding the vascular changes that occur in the intraovarian milieu using transvaginal pulsed color Doppler may improve our understanding of the peripheral circulatory conditions that reflect the hormonal changes that occur during spontaneous and induced cycles. The combination of real-time ultrasound, pulsed Doppler, and color flow mapping in studying the female reproductive system on an anatomic and physiological basis has been successfully used to assess the hemodynamic changes in various physiological and pathological entities.

Vascular supply of the ovaries

The ovary receives its arterial vascularity from two sources: the ovarian artery and the utero-ovarian branch of the uterine artery. These arteries anastomose to form an arch parallel to the ovarian hilus and constitute the vascular genital arcade (Figure 14.1). From the ovarian hilus, the arterial branches penetrate the stroma and acquire a tortuous and helical pathway, termed the spiral or helical arteries, *demonstrating high resistance to flow*. This facilitates the accommodation to changes in size with development of the follicle [1].

Transvaginal ovarian color Doppler imaging

After visualization of the pelvic anatomy by B-mode and color Doppler sonography, the color flow of the ovaries can be explored with Doppler sample volume until the typical spectral waveform is seen. As the ovarian artery traverses the broad ligament, entering the ovary at an angle of approximately 90 degrees to the insinuating vaginal ultrasound beam (Figure 14.2), satisfactory ovarian Doppler signals are difficult to obtain vaginally. However, intraovarian vessels traverse the ovary at varying angles of orientation. With the increased blood supply to the ovary containing the corpus luteum, vessels are relatively easily identified with a color system at low angles of insinuation. It is additionally difficult to visualize ovarian

vessels because the color flow is usually not prominent, velocity is low, and the resistance varies according to the day of the menstrual cycle (Figure 14.3). Nevertheless, it should be emphasized that the information obtained by color Doppler sonography is rarely diagnostic by itself. It should also be noted that blood flow demonstrated with color Doppler images that depends on flow velocity is not directly dependent on the amount of blood flow and the diameter of a vessel. Therefore, the vascularity seen on a color flow image does not always correlate with that assessed by angiography or dynamic computed topography.

Blood flow during the follicular, periovulatory, and mid-luteal period in spontaneous and induced cycles

The ovarian blood flow of an ovulatory cycle is more or less at constant level throughout the follicular phase and then shows a steady decline to reach a nadir on the approach to ovulation. These blood flow changes are not seen in anovulatory cycles. The blood flow changes that occur before ovulation indicate the complexity of changes that involve angiogenesis as well as hormonal factors. Furthermore, corpus luteum blood flow is characterized by low impedance [2] and high flow pattern [3] that can easily be detected (Figure 14.4). One study measured the resistance index (RI) of the flow velocity waveforms of the uterine and the ovarian arteries during the menstrual cycle in 100 infertile anovulatory women compared with 150 fertile spontaneously ovulating women. The authors recognized that the RI of the uterine arteries was around 0.88 until day 13 of a 28-day cycle. Then a significant decline began, reaching 0.84 at day 16 [4]. These changes did not occur in anovulatory cycles; in contrast there was an increase in the RI. However, ovarian flow velocity differs somewhat from the uterine vasculature, where the resistance index is approximately 0.54 until ovulation approaches, after which a decline begins 2 days before ovulation and reaches a nadir at ovulation (0.44). Thereafter it remains at this low level for four more days and gradually climbs to a level of 0.50. Another study [5] has looked at the

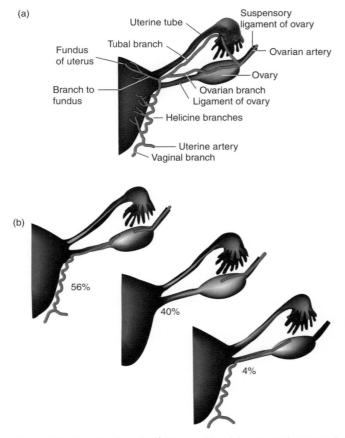

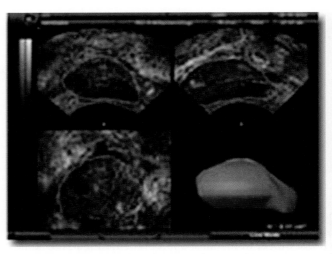

Figure 14.3. Stromal blood flow of the ovary determined by 3D power Doppler ultrasound.

Figure 14.1. The arterial supply of the ovary (a) and the various aberrations that occur (b). In 56% of cases the ovarian arterial blood supply comes from both the ovarian and uterine arteries, in 40% from the ovarian artery alone, and in 4% from the uterine artery only.

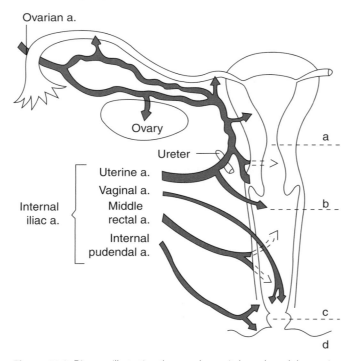

Figure 14.2. Diagram illustrating the vascular genital arcade and the ovarian blood supply from both the ovarian and uterine arteries.

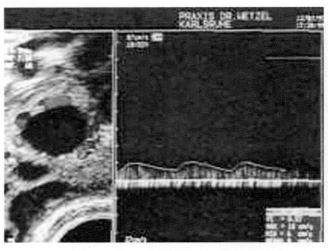

Figure 14.4. Blood flow characteristics of the corpus luteum. Note that corpus luteum blood flow is of low impedance and high flow pattern.

intraovarian blood flow during the early follicular, periovulatory, and mid-luteal phases in spontaneous and induced ovarian cycles. The researchers measured the pulsatility index (PI) in 8 women with spontaneous cycles, 20 women undergoing induction of ovulation with clomiphene citrate, and 11 women undergoing controlled ovarian stimulation for in-vitro fertilization with gonadotropin-releasing hormone agonists (GnRH-a), human menopausal gonadotropin (hMG), and human chorionic gonadotropin (hCG). Although statistically nonsignificant, the intraovarian PI showed a gradual decrease from the early follicular (1.05) through the periovulatory (0.99) to the mid-luteal phase (0.85). Intraovarian blood flow velocity waveforms were found in 20% of cases at the early follicular phase, in 56% of cases during the periovulatory phase, and in 85% during the mid-luteal phase.

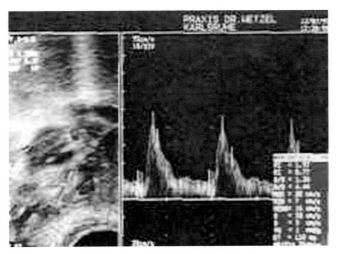

Figure 14.5. Increased blood flow indices and the peak velocity of the growing follicles in super-stimulated cycles during an in-vitro fertilization program.

Role of transvaginal pulsed color Doppler in assisted conception

In the in-vitro fertilization-embryo transfer (IVF-ET) program, the oocyte quality and recovery, the embryo quality, and the receptivity of the endometrium are among the most important parameters that determine the success rate. Several studies noted that the perifollicular peak velocity values increase gradually with the increase in size of the growing follicles. In addition, there is a strong positive correlation between the size of the ovarian follicles and their peak velocity (Figure 14.5), which suggests an increase of blood flow around developing follicles in the course of the follicular phase. Moreover, hCG plays an important role in inducing an influx of blood within the follicles. However, it appears that the resistance index is not a useful parameter for characterization of the intrafollicular flow. Color Doppler assessment of folliculogenesis in IVF-ET patients was studied in 52 patients undergoing hormonal stimulation for IVF [8]. A highly significant elevation of the peak velocity was observed, especially after hCG injection. Such rapid rise of blood velocity was greater in the right ovary than in the left.

The role of transvaginal pulsed color Doppler ultrasound in the prediction of the outcome of an in-vitro fertilization program has been assessed in several studies. In one study [9] 30 patients were followed longitudinally during stimulated cycles and the PI and the maximum peak systolic velocity of the intra-ovarian and the uterine blood flow were measured. There were no detectable changes in Doppler measurements affecting the intra-ovarian blood flow. All flow velocity waveforms obtained from intra-ovarian vessels [10] showed a low resistance with continuous end-diastolic component. The highest individual PI value was less than 1.1. It is suggested that the plateau seen in the Doppler parameters of the intra-ovarian blood flow may be explained by the small perifollicular vessels in the ovary that appear to offer minimal resistance to blood flow. This operates as if they are maximally dilated [11] and consequently, once the optimal flow conditions are achieved, further changes in endocrine profile may not be reflected in the Doppler parameters of the ovarian blood flow. Secondly, the endocrine profile in IVF therapy with GnRH-a differs from that in spontaneous cycles, the most important feature being the lack of the physiological LH surge prior to the follicular aspiration; therefore the cyclic changes seen in Doppler parameters taken during spontaneous cycles do not necessarily occur during the stimulation protocol used in IVF. Thus, the PI and PSV (peak systolic velocity) values of the blood flow [12] in these arteries were much lower than those of the uterine artery. In addition, as a consequence of angiogenesis, the perifollicular blood vessels have a different vessel wall structure [13] from that of uterine artery. It was noted [14] that the detection rate of blood vessels around the developing follicles was 34% during suppression with GnRH-a compared with 86% at the time of follicular aspiration. The low detection rate of the intra-ovarian vascularity during the suppression period shows a novel effect

In addition, the indices of the blood flow at a given site within the leading follicle have been monitored by transvaginal color Doppler imaging over the periovulatory period. Campbell and his colleagues assessed the intraovarian blood flow in relation to ovarian morphology and function during the periovulatory period [6]. They studied 10 women with apparently normal ovarian function awaiting treatment for infertility by IVF-ET during subsequent natural cycles. The main outcome measures were the PI and the maximum peak systolic velocity from vessels within the dominant follicle, the maximum follicular diameters, and serum FSH, LH, and progesterone levels. There was an apparent increase in the intrafollicular blood flow over the periovulatory period, with an insignificant trend toward lower values for the mean PI and a significant increase in the peak systolic velocity. These changes appeared to follow the rise in circulating LH. The increase in the peak systolic velocity and the relatively constant PI suggested a marked increase in blood flow at this time during the ovarian cycle and might herald impending ovulation.

Others have examined the uterine and ovarian perfusion during the periovulatory period [7]. The researchers measured the flow velocity of the uterine, radial, spiral, and ovarian arteries during the periovulatory period in spontaneous and induced ovarian cycles with confirmed ovulation in 78 patients attending an infertility clinic because of a male factor of infertility. They demonstrated that ovarian flow velocity had a RI of 0.52 on the day before ovulation in the group with spontaneous cycles and 0.51 in the group with stimulated cycles. The value for the RI tended to decrease, whereas blood velocity tended to increase during the day after ovulation. A nadir of 0.46 was reached one day after ovulation in the group with spontaneous cycles and of 0.43 in the group with stimulated cycles. However, there were no statistically significant differences in the results between spontaneous and stimulated cycles.

of the pituitary desensitization when ovaries are in a resting state with no folliculogenesis.

The basic keystone of the hemodynamic regulation of the intra-ovarian blood flow is the accentuation of the blood perfusion of the ovaries during hormonal stimulation. This augmentation in perfusion is demonstrated by an increasing number of vessels around the developing follicles and the acceleration in the peak velocity of the blood flow in the uterine and intra-ovarian arteries [15]. Some authors proposed correlating the ultrasound-derived indexes of the blood flow in individual follicles (PSV and PI) on the day of but before the administration of hCG with the subsequent recovery of the oocytes and the production of preimplantation embryos. Nargund and colleagues [16] studied data obtained from 20 women undergoing IVF-ET. The peak systolic velocity was higher (12.7 cm/s) in follicles that were associated with the production of an embryo than in those that were not (8.5 cm/s). The probability of producing a grade I or II embryo was 75% if the PSV was more than 10 cm/s, 40% if it was less than 10 cm/s, and 24% if blood flow was not detected. They concluded that the value for PSV before the administration of hCG can be used to identify follicles with a high probability of producing an oocyte and a high-grade preimplantation embryo. They also emphasized that this information may also be used to time the administration of hCG to achieve the optimum number and quality for patient management. However, there was no clear difference in either PI or PSV [17] values between pregnant and nonpregnant women, making prediction of the outcome of the treatment not feasible with Doppler.

The detection and quantification of follicular vascularity with pulsed color Doppler can be used to predict oocyte recovery rate and hence may be useful in determining the most appropriate time to administer hCG. In order to optimize oocyte recovery rates Oyesanya and colleagues [18] have studied the intraovarian blood flow in a prospective longitudinal study of women undergoing IVF-ET and having at least 20 follicles between the two ovaries on the day of hCG administration, aiming to detect and qualify the follicular vascularity before hCG administration and then correlate this vascularity with oocyte recovery rate. They used "the follicular vascularity index," which is the ratio of the number of follicles demonstrating pulsatile vascularity to the total number of follicles, and also measured the intraovarian PSV, PI, and follicular diameter. The follicular vascularity index correlated positively with oocyte recovery rate, while the PSV and the PI did not show any significant changes and did not correlate with the oocyte recovery.

It was assumed that high-grade follicular vascularity is associated with increased pregnancy rate and that there is a possible link between follicular vascularity and implantation potential. Moreover, the pregnancy rate in women undergoing IVF would be expected to be increased by selection for transfer of embryos derived from follicles with high PSV. Conversely, pregnancy rates would be expected to decrease in cycles where the follicular PSV is universally poor. Chui et al. [12], in their prospective study on 38 women undergoing IVF-ET, tested the ability of power Doppler ultrasonography to assess the relationship between follicular vascularity and outcome in women undergoing IVF-ET, in addition to measuring the conventional PI of the uterine and intraovarian arteries. They assessed the vascularity of the individual follicles by power Doppler on the day of oocyte collection using a subjective grading system. The grading system consisted of assessing the percentage of the follicular circumference in which most flow was identified from a single cross-area slice, and the quality of follicular flow was graded from 1 to 4 according to the amount of visible color flow around the follicle. The grading is lowest if the flow is detected in <25% of the circumference and highest if flow is identified in 100% of the circumference. Pregnancies that were observed in the study were confined to those women whose embryos were derived from follicles with grades 3 and 4 vascularity. Coulam et al. [19], in an attempt to predict the factors affecting pregnancy after IVF-ET, studied 106 women undergoing IVF treatment for infertility who were considered to be at risk of failure (more than 37 years old, history of low response to gonadotropin stimulation, or multiple failed IVF cycles). They measured the PSV from the largest three follicles on the day of hCG administration. Clinical pregnancies resulted in 10% of the 106 high-risk women. Women who had PSV more than 10 cm/s in at least one follicle on the day of hCG administration more often became pregnant than those with PSV less than 10 cm/s. All pregnancies occurred in women with grade 3 or 4 follicular blood flow.

It is evident that there is a developmentally relevant association between follicular oxygen content and embryo implantation potential, in which a significant increase in pregnancy rate occurred when morphologically equivalent 6- to 10-cell-stage embryos were selected for uterine transfer on the basis of either the dissolved oxygen content of the follicles or color Doppler ultrasonographic characteristics of the follicle suggestive of a well-developed perifollicular microvasculature. This may aid in identification of healthy follicles with a high probability of containing oocytes free of cytoplasmic or chromosomal/spindle defects. Van Blerkom et al. [20] looked at the association between the chromosome/spindle normality of the mature oocyte and the dissolved oxygen content, vascular endothelial growth factor concentration, and perifollicular blood flow characteristics of the corresponding ovarian follicles. The findings from more than 1000 samples of follicular fluid show that developmentally significant differences in dissolved oxygen occur in follicular fluids aspirated from follicles of equivalent size and sonographic appearance. Oocytes from severely hypoxic follicles were associated with high frequencies of abnormalities of the organization of the chromosomes on the metaphase spindle that could lead to segregation disorders and catastrophic mosaics in the early embryo. After measuring the RI, peak systolic velocity, and the pattern of vascularity around each follicle, they divided the follicles into two types, "A" or "B." Type A follicles had well-developed perifollicular vasculature with RI <0.5 and dissolved oxygen content more than 3%. The oocytes resulting from these follicles displayed significantly lower frequency of abnormalities in chromosomal organization on the metaphase II (MII) spindle, and the resulting embryos exhibited a higher capacity to develop to the 6- to 8-cell stages after 54–60 hours of culture. Type B follicles demonstrated no measurable blood flow with RI >0.65 and the dissolved oxygen content was <1.5%. These oocytes displayed significantly higher frequency of abnormalities in chromosomal organization on the MII spindle, and the resulting embryos exhibited a lower capacity for development beyond the 4-cell stage in vitro. The hypoxic intrafollicular conditions that result from the failure of an appropriate microvasculature to develop around the growing or preovulatory follicle could be the proximate cause of the maternal age-related increase in the incidence of trisomic conditions [21]. In addition, when compared with oocytes with normal cytoplasm, MII oocytes with severe cytoplasmic disorganization have a lower pH and ATP content [22] and exhibited comparatively high frequencies of chromosomal and scattering aneuploidy.

Key points in clinical practice

- The display of blood flow across the whole scanning plane of the pelvis is probably the most important advantage of transvaginal color Doppler. As such the pulsed Doppler sample volume can be placed very precisely on the color flow of interest and spectral waveform analysis easily achieved.

- Studying the intraovarian blood flow may be of value in prediction of the ovulation process and can increase the precision and efficacy of some of the assisted reproductive techniques.

- Measuring the RI, the PI, and blood flow of the uterine arteries during the menstrual cycle can provide a better tool for prediction of good-quality follicles.

- The noninvasive Doppler technique offers great potential in the assessment of the physiology of hemodynamic regulation of spontaneous and induced cycles; its clinical impact on daily practice in IVF programs is variable.

- Oocyte/embryo selection for transfer may benefit from a brief color Doppler examination of each follicle at aspiration and pooling of oocytes with respect to follicles with type A to C characteristics.

Conclusion

Indices of the intraovarian blood flow at a given site within the leading follicle can be monitored by transvaginal color Doppler imaging during the periovulatory period. The increase in the peak systolic velocity and the relatively constant PI suggest a marked increase in blood flow at this time during the ovarian cycle, and this might herald impending ovulation. The blood flow changes that occur before ovulation indicate the complexity of the changes and may involve angiogenesis as well as hormonal factors. Nevertheless, the general consensus of studies of the intraovarian blood flow by color

Doppler using various parameters shows that the blood flow indexes alone (PI and RI) are of very significant value, and that there is a physiological relationship between follicular vascularity and oocyte recovery and the production of a high-grade preimplantation embryo. Ovarian blood flow correlates well with oocyte recovery rates and hence may be useful in determining the most appropriate time to administer hCG in order to optimize oocyte recovery rate. Furthermore, high-grade follicular vascularity also correlates well with high-grade preimplantation embryos, so it might represent a new parameter for predicting the outcome of assisted conception therapy by selecting for transfer those embryos derived from follicles with the highest grade of vascularization. Likewise, it may be appropriate to counsel patients as to the advisability of proceeding with oocyte collection in cycles where the follicular vascularity is universally poor.

References

1. Coveney D, Cool J, Oliver T, Capel B. Four-dimensional analysis of vascularisation during primary development of an organ, the gonad. *Proc Natl Acad Sci USA* 2008; **105**(20): 7212–17.

2. Guerriero S, Ajossa S, Melis G. Luteal dynamics during the human menstrual cycle: new insight from imaging. *Ultrasound Obstet Gynecol* 2005; **25**(5): 425–7.

3. Ottander U, Solensten N, Bergh A, Olofsson J. Intra-ovarian blood flow measured with color Doppler ultrasonography inversely correlates with vascular density in the human corpus luteum of the menstrual cycle. *Fertil Steril* 2004; **81**(1): 154–9.

4. Jokubkiene L, Sladkevicius P, Rovas L, Valentin L. Assessment of changes in volume and vascularity of the ovaries during the normal menstrual cycle using three-dimensional power Doppler ultrasound. *Hum Reprod* 2006; **21**(10): 2661–8.

5. Tekay A, Martikainen H, Jouppilas P. Blood flow changes in uterine and ovarian vasculature and predictive value of transvaginal pulsed

color Doppler ultrasonography in an in vitro fertilization program. *Hum Reprod* 1996; **10**: 688–93.

6. Campbell S, Bourne TH, Waterstone J, et al. Transvaginal color flow imaging of the peri-ovulatory follicle. *Fertil Steril* 1993; **60**(3): 433–8.

7. Kurjak A, Kupesic S, Schulman H, et al. Transvaginal color flow Doppler in the assessment of ovarian and uterine blood flow in infertile women. *Fertil Steril* 1991; **56**: 870–3.

8. Lunenfeld E, Schwartz I, Meizner I, Potashnik G, Glezerman M. Intra-ovarian blood flow during spontaneous and stimulated cycles. *Hum Reprod* 1996; **11**(11): 2481–3.

9. Kupesic S, Kurjak A. Uterine and ovarian perfusion during the peri-ovulatory period assessed by transvaginal color Doppler. *Fertil Steril* 1993; **60**(3): 439–43.

10. Balakier H, Stronell RD. Color Doppler assessment of folliculogenesis in vitro fertilization patients. *Fertil Steril* 1994; **62**(6): 1211–16.

11. Tekay A, Martikainen H, Jouppilas P. The clinical

value of transvaginal color Doppler ultrasound in assisted reproductive technology procedure. *Hum Reprod* 1996; **11**: 1589–93.

12. Chui D, Pugh N, Walker S, Gregory L, Shaw R. Follicular vascularity – the predictive value of transvaginal power Doppler ultrasonography in an in vitro fertilization program: A preliminary study. *Hum Reprod* 1997; **12**(1): 191–6.

13. Wiltbank M, Gallagher K, Christensen A, Brabec R, Keyes P. Physiological and immunocytochemical evidence for a new concept of blood flow regulation in the corpus luteum. *Biol Reprod.* 1990; **42**(1): 139–49.

14. Bassil S, Wyns C, Toussaint-Demylle D, Nisolle M, Gordts S, Donnez J. The relationship between ovarian vascularity and the duration of stimulation in in-vitro fertilization. *Hum Reprod* 1997; **12**(6): 1240–5.

15. Nakagawa K, Ohgi S, Kojima R, et al. Reduction of perifollicular arterial blood flow resistance after hCG administration is a good indicator of the recovery of mature oocytes in ART treatment. *J Assist Reprod Genet.* 2006; **23**(11–12): 433–8.

16. Nargund G, Doyle PE, Bourne TH, et al. Ultrasound derived indices of follicular blood flow before HCG administration and prediction of oocyte recovery and pre-implantation embryo quality. *Hum Reprod* 1996; **11**(11): 2512–17.

17. Costello M, Shrestha S, Sjoblom P, et al. Power Doppler ultrasound assessment of ovarian perifollicular blood flow in women with polycystic ovaries and normal ovaries during in vitro fertilization treatment. *Fertil Steril* 2005; **83**(4): 945–54.

18. Oyesanya O, Parsons J, Collins W, Campbell S. Prediction of oocyte recovery rate by transvaginal and color Doppler imaging before human chorionic gonadotropin administration in in-vitro fertilization cycles. *Fertil Steril* 1996; **65**(4): 806–9.

19. Coulam C, Goodman C, Rinehart J. Color Doppler indices of follicular blood flow as predictors of pregnancy after in vitro fertilization and embryo transfer. *Hum Reprod* 1999; **14**(8): 1979–82.

20. Van Blerkom J, Antezak M, Schrader R. The developmental potential of the human oocyte is related to the dissolved oxygen content of follicular fluid: association with vascular endothelial growth factor levels and perifollicular blood flow characteristics. *Hum Reprod* 1997; **12**(5): 1047–55.

21. Gaulden M. Maternal age effect: the enigma of Down syndrome and other trisomic conditions. *Mutat Res* 1992; **296**(1–2): 69–88.

22. Van Blerkom J, Davis P, Alexander S. Inner mitochondrial membrane potential (DeltaPsim), cytoplasmic ATP content and free Ca^{2+} levels in metaphase II mouse oocytes. *Hum Reprod* 2003; **18**(11): 2429–40.

Chapter 15

Ultrasonography of pelvic endometriosis

Juan A. Garcia-Velasco, Maria Cerrillo and Lia Ornat

Introduction

Endometriosis is a benign disease, although chronic in its development, characterized by the presence of ectopic endometrium outside of the uterine cavity. The prevalence may vary according to the population studied as well as the method used to diagnose it. Basically, we may say that endometriosis affects 12% of the female population during their fertile age [1]. Several factors seem to favor development of the disease, such as early menarche, nulliparity, Asian or European ethnic origin, or a family history of endometriosis [2].

There are two distinct clinical entities regarding uterine involvement:

1. Internal endometriosis or adenomyosis (endometrial tissue within the myometrial wall).

2. External endometriosis (endometriotic foci outside of the uterine cavity), the ovaries and the peritoneal serosa (utero-sacral ligaments, plica vesicouterine, and the Douglas pouch) being the most frequent locations; less frequent locations are the vagina, urinary tract, gastrointestinal tract – most commonly in the lower intestine – lungs, brain, and skin.

Clinical symptoms

From the clinical point of view, endometriosis is characterized by the lack of correlation between intensity of the symptoms and the extent and severity of the endometriotic lesions.

Pain is the main clinical symptom of endometriosis, which may be present as dysmenorrheal pain (50–91%), dyspareunia (25–40%), chronic pelvic pain (10–25%), and/or dyschezia (5–10%). Pain may be associated or not with infertility.

At physical examination we may find a painful bimanual exploration, with induration of the pouch of Douglas, adnexal masses, and a fixed uterus.

The most common symptoms associated with unusual locations of endometriosis are thoracopleural pain, pleural effusion, pneumothorax or hemoptisis due to lung implants, headaches due to brain lesions, sciatic pain from retroperitoneal implants, cyclic pain in the umbilicus or the episiotomy area if there are cutaneous implants, or cyclic rectorrhagia when the gastrointestinal tract is affected.

The risk of malignant transformation of endometriotic lesions is thought to be less than 1%.

Classification

Endometriosis requires laparoscopy for a final diagnosis and classification. From the laparoscopy, the disease will be classified according to the 1985 American Fertility Society (AFS) classification into four stages, from stage I to stage IV, which is the most severe with the highest impact on fertility. The AFS was renamed the American Society for Reproductive Medicine (ASRM) in 1995, and in 1996 it revised the classification again [3]. This classification is based on the number of implants visible in the ovaries and the peritoneum (both superficial and deep implants), as well as on the presence of adhesions and obliteration of the posterior pouch; in addition, the appearance of the endometrial implants is classified as red, white, or black. However, this classification, though useful for describing the disease among physicians, was designed to estimate the probabilities of future fertility; its score does not correlate with pain or prognosis [4]. Even more, it does not consider the activity of the endometriotic lesions. Table 15.1 shows the ASRM classification.

Types

- **Peritoneal endometriosis:** Endometriotic foci in the peritoneal serosa that, according to their activity, may present as purple spots, red lesions, adhesions, yellowish dots, or hypervascularization areas.

- **Cystic endometriosis** (so-called "chocolate cysts"; also known as endometrioma): Hemorrhagic ovarian cysts with an inner wall of endothelial mucosa of normal appearance. It is one of the most frequent findings, and ultrasound here is an extremely useful tool to objectively establish the diagnosis (Figure 15.1).

- **Deep, infiltrating, nodular endometriosis:** Endometriotic lesions that penetrate at least 5 mm in the retroperitoneal space.

Diagnosis of endometriosis

The basis for a correct medical diagnosis including endometriosis is a detailed anamnesis and physical examination. However,

Ultrasonography in Reproductive Medicine and Infertility, ed. Botros R. M. B. Rizk. Published by Cambridge University Press. © Cambridge University Press 2010.

imaging technologies and specifically transvaginal ultrasound help tremendously in the diagnosis of gynecologic conditions as well as in disregarding normal physiological changes.

Although laparoscopy is still the "gold standard" for a definitive diagnosis of endometriosis [5] – as it requires visualization and biopsy of the lesions – imaging techniques such as ultrasound and magnetic resonance imaging (MRI) provide a great contribution to both diagnosis and follow-up of endometriosis. Transvaginal sonography (TVS) associated with color Doppler techniques offers a very precise diagnosis of ovarian endometriomas and bladder endometriotic foci. On the other hand, MRI has proven to be more precise in other locations, such as uterosacral ligaments, the vagina, and the intestinal tract [6].

For the diagnosis of ovarian endometrioma some authors [7] report very high sensitivity and specificity with TVS (92% and 97%, respectively), although some others [8] report lower values (81% and 91%, respectively). Table 15.2 summarizes the diagnostic capacity of TVS associated or not with color

Doppler [8,9,10]. Computerized tomography (CT) does not improve the diagnostic value of ultrasound. However, MRI allows a global evaluation of the pelvis and is especially attractive in deep lesions, although these can also be observed with the new high-resolution transrectal probes with 360° annular field. When ultrasound does not reach a conclusive result, MRI is indicated, if possible with IV contrast to differentiate between a solid mass and a hemorrhagic cyst. Contrast MRI will be able to distinguish benign lesions, avoiding the misdiagnosis of atypical endometriomas with ovarian cancer [11]. Bazot et al. [12] compared the accuracy of MRI and rectal endoscopic sonography (RES) for the diagnosis of deep pelvic endometriosis. They performed a longitudinal study of 88 patients referred for surgical treatment of deep endometriosis who had MRI and RES previous to surgical intervention. The authors found a higher sensitivity, specificity, and positive and negative predictive values of MRI compared with RES, except in colorectal endometriosis where they found no difference between the two imaging techniques. Recent new technology such as 3D ultrasound still has not improved the diagnostic capacity of conventional TVS, with similar sensitivity and specificity, although it may offer new possibilities in the near future [13] (Figures 15.2 and 15.3).

CA 125 is a nonspecific serum marker of pelvic inflammation. There have been efforts to correlate serum CA 125 levels with endometriosis, finding higher levels in women with endometriosis. However, in the early stages of the disease it has a very low sensitivity as a diagnostic test [14]. In a meta-analysis summarizing the results of 23 studies that compared serum levels of CA 125 with laparoscopic findings in women with endometriosis, it was concluded that serum CA 125 analysis has a poor diagnostic value in early disease stages. Thus, it is a poor diagnostic test, although some authors have claimed that it may be useful in monitoring treatment response as well as in the differential diagnosis from various ovarian cysts when ultrasound findings are not clear enough [15].

Table 15.1. ASRM Classification (Revised in 1996)

Stages:					
I	1–5				
II	6–15				
III	16–40				
IV	>40				
Peritoneum		Endometriosis	<1 cm	1–3 cm	>3 cm
		Superficial	1	2	4
		Deep	2	4	6
Right ovary		Superficial	1	2	4
		Deep	4	16	20
Left ovary		Superficial	1	2	4
		Deep	4	16	20
Cul-de-sac obliteration			Partial	4	
			Complete	40	
Ovary		Adherens	<1/3	1/3–2/3	>2/3
			Enclosure	Enclosure	Enclosure
	Right	Filmy	1	2	4
		Dense	4	8	16
	Left	Filmy	1	2	4
		Dense	4	8	16
Tube	Right	Filmy	1	2	4
		Dense	4	8	16
	Left	Filmy	1	2	4
		Dense	4	8	16

Table 15.2. Accuracy of TVS (%) in the diagnosis of endometriotic cyst with and without color Doppler

	Gray scale		Color Doppler	
	Sensitivity	Specificity	Sensitivity	Specificity
Kurjak (1994) [8]	84%	97%	99%	99%
Alcazar (1997) [9]	89%	91%	76%	89%
Guerriero (1998) [10]	81%	91%	90%	97%

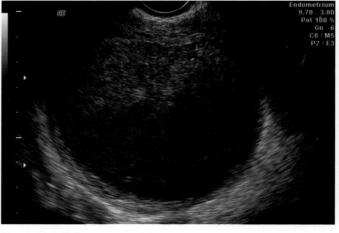

Figure 15.1. Endometrioma with homogeneous content.

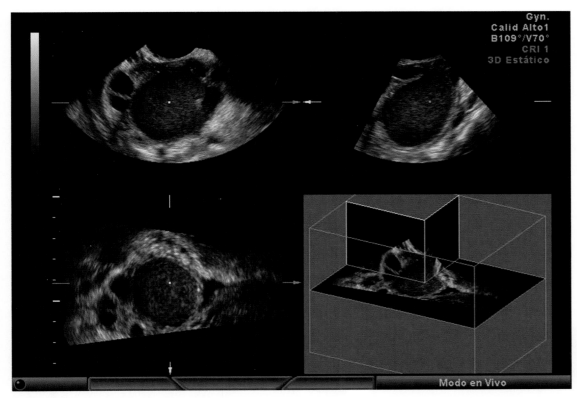

Figure 15.2. 3D image of ovary with endometriosis.

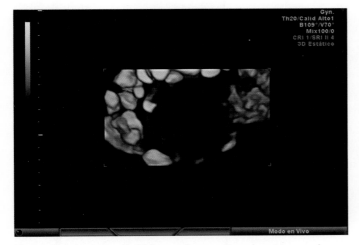

Figure 15.3. Inverse-mode 3D image of ovary with endometrioma and surrounding antral follicles.

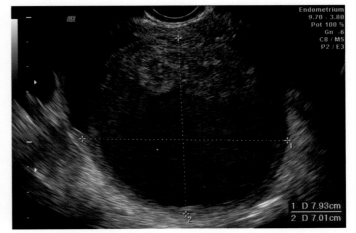

Figure 15.4. Endometrioma with inhomogeneous content.

Ultrasonographic characteristics of ovarian endometrioma

Ovarian cystic endometriosis – endometrioma – may present on ultrasonography as an easily identifiable hyper-refringent adnexal mass and the most frequent variation; as a cyst with heterogeneous, diffuse, low-level internal echoes and absence of particular neoplastic features (Figure 15.4); and with no

features of acute hemorrhage, multilocularity, or hyperechoic wall foci. We may find internal fluid levels, or even a cystic appearance with regular margins, precise limits, and absolutely sonolucent interior (the least frequent variation), which is difficult to diagnose as it may easily be misdiagnosed as functional ovarian cysts (16), such as luteinized unruptured follicle, hemorrhagic follicles, and/or corpus luteum (Figures 15.5, 15.6, 15.7, 15.8).

The characteristics of endometrioma are summarized in Table 15.3:

- Mostly unilocular cysts, sometimes multilocular, although not truly septate
- Sharp margins with the surrounding stroma
- Absence of papillae
- Absent or very limited color Doppler map in the interior
- Dense content without lineal tracts in the interior
- Very variable in size

Table 15.3. Typical features of ultrasound morphology of endometriomas

Oval mass
Hypoechoic content
Hyperechogenic wall
Absence of papillae

Generally speaking, a unilocular image in the ovary, especially if it is monolateral, under 5 cm in diameter, without septa or papillae, with very sparse vascularization independently of the density of the content, has very little possibility of being malignant. Doppler ultrasound is of great help in the differential diagnosis, as most endometriomas show the typical peripheral vascularization [7] whereas other show the "hilus sign" described by Kurjak [8], which is the presence of vessels between the cyst capsule and the ovarian parenchyma.

It has been demonstrated that, with gray scale, ultrasound can achieve a high degree of accuracy in the diagnosis of endometrioma. An adnexal mass with diffuse low-level internal echoes and absence of neoplastic features is highly likely to be an endometrioma if there are no features of acute hemorrhage. In one study [17] authors advised that in patients with suspected endometriomas and masses with low-level internal echoes, follow-up ultrasound appeared most useful when the mass did not have wall nodularity, when it was unilocular, and did

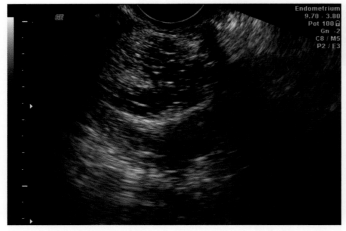

Figure 15.5. Dermoid cyst.

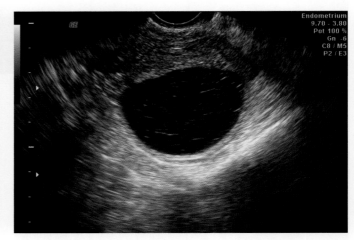

Figure 15.7. Luteinized unruptured follicle: luteinization signs.

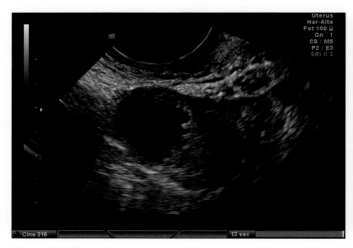

Figure 15.6. Corpus luteum.

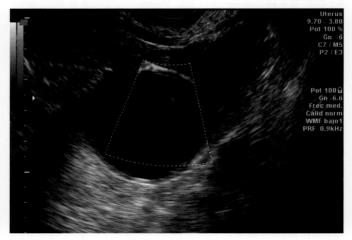

Figure 15.8. Hemorrhagic cyst.

Table 15.4. Atypial features of endometriomas

Septae
Inhomogeneous content
Irregular internal wall
Papillary projections

Table 15.5. Differential diagnosis of endometriotic cyst

	Endometrioma	Corpus luteum	Cystadenoma	Dermoid
Septae	Infrequent	No	Frequent	Infrequent
Inhomogeneous content	Infrequent	Present	Rare	Frequent
Posterior reinforcement	No	No	No	Frequent
Hyperechogenic dots	Frequent	No	No	No

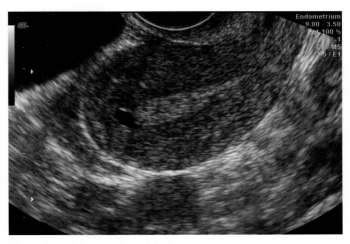

Figure 15.9. Adenomyosis: nodular image.

not possess hyperechoic wall foci, while MRI might be useful in discriminating between endometriomas and neoplasms when wall nodularity is present. Although all of these are typical characteristics of endometrioma, they sometimes may show atypical characteristics, as illustrated in Table 15.4.

The heterogeneous image of the ovarian endometrioma on TVS may require a careful differential diagnosis from other benign or malignant conditions of the ovary. For instance, dermoid cysts, cystoadenomas, or simple corpus luteum have to considered in the differential diagnosis, as these sometimes may share some of the characteristics shown in Table 15.5.

Endometriosis in atypical locations

Peritoneal implants are difficult to diagnose with TVS, especially if they are <1 cm, although on occasion they may be observed as hypoechogenic, avascular areas with poorly defined margins in the pouch of Douglas, in the bladder, or in the intestinal wall [10]. As mentioned previously, the evaluation of these lesions with TVU is quite complex, and MRI here shows markedly higher sensitivity and specificity.

The most frequent location in the pelvis is the posterior pelvis in the rectovaginal septum, although it may be present from the cervix to the rectum, invading parametrium and uterosacral ligaments. Different studies have tried to evaluate the diagnostic capacity of TVS in deep endometriosis. When ultrasonographic findings were compared with surgical findings and pathology reports, a low sensitivity (around 30%) was reported for vaginal or rectovaginal septum endometriosis, with a high rate of false negatives [18]. However, acceptable sensitivity and specificity were reported for bladder endometriosis (71% and 100%, respectively).

Different strategies have been implanted with the intention of improving the diagnostic efficacy of TVS, such as instilling serum into the vagina to distend it to allow proper evaluation

of its walls. Other authors have combined TVS with rectal contrast for the adequate diagnosis of rectovaginal endometriosis [19]. Comparing the ultrasonographic findings with surgical and pathology findings, sensitivity for detection of infiltration of the muscular wall of the rectum 100%, with a specificity of 85.7%, yielding a positive predictive value of 91.3% and negative predictive value of 100%. Although in 80% of the cases evaluated with TVS and rectal contrast the grade of rectal infiltration was underestimated, these authors consider that this may be an efficient method that is well tolerated by patients.

Adenomyosis

Ultrasound diagnosis of adenomyosis is not an easy task. We can differentiate two different types of ultrasound images, diffuse and nodular:

1. **Diffuse image:** this is the most frequently observed and it has some identifiable characteristics, such as

   - Widening of the anteroposterior uterine diameter, which mainly affects its posterior wall
   - Hypoechogenic striations that alternate with hyperechogenic striations from the endometrium to the myometrium
   - Loss of endometrium–myometrium border
   - Pain and hypersensitivity during ultrasound scan

2. **Nodular image:** this can be identified with more clarity and shows as hypoechogenic nodules in the myometrium (Figure 15.9).

The characteristic ultrasonographic images of adenomyosis are of hypoechogenic, heterogeneous areas within the myometrium. These areas may appear with or without anechoic lacunas of varying diameter. Power Doppler ultrasound shows an absence of vascularization in the interior, which helps in the differential diagnosis of possible vessels or uterine vascular dilations; also uterine leiomyomas with a

Table 15.6. Accuracy (%) of transvaginal sonography (TVS) and magnetic resonance imaging (MRI) in the diagnosis of adenomyosis

	Reinhold et al. [21,24]	Bazot et al. [22]	Dueholm et al. [23]	Total
TVS				
Sensitivity	89	65	68	74
Specificity	89	98	65	87
MRI				
Sensitivity	86	78	70	78
Specificity	86	93	86	88

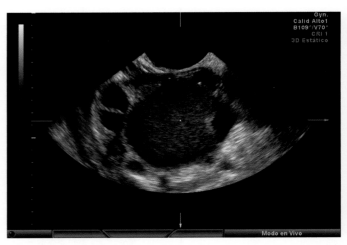

Figure 15.10. Endometrioma with healthy antral follicles in the periphery.

well-defined vascular ring around them are easily distinguishable from adenomyosis, where vessels are perpendicular to the myometrial wall.

The accuracy of ultrasound in the diagnosis of adenomyosis varies widely among operators, with sensitivity around 53–89% and specificity 50–99%. This great variability among studies and operators is due to the lack of universal diagnostic criteria of the disease. TVS is a good technique for diagnosis of adenomyosis in patients with clinical symptoms, although not so good for symptom-free patients with fibroids [20].

MRI has been compared with TVS to test their diagnostic capacity in three different studies [21,22,23] (Table 15.6). These studies enrolled patients undergoing hysterectomy immediately after the diagnosis, so that the diagnosis could be ratified by the pathologist. MRI proved to be superior, with lower interobserver variability than TVS, specially in premenopausal women.

Nevertheless, transvaginal ultrasonography carried out by experienced physicians was as effective as MRI, and it had the additional advantage of being lower in cost and more easily available than MRI [24].

Endometriosis and infertility

Recent reports suggest that 30–50% of women with endometriosis suffer from infertility, and endometriosis is associated with sterile patients in 25–50%.

We should remember that infertile women with endometriosis have a higher prevalence of associated functional images, such as unruptured luteinized follicles, hydrosalpinges, adenomyosis, and/or intraovarian endometriosis that may interfere with oocyte retrieval.

While doing the ultrasound evaluation of an infertile woman with endometriosis, we should pay special attention to the antral follicle count, which will very accurately reflect the status of her ovarian reserve, as endometriosis by itself may reduce it. We should also focus on the presence and localization of the endometriomas, considering whether they may complicate follicular development and later ovum pick-up (Figure 15.10). If possible, rule out pelvic adhesions due to advanced stages of the disease or previous surgery, which are

visualized as hyper- and hypoechogenic images with anechoic areas. In this type of patient, tubal involvement may be present, with tubal blockage or even hydrosalpinges, and impaired embryo implantation.

Postsurgical medical treatment is not recommended, as the first few months after surgery are the optimum for a higher monthly fecundity rate, and most treatment will inhibit ovulation.

There are no studies comparing surgical treatment with IVF as a primary treatment of women with advanced stages of the disease. Some studies have reported a lower ovarian response, with a higher dose of gonadotropins needed, in those women who underwent surgery for ovarian endometrioma compared with tubal surgery, but pregnancy and live birth rate were comparable [25]. Large endometriomas (>4 cm) may impede follicular growth, complicate egg retrieval, and have a higher risk of infectious complications in case of accidental puncture at ovum pick-up [26].

Key points in clinical practice

- A final diagnosis of endometriosis requires endometriotic lesion biopsy and pathology report.
- TVS offers a highly suggestive endometrioma diagnosis, with very high sensitivity and specificity.
- TVS is a first-line diagnostic technique, with enough capacity to differentiate the endometrioma from other adnexal masses.
- The role of TVS in the diagnosis of extraovarian endometriosis, an area where MRI has proved to be much more beneficial, is yet to be established.
- 3D ultrasound still requires further research to determine its role in the diagnosis of this disease.
- MRI offers a better suggestive diagnosis of adenomyosis than TVS due to its lower interobserver variability.

References

1. Barbieri RL. Etiology and epidemiology of endometriosis. *Am J Obstet Gynecol* 1990; **162**: 565–7.

2. Nargund G. Ovarian pathology. In: Nargund G, ed. *Avanced Ultrasound in Reproductive Medicine: A Theoretical and Practical Workshop.* London; HER Trust, 2006; 10–14.

3. Revised American Society for Reproductive Medicine Classification of Endometriosis: 1996. *Fertil Steril* 1997; **67**: 817–21.

4. Olive DL, Pritts EA. Treatment of endometriosis. *N Engl J Med* 2001; **345**: 266–75.

5. Brosens I, Puttemans P, Campo R, Gordts S, Kinkel K. Diagnosis of endometriosis: pelvis endoscopy and imaging techniques. *Best Pract Res Clin Obstet Gynaecol* 2004; **18**: 285–303.

6. Bazot M, Darai E, Hourani R, et al. Deep pelvis endometriosis: MR imaging for diagnosis and prediction of extension of disease. *Radiology* 2004; **232**: 379–89.

7. Valentin L. Imaging in gynecology. *Best Pract Res Clin Obstet Gynaecol* 2006; **20**: 881–906.

8. Kurjak A, Kupesic S. Scoring system for prediction of ovarian endometriosis based on transvaginal color and pulsed Doppler sonography. *Fertil Steril* 1994; **62**: 81–8.

9. Alcázar JL, Laparte C, Jurado M, López-García G. The role of transvaginal ultrasonography combined with color velocity imaging and pulsed Doppler in diagnosis of endometrioma. *Fertil Steril* 1997; **67**: 487–91.

10. Guerriero S, Ajossa S, Mais V, Risalvato A, Lai MP, Melis GB. The diagnosis of endometriomas using colour Doppler energy imaging. *Hum Reprod* 1998; **13**: 1691–5.

11. Wu TT, Coakley FV, Qayyum A, Yeh BM, Joe BN, Chen LM. Magnetic resonance imaging of ovarian cancer arising in endometriomas. *J Comput Assist Tomogr* 2004; **28**: 836–8.

12. Bazot M, Bornier C, Dubernard G, Roseau G, Cortez A, Darai E. Accuracy of magnetic resonance imaging and rectal endoscopic sonography for the prediction of location of deep pelvic endometriosis. *Hum Reprod* 2007; **22**: 1457–63.

13. Raine-Fenning N. Three-dimensional ultrasonographic characteristics of endometrioma. *Ultrasound Obstet Gynecol* 2008; **31**: 718–24.

14. Hornstein MD, Harlow BL, Thomas PP, Check JH. Use of a new CA 125 assay in the diagnosis of endometriosis. *Hum Reprod* 1995; **10**: 932–4.

15. Mol BW, Bayram N, Lijmer JG, et al. The performance of CA-125 measurement in the detection of endometriosis: a meta-analysis. *Fertil Steril* 1998; **70**: 1101–8.

16. Shwayer JM. Pelvic pain, adnexal masses, and ultrasound. *Sem Reprod Med* 2008; **26**: 252–65.

17. Patel M, Feldstein V, Chen D, Lipson S, Filly R. Endometriomas: diagnostic performance of US radiology 1999; **3**: 739–45.

18. Bazot M, Thomassin I, Hourani R, Cortez A, Darai E. Diagnostic accuracy of transvaginal sonography for deep pelvic endometriosis. *Ultrasound Obstet Gynecol* 2004; **24**: 180–5.

19. Menada MV, Remorgida V, Abbamonte LH, Fulcheri E, Ragni N, Ferrero S. Transvaginal ultrasonography combined with water-contrast in the rectum in the diagnosis of rectovaginal endometriosis infiltrating the bowel, *Fertil Steril* 2008; **89**: 699–700.

20. Dueholm M. Transvaginal ultrasound for diagnosis of adenomyosis: a review. *Best Pract Res Clin Obstet Gynaecol* 2006; **20**: 569–82.

21. Reinhold C, McCarthy S, Bret PM, et al. Diffuse adenomyosis: comparison of endovaginal US and MR imaging with histopathologic correlation. *Radiology* 1996; **199**: 151–8.

22. Bazot M, Cortez A, Darai E, et al. Ultrasonography compared with magnetic resonance imaging for diagnosis of adenomyosis. *Hum Reprod* 2001; **16**: 2427–33.

23. Dueholm M, Lundorf E, Hansen ES, Sørensen JS, Ledertoug S, Olesen F. Magnetic resonance imaging and transvaginal ultrasonography for the diagnosis of adenomyosis. *Fertil Steril* 2001; **76**: 588–94.

24. Reinhold C, Atri H, Mehio A, Akarian R, Ildis A, Bret P. Difusse uterine adenomiosis: morphologic criteria and diagnostic accuracy of endovaginal sonography. *Radiology* 1995; **197**: 609–14.

25. Al-Azemi M, Bernal AL, Steele J, Gramsbergen I, Barlow D, Kennedy S. Ovarian response to repeated controlled stimulation in in-vitro fertilization cycles in patients with ovarian endometriosis. *Hum Reprod* 2000; **15**: 72–5.

26. Garcia-Velasco JA, Somigliana E. Management of endometriomas in women requiring IVF: to touch or not to touch. *Hum Reprod* 2009; **24**(3): 496–501.

Chapter 16

Adenomyosis

Edward A. Lyons

Introduction

Adenomyosis is a common disorder defined by the presence of ectopic endometrial glands and stroma within the myometrium, as well as adjacent myometrial hyperplasia. It most typically presents with one or all of excessive menstrual bleeding, pelvic pain, or tenderness.

Pelvic pain and abnormal uterine bleeding are commonly seen in office and hospital gynecologic practices. The exact cause may be difficult to determine. Adenomyosis is a very common cause and must always be considered in the differential diagnosis. In a limited survey of our patients presenting with pelvic pain, adenomyosis based on established ultrasound criteria was the diagnosis in over 50% of cases.

Ultrasound in our university hospital referral practice has been very helpful in establishing the diagnosis of adenomyosis. Adenomyosis is a most frequent cause of pelvic pain and abnormal bleeding and is generally underdiagnosed and therefore not appropriately treated. Many women suffer for years because this diagnosis was not considered and because the diagnostic features on ultrasound are not well appreciated. In 2006 Bordman and Jackson [1] stated that the most common causes of chronic pelvic pain (CPP) were endometriosis, adhesions, interstitial cystitis, and irritable bowel syndrome. There was no mention of adenomyosis. Adenomyosis is only today emerging as a significant cause of CPP. I suspect but cannot prove that many cases of adenomyosis were misdiagnosed and subsequently treated as interstitial cystitis and irritable bowel, with little or no relief.

The cause of pelvic pain is best assessed during the ultrasound scan by the individual performing the scan. Only at that time can the tender organ be identified and the diagnosis established. Specific questioning of the patient is also essential in confirming the problematic symptoms and connecting them with the sonographic features. Unfortunately most physicians do not scan the patient themselves and have the procedure performed exclusively by a sonographer. Sonographers in general are limited in their skills of identifying organ tenderness and then asking the most appropriate questions to confirm the diagnosis. I have had many years of experience working closely with a large number of sonographers and have a good sense of who can or cannot do a complete study. There is an increasing trend for gynecologists to scan their own patients, but at present their ultrasound expertise varies widely. This may change over time with more experience.

Chronic pelvic pain is an unusually common problem in women. The usual criteria for CPP include pain of at least 6 months' duration, including pain within the last 3 months. Usually pregnant or postmenopausal patients and patients with pain related to menstruation or intercourse are excluded. In 2002, Stones and Price [2] reported an incidence of CPP of 14.7% (773/5263) from a telephone survey [3] of American women aged 18–50 and of 24% (483/2016) from a British postal survey from the Oxfordshire Health Authority [4]. There is seldom mention of adenomyosis as a possible diagnosis and consequently the opportunities for treatment are not even explored.

Ultrasound, and in particular endovaginal ultrasound, is a great tool for the identification of the cause of pelvic pain. The exception to this is the diagnosis of endometriosis, which is recognized only if there is an endometrioma presenting as a mass with typical sonographic features. The small superficial lesions seen throughout the peritoneal cavity on laparoscopy are not seen with the endovaginal probe because of a lack of contrasting density. The solid tissues of the bladder wall, bowel, and uterus do not provide any contrasting background for recognition of the endometriotic deposits. One sign that has been described but is not frequently used is the "sliding organ sign." In the presence of pelvic adhesions the pelvic organs do not slide freely over one another, whereas normally they do.

Diagnosis of adenomyosis

Clinical features

Clinically, adenomyosis is usually seen in women in their thirties but has been seen from the early twenties into the postmenopausal period. It can also be seen during pregnancy. It usually presents with pelvic pain that may be constant or associated with menses or intercourse. Bleeding is common, with most women having menorrhagia with clots and some metrorrhagia or postcoital bleeding.

The uterus on clinical examination is soft, tender, and bulky depending on the extent of the myometrial involvement.

Pathology

Pathologically, adenomyosis is confirmed if there are ectopic endometrial glands and stroma in the myometrium. This induces hyperplasia and hypertrophy of the adjacent smooth muscle, causing uterine enlargement. There is a spectrum of disease. It can be localized (adenomyoma) or generalized (adenomyosis) within the junctional zone or can extend right through to the serosal surface. Striations can be seen on the serosal surface at laparoscopy. The diagnosis is confirmed only if there is careful dissection of the uterus by the pathologist. We have followed several cases in which the ectopic glands were overlooked and only found after the specimen was scanned with ultrasound and the tissue re-sectioned in the area of interest. The incidence of adenomyosis is said to be between 8% and 40%, but may be even higher with careful and extensive sectioning at pathology.

The junctional zone or area just beneath the endometrium is the area most commonly found to have adenomyosis, and it is this area that is focused on by magnetic resonance imaging (MRI) to make the diagnosis. Tocci et al. [5] state that thickening of the junctional zone alone may be a new entity with specific and significant relation to infertility.

There is an association with pelvic endometriosis, but the contribution of each to the clinical symptoms is poorly understood [6].

Sonographic features of fibroids and adenomyosis.

The sonographic diagnosis of fibroids has long been confused with that of adenomyosis. For a better understanding of the distinctive differences, the sonographic features of each are outlined.

Typical sonographic features of fibroids

- More common in nulliparous women but seen in parous ones
- Distinct mass
- Hypoechoic periphery due to compressed myometrium
- Echogenicity will vary from hypoechoic, iso- or hyperechoic
- Cystic areas within the fibroid are uncommon
- Peripheral vascularity in general but some also have central vascularity
- Rarely tender to palpation except in pregnancy, torsion, and infarction
- Calcification

Typical sonographic features of adenomyosis

- Usually found in multiparous women
- Ill-defined areas
- Asymmetrical myometrial thickening

- Mixed echogenicity
- Cysts are common, often 3 mm in size in the endo-myometrial junction
- Central vascularity
- Irregular or streaky shadows
- Focal myometrial tenderness
- No calcification
- Obscure endo-myometrial junction

Fibroids

Leiomyomata or fibroids are common in women, with an increased incidence of 7 times in blacks and nulliparous women. They present more commonly with menorrhagia or symptoms of a pelvic mass. The diagnosis is made with ultra-sonography or MRI, although ultrasound is more common, more widely available, and less expensive. On endovaginal scanning the smaller fibroid is best detected during palpation of the uterus. The fibroid is firmer than the surrounding normal myometrium and stands out. Isoechoic fibroids can be overlooked if one is only viewing images after the scan and not involved in the actual scan. The hypoechoic periphery of compressed myometrium is best and sometimes only appreciated on endovaginal scans. Deep to the fibroid there is dense shadowing posterior to the mass (Figure 16.1).

Cystic changes in the fibroid are not common, and even when present may be overlooked if there is echogenic debris within the cyst. During the scan one can see movement of the echogenic debris by applying gentle pressure and release over the area.

Vascularity is usually seen to be peripheral. There are central vessels in fibroids that have a tendency to grow more rapidly.

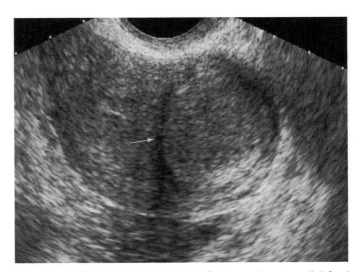

Figure 16.1. Fibroid. In this transverse scan of the uterus there is a well-defined mass on the left that has a typical hypoechoic zone at the periphery of the fibroid. This represents compressed myometrium or a pseudo-capsule.

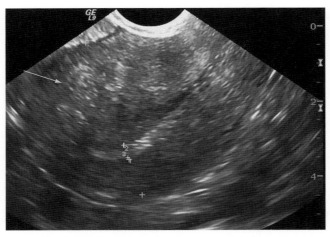

Figure 16.2. Asymmetrical myometrial thickening. In the body of the uterus in this sagittal scan, the anterior myometrium is twice the thickness of the posterior myometrium. Anteriorly the myometrium is more heterogeneous as well, with areas of increased density. (arrow).

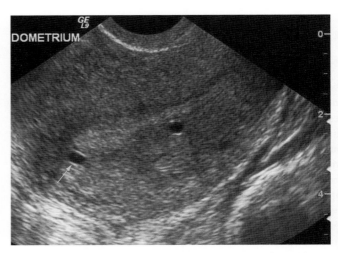

Figure 16.4. Small myometrial cysts (arrow) in the junctional zone. The myometrium is also heterogeneous.

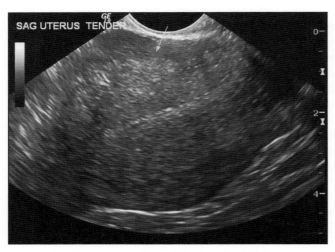

Figure 16.3. Myometrial heterogeneity. Areas of increased echodensity are seen anteriorly in the middle myometrium (arrow) extending down to the endometrium. This is also an area of focal tenderness. Changes are also seen posteriorly.

best appreciated with higher-resolution ultrasound scanners. There may also be areas of mixed echogenicity with or without cystic changes. Cysts are most commonly small and near the endo-myometrial junction (Figure 16.4). Typically they are 2–3 mm in diameter and may easily be overlooked. Larger cysts of 4–5 cm have been seen and followed for years as they enlarge further (Figure 16.5). Myometrial cysts that are not distended with fluid look like small nonshadowing echodensities. They are typically situated in the junctional zone but can also be seen in the middle layer of myometrium. With high-resolution imaging the front and back wall of the collapsed cyst may be demonstrated (Figure 16.6). The densities do not, as has previously been reported, represent scarring from previous intervention such as a dilatation and curettage.

Vascularity is seen throughout the abnormal area and, although we do not use its features for diagnosis, some have described an abnormal or distorted pattern of vascularity. This would be expected with the infiltrative nature of the disease process. The central vascular pattern is different from the peripheral one seen in fibroids.

Deep to the area of adenomyosis there are streaky shadows as opposed to the dense block of shadow of the fibroid. On the extreme lateral aspect of the uterus one may see a similar appearance of streaky shadowing that may not be due to adenomyosis (Figure 16.7).

The adenomyotic tissue is not known to calcify, so that the presence of calcification would not be expected and may be due to an associated fibroid.

The uterus is usually but not always tender in patients with adenomyosis. This tenderness is usually localized over the area of involvement but if it is extensive it may be quite generalized. In patients who also report dyspareunia, the tenderness elicited by the examining probe should approximate the same pain as felt during intercourse.

Finally, the endo-myometrial junction or junctional zone is thickened and may be obscured on ultrasound (Figure 16.8). This sign is also used in MRI.

Calcification may be central or peripheral and has been described as flocculent.

It is important to identify focal tenderness and the tender organ in patients presenting with pelvic pain. Fibroids in my experience are *not* the source of tenderness except in rare cases of infarction or with a more common red degeneration of pregnancy.

It is important to know the sonographic features of both fibroids and adenomyosis.

Adenomyosis

Adenomyosis is a diffuse infiltrative process and appears as asymmetrical myometrial thickening often in the body of the uterus (Figure 16.2). The myometrium has areas of increased echogenicity (Figure 16.3) that may be subtle and

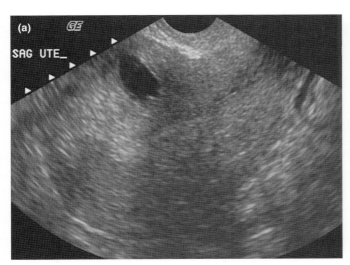

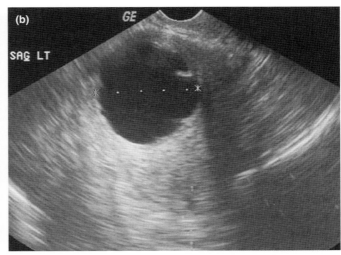

Figure 16.5. Large irregular myometrial cyst in the anterior uterine body. It was seen as an irregular 2 cm cyst (a) and grew over a 3-year period to 4 cm. (b). It was proven at hysterectomy to be an adenomyotic cyst. The patient also had pain, tenderness, and menorrhagia.

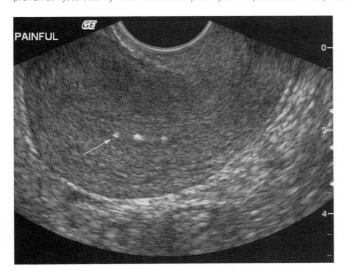

Figure 16.6. Collapsed cysts appear as focal densities (arrow) at the endo-myometrial junction.

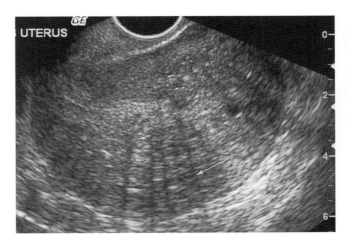

Figure 16.7. Streaky shadows are typical of adenomyosis. They appear posterior to the affected area, as in this sagittal scan of a retroverted uterus.

Sonohysterography in adenomyosis

In a recently reported study by Verma et al. [7], the authors reviewed a group of patients who had had MRI as well as saline sonohysterography (SIS). They saw tracks of fluid extending from the endometrial canal into the myometrium in 26% of cases and attributed the tracks to the dilated ducts of ectopic endometrial glands that communicate with the cavity (Figure 16.9). These tracks may be more apparent during an SHS because of the increased intrauterine pressure that is created using a balloon catheter. I personally have seen small tracks in only one case but do not doubt their results or interpretation.

The diagnosis of adenomyosis

The diagnosis should not depend only on the sonographic appearance but must rather consider the whole picture or triad of history, sonographic features, and signs of tenderness.

A positive history of bleeding, especially with clots, pain, and uterine tenderness is important to the diagnosis and to whether or not treatment is required. The demonstration of focal uterine tenderness with the endovaginal probe is also very helpful if present but does not rule out the diagnosis if it is absent. Over 80% of patients in our pathological study had a positive history, sonographic features, and physical findings of tenderness. Remember that the treatment is only to manage the symptoms.

If a patient has never had any symptoms but has the typical sonographic features of adenomyosis, does she actually have the condition? She would not require therapy as she is asymptomatic. Will she eventually develop symptoms? Should she be labeled as having adenomyosis and if so will it have any adverse effect? I have recently seen two women who had sonography as part of a research study on pelvic ultrasound (Figure 16.10). Both are 40–45 years old and have similar sonographic features of adenomyosis. One has had two children and has never had any symptoms or menstrual irregularities at all, while the other has had three children and has had such severe pain and

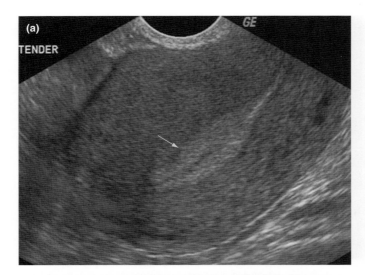

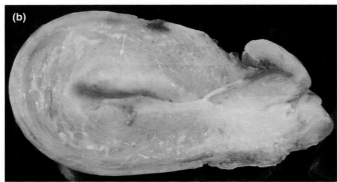

Figure 16.8. Obscured endo-myometrial junction (arrow) on sagittal sonography. (a) This 33-year-old with menorrhagia, hypermenorrhea, and pelvic pain also had thickening of the junctional zone seen in the bisected uterus (b) (arrow).

menorrhagia that she required a hysterectomy to provide complete symptom relief.

The modality of choice

Ultrasonography could and should be the imaging modality of choice for the diagnosis of adenomyosis. This is a rather bold statement but one that I strongly feel is true. There is a caveat, however, and that involves the person doing the scan and the equipment being used. The scan must be performed using the transvaginal probe. The probe must use a frequency at or above 5 MHz. The person doing the scan and the one reporting it must be trained and knowledgeable about the sonographic features of adenomyosis.

The MRI diagnosis of adenomyosis is reported in the literature and is generally considered to be the gold standard, with thickening of the junctional zone as the hallmark. The key to MRI is that it is more objective and therefore not as operator-dependent as is transvaginal ultrasound.

Uterine tenderness is a hallmark of adenomyosis and can only be assessed using endovaginal ultrasound and not by MRI. It is most important that the one doing the scan must examine the uterus with the probe, looking specifically for areas of focal

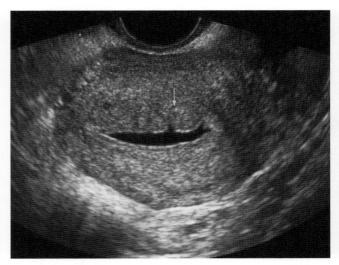

Figure 16.9. Distended ectopic endometrial gland duct tracks. Transverse scan of the body of the uterus with the endometrial canal distended with saline under pressure. A dilated duct is seen anteriorly (arrow); others may also be present on the lateral aspect of the canal.

uterine tenderness. You must ask "Does this hurt?" as you are probing the uterus. This cannot be done without a vaginal probe and without actually talking to the patient. It is insufficient for the sonographer simply to infer that the uterus was not tender because the patient did not volunteer the information. You must also differentiate actual pain and tenderness from a sense of deep pressure, which is a normal response. Remember that apparent tenderness of the uterus can be due to a generalized pelvic tenderness from a variety of causes, including inflammation of the bowel behind the uterus or even tenderness of the pelvic floor muscles. Uterine tenderness is a hallmark of adenomyosis, but uterine tenderness may be due to endometritis in certain clinical situations, and a nontender uterus does not rule out adenomyosis.

Accuracy of diagnosis

In an unpublished ultrasound-pathology study of 28 patients by our group, the accuracy of diagnosis of adenomyosis was 93%. This was achieved by doing ultrasound on the excised uterus and directing the pathologist to the suspicious areas. In several cases the adenomyosis was missed and only appreciated once the specimen was re-scanned and further sections obtained. In 1996 Reinhold et al. reported an ultrasound sensitivity of 89% [8]. In a recent meta-analysis of the accuracy of diagnosis, Meredith et al. showed a likelihood ratio of 4.67 (95% CI) and an overall probability of adenomyosis with an abnormal scan of 66.2% [9].The problem with this analysis is that it collected studies done from 1966 to 2007, when there was not widespread acceptance of the true value of ultrasound diagnosis of adenomyosis.

Prevalence of adenomyosis

A prospective pathological study by Yeniel et al. from Turkey found an incidence of adenomyosis on histopathology of 36.2% of all 298 cases [10]. There was a higher incidence of pelvic pain,

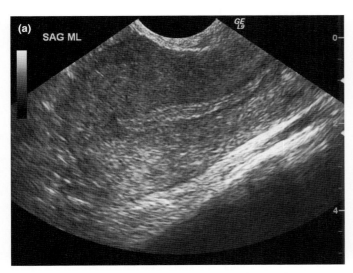 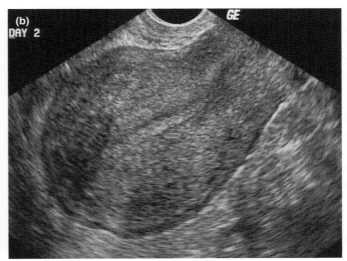

Figure 16.10. Comparison of two patients. Mid-sagittal scans of two women with similar sonographic changes of areas of increased echodensity in the body anteriorly. The patient in (a) was completely asymptomatic while the one in (b) had all the classical symptoms and required hysterectomy.

dysmenorrhea, and dyspareunia compared with the non-adenomyosis group. Both groups had a high incidence of fibroids but with no difference between the groups.

Gordts et al., in *Reproductive Biomedicine Online* [6], suggest that recent studies indicate that adenomyosis is a progressive disease that changes in appearance during the reproductive years. They also call for a consensus classification of uterine adenomyosis that is urgently required.

There is a familial incidence of endometriosis of 7 times compared with controls [11]. Does this also hold true with adenomyosis? We have seen several families, some symptomatic and others not, but all with sonographic evidence of adenomyosis. I suspect there is an increased incidence.

The incidence of adenomyosis in the adolescent and pediatric population is unknown but it is presumably uncommon. Ho et al. reported a case of an 18-year-old with pelvic pain who had MRI and pathological features of an adenomyotic cyst [12].

Gerson Weiss et al. [13] even go so far as to say in a recent article that adenomyosis is not a disease but a variant. They also report an incidence that ranges from 8.8% to 61.5%, although these studies were based on pathology. In their 10-year multisite, multiethnic, community-based follow-up study, from 239 of the 3103 study patients who had incidental hysterectomies, 137/239 (57%) provided consent and had information about the surgical pathology. Of these patients 48% (66/137) had evidence of adenomyosis. Extent of the adenomyosis was not recorded. Pathological detection of adenomyosis depends on a scrupulous search for foci of involvement, not something that is commonly done. We have scanned uteri after the initial sectioning and have found areas that would not have been detected without further cuts. My concern is that the range of community-based pathologists may not have been able to detect the true incidence and extent of adenomyosis. These patients had surgery for a reason, so that the conclusion should

have been that "in women with symptoms severe enough to require hysterectomy, the incidence of adenomyosis was 46%."

Gerson Weiss also states that "adenomyosis is not a determinant of chronic pelvic pain in patients with or without fibroids." I cannot agree. In our experience, fibroids are not tender, with the exception of fibroids in pregnancy or the rare case of infarction. This is based on actually palpating the fibroid with the endovaginal probe during the ultrasound examination and asking the question, "Does this hurt?" I personally have seen only one case of a painful fibroid in hundreds of patients aged over 40 years.

The true incidence of adenomyosis in humans of all ages has yet to be determined. There is also the question whether it exists in other species. A recent case was reported of an orangutan with menorrhagia and proven adenomyosis following subtotal hysterectomy [14]. There was no mention, nor is there likely any way of knowing, whether she also had dysmenorrhea or dyspareunia.

Adenomyosis and infertility

Not much has been written about adenomyosis and infertility in the absence of endometriosis. The diagnosis of adenomyosis by ultrasound is relatively recent. Adenomyosis has been suspected as a cause of infertility. We have studied myometrial contractility in normal patients as well as in those with adenomyosis. We have found a distorted pattern of contractility in adenomyosis where the contraction wave begins at mid-cycle at the cervix but then travels into the middle layer of the myometrium at a site of adenomyosis rather than extending up to the fundus and then down the fallopian tube. We have recorded contraction waves in the uterus but not actually down the tube [15]. There is evidence that it is these contraction waves that transport the sperm from the vaginal vault to the distal third of the fallopian tube and not the action of the tail of the sperm. Most notably, a sperm will reach the distal tube in vivo in 5–15 minutes, whereas in the excised uterus this takes 70 minutes. This is a speed of 2.5 mm/min, which is the same rate of travel seen with a sperm on a glass slide. In addition, carbon particles [16] and radio-labeled albumin macroaggregates will also be seen in the distal tube within 20–28 minutes and they clearly do not possess any means for independent motion. It must then be the action of the myometrial contraction waves that propels inert objects as well as sperm. An interruption of this action should therefore have an adverse effect on sperm travel and their success in fertilization.

Treatment of adenomyosis

Medical treatment

The treatment of adenomyosis is mainly symptomatic. That is "treat the patient not the "disease." There are patients with classical imaging findings of adenomyosis who have absolutely no symptoms and no pain, excess bleeding, or tenderness. These obviously do not need therapy. Will they ever need treatment? Will the condition progress or regress and if so what are the influences that will promote this? These are all good questions that need to be answered so as to better understand whether adenomyosis is actually a "disease." If it is so prevalent, how can it be abnormal? What is the true incidence of symptomatic and asymptomatic adenomyosis in different countries and different regions and in different groups of within country?

In treating the symptoms of excess bleeding, more physicians are relying on a levonorgestrel-releasing intrauterine system, (LNg-IUS), even though it is not formally recognized and approved for this use today [17]. Its approval is actually based on its contraceptive capability. The levonorgestrel acts locally within the myometrium to shrink the ectopic endometrial tissue and decrease the symptoms of bleeding and pain. This may also decrease the need for hysterectomies that are being done solely as a treatment for menorrhagia. In a group of 47 patients with a *clinical* diagnosis of adenomyosis followed for 36 months, Cho et al. found that "the LNg-IUS is effective for the reduction of uterine volume with improvement of vascularity and relief of symptoms. However, the efficacy of LNg-IUS on uterine volume may begin to decrease 2 years after insertion." [18].

For years clinicians have used androgens to suppress ovarian function and reduce the symptoms of adenomyosis. Oral Danazol (Danocrine) and the injectable form of a GnRH agonist such as leuprolide acetate (Lupron depot; Abbott Pharmaceuticals, Mississauga, Ontario, Canada) were also commonly used. This has been successful but is not without its side effects of weight gain and excessive hair growth. Women often take the medication until the symptoms subside and then stop.

Oral contraceptives can also be used to decrease the bleeding. Some herbal remedies have also been used but there are no good studies of the dose or monitoring with imaging.

None of these therapeutic approaches will help the patient who is trying to conceive. They may provide temporary relief, but how that will affect future fertility has not been well studied.

Surgical treatment

For years before the diagnosis could be made with ultrasound or MRI, the definitive treatment was hysterectomy, with the diagnosis being established at pathology.

There are those who have treated adenomyosis with laparoscopic resection of areas of affected myometrium. The series are small and long-term follow-up is not generally reported.

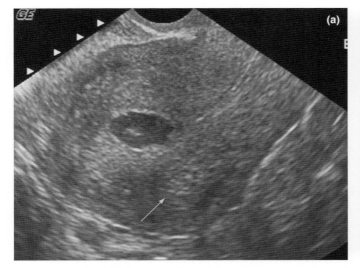
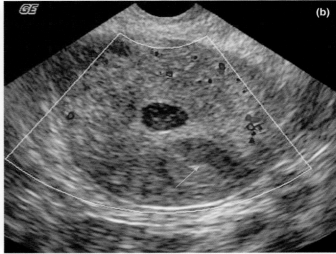

Figure 16.11. Blood-filled myometrial cyst. (a) Sagittal scan one year post endometrial ablation with an irregular cyst that is eccentric with the long axis oriented obliquely to the axis of the endometrial canal. The myometrium has focal areas of increased echodensity (arrow) typical of adenomyosis. At hysteroscopy no collection was seen. Transabdominal ultrasound was used to guide a scalpel hysteroscopically into the collection and drain it.. (b) This transverse section of the fundus also demonstrates blood in a distended intramural portion of the fallopian tube (arrow).

Endometrial ablation is still used today to control menorrhagia. This may make sense if the disease is limited to the superficial myometrium that is removed or destroyed by the ablation. In our experience the adenomyosis extends more than 3 or 4 mm beyond the endo-myometrial junction and often into the middle or outer layers of myometrium. Ablation would have no effect on the bleeding or on the associated pain that is so often the predominant symptom. We have also seen the development of collections of blood just beneath the scarred surface. They are not symmetrical or central within the uterus, but rather eccentric and irregular in shape (Figure 16.11). These are by definition not hematometra in that they are outside of the endometrial canal. On several occasions I have been called to the operating room to do a transabdominal ultrasound scan during hysteroscopy. We had reported a "hematometra" and none could be seen. In reality the collection was concealed by scar tissue. It was readily apparent sonographically and the hysteroscopist could then be guided into the collection for successful drainage.

There are gynecologists who will not do an ablation if they feel a boggy, tender uterus; now, with good evidence from imaging, ablation would seem to be a less useful approach.

Uterine artery embolization can reduce the symptoms in patients with adenomyosis. Kitamura studied 19 patients with a 12-month follow-up; 25% had a reduced uterine volume, with 88.9% reporting improvement in their symptoms [19].

In conclusion, adenomyosis has burst onto the horizon of female pelvic pathology. We must stop to ask ourselves some questions. Why is adenomyosis now so common? Has the incidence always been the same that we are now seeing or is it increasing and why should that be? Is it all clinically significant? Many cases seen have none of the classical symptoms, but do these have other symptoms of which we are not aware? Did they have symptoms that resolved spontaneously? Will they develop symptoms in the future? Is adenomyosis really a disease or not? For those women with symptoms, our ability to make this diagnosis and institute therapy can truly be life-altering.

References

1. Bordman R, Jackson, B. Below the belt: approach to chronic pelvic pain. *Can Fam Physician* 2006; **52**: 1556–62.

2. Stones RW, Price C. Health services for women with chronic pelvic pain. *J R Soc Med* 2002; **95**: 531–5.

3. Mathias SD, Kuppermann M, Liberman RF, Lipschutz RC, Steege JF. Chronic pelvic pain: prevalence, health-related quality of life, and economic correlates. *Obstet Gynecol* 1996; **87**: 321–7.

4. Zondervan KT, Yudkin PL, Vessey MP, et al. The community prevalence of chronic pelvic pain in women and associated illness behaviour. *Br J Gen Pract* 2001; **51**: 541–7.

5. Tocci A, Greco E, Ubaldi FM. Adenomyosis and "endometrial-subendometrial myometrium unit disruption disease" are two different entities. *Reprod Biomed Online* 2008; **17**: 281–91.

6. Gordts S, Brosens JJ, Fusi L, et al. Uterine adenomyosis: a need for uniform terminology and consensus classification. *Reprod Biomed Online* 2008; **17**: 244–8.

7. Verma SK, Lev-Toaff AS, Baltarowich OH, et al. Adenomyosis: sonohysterography with MRI correlation. *AJR* 2009; **192**: 1112–16.

8. Reinhold C, McCarthy S, Bret PM, et al. Diffuse adenomyosis: comparison of endovaginal US and MR imaging with histopathologic correlation. *Radiology* 1996; **199**: 151–8.

9. Meredith SM, Sanchez-Ramos L, Kaunitz AM. Diagnostic accuracy of transvaginal sonography for the diagnosis of adenomyosis: systematic review and metaanalysis. *Am J Obstet Gynecol* 2009; **200**: 107.e1–6.

10. Yeniel O, Cirpan T, Ulukus M, et al. Adenomyosis: prevalence, risk factors, symptoms and clinical findings. *Clin Exp Obstet Gynecol* 2007; **34**: 163–7.

11. Simpson JL, Elias S, Malinak LR, Buttram VCJr. Heritable aspects of endometriosis. Genetic studies. *Am J Obstet Gynecol* 1980; **137**: 327–31.

12. Ho ML, Raptis M, Hulett R, et al. Adenomyotic cyst of the uterus in an adolescent; a case report. *Pediatr Radiol* 2008; **38**: 1239–42.

13. Gerson Weiss MD, Maseelall P, Schott LL, et al. Adenomyosis a variant, not a disease? Evidence from hysterectomized menopausal women in the Study of Women's Health Across the Nation (SWAN) *Fertil Steril* 2009; **91**: 201–6.

14. Graham KJ, Hulst FA, Vogelnest L, Fraser IS, Shilton CM. Uterine adenomyosis in an orang-utan (*Pongo abelii/pygmaeus*). *Aust Vet J* 2009; **87**: 66–9.

15. DeVries K, Lyons EA, Ballard G, Levi CS, Lindsay DJ. Contractions of the inner third of the myometrium. *Am J Obstet Gynecol* 1990; **612**: 679–82.

16. Egli GE, Newton M. The transport of carbon particles in the human female reproductive tract. *Fertil Steril* 1961; **12**: 151–5.

17. Laoag-Fernandez JB, Maruo T, Pakarinen P, Spitz IM, Johansson E. Effects of levonorgestrel-releasing intra-uterine system on the expression of vascular endothelial growth factor and adrenomedullin in the endometrium in adenomyosis. *Hum Reprod* 2003; **18**: 694–9.

18. Cho S, Nam A, Kim H, et al. Clinical effects of the levonorgestrel-releasing intrauterine device in patients with adenomyosis. *Am J Obstet Gynecol* 2008; **198**: 373.

19. Kitamura Y, Allison SJ, Jha RC, et al. MRI of adenomyosis. Changes with uterine artery embolization. *AJR* 2006; **186**: 855–64.

Congenital uterine malformations

Mona Aboulghar

Embryological development of the uterus

The uterus develops from fusion of the paramesonephric ducts, which join in the midline at about the 10th week of gestation to form the unified body of the uterus (Figures 17.1, 17.2). Abnormalities in the resorption of the fused midline tissues occur by the 20th week and can result in the formation of septa of variable length and position. Apoptosis has been proposed as a mechanism by which the uterine septum regresses [1]. The protein Bcl-2 had been suggested to be absent in cases with failure of regression [1].

The American Fertility Society [2], on the basis of the previous work of Buttram and Gibbons [3], classified the anomalies of the female reproductive tract into groups according to the degree of failure of normal development with similar clinical manifestations, treatment, and possible prognoses for their reproductive performance. The various müllerian anomalies are the consequence of four major disturbances in the development of the female genitalia system during fetal life:

1. Failure of one or more müllerian duct to develop (agenesis, unicornuate uterus without rudimentary horn)

2. Failure of the ducts to canalize (unicornuate uterus with rudimentary horn without proper cavities)

3. Failure to fuse or abnormal fusion of the ducts (uterus didelphys, bicornuate uterus)

4. Failure of resorption of the midline uterine septum (septate uterus, arcuate uterus)

Incidence of müllerian uterine anomalies

Incidence of müllerian uterine anomalies in the general population is reported at around 5% [4]. Raga et al. reported an incidence of 0.1–3.8% in normal fertile females, which reached 6.7% in infertile patients (5). A study using ultrasound examination done for various reasons in women and girls ranging in age from 8 to 93 years gave a prevalence of 1 in 250 [6].

Müllerian uterine anomalies have been reported to be higher in infertile patients. A recent report by Mazouni et al. [7] indicated that the main reasons for discovery of müllerian anomalies were infertility (33.6%) and repeat miscarriage (18.2%).

With hysterosalpinography (HSG) the incidence was found to be 10%, with arcuate uterus being the most common (57.6%), followed by subseptate uterus (18.2%), bicornuate uterus (10.6%), uterus didelphys (3%), septate uterus (6%), and unicornuate uterus (3%) [8].

An association has been reported between polycystic ovaries and uterine müllerian anomalies, Appelman et al. [9] gave a 44% incidence in polycystic ovary patients compared with 18% in the normal ovary group ($P < 0.001$).

Investigations of patients with müllerian anomalies should include searching for other associated anomalies, mainly renal, as a high degree of association has been found in up to 36% of patients [10].

Müllerian anomalies have been implicated in female subfertility, implantation failure, miscarriages, and preterm labor [7].

Thus, accuracy of diagnosis is important for planning of management and assessment of the need for intervention. Multiple imaging techniques are usually needed to reach final diagnosis and confirmation and this often delays diagnosis [7]. Ideally, a technique with the highest accuracy and lowest rate of false-positive results is needed.

Many diagnostic modalities are available: 2D ultrasound (2D US), 3D ultrasound (3D US), with or without saline instillation; sonohysterography, HSG, magnetic resonance imaging (MRI), hysteroscopy, laparoscopy. Hysterosalpingography, hysteroscopy, and laparoscopy are invasive procedures and diagnosis is based on the subjective impression of the operator.

Hysterosalpingography (HSG)

Hysterosalpingography is the first diagnostic test used for patients with suspected müllerian anomalies, but it has a low reported sensitivity of 44% [11].

HSG can detect a two-chambered uterus and allow assessment of the size and extent of a septum [12]. It reveals an image of two hemicavities with a clear central division showing a typical "Y" shape. With bicornuate and didelphic uteri the hemicavities have convex medial walls and the angle between them is generally >90°, whereas with septate uteri the medial walls are straighter and the resulting angle is generally <90° [Figures 17.3, 17.4]. However, the main drawback of this measurement is that it

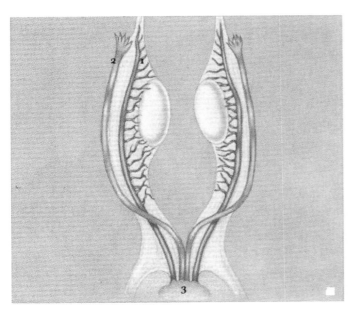

Figure 17.1. Embryology of the müllerian system.

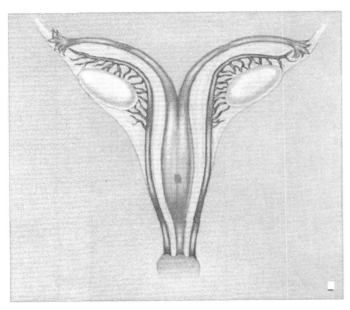

Figure 17.2. Unified müllerian ducts.

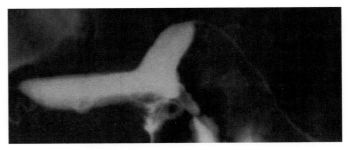

Figure 17.3. Hysterosalpingography of septate uterus.

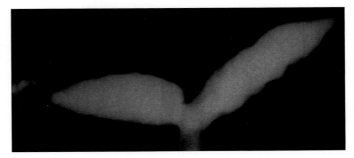

Figure 17.4. Hysterosalpingography of septate uterus.

cannot reliably differentiate between septate and bicornuate uterus. Reuter et al. revealed a diagnostic accuracy of only 55% for HSG in differentiating between septate and bicornuate uterus [13]. It may miss small septal defects [14].

In a study of 110 patients with müllerian anomalies, including 73 septate uterus, 20 bicornuate, 10 hypoplastic, 4 unicornuate, and 3 müllerian agenesis, comparing HSG with other imaging modalities, HSG diagnosed uterine hypoplasia in 70% and ultrasonography (US) in 30%. Diagnosis of bicornuate uterus was confirmed by US in 85% and by HSG in the remaining 15%. Diagnosis of unicornuate uterus was confirmed by HSG in one case and by US in the remaining three. All cases of müllerian agenesis were diagnosed by US. For women with septate uterus, diagnosis was suspected by HSG in 21.5% and by hysteroscopy in 19.6%. For septate uterus, standard US technique gave a false diagnosis in 80.8% of cases [7].

HSG is considered an invasive test; it necessitates injection of a contrast medium and exposure to irradiation, in addition to risk of pain and infection. However, HSG offers the advantage of the ability to assess tubal patency, which is not possible with routine ultrasonography.

Two-dimensional ultrasonography

Two-dimensional (2D) ultrasonography was previously done by the transabdominal route, but transvaginal ultrasonography (TVS) is superior to the transabdominal route and is now the standard imaging technique for the uterus [15]. It avoids obesity and abdominal fat, lies closer to pelvic structures, and uses higher-frequency probes.

Pellerito et al. reported an accuracy of 92% for ultrasound detection of müllerian anomalies, as compared with 100% accuracy with MRI [16]; however, ultrasound has a reported difficulty in distinction between various types of uterine anomalies [17]. 2D TVS has a reported sensitivity of 100% and specificity of 80% in diagnosing septate uterus [16].

Three-dimensional ultrasonography

The main advantage of three-dimensional (3D) ultrasonography over 2D is the ability to image the three orthogonal planes of the uterus, of which the coronal view is the most important. This view is essential for assessing the external uterine contour and viewing the fundus, endometrium, and myometrium – i.e. the whole length of the uterus down to the cervix – and consequently for determining the exact type of uterine anomaly. It also enables the measurement of the length of a uterine septum

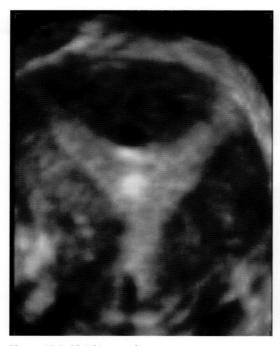

Figure 17.5. 3D US image of arcuate uterus.

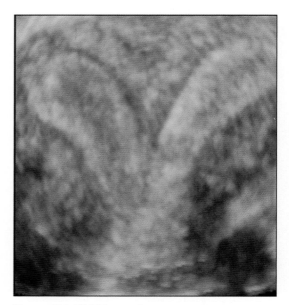

Figure 17.7. 3D US image of septate uterus.

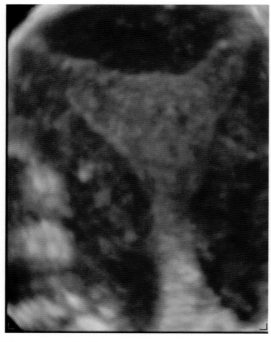

Figure 17.6. 3D US image of arcuate uterus.

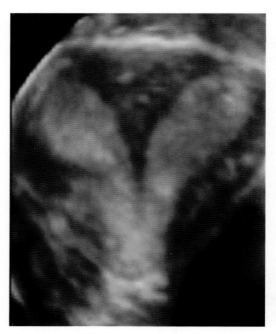

Figure 17.8. 3D US image of septate uterus.

and depth of fundal cleft. Another advantage of 3D ultrasound is the possibility to store the images and re-evaluate the volumes later, possibly pooling the data in a database for review by another sonographer. Disadvantages of 3D ultrasound include the time needed for learning manipulation of the volumes and poor visualization in cases of shadowing by fibroids.

Several studies have reported high sensitivity and specificity with 3D ultrasound in diagnosis of major müllerian anomalies.

In a study that included 61 patients, Jurkovic et al. [18] reported 100% sensitivity and specificity, compared with 100% and 95%, respectively, with 2D TVS. There were no false-negatives or false-positives for the 3D technique in diagnosing uterine müllerian anomalies. Three-dimensional ultrasound was compared with HSG and had a higher accuracy.

In this study criteria for diagnosis of an arcuate uterus were normal appearance of the cervix and myometrium, absence of fundal cleft, and a rounded appearance of the fundal portion of the uterine cavity (Figures 17.5, 17.6) [18]. In cases of subseptate uterus, the proximal part of the uterine cavity was

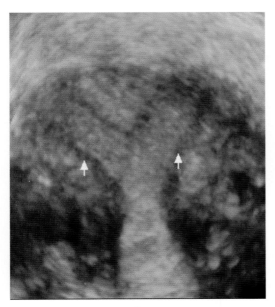

Figure 17.9. 3D US image of small uterine septum.

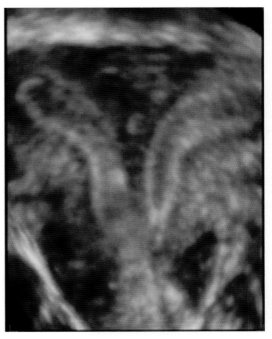

Figure 17.11. 3D US image of long uterine septum.

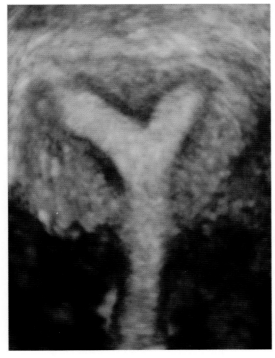

Figure 17.10. 3D US image of small uterine septum.

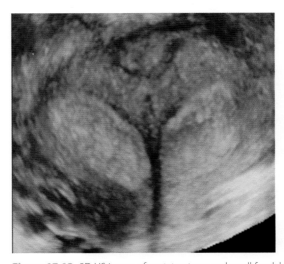

Figure 17.12. 3D US image of septate uterus and small fundal cleft.

partially divided by a septum and the myometrium appeared normal. However, if a fundal indentation was present, it had to be less than 1 cm in depth to allow classification as a subseptate uterus (Figures 17.7, 17.8, 17.9, 17.10, 17.11, 17.12). The diagnosis of bicornuate uterus was made when divergent, well-formed cornua were seen separated by a large fundal cleft (>1 cm).

Raga et al. studied 42 patients with a history of infertility, of whom 12 had müllerian anomalies that were all detected by 3D ultrasound, while 11 were correctly classified [5].

In a study by Wu et al. [19], 40 patients with a history suggesting müllerian anomaly were included, out of whom 28 women were confirmed to have Müllerian anomalies (by laparoscopy and/or hysteroscopy). These comprised 3 unicornuate uteri, 3 bicornuate uteri, 12 cases with complete or partial septate uterus, 9 cases of arcuate uterus, and one case of didelphic uterus. Three-dimensional sonography demonstrated all congenital uterine abnormalities with a sensitivity and specificity of 100%. Septate uterus and bicornuate uterus could be

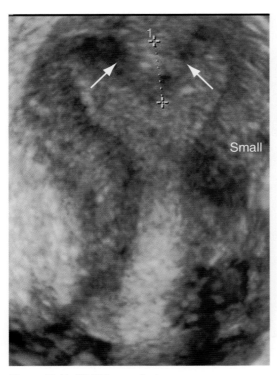

Figure 17.13. 3D US image of subseptate uterus.

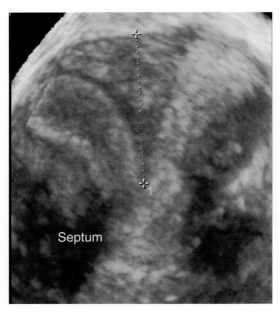

Figure 17.14. 3D US image of long uterine septum.

correctly diagnosed using 3D sonography in 11 of 12 cases (92%) and 3 of 3 cases (100%), respectively.

Use of 3D ultrasound to examine patients with recurrent miscarriage as compared with normal controls showed no difference in the relative proportions of congenital uterine anomalies in the two groups of women; arcuate and septate uterus were the most common anomalies prevalent (90%). The measurement of depth of the uterine septum and residual cavity depth showed

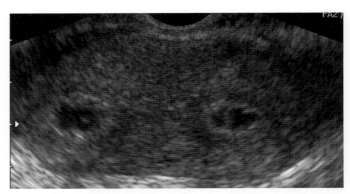

Figure 17.15. Sonohysterographic image of two uterine cavities in transverse section.

that in both arcuate and subseptate uteri the length of remaining uterine cavity was significantly shorter ($P < 0.01$) and the distortion ratio was significantly higher ($P < 0.01$) in patients with recurrent miscarriage [20] (Figures 17.13, 17.14).

Three-dimensional ultrasound has been found to be a reproducible method in diagnosing uterine congenital malformations (20).

Sonohysterography

Sonohysterography is an ultrasound-aided technique that entails injection of normal saline into the uterine cavity; in some situations contrast medium could be injected to allow visualization of the external contour of the uterus and could aid in diagnosis of the type of müllerian anomaly.

Soares et al. compared HSG with TVS and with sonohysterography using hysteroscopy as the gold standard [11]. Out of 65 patients, 9 had uterine malformations. The sensitivity, specificity, positive predictive value (PPV), and negative predictive value (NPV) of sonohysterography were, respectively, 77.8%, 100%, 100%, 96.6% compared with values for HSG of 44%, 96.4%, 66.7%, 91.5%, and with values for TVS of 44.4%, 100%, 100%, 91.5%. Thus, in this study sonohysterography performed better in the diagnosis of müllerian anomalies. Sonohysterography and TVS had no false-positive diagnoses (Figure 17.15).

Septate uterus is the most common müllerian anomaly and is known to result in adverse obstetric outcomes; it is therefore of great importance to differentiate septate from bicornuate uterus, which is much less common, so that hysteroscopic septum excision can be performed [21]. Surgery has reportedly improved pregnancy rate from 3–20% to 70–90% [22].

Valenzano et al. reported on 54 patients included in a study in which sonohysterography was compared with the standard investigation of hysteroscopy (though patients also had undergone TVS & HSG investigations) [23]. Sonohysterography was able to detect all the anomalies. The sensitivity and specificity of sonohysterography were the same as for hysteroscopy. However, although there was no significant difference between the diagnostic capabilities of the methods analyzed, the authors recommended that, because it is an easy and cheap technique, it should be the first used in infertile patients as well as in those with recurrent miscarriage.

Table 17.1. The sensitivity, specificity, and positive (PPV) and negative (NPV) predictive values of various imaging modalities for the diagnosis of septate uterus in 420 patients with history of infertility and recurrent miscarriage

Imaging modality	Sensitivity (%)	Specificity (%)	PPV (%)	NPV (%)
Transvaginal sonography	95.21	92.21	95.86	91.03
Transvaginal color Doppler	99.29	97.93	98.03	98.61
Saline contrast sonography	98.18	100.00	100.00	95.45
Three-dimensional ultrasound	98.38	100.00	100.00	96.00

Reproduced from Kupesic and Kurjak [27] with permission from the American Institute of Ultrasound in Medicine.

Lev-Toaff et al. compared 2D sonohysterography with 3D sonohysterography and x-ray HSG and found 3D to be advantageous over the other two techniques, with the coronal plane being the most important in providing information [24].

Addition of sonohysterography to 3D imaging allows precise recognition and localization of the lesion; therefore if 2D and 3D SHG are normal, invasive diagnostic procedures such as hysteroscopy can be avoided [25].

Guimarães Filho et al. compared sonohysterography with HSG and hysteroscopy (as the gold standard), in investigating patients with recurrent miscarriage [26]. The accuracy of sonohysterography and HSG was 90.9 and 85.2%, respectively; the general sensitivity of sonohysterography was superior to that of HSG (90.5 vs. 75%), and it also had a higher degree of agreement with hysteroscopy (Kappa = 0.81 vs. 0.68). Pain was significantly less with sonohysterography than with the other two methods.

The main disadvantage of 2D ultrasound and sonohysterography is that the techniques are operator dependent.

Kupesic and Kurjak compared four imaging techniques – transvaginal 2D ultrasound, color and pulsed Doppler, sonohysterography, and 3D ultrasound – preoperatively in diagnosing septate uterus [27]. Four hundred and twenty infertile patients undergoing hysteroscopy were examined. Of these 278 patients had an intrauterine septum, all complaining of adverse obstetric complications, of which 43 had repeated spontaneous miscarriage; 71 had one spontaneous miscarriage; 81 had primary infertility; and 20 had preterm deliveries. The highest sensitivity and specificity were demonstrated with 3D ultrasound (Table 17.1).

In this study the height and thickness of the septum did not correlate with the obstetric outcome, which contrasts with a previously mentioned study [20] that reported that in patients with recurrent miscarriage the degree of residual uterine cavity distortion was higher. However, septal vascularity correlated well. Patients with vascularized septa had significantly higher prevalence of early and late pregnancy complications than those with avascular septa, and this may reflect an increased amount of muscle in the septum, producing local uncoordinated myometrial contractility.

Magnetic resonance imaging

Many magnetic resonance imaging (MRI) studies have shown a very high sensitivity of 100% [16], and more recently values of 95% have been reported in cases of müllerian anomalies [7]. The main disadvantage of MRI is high cost, in addition to lack of information as regards tubal patency.

Conclusion

Uterine müllerian anomalies have a high frequency of adverse obstetric implications. Diagnostic modalities for detection of uterine anomalies are many, with varying sensitivities and specificities. Three-dimensional ultrasound seems very encouraging; it delivers good sensitivity, it is easy and is noninvasive, and it is becoming more available.

References

1. Lee DM, Osathanondh R, Yeh J. Localization of Bcl-2 in the human fetal Müllerian tract. *Fertil Steril* 1998; **70**: 135–40.

2. The American Fertility Society classifications of adenexal adhesions, distal tubal occlusion, tubal occlusion secondry to tubal ligation, tubal pregnancies, Mullerian anomalies and intrauterine adhesions. *Fertil Steril* 1998; **49**: 944–55.

3. Buttram VC, Gibbons WE. Mullerian anomalies: a proposed classification (an analysis of 144 cases); *Fertil Steril* 1979; **32**: 40–8.

4. Nahum GG. Uterine anomalies. How common are they and what is their distribution among subtypes? *J Reprod Med* 1998; **43**: 877–87.

5. Raga F, Bonilla-Musoles F, Blanes J. Congenital Mullerian anomalies: diagnostic accuracy of three-dimensional ultrasound. *Fertil Steril* 1996 Mar; **65**(3): 523–8.

6. Byrne J, Nussbaum-Blask A, Taylor WS. Prevalence of Mullerian duct anomalies detected at ultrasound. *Am J Med Genet* 2000; **94**: 9–12.

7. Mazouni C, Girard G, Deter R. Diagnosis of Mullerian anomalies in adults: evaluation of practice. *Fertil Steril* 2008; **89**(1): 219–22

8. Braun P, Grau FV, Pons RM. Is hysterosalpingography able to diagnose all uterine malformations correctly? A retrospective study. *Eur J Radiol* 2005; **53**: 274–9.

9. Appelman Z, Hazan Y, Hagay Z. High prevalence of Mullerian anomalies diagnosed by ultrasound in women with polycystic ovaries. *J Reprod Med.* 2003; **48**(5): 362–4.

10. Oppelt P, vonHave M, Paulsen M. Female genital malformations and their associated abnormalities. *Fertil Steril* 2007 Feb; **87**(2): 335–42.

11. Soares SR, Barbosa dos Reis MB, Camargos AF. Diagnostic accuracy of sonohysterography, transvaginal sonography and hysterosalpingography in patients with uterine cavity diseases. *Fertil Steril* 2000; **73**: 406–11.

12. Barbot J. Hysteroscopy and hysterography. *Obstet Gynecol Clin North Am* 1995; **22**: 591–603.

13. Reuter KL, Daly DC, Cohen SM. Septate versus bicornuate uteri: errors in imaging diagnosis. *Radiology* 1989; **172**: 749–52.

14. Golan A, Ron-El R, Herman A. Diagnostic hysteroscopy: its value in an in vitro fertilization/embryo transfer unit. *Hum Reprod* 1992; **7**: 1433–4.

15. Qureshi IA, Ullah H, Akram MH, Ashfaq S, Nayyar S. Transvaginal versus transabdominal sonography in the evaluation of pelvic pathology. *J Coll Physicians Surg Pak* 2004; **14**(7): 390–3

16. Pellerito JS, Mc Carthy SM, Doyle MB. Diagnosis of uterine anomalies: relative accuracy of MR imaging, endovginal sonography and hysterosalpingography.

Radiology 1992; **183**: 795–800.

17. Nicolini U, Bellotti M, Bonazzi B. Can ultrasound be used to screen uterine malformations? *Fertil Steril* 1987; **47**; 89–93.

18. Jurkovic D, Geipel A, Gruboek K. Three-dimensional ultrasound for the assessment of uterine anatomy and detection of congenital anomalies: a comparison with hysterosalpingography and two-dimensional sonography. *Ultrasound Obstet Gynecol* 1995; **5**(4): 219–21.

19. Wu MH, Hsu CC, Huang KF. Detection of congenital mullerian duct anomalies using three-dimentional ultrasound. *J Clin Utrasound* 1997; **25**(9): 487–92.

20. Salim R, Woelfer B, Backost M. Reproducibility of three-dimensional ultrasound diagnosis of congenital uterine anomalies. *Ultrasound*

Obstset Gynecol 2003; **21**: 578–82.

21. Alborzi S, Dehbashi S, Parsanezhad ME. Differential dagnosis f septate and bicornuate uterus by sonohysterography eliminates the need for laparoscopy. *Fertil Steril* 2002; **78**: 176–8.

22. Fedele L, Arcaini L, Parazzini F. Reproductive prognosis after hysteroscopic metroplasty in 102 women: life table analysis. *Fertil Steril* 1993; **59**: 768–72.

23. Valenzano MM, Mistrangelo E, Lijoi D. Transvaginal sonohysterographic evaluation of uterine malformations. *Eur J Obstet Gynecol Reprod Biol* 2006 Feb; **124**(2): 246–9.

24. Lev-Toaff AS, Pinheiro LW, Bega G. Three-dimensional multiplanar sonohysterography: comparison with conventional two-dimensional

sonohysterography and X-ray hysterosalpingography. *J Ultrasound Med* 2001; **20**(4): 295–306.

25. Sylvestre C, Child TJ, Tulandi T. A prospective study to evaluate the efficacy of two- and three-dimensional sonohysterography in women with intrauterine lesions. *Fertil Steril* 2003; **79** (5): 1222–5.

26. Guimarães Filho HA, Mattar R, Pires CR. Comparison of hysterosalpingography, hysterosonography and hysteroscopy in evaluation of the uterine cavity in patients with recurrent pregnancy losses. *Arch Gynecol Obstet* 2006; **274**(5): 284–8.

27. Kupesic S, Kurjak A. Septate uterus: Detection and prediction of obstetrical complications by different forms of ultrasonography. *J Ultrasound Med* 1998; **17**: 631–6.

Chapter 18

Uterine septum

Mohamed F. M. Mitwally and Mostafa Abuzeid

Introduction

There is no doubt that contemporary developments in the technology of ultrasonography (US), including enhanced resolution with increased ability to differentiate among various tissues and structures, have made ultrasonography a strong armamentarium for the diagnosis and management of uterine septum and various other congenital malformations of the uterus. This chapter discusses the role of ultrasonography in the evaluation and management of uterine septum. We recently published a comprehensive review of the diagnosis and management of uterine septum, as well as of the reproductive problems that could be associated with various types of uterine septi [1]. For the convenience of the reader and by permission of the editor, a great proportion of that original chapter is included here.

We believe that this topic generates significant controversy regarding diagnosis and treatment because of the paucity of comprehensive evidence-based data on female congenital anomalies, in particular, uterine septum. This has resulted in the lack of a consensus on how the presence of a uterine septum might affect female reproduction. We will discuss the available data, aiming to provide a balanced appraisal that can help reproductive medicine specialists to better counsel patients about their reproductive potential when a uterine septum is discovered.

Embryology of uterine septum

Around the 10th week of gestation, the uterus forms from fusion of the paramesonephric ducts (müllerian ducts), which join in the midline in the absence of müllerian-inhibiting substance [2]. It is interesting that the müllerian ducts can develop into two distinct types of tissue: the smooth-muscle tissue of the uterus and the fibrous tissue of the cervix. This could explain the various structural subtypes of uterine septum containing different proportions of fibrous and muscle structure. Such structural disparity might have implications for the mechanism of reproductive failure associated with uterine septum [2].

A uterine septum results when there is incomplete resorption of the adjacent walls of the two müllerian ducts. The resulting fibromuscular structure can range from a slight midline septum in the fundus of the uterus to complete midline division of the endometrial cavity. Even segmental septa can exist, resulting in partial communications of a partitioned uterus [2].

Reports of cases of complete vaginal septum associated with different degrees of uterine septum ranging from complete uterine septum with cervical duplication [3,4] to incomplete septum (subseptate uterus) [5] challenged the classic theory of unidirectional (caudal to cranial) müllerian development. Accordingly, an alternative "bidirectional" theory was proposed, which suggested that fusion and resorption begin at the isthmus of the uterus and proceed simultaneously in both the cranial and caudal directions [6].

Prevalence of uterine septum

Although uterine anomalies have been reported in 0.1–2.0% of all women, in 4% with infertility, and in up to 15% of those with recurrent miscarriage, their true incidence is not known [4]. Pedro Acien suggested that the variability in the reported incidence of uterine anomalies is due to five factors: (1) the population studied; (2) the study design and physician's interest and awareness in finding or rejecting a uterine anomaly; (3) the diagnostic method used; (4) the classes included as congenital uterine anomalies in the different studies – e.g., hypoplastic uterus, T-shaped anomalies, and arcuate uterus frequently not included; (5) the criteria and diagnostic tools used to classify the different types of uterine malformation [7].

In a selected group of women undergoing hysteroscopy for abnormal uterine bleeding, Maneschi et al. [8] assessed the prevalence of uterine anomalies and compared the reproductive outcome in women with müllerian anomalies with that in women with a normal uterine cavity. The authors found müllerian anomalies in about 10% of women. Their findings were similar to those reported in studies dealing with the frequency of diagnosis of uterine anomalies in women undergoing tubal sterilization investigated by hysterosalpingography (HSG), when septate, bicornuate, and arcuate uteri were found in 1.9%, 3.6%, and 11.5%, respectively, of women with no history of reproductive problems [9].

Uterine septum (complete or partial) has been the most common (34–48%) type of structural uterine anomaly [10,11,12,13]. The significance of the uterine septum comes from the fact that it is the form of müllerian anomaly that is believed to be associated with the poorest reproductive outcome, including low fetal survival rates of 6–28% and high rates of spontaneous miscarriage [12,13,14].

Types

The classification of uterine anomalies divides the uterine septum into complete (septate) or partial (subseptate) groups according, respectively, to whether the septum approaches the internal os or does not. The complete septum that divides both the uterine cavity and the endocervical canal may be associated with a longitudinal vaginal septum. However, the presence or absence of a longitudinal vaginal septum is not considered in the classification [15]. Different classification systems have been proposed for müllerian anomalies, with the early classification systems being criticized for their confusion, incompleteness, or irrelevant details. In 1979, Buttram and Gibbons [15] introduced the classification system of müllerian anomalies shown in Table 18.1. The American Fertility Society (currently known as the American Society for Reproductive Medicine or ASRM)

revised the Buttram and Gibbons classification [16] with the aim to make it an easy-to-use reporting system that would allow clinicians to classify patients better, so that data could be accumulated more readily concerning the incidence of fetal wastage and obstetric complications for these malformations (see Box 18.1 and Figure 18.1).

As shown in Figure 18.2, the uterine septum has three parts: the *base* (where it attaches to the fundus); the *body* of the septum that extends down from the fundus all the way toward the cervix (complete septum), as shown in Figure 18.3, or stops somewhere between the fundus and the cervix (subseptate or incomplete or short septum), as shown in Figures 18.4 and 18.5; and the *apex* of the septum (the cervical end of the septum).

In addition to the regular classification into long (complete) or short (incomplete) subtypes, as shown in Figures 18.3 and 18.4,

Table 18.1. The Buttram and Gibbons classification of müllerian anomalies [15]

Uterine morphology	Fundal contour	External contour
Normal	Straight or convex	Uniformly convex or with indentation <10 mm
Arcuate	Concave fundal indentation with central point of indentation at obtuse angle	Uniformly convex or with indentation <10 mm
Subseptate	Presence of septum that does not extend to cervix, with central point of septum at an acute angle	Uniformly convex or with indentation <10 mm
Bicornuate	Two well-formed uterine cornua, with a convex fundal contour in each	Fundal indentation >10 mm dividing the two cornua

Box 18.1 American Fertility Society classification of congenital uterine anomalies [16] (see Figure 18.1)

I. **Agenesis: vagina, cervix, uterine fundus, fallopian tube, or any combination thereof**

II. **Unicornuate uterus**
- Connected
- Not connected
- Without a cavity
- Without a horn

III. **Uterus didelphys (double uterus and cervix)**

IV. **Bicornuate uterus (complete, partial, arcuate)**

V. **Septate uterus**
- Complete
- Partial

VI. **Arcuate**

VII. **DES drug related, e.g., T-shaped uterus resulting from diethylstilbestrol exposure**

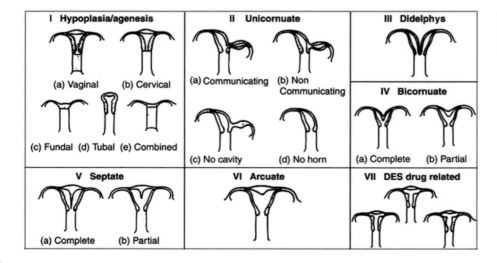

Figure 18.1. The American Fertility Society (subsequently the American Society for Reproductive Medicine) classification of congenital uterine anomalies [16].

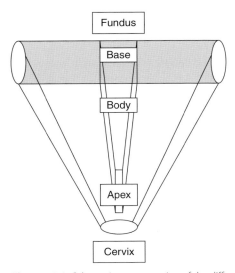

Figure 18.2. Schematic representation of the different parts of the uterine septum in relation to the uterine walls: *base* of the septum where it meets the fundus; *body* of the septum that extends down, dividing the uterine cavity into two sides; and *apex* of the septum, which is the lowermost part of the septum.

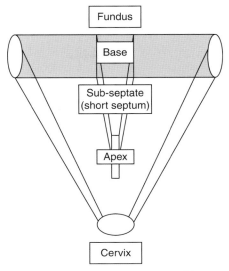

Figure 18.4. Schematic representation of the incomplete-short type of uterine septum (subseptate uterus). In this type, the apex of the septum stops somewhere below the fundus before reaching the cervix.

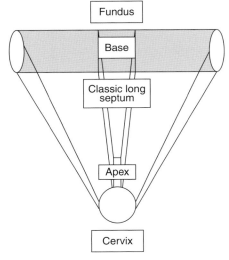

Figure 18.3. Schematic representation of the complete or long septum type (septate uterus). In this type of uterine septum, the body of the septum extends all the way down from the fundus to the cervix, completely separating the uterine cavity into two sides.

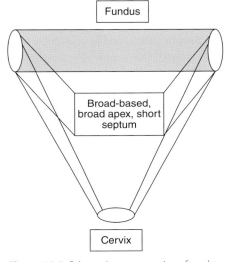

Figure 18.5. Schematic representation of a subtype of the short septum. We term it the broad-based short septum because in this type the base of the septum is very broad, extending between almost the whole distance between the two tubal ostia.

in our experience we observed two different subtypes of the short uterine septum based on the width of the uterine septum and the symmetry between the two uterine cavities on either side of the septum: broad-based (sometimes has a broad apex too) and asymmetrical (unequal-sided) septum, as shown in Figure 18.5 (usually has a broad base too), and Figures 18.6 and 18.10, respectively We note those subtypes to be frequently encountered in infertile patients and in patients with poor reproductive outcomes, including assisted reproductive technology (ART) failure and pregnancy loss (unpublished data). Another investigator using three-dimensional (3D) US and saline sonogram with 3D US has observed similar subtypes of the short uterine septum,

which he named "wide-shallow septum" and "irregular septum." This author also reported a special type, which he called "T-shaped-shallow septum." The latter type was also observed by our group using 3D US (unpublished data).

We believe that the diagnosis of these two subtypes of short septum (broad-based and asymmetrical) may be missed or at least confused with the diagnosis of arcuate uterus. This is particularly true when only HSG is relied upon without further evaluation by ultrasonography, especially 3D US and hysteroscopy. This confusion could explain the controversy in the literature regarding the association of reproductive problems (pregnancy loss and preterm labor) and arcuate uterus, as will be discussed later.

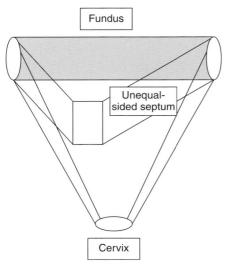

Figure 18.6. Schematic representation of another subtype of the short septum (asymmetrical). In this type, the two sides of the uterine cavity are unequal. The apex of the septum is deviated more toward one side.

Structure

The high rate of spontaneous abortion in patients with uterine septum has been related to a specific histological feature of the septum, in which there is less vascularity and inadequate endometrial development that results in abnormal placentation [17]. It has also been claimed that, during hysteroscopic excision of the septum when bleeding appears, the natural wall of the uterus (because of its increasing vascularity) has been reached and further division is not needed [17,18].

Classically, the uterine septum structure has been described as a "fibroelastic" tissue that has three main features: first, a very small amount of muscle tissue [17,18]; second, it is mainly formed of fibroelastic tissue [19]; third, very scanty vasculature (avascular) [20,21].

Interestingly, contrary to the classic description of the uterine septum, Dabirashrafi et al. [22] reported opposite findings of significantly less connective tissue in the septum and a higher amount of muscle tissue and vasculature when compared with posterior uterine muscle away from the septum. The authors concluded that their findings challenged the classical theory of the cause of fetal wastage associated with uterine septum (avascularity of the septum). They proposed two other mechanisms for the increased pregnancy loss: first, the poor decidualization and placentation due to reduced connective tissue; and second, the higher noncoordinated contractility in the uterine septum due to the higher amounts of interlacing muscle tissue [22]. Kupesic and Kurjak, using color and pulsed Doppler sonographic studies of the septal areas, reported vascularity in 71% of patients. This study therefore suggests that a uterine septum can be formed of muscular tissue in some patients and primarily of fibroelastic tissue in others [23].

Diagnosis of uterine septum and the role of ultrasonography

It is important to distinguish between the bicornuate uterus and the septate uterus. This is crucially important because the bicornuate uterus is infrequently associated with reproductive failures, whereas the septate uterus is frequently associated with reproductive problems, such as pregnancy failure, that usually require further intervention [24]. It is also important to differentiate between arcuate uterus and short incomplete septum, and between complete septum with cervical duplication and longitudinal vaginal septum and uterus didelphys. In addition, in cases of subtle short uterine septum and arcuate uterus, physicians often fail to acknowledge the presence of such anomalies, as these cases are being interpreted as variants of normal. We believe that it is imperative to diagnose such cases, although we acknowledge that there is a controversy regarding the effect of such anomalies on reproductive potential.

Imaging

Although surgery (hysteroscopy, alone or with laparoscopy), constitutes the gold standard for the diagnosis of uterine septum, various imaging tools including hysterosalpingography (HSG), ultrasonography, and magnetic resonance imaging (MRI) have great value in the diagnosis, with high levels of accuracy.

Hysterosalpingography (HSG)

Hysterosalpingography provides valuable information about tubal patency, in addition to some information about the uterine cavity. However, its usefulness is limited in identifying uterine anomalies, including the uterine septum, because it does not provide definitive information about the external contour of the uterus. Other imaging modalities, including ultrasonography and MRI, have been shown to be useful complementary tools in characterizing and delineating more clearly the exact nature of the müllerian anomalies [25]. This is particularly true for the distinction between uterine septum and bicornuate uterus, which cannot be made definitively by examination of a hysterogram (during HSG) because the images of the cavities may be exactly the same [24]. Figure 18.7a is a hysterosalpingogram showing a significant incomplete septum versus incomplete bicornuate uterus. Figure 18.7d is a hysterosalpingogram of a variant of subtle incomplete septum with flat apex. Figure 18.9a illustrates a complete uterine septum versus complete bicornuate uterus. Figure 18.10a is a hysterosalpingogram of a variant of subtle incomplete septum with asymmetrical sides (right side more prominent than left side).

Hysterosalpingograms of an acutely anteverted/anteflexed or retroverted/retroflexed uterus are shown in Figure 18.11a and 18.11b, and of a uterus rotated to the side in Figure 18.11c. Such acute angulations of the uterus against the vaginal axis (anteverted or retroverted) or against its axis (anteflexed or retroflexed), or rotation against its longitudinal axis, i.e. levo- or dextro-rotated, all may cause problems in interpretation of the hysterosalpingogram.

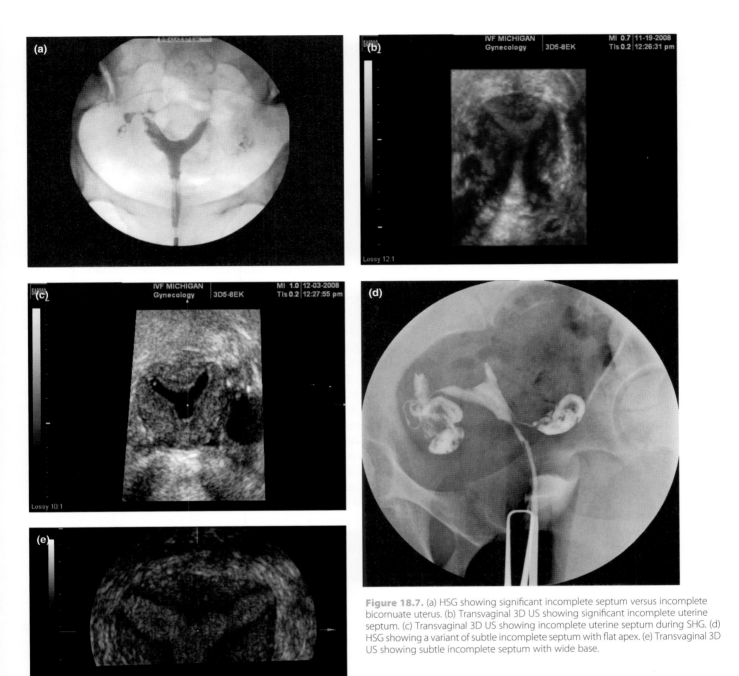

Figure 18.7. (a) HSG showing significant incomplete septum versus incomplete bicornuate uterus. (b) Transvaginal 3D US showing significant incomplete uterine septum. (c) Transvaginal 3D US showing incomplete uterine septum during SHG. (d) HSG showing a variant of subtle incomplete septum with flat apex. (e) Transvaginal 3D US showing subtle incomplete septum with wide base.

It is advisable in those cases to adjust the position of the uterus by applying pressure and/or traction in the right direction to ensure a straightened alignment of the hysterogram. This can be done by manipulating the tenaculum applied on the cervix and the HSG catheter applied to the cervix. In such cases it is sometimes difficult to rule out subtle, incomplete uterine septum

Ultrasonography (US)

Ultrasonography has the advantages of minimal invasiveness, relatively low cost, and ease of performance. Although transabdominal two-dimensional ultrasonography (2D US) was the first ultrasound technique used for identifying uterine cavity disorders, transvaginal US has become the modality of choice, replacing the transabdominal approach. This is

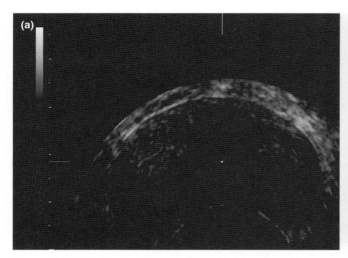
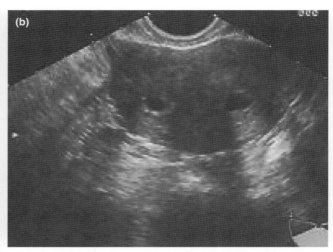

Figure 18.8. (a) Transvaginal 2D US showing a transverse section in the upper uterine segment, illustrating endometrial separation and suggesting uterine septum versus bicornuate uterus. (b) Transvaginal 2D US showing a transverse section in the upper uterine segment, illustrating endometrial separation during SHG in a patient with uterine septum versus bicornuate uterus.

because of its ability to be closer to the uterus, which allows better anatomic delineation, in addition to its higher resolution associated with high frequency of the ultrasound beam, which provides images with better contrast and resolution [26].

Despite the advantages of transvaginal 2D US, it has a fairly low sensitivity as a screening test of uterine anomalies (~70%) [27]. In addition, sometimes it is impossible to distinguish between different types of anomalies. Another problem is that a transverse or oblique transverse view of the uterus is not optimal in diagnosing uterine abnormalities, particularly when the uterine body has a *retroverted* position. Furthermore, 2D ultrasound is operator-dependent and hardcopy images can be difficult for a third party to interpret [26]. Figure 18.8a is a transvaginal 2D US picture showing the phenomenon of endometrial separation in a transverse section of the upper uterine segment, suggesting uterine septum versus bicornuate uterus.

Sonohysterography (SHG)

Optimal imaging of the endometrium and myometrium may require distension of the uterine cavity with saline to separate the walls of the uterus to make clear the outline of the endometrial contour, and to detect endoluminal lesions, i.e., lesions protruding into the uterine cavity or uterine septum. This procedure is frequently called sonohysterography (SHG) or saline infusion sonohysterography (SIS).

Preparation of the patient for SHG is more or less similar to that for HSG, i.e., ensure that the patient is not pregnant and that there is no evidence of active pelvic infection or other less likely contraindications to the procedure such as allergy to the ultrasound contrast medium. In addition, conventional transvaginal ultrasound examination should be done before SHG to assess the appearance of the uterus before instillation of fluid into the uterine cavity and to

determine the orientation of the uterus to facilitate insertion of a catheter into the cervical canal for instillation of the saline or the ultrasound contrast medium [26]. Performing the procedure during the follicular phase has the advantage of avoiding the risk of disturbing an early pregnancy. It is preferable to use a balloon-bearing catheter to occlude the internal os so as to allow adequate distension of the uterine cavity [26]. This has the disadvantages of being more uncomfortable for the patient and the fact that its shadow might obscure lesions present in the lower uterine segment or the cervical canal. However, in the majority of cases, an adequate distension of the uterine cavity can be achieved without the need to inflate a balloon, with the use of balloon-free catheters such as those used for intrauterine insemination.

Sonohysterography is thought to have almost 100% sensitivity and specificity when compared with the gold standard of surgery [28]. Another study [29] found SHG to have the same diagnostic accuracy as the gold standard for polypoid lesions and endometrial hyperplasia. The consensus by the experts in the area of ultrasonography of uterine cavity disorders is that SHG and HSG are highly sensitive in the diagnosing of major uterine malformations. However, SHG is not sufficiently sensitive in the diagnosis of minor uterine abnormalities [26]. A recent report suggests the use of a very small volume of viscous gel, with impressive results [30]. Figure 18.8b is a transvaginal 2D ultrasonogram during SHG showing a transverse section in the upper uterine segment, illustrating endometrial separation in a patient with uterine septum versus bicornuate uterus.

Three-dimensional ultrasonography (3D US)

Transvaginal 3D US is a noninvasive imaging technique with the ability to generate accurate images of both the endometrial cavity and the external contour of the uterus [31,32]. A major advantage of 3D US is the ability to obtain coronal views of the uterus, which are usually not obtainable by 2D US because of anatomic limitations (the vaginal probe has limited mobility within the confines of the vagina). Coronal views show the relationship between the endometrium and the myometrium at the uterine fundus, delineate the entire cervical canal, and depict the corneal angles. This enables the operator to measure the depth of the uterine septum and the distance between the apex of the septum and the internal os. In addition, the use of 3D US enables us to diagnose new types of the uterine septum, such as unequal sides [33,34]. Furthermore, 3D US can differentiate between arcuate uterus and a short, incomplete septum.

Another major advantage is that with 3D US a volume of ultrasonographic data are rapidly stored and made available for later analysis. This is particularly helpful in case of SHG. The ability to store data would shorten the amount of time during which the uterine cavity must remain distended [35]. Obviously this is major advantage of 3D US because all of the original ultrasonographic data are contained in the saved volume without loss of information, as might occur when only selected static images are available for interpretation, which is the case with 2D US [36]. Even if the ultrasonographic procedure is videotaped, findings remain operator-dependent, and any observation not clearly documented on the tape would be lost. The multiplanar capability of 3D US permits an unlimited number of scan planes to be obtained from the original data set, an advantage that should significantly reduce operator-dependent bias. This data set is available for interactive review at any time after the patient has been discharged or before surgical intervention. Additional findings not initially detected during the real-time examination can be made by "scrolling" through the volume data. Clearly, this can be accomplished without inconveniencing the patient by prolonged or repeated vaginal scanning [36]. Clearly, combining SHG with 3D US can add to the accuracy of both procedures [37].

One limitation of 3D US is the time required to learn to manipulate the 3D volume data, although this decreases with experience. Also, shadowing caused by uterine fibroids, irregular endometrial lining, or thickened endometrial lining (as seen during the periovulatory period), as well as the decreased volume of the uterine cavity (in cases of intrauterine adhesions) are obvious limitations of 3D US [26]. Furthermore, we have observed that when the uterus is retroverted in position some difficulty is encountered in making the diagnosis of subtle uterine septum or arcuate uterus by 3D US.

3D US has been reported to have a sensitivity and specificity of 100% in diagnosing arcuate uteri compared with 67% and 94%, respectively, for transvaginal 2D US. Interestingly, in diagnosing major müllerian anomalies, while the sensitivity and specificity of transvaginal 3D US were both 100% compared with 100% sensitivity and 95% specificity for transvaginal 2D US, the positive predictive value was 100% for 3D US but only 50% for 2D US [34]. Because of the higher accuracy of the 3D US in diagnosing müllerian disorders, higher prevalence (~6%) was reported when 3D US was applied for detecting

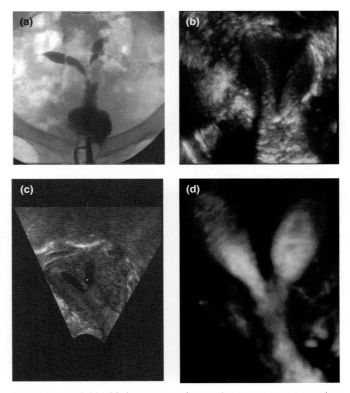

Figure 18.9a–d. (a) HSG showing complete uterine septum versus complete bicornuate uterus. (b) Transvaginal 3D US showing complete uterine septum. (c) Transvaginal 3D US showing complete uterine septum during SHG. (d) Transvaginal 3D US showing bicornuate uterus.

those disorders [32]. Figure 18.7b is a transvaginal 3D US picture showing significant incomplete uterine septum. Figure 18.7c is a transvaginal 3D US image showing incomplete uterine septum during SHG. Figure 18.7e is a transvaginal 3D US picture showing subtle incomplete septum with wide base. Figures 18.9b and 18.9c illustrate a transvaginal 3D US picture showing complete uterine septum and SHG of complete uterine septum, respectively. Figure 18.9d illustrates how the diagnosis of bicornuate uterus can be made by transvaginal 3D US. Figures 18.9b and 18.9d illustrate how 3D US can differentiate between uterine septum and bicornuate uterus by allowing evaluation of the external contour of the fundal region. Figures 18.10b and 18.10c are, respectively, transvaginal 3D US pictures showing a subtle incomplete septum of the asymmetrical variant, and the same phenomenon during SHG. Notice that the left side is more prominent than the right side. Figure 18.12 is a transvaginal 3D US image showing a typical T-shaped uterus with an arcuate appearance of the fundal region (T-shaped shallow septum).

Doppler ultrasonography

Evaluation of the vascularity of the septum by Doppler ultrasonography is believed to provide important information about its structure and the risk of reproductive problems. Kupesic and

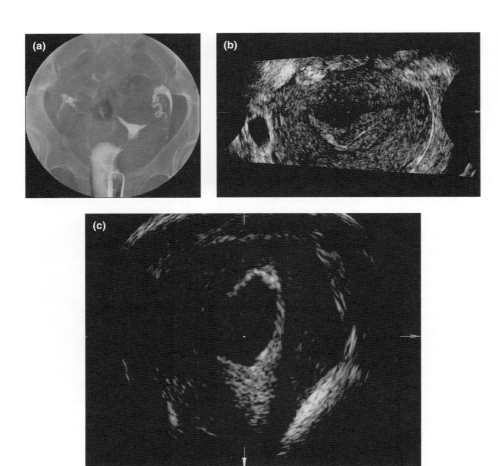

Figure 18.10. (a) HSG picture of a variant of subtle incomplete septum with asymmetrical sides (right side more prominent than left side). (b) Transvaginal 3D US showing a subtle incomplete uterine septum. (c) SHG showing a subtle asymmetrical uterine septum.

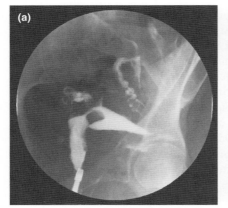
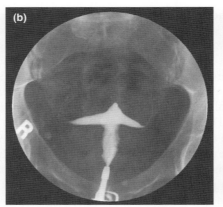
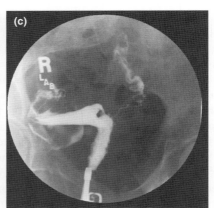

Figure 18.11. HSG images showing an acutely anteverted/anteflexed (a) and retroverted/retroflexed uterus (b), and a uterus rotated to one side (c).

Kurjak [38] attempted to evaluate the combined use of transvaginal 2D US, transvaginal color and pulsed Doppler ultrasonography, HSG, and transvaginal 3D US in the preoperative diagnosis of uterine septum in a group of 420 infertile patients undergoing operative hysteroscopy. Of these, 278 patients had an intrauterine septum (66.2% of all patients) that was corrected surgically. In 43 patients with a uterine septum, there was a history of repeated spontaneous miscarriage, and 71 had had one spontaneous miscarriage (56 in the first trimester, and 15 in

the second trimester). Each patient underwent transvaginal ultrasound and transvaginal color Doppler examination during the luteal phase of their cycle. Color and pulsed Doppler were superimposed to visualize intraseptal and myometrial vascularity in each patient. It is interesting that, although the authors did not find correlation between septal length or the septal thickness and occurrence of obstetric complications, they found the septal vascularity to correlate significantly with those complications. The authors extrapolated from those data that this

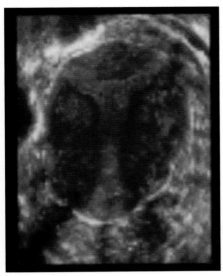

Figure 18.12. Transvaginal 3D US showing a typical T-shaped uterus with an arcuate appearance of the fundal region (T-shaped shallow septum).

might reflect an increased amount of muscle in the septum, producing local uncoordinated myometrial contractility that resulted in adverse obstetric outcomes [39].

Magnetic resonance imaging (MRI)

MRI can delineate both internal and external uterine architecture, which provides an interesting alternative diagnostic method for the evaluation of müllerian tract anomalies. However, several disadvantages make it difficult to apply in routine practice, including high cost, unsuitability for office practice, and most importantly, the extremely high accuracy of 3D US, which can provide very comparable information to that from MRI while having the advantages of low cost, suitability for office practice, and even more information, including Doppler examination of the vascularity. However, MRI is mandatory for differentiating between uterus didelphys and long complete uterine septum with cervical duplication and a vertical vaginal septum.

Surgery

Hysteroscopy allows both direct visualization of the uterine cavity and operative intervention when uterine septa are encountered. As is the case with HSG, hysteroscopy cannot evaluate the external contour of the uterus. However, advantages of hysteroscopy are the direct visualization of the endometrium and the fact that it can be performed as an outpatient procedure, though one should be aware of the risk of surgical complications, e.g., perforation, infection, and bleeding. Concurrent laparoscopy is essential for evaluation of the external contour of the uterus, mainly to differentiate between uterine septum and bicornuate uterus, which cannot be surgically corrected through the hysteroscopic approach if even surgical correction is warranted. In addition, laparoscopy is helpful for assessing the extent of hysteroscopic resection of

uterine septa, and identifying and repair of uterine perforation promptly should it occur [26]. Furthermore, laparoscopy should be mandatory if hysteroscopic metroplasty is performed in a patient with a history of infertility, to rule out endometriosis, pelvic adhesions, and subtle fimbrial pathology [40]. This is particularly the case in view of recent data suggesting an association between uterine septum and endometriosis [41].

Reproductive problems associated with uterine septum

Various clinical problems have been reported, including pregnancy failure and other obstetric complications, e.g., preterm labor and placental abruption. Other reproductive problems, especially infertility, have been suggested, thought not universally accepted. Other conditions, e.g., endometriosis, and urinary tract anomalies and even malignancy, have been thought to be associated with congenital uterine malformation. For a comprehensive review of the various reproductive problems associated with uterine septum, and reproductive outcome of uterine septum treatment, refer to our chapter in the earlier work mentioned in the introduction [1].

Management of uterine septum and the role of ultrasonography

Treatment of uterine septum has come full circle, from its start in 1919 with successful transcervical therapy [42,43] to be replaced by the abdominal approach (e.g., Jones and Tompkins procedures). This latter approach has become almost obsolete, with the consensus now back to the transcervical approach (hysteroscopic metroplasty). Hysteroscopic resection is favored because of its simplicity compared with the abdominal metroplasty that is performed through a laparotomy [44]. The abdominal approach has been proposed for extremely wide uterine septum, but the transcervical approach can still be accomplished in most cases, although a second attempt might be necessary in certain instances to completely incise the septum [24].

Which septum needs resection?

The answer to which septum needs resection depends primarily on the reproductive history rather than the type of the septum itself; for example, hysteroscopic metroplasty is obviously recommended for patients with a history of recurrent pregnancy loss. However, it is important to evaluate patients with pregnancy loss who also have uterine septa, to rule out additional underlying etiologies.

Other reasonable indications include a history of adverse obstetric outcomes, including second-trimester losses, abnormal presentation, preterm deliveries, or antepartum hemorrhage when associated with a uterine septum. Again, it is important to reiterate that it is the history of reproductive problems rather than the extent of the uterine septum that should determine the decision whether to resect or not. Age is another consideration, because older women may benefit from prompt treatment to optimize outcome. Choe and Baggish [45] suggested that the uterine septum should be corrected as early as possible, especially in patients >35 years of age, to increase fecundity.

When a uterine septum is an incidental finding in a woman without a history of reproductive problems that are known to be associated with uterine septum, it is still a controversial issue whether prophylactic metroplasty should be done to prevent those complications. Limited data suggest that metroplasty is not indicated for treatment of infertility, because primary infertility patients conceived after metroplasty at a similar rate to that in infertile counterparts without septa [18]. In women with the incidental diagnosis of uterine cavity disorders at the time of abdominal or pelvic surgery performed for other reasons, successful pregnancy was achieved in the majority of patients with didelphys, bicornuate, and septate uteri, with success rates of 93%, 84%, and 78%, respectively [46].

We have extensive experience (unpublished data) with a large number of cases (more than 300) in which short uterine septum was diagnosed as an incidental finding during routine infertility work-up (~50% with primary infertility). After diagnosis patients with primary infertility were counseled regarding the two options of prophylactic metroplasty versus proceeding with infertility interventions (ovarian hyperstimulation with intrauterine insemination [COH + IUI] and ART when insemination is not successful) without surgical correction of the uterine septum. The majority of these patients opted to undergo hysteroscopic metroplasty. We observed an increased spontaneous fecundity rate, excellent pregnancy rates after COH + IUI and ART, and excellent obstetric outcome [47]. Interestingly in patients with secondary infertility, hysteroscopic metroplasty has reversed previous poor outcomes and the majority of those patients achieved full-term deliveries spontaneously or after receiving their infertility intervention following hysteroscopic metroplasty (unpublished data). These findings prompted us to favor and to recommend routine resection of uterine septum (irrespective of its extent) before infertility interventions (ovarian stimulation with insemination or ART), or even when patients want to continue to try to achieve pregnancy spontaneously [46]. Moreover, the simplicity of hysteroscopic treatment and low morbidity have advanced the argument for prophylactic hysteroscopic metroplasty, particularly in women with unexplained infertility, before ART treatment, or even for removal of the septum at the time of diagnosis to increase fecundity and to prevent miscarriages and obstetric complications [48].

Preoperative preparation

It is advisable to perform surgery early during the follicular phase, or alternatively patients are treated preoperatively with a gonadotropin-releasing hormone analog, to eliminate the possibility of thick endometrium diminishing the clarity of view during surgery. We have fairly good experience of endometrial preparation with a few weeks of combined oral contraceptives.

It is interesting to mention here the approach for preparing the endometrial cavity before hysteroscopic metroplasty and other forms of hysteroscopic surgery that benefit from achieving a thin endometrium, namely, using one of the new third-generation aromatase inhibitors anastrozole or letrozole. By shutting off estrogen production, the use of aromatase inhibitors for few days before hysteroscopic surgery is expected to result in a thin endometrium that will facilitate the performance of the surgery [45].

Preoperative antibiotics are often given empirically, despite the lack of strong evidence to support their use [24]. In our practice we do not routinely administer any antibiotics either preoperatively or postoperatively.

Operative technique

Before we proceed to the detailed description of the surgical management of uterine septum (septum resection), it is important to clarify the misnomer of the term "resection." Surgical management of the uterine septum actually involves its "incision" and not "resection." Some prefer the word "lyse" rather than "resect" to describe the surgical management of the uterine septum.

As explained earlier, uterine septum results from the incomplete fusion between the two müllerian ducts. Anatomically the two ducts are side by side. Incomplete fusion results in the persistence of the wall between the two tubes (the uterine septum) that extends anteroposteriorly (sagittal axis). For that reason, the uterine septum extends between the "anterior" and "posterior" walls of the uterus. Hence the septum should be incised transversely. Every effort should be made that the transverse incision be equidistant between the anterior and posterior uterine wall up to the fundus, without entering the fundal myometrium. The septum should be transected systematically in the midline, avoiding drifting to the posterior or anterior wall.

There are three important tools to help navigate the systematic resection of the septum in the midline (as illustrated in Figure 18.13): (1) following the symmetry of both uterine tubal openings; (2) observing the rich myometrial vascularization when cutting through the uterine wall; (3) observing the uniform translucency of the hysteroscopic light laparoscopically.

At the completion of the procedure, the intrauterine pressure produced by the distending fluid may be lowered to less than 50 mmHg. This helps in identifying areas of bleeding. Usually, small bleeders stop on their own, but if the number of active arterial bleeders is significant, these can be individually coagulated with a pinpoint electrode [21,46,47,48].

Postoperative care

After the procedure, uterine bleeding may be controlled using a Foley catheter to tamponade the cavity. It is important to ensure the patient's ability to void on her own before discharge home. Pain medications are usually administered in the form of mild analgesics. The use of strong analgesics is particularly important when a Foley catheter is left inside the uterine cavity. Some may

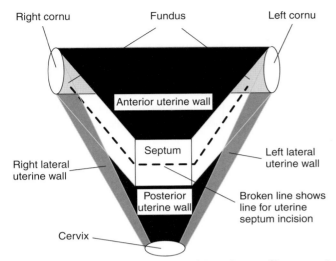

Right cornu — Fundus — Left cornu

Anterior uterine wall

Septum — Left lateral uterine wall

Right lateral uterine wall

Posterior uterine wall — Broken line shows line for uterine septum incision

Cervix

Figure 18.13. Schematic representation of the technique of hysteroscopic incision of the uterine septum. The hallmark of success of this procedure lies in incising the septum in the right plane., i.e., the middle of the septum (as shown by the broken line), avoiding too much interference with the anterior or the posterior wall of the uterus or the fundus.

insert an intrauterine device to prevent formation of intrauterine adhesions (synechiae). However, other surgeons may opt to leave the uterine cavity empty. Hormonal therapy is often prescribed after the procedure to promote rapid epithelialization and decrease the risk of intrauterine synechiae. Estrogens are usually given in the form of conjugated estrogens and progesterone, such as medroxyprogesterone acetate, after the estrogen course is completed. At the completion of hormonal treatment and withdrawal bleeding, SHG with 3D US is performed to assess the results of the hysteroscopic treatment by evaluating the uterine cavity. If the uterine cavity is satisfactory, the patient is allowed to conceive. Once pregnancy is achieved, consideration should be given to cervical cerclage versus careful monitoring of the cervical length with frequent transvaginal ultrasound. Attempts at pregnancy should be postponed for 2 months after surgery, because postoperative hysteroscopy with biopsy has shown the uterine cavity to be normal at 8 weeks after surgery [48].

Role of ultrasonography in the management of uterine septum

In addition to the role of ultrasonography in the diagnosis of uterine septum, we believe it to have a significant role in its management before, during, and after hysteroscopic resection.

Preoperative ultrasonography

We strongly recommend ultrasonographic evaluation of the endometrium to confirm that the endometrium is thin enough within a few days prior to the surgery. An endometrial thickness less than 6 mm should be suitable and a thickness less than 4 mm would be ideal. There are no significant data in the literature regarding the optimal endometrial thickness prior to hysteroscopic incision of uterine septum.

Intraoperative ultrasonography

We recommend performing hysteroscopic incision of the uterine septum under ultrasonographic guidance. The use of intraoperative transvaginal ultrasonography helps in ensuring complete incision of the septum all the way to the level of the uterine fundus, as well as the perfect placement of the uterine stent (intrauterine balloon) after completing surgery to prevent formation of intrauterine synechiae.

With the help of an assistant, it is usually technically feasible to perform transvaginal ultrasonography during operative hysteroscopy. Interestingly, we found also that a transrectal approach (by placing the vaginal ultrasound probe into the rectum) provides an excellent view of the uterine wall and uterine cavity. Such an approach provides help in determining the extent of hysteroscopic dissection for various hysteroscopic procedures. This might reduce the risk of uterine perforation and helps ensure adequate resection of uterine cavity lesions, including uterine septi and others such as submucous leiomyomas. We adopted the approach of transrectal ultrasonography by extrapolation from the approach of transesophageal intraoperative ultrasonography during cardiac surgery.

Postoperative ultrasonography

There have been some pathological studies showing that residual septa on the anterior and posterior walls, after septal incision, retract underneath the endometrium and the endometrium then overgrows the area [26]. Traditionally, most gynecologists are very conservative while performing hysteroscopic metroplasty for fear of uterine perforation or subsequent uterine rupture during pregnancy. Some have noted that postoperative HSG always showed a residual septum [49]. Others have found that the reproductive performance was not adversely affected by a residual septum of up to 1 cm [50]. A recent report suggests that women with a residual uterine septum have an increased chance of successful pregnancy with improved obstetric outcome after normalization of the uterine cavity [51].

Grimbizis et al. [52] reported that all patients with recurrent miscarriage and normal fertility who were trying to become pregnant conceived spontaneously at least once after their treatment. Daly et al. [53] have reported normal postoperative monthly fecundity rates. This confirms that hysteroscopic metroplasty does not impair the fertility potential of women with a history of recurrent miscarriages.

Grimbizis et al. [52] found significant improvement in pregnancy outcomes following hysteroscopic resection of the uterine septum, including a drop in the miscarriage rate to 25% and increase in term delivery rate to 63.7% (although 4.5% of the pregnancies were still ongoing at the time of their publication). Other investigators have also described a significant improvement in pregnancy outcome after hysteroscopic metroplasty. Postoperative miscarriage rates between 5% and 20% and live birth rates between 73% and 87% were reported [17,18,21,54,55]. However, the studies reported had significant limitations, including the retrospective design and absence of control groups (patients served as their own historical control in some). Interestingly, data are more impressive in women with uterine septum undergoing ART. While pregnancy rates achieved after ART treatment done before and after hysteroscopic resection of the septum were comparable, the improvement of pregnancy outcome was very impressive [26]. A review of the literature indicates an overall term delivery rate of about 50% in patients with untreated uterine malformations, while the term delivery rate after hysteroscopic treatment is about 75%. The rate of pregnancy wastage in the post-treatment group was 15% compared with 96.3% in the pretreatment group. The authors concluded that hysteroscopic septum resection can be applied as a therapeutic procedure in symptomatic patients, and also as a "prophylactic" procedure in asymptomatic patients in order to improve their chances of a successful delivery [52,56].

Patients with a previous hysteroscopic metroplasty or complicated hysteroscopy should be aware of the potential risks of uterine rupture during pregnancy. In a recent review of the literature to identify predictors of uterine rupture following operative hysteroscopy, the authors found that a history of uterine perforation and/or the use of electrosurgery increase this risk but were not considered an independent risk factor. The authors concluded that uncomplicated hysteroscopic surgery did not alter obstetric outcome and, apart from use of scissors being favorable for hysteroscopic metroplasty, no accurate methods to prevent or detect impending ruptures in subsequent pregnancies were found [57]. In another series, two cases of uterine rupture during the delivery of twin pregnancies after hysteroscopic metroplasty led the investigators to suggest that cesarean section be performed for multiple pregnancy [58]. In our experience, we had no patients who experienced uterine rupture in a subsequent pregnancy following hysteroscopic resection of the uterine septum (unpublished data).

Summary and future research

There is significant controversy concerning the diagnosis and management of uterine septum. The technology of 3D US constitutes a major breakthrough in evaluating the uterine cavity. This is particularly true when the assessment is complemented by both color Doppler examination and distension of the uterine cavity with saline or ultrasound contrast medium (SHG).

There are enough data to support the routine surgical excision of uterine septa, irrespective of their types, in women with poor reproductive history and in particular recurrent pregnancy loss. However, in asymptomatic patients, the prophylactic excision of incidentally discovered uterine septum in asymptomatic patients is still controversial. In women undergoing ART treatment, surgical excision of an incidentally discovered uterine septum is more universally accepted. In infertility patients we believe that incidentally discovered uterine septum and even arcuate uterus should be corrected hysteroscopically prior to any infertility treatment, to enhance reproductive outcome

The hysteroscopic approach for surgical resection of uterine septum is a safe and effective approach. While generally it is an operator preference whether to utilize ablative energy, e.g., electrical diathermy or laser, or to utilize sharp scissors without energy, the outcome of treatment is comparable as regards complication and reproductive performance after surgery.

For women with incidentally discovered uterine septum, there is a need for randomized prospective trials comparing pregnancy rate and pregnancy outcome in a treated and an untreated group. In such studies, accurate diagnosis of the extent and structure of the uterine septum can provide extremely valuable information about which septum subtypes correlate significantly with the different reproductive outcomes.

Key points in clinical practice

- The reproductive implications associated with the presence of uterine septa are a matter of significant controversy in the literature.

- There is consensus on a relationship between uterine septa and various reproductive problems. However, the nature and extent of this relationship is still a big dilemma.

- A significant part of this dilemma is due to variation in the literature regarding the methods of diagnosis, treatment, and follow-up of women with uterine septa.

- The technology of 3D US constitutes a major breakthrough in evaluating the uterine cavity disorders, including uterine septa.

- While there are data supporting the routine surgical excision of uterine septa, irrespective of their types, in women with recurrent pregnancy loss, in asymptomatic patients the prophylactic excision of incidentally discovered uterine septum is still controversial. However, prior to assisted reproduction, surgical excision of an incidentally discovered uterine septum is more universally accepted.

- In infertility patients we believe that incidentally discovered uterine septum and even arcuate uterus should be corrected hysteroscopically prior to any infertility treatment to enhance reproductive outcome.

- While the hysteroscopic approach for surgical resection of uterine septum is safe and effective, the choice of surgical technique (using sharp scissors or electrocautery) is an operator preference.

- For women with incidentally discovered uterine septum, there is a need for randomized prospective trials comparing reproductive performance in a treated and an untreated group.

References

1. Mitwally M, Abuzeid M. Operative hysteroscopy for uterine septum. In: Rizk B, Garcia Velasco JA, Sallam H, Makrigiannakis A, eds. *Infertility and Assisted Reproduction*, chapter 13. Cambridge: Cambridge University Press, 2008; 115–31.

2. Patton PE. Anatomic uterine defects. *Clin Obst Gynecol* 1994; **37**: 705–21.

3. McBean JH, Brumsted JR. Septate uterus with cervical duplication: a rare malformation. *Fertil Steril* 1994; **62**: 415–17.

4. March ChM. Mullerian anomalies. Fertil News 24/1. *Endocrine Fertil Forum* 1990; **13**: 1–5.

5. Ergun A, Pabuccu R. Atay V, et al. Three sisters with septate uteri: another reference to bidirectional theory. *Hum Reprod* 1997; **12**: 140–2.

6. Muller PP, Musset R, Netter A, et al. État du haut appareil urinaire chez les porteuses de malformations uterines: etude de 133 observations. *La Presse Med* 1967; **75**: 1331–6.

7. Acien P. Incidence of Müllerian defects in fertile and infertile women. *Hum Reprod* 1997; **12**: 1372–6.

8. Maneschi F, Zupi E, Marconi D, et al. Hysteroscopically detected asymptomatic Müllerian anomalies. *J Reprod Med* 1995; **40**: 684–8.

9. Ashton D, Amin HK, Richart RM, et al. The incidence of asymptomatic uterine anomalies in women undergoing transcervical tubal sterilization. *Obstet Gynecol* 1988; **72**: 28–30.

10. Raga F, Bauset C, Remohi J et al. (1997). Reproductive impact of congenital Müllerian anomalies. *Hum Reprod* **12**: 2277–81.

11. Nasri MN, Setchell ME, Chard T. Transvaginal ultrasound for the diagnosis of uterine malformations. *Br J Obstet Gynecol* 1990; **97**: 1043–5.

12. Heinonen PK. Reproductive performance of women with uterine anomalies after abdominal or hysteroscopic metroplasty or no surgical treatment, *J Am Assoc Gynecol Laparosc* 1997; **4**: 311–17.

13. Grimbizis GF, Camus M, Tarlatzis BC, et al. Clinical implications of uterine malformations and hysteroscopic treatment results. *Hum Reprod Update* 2001; **7**: 161–74.

14. Homer HA, Cooke TC Li, ID. The septate uterus: a review of management and reproductive outcome. *Fertil Steril* 2000; **73**: 1–14.

15. Buttram VC, Gibbons WE. Muellerian anomalies: a proposed classification (an analysis of 144 cases). *Fertil Steril* 1979; **32**: 40–6.

16. The American Fertility Society. The American Fertility Society classifications of adnexal adhesions, distal tubal occlusion, tubal occlusion secondary to tubal ligation, tubal pregnancies, Müllerian anomalies and intrauterine adhesions. *Fertil Steril* 1988; **49**: 944–55.

17. Fayez JA. Comparison between abdominal and hysteroscopic metroplasty. *Obstet Gynecol* 1986; **68**: 399–403.

18. Daly DC, Maier D, Soto-Albors C. Hysteroscopic metroplasty: six years' experience. *Obstet Gynecol* 1989; **73**: 201–5.

19. March CM. Hysteroscopy as an aid to diagnosis in female infertility. *Clin Obstet Gynecol* 1983; **26**: 302–12.

20. Worthen N, Gonzalez F. Septate uterus: sonographic diagnosis and obstetric complications. *Obstet Gynecol* 1984; **64**: 345–85.

21. Perino A, Mencaglia L, Hamou J, et al. Hysteroscopy for metroplasty of uterine septa: report of 24 cases. *Fertil Steril* 1987; **48**: 321–3.

22. Dabirashrafi H, Bahadori M, Mohammad K, et al. Septate uterus: New idea on the histologic features of the septum in this abnormal

uterus. *Am J Obstet Gynecol* 1995; **172**: (1 pt 1): 105–7.

23. Kupesic S, Kurjak A. Septate uterus: detection and prediction of obstetrical complications by different forms of ultrasonography. *J Ultrasound Med* 1998; **17**: 631–6.

24. Baramki T. Congenital uterine malformations. In: Rizk B, Garcia Velasco JA, Sallam H, Makrigiannakis A, eds. *Infertility and Assisted Reproduction*. Chapter 35. Cambridge: Cambridge University Press, 2008; 327–31.

25. Carrington BM, Hricak H, Nuruddin RN, et al. Müllerian duct anomalies: magnetic resonance imaging evaluation. *Radiology* 1990; **176**: 715.

26. Kupesic S. Clinical implications of sonographic detection of uterine anomalies for reproductive outcome. *Ultrasound Obstet Gynecol* 2001; **18**: 387–400.

27. Nicolini U, Bellotti M, Bonazzi B, et al. Can ultrasound be used to screen uterine malformations? *Fertil Steril* 1987; **47**: 89–93.

28. Keltz MD, Olive DL, Kim AH, et al. Sonohysterography for screening in recurrent pregnancy loss. *Fertil Steril* 1997; **67**: 670–4.

29. Soares SR, Barbosa dos Reis MMB, Camargos AF. Diagnostic accuracy of sonohysterography, transvaginal sonography, and hysterosalpingography in patients with uterine cavity diseases. *Fertil Steril* 2000; **73**: 406–11.

30. Exalto N, Stappers C, van Raamsdonk LA, Emanuel MH. Gel instillation sonohysterography: first experience with a new technique. *Fertil Steril* 2007; **87**: 152–5.

31. Jurkovic D, Geipel A, Gruboeck K, et al. Three-dimensional ultrasound for the assessment of uterine anatomy and detection of congenital anomalies: a comparison with hysterosalpingography and two-dimensional sonography. *Ultrasound Obstet Gynecol* **5**: 1995; 233–7.

32. Jurkovic D, Gruboeck K, Tailor A, et al. Ultrasound screening for congenital uterine anomalies. *Br J Obstet Gynaecol* 1997; **104**: 1320–1.

33. Abuzeid OM, Sakhel K, Abuzeid MI. Diagnosis of various types of uterine septum in infertile patients. *J Minim Invasive Gynecol* 2005; **12**(5): 117.

34. Hartman A. Uterine imaging – malformations, fibroids and adenomyosis. *Thirty-Ninth Annual Postgraduate Program, Course 17 Reproductive Imaging – How to Improve the Outcome of Assisted Reproductive Technology.* New Orleans, Louisana; sponsored by ASRM, October 22, 2006.

35. Weinraub Z, Maymon R, Shulman A, et al. Three-dimensional saline contrast hysterosonography and surface rendering of uterine cavity pathology. *Ultrasound Obstet Gynecol* 1996; **8**: 277–82.

36. Lev-Toaff AS, Pinheiro LW, Bega G, et al. Three-dimensional multiplanar sonohysterography. *J Ultrasound Med* 2001; **20**: 295–306.

37. Ayida G, Kennedy S, Barlow D, et al. Contrast sonography for uterine cavity assessment: a comparison of conventional two-dimensional with three-dimensional transvaginal ultrasound: a pilot study. *Fertil Steril* 1996; **66**: 848–50.

38. Kupesic S, Kurjak A. Diagnosis and treatment outcome of the septate uterus. *Croat Med J* 1998; **39**: 185–90.

39. Toaff ME, Lev-Toaff AS. Communicating uteri: review and classification of two previously unreported types. *Fertil Steril* 1984; **41**: 661–79.

40. Abuzeid M, Mitwally MF, Ahmed A, et al. The prevalence of fimbrial pathology in patients with early stages of endometriosis. *J Minim Invasive Gynecol* 2007; **14**: 49–53.

41. Abuzeid MI, Sakhel K, Khedr M, et al. The association of endometriosis and uterine septum. *Hum Reprod Suppl* 2003; **1**: P-610.

42. Hirst BC. The operative treatment of uterus subseptus or semipartus with a case report. *Trans Obstet Soc Phila* **1919**: 891–2.

43. Luikart R. Technique of successful removal of the septum uterine septus and subsequent deliveries at term. *Am J Obstet Gynecol* 1936; **31**: 797–9.

44. Rock JA. Surgery for anomalies of the Müllerian ducts. In: Thompson JD, Rock JA, eds. *Te Linde's Operative Gynecology*, 7th edn. Philadelphia, PA: Lippincott, 1992; 603–46.

45 Choe KJ, Baggish SM. Hysteroscopic treatment of septate uterus with neodymium-YAG laser. *Fertil Steril* 1992; **57**: 81–4.

46. Abuzeid M, Sakhel K, Imam M, Mitwally MF, Ashraf M, Diamond MP. Reproductive outcome after hysteroscopic metroplasty in women with primary infertility. *J Minim Invasive Gynecol* 2008; **15**: 80S.

47. Lin BL, Iwata Y, Miyamoto N, et al. Three contrast methods: an ultrasound technique for monitoring transcervical operations. *Am J Obstet Gynecol* 1987; **56**: 469–72.

48. Mencaglia L, Tantini C. Hysteroscopic treatment of septate and arcuate uterus. *Gynaecol Endosc* 1996; **5**: 151–4.

49. Nisolle M, Donnez J. Endoscopic treatment of uterine malformations. *Gynaecol Endosc* 1996; **5**: 155–60.

50. Fedele L, Bianchi S, Marchini M, et al. Residual uterine septum of less than 1cm after hysteroscopic metroplasty does not impair reproductive outcome. *Hum Reprod* 1996; **11**: 727–9.

51. Kormanyos Z, Molnar BG, Pal A. Removal of a residual portion of a uterine septum in women of advanced reproductive age: obstetric outcome. *Hum Reprod* 2006; **4**: 1047–51.

52. Grimbizis G, Camus M, Clasen K, et al. Hysteroscopic septum resection in patients with recurrent abortions or infertility. *Hum Reprod* 1998 **13**: 1188–93.

53. Daly DC, Maier D, Soto-Albers C. Hysteroscopic metroplasty: six years' experience. *Obstet Gynecol* 1989; **73**: 201–5.

54. Fedele L, Arcaini L, Parazzini F, et al. Reproductive prognosis after hysteroscopic metroplasty in 102 women: lifetable analysis. *Fertil Steril* 1993; **59**: 768–72.

55. Jacobsen IJ, DeCherney A. Results of conventional and hysteroscopic surgery. *Hum Reprod* 1997; **12**: 1376–81.

56. Preutthipan S, Linasmita V. Reproductive outcome following hysteroscopic treatment of the septate uterus: a result of 28 cases at Ramathibodi Hospital. *J Med Assoc Thai* 2001; **84**: 166–70.

57. Sentilhes L, Sergent F, Roman H, et al. Late complications of operative hysteroscopy: predicting patients at risk of uterine rupture during subsequent pregnancy. *Eur J Obstet Gynecol Reprod Biol* 2005; **120**: 134–8.

58. Nisolle L, Donnez J. Endoscopic treatment of uterine malformations. *Gyaecol Endosc* 1996; **5**; 155–60.

Chapter 19

Ultrasonography and incidental ovarian pathology

Dimitrios Siassakos, Valentine Akande and Luciano G. Nardo

Introduction

Ultrasonography is an invaluable tool in the noninvasive assessment and monitoring of treatment in infertile women. Incidental adnexal pathology is identified in 5–18% of such women when using ultrasound (US). Transvaginal high-resolution ultrasonography in particular has gained widespread use in infertile women because of the detail that can be visualized when examining the pelvis and reproductive organs. Incidental adnexal masses may be seen when pelvic ultrasound or hysterosalpingo-contrast-ultrasonography (HyCoSy) is performed with the intention of evaluating uterine pathologies potentially associated with subfertility, such as adhesions, polyps, submucous leiomyomas, and septae [1].

Adnexal pathology may also be seen when monitoring ovarian response to stimulation with gonadotropins or ovulation induction with clomiphene citrate, during oocyte retrieval, or at the time of US-guided embryo transfer. A functional ovarian cyst is also a relatively common finding with the widespread use of gonadotropin-releasing hormone (GnRH) agonists, which initially provoke an initial follicle-stimulating hormone (FSH) surge [2]. In addition, women undergoing ovarian stimulation may present with acute pelvic pain because of ovarian hyperstimulation syndrome (OHSS), pelvic infection, or ovarian accident.

In this chapter we will discuss a range of incidental adnexal findings in nonacute presentations, their significance for reproduction and assisted reproductive technologies (ART), and how to approach them once found.

Differential diagnosis

Imaging artifacts

Artifacts found during ultrasonography can be the result of either operator technique or patient characteristics, for example, increased subcutaneous fat.

"Reverberation" occurs when reflections from a highly reflective structure bounce back and forth within adjacent tissue before returning to the ultrasound probe, resulting in the system recording each of these bounced reflections as a separate structure. These can present as false septae within cysts.

"Refraction" occurs when sound is bent as a result of adjacent tissues with dissimilar sound propagation velocities. This results in the position of a lesion being demonstrated as displaced' e.g., a mass may be seen within the adnexae when it actually belongs to another structure.

"Mirror image" occurs when strong reflectors send the beam off the scan plane toward another lateral structure, and the reflection of that structure returns via the same path all the way back to the transducer. The system assumes that propagation occurred in an entirely linear fashion, and places the structure straight behind the strong reflector, as well as in its original lateral position as scanned by another part of the beam.

To decrease the likelihood of such artifacts, one should aim for achieving a perpendicular direction of the ultrasound beam relative to the structure or organ under observation.

Physiological artifacts

The ability to identify abnormality relies on the operator's knowledge of normality, but also on recognition of the physiological changes that occur in the menstrual cycle or in response to treatment or pregnancy. For example, fluid in the pouch of Douglas is a common feature and may relate to the phase of the menstrual cycle. As such, there is almost always a small amount present after ovulation. A rule of thumb is that it should never be more than 2 cm in depth, or more than two-thirds of the length of the uterus in the sagittal plane. Increasing density or volume of hyperechoic particles or strands is suggestive of pathology, for example, bleeding, inflammation, or infection.

The ovary is a dynamic structure of utmost endocrine importance for fertility, where follicles are noted to grow, regress, or ovulate. When ovulation is impending, the mature follicle can present as a simple cyst with a small internal protrusion, which represents the cumulus oophorus.

Multiple, unilateral, or bilateral ovarian peripheral echogenic foci are common and can be found in up to 49% of women; these usually have a punctuate pattern and may represent psammomatous calcifications associated with superficial epithelial inclusion cysts [3]. It must be noted, however, that

Ultrasonography in Reproductive Medicine and Infertility, ed. Botros R. M. B. Rizk. Published by Cambridge University Press. © Cambridge University Press 2010.

calcifications are also a feature of serous cystadenomas and dermoids, and when uncertain further diagnostics should be considered.

Bowel masses

Bowel masses are identified by the presence of multiple wall layers (2–5 visible, "target" sign) and usually peristalsis. Fecal matter can make diagnosis more difficult and necessitate the use of enemas. If bowel shadowing makes the visualization of the pelvic organs difficult, placing the patient in the Trendelenburg position may improve the ultrasound picture.

Adnexal masses

Table 19.1 describes some of the incidental pathologies that can be found while scanning the adnexal area. Sometimes these can be difficult to visualize and may require positioning the patient in a favorable position for adequate pelvic images to be obtained; for example, placing the patient in a semi-lithotomy position, with the pelvis raised by placing a pillow and/or fists under the buttocks, for a transvaginal ultrasound scan.

Diagnostic approach to masses

The size of the mass in three dimensions, its location, consistency, and borders (well-/ill-defined) should be determined. With regard to cysts, it is important to note wall thickness, whether they are unilocular or multilocular, the presence, regularity and thickness of septae, the presence of nodules or projections, or any other solid components. One should always check the contralateral adnexum and the pouch of Douglas, as well as around both adnexae for free fluid. The more abnormalities, the higher the index of suspicion of abnormal pathology such as malignancy.

Generally, most diagnoses can be made by transvaginal ultrasonography; however, a combination of transabdominal and transvaginal scan should be considered as they have different advantages and disadvantages (Table 19.2). Color and power Doppler ultrasound examination may be a useful adjunct for assessing blood flow around cysts as well as within masses and septae. Further examination with computed tomography (CT) or magnetic resonance imaging (MRI) may be indicated in selected cases.

The patient's age is important: young women (with infertility due to congenital anomalies) are more likely to have germ cell tumors than women who are older than 40 years. For the latter, the possibility of malignancy is increased.

History may elicit diagnostic clues: long-standing dyspareunia and dysmenorrhea in a patient with a thick-walled cyst with internal echoes on ultrasound suggests an endometrioma rather than a hemorrhagic corpus luteum, whereas a family history of ovarian cancer should lower the threshold for further investigation of any ovarian mass.

Selected laboratory tests such as CA-125 may be useful, but also consider additional investigations if malignancy is highly suspected or if there is concern about ureteric compression, particularly with large or retroperitoneal masses. It should be noted that the clinical interpretation of tumor marker levels may be difficult in patients who have had fertility treatment or have endometriosis, as these are often elevated in such cases.

Specific conditions

Functional cysts

Follicular ovarian cysts (Figure 19.1) comprise the most common cystic adnexal mass seen in women of reproductive age. They are lined by granulosa cells, are usually an incidental finding, and rarely reach a size larger than 8 cm. The cysts tend to regress after one or two menstrual cycles.

Luteal cysts are characterized by peripheral blood flow at Doppler examination ("ring" sign) and menstrual disturbances, and are found in women with delayed menses. They are usually irregular with thick echogenic walls, and can bleed internally and assume an appearance similar to endometriomas. Sometimes a fluid level can be seen within the cyst, representing blood or clot.

Table 19.1. Differential diagnosis of incidental adnexal masses

Origin	Usually cystic	Solid or complex
Adnexal	Functional cysts (follicular, luteal, etc.) Luteinized unruptured follicle syndrome Ovarian cystadenoma Borderline ovarian tumor Endometrioma Dermoid Embryological remnants Hydrosalpinx Ectopic pregnancy	Uterine leiomyoma (subserosal, broad ligament) Sex-cord tumors (fibroma, granulosa cell) Metastatic tumors
Nonadnexal	Round ligament cyst Peritoneal inclusion cyst Bowel loops	Pelvic kidney Retroperitoneal masses

Table 19.2. Comparison of transabdominal (TAS) versus transvaginal (TVS) ultrasound scanning for incidental adnexal masses

Modality	TAS	TVS
Advantages	Better penetration, offers global view, and can evaluate masses that lie higher in the abdomen, particularly in the presence of adhesions or fibroids Good for assessing moderate or significant ascites Can identify hydronephrosis	Can assess adnexal/mass tenderness with the probe Higher resolution, good for assessing pelvic anatomy
Disadvantages	Low resolution; differentiating masses from bowel gases may be a problem	Not good for masses that lie high, as a result of its poor penetration

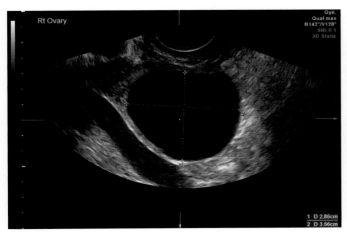

Figure 19.1. Transvaginal image of simple (follicular) ovarian cyst.

Theca-lutein cysts are large, multiple, bilateral and can be seen in association with ovulation induction, multiple pregnancy, or molar pregnancy.

Diagnostic approach and reproductive significance

Conservative management is the usual option. Ultrasound follow-up after two to three menstrual cycles is indicated for all simple cysts less than 5 cm in diameter. Surgery is reserved for persistent cysts, particularly if they are more than 5 cm in size and/or if symptomatic [4].

Ovulation induction may have to be postponed for women with multiple theca-lutein cysts, but not for presumed follicular or corpus luteum cysts. The effect of the latter on treatment cycles remains controversial. It is important to record any cysts before ovarian stimulation in order to monitor accurately the development of follicles, or of any de novo cysts.

In the presence of anovulation these cysts are likely to be hormonally active. It is good practice to commence stimulated cycles only after spontaneous menstruation indicates that hormonal levels are back to baseline. Should menstruation not occur, further diagnostics should be arranged.

Endometriomas

US appearance

Endometriosis is a very common finding in subfertile women, and endometriotic cyst formations within the ovary are known as endometriomas. They can be bilateral and cause significant pelvic pain symptoms; they are often found to be adherent to surrounding structures such as bowel. They are cystic with hazy, uniform hyperechoic content similar to blood seen within hemorrhagic cysts (Figure 19.2a, b) and the two can be difficult to distinguish on ultrasonography.

Diagnostic approach

The sonographic appearance of endometriomas is usually nonspecific, but includes having a homogeneous hyperechoic carpet of low-level echoes [5] (Figure 19.3). MRI is a good diagnostic test, with sensitivity and specificity comparable to those of laparoscopy.

Reproductive significance

Severe cases of endometriosis should be referred to units with the necessary expertise to offer all available treatments in a multidisciplinary context, including advanced laparoscopic surgery before ART [6].

There is no evidence to support the use of ovarian suppression agents in the treatment of endometriosis-associated infertility, and such use should be avoided because of adverse effects and the lost opportunity to conceive.

Subsequent spontaneous pregnancy rates may be improved with laparoscopic cystectomy. Some physicians offer laparoscopic ovarian cystectomy if an ovarian endometrioma of more than 4 cm diameter is found. Theoretically, the surgery aims to confirm the diagnosis histologically, reduce the risk of infection, improve access to follicles during oocyte retrieval for IVF, possibly improve ovarian response, and prevent progression of endometriosis. Nevertheless, a recent meta-analysis of five studies showed that surgical management of endometriomas has no significant effect on IVF pregnancy rates and ovarian response to stimulation compared with no treatment [7].

If an endometrioma is seen during oocyte retrieval, it is important to avoid aspirating it as there is a high risk of ovarian infection.

Germ-cell tumors, including dermoids

The increased resolution capabilities provided by transvaginal ultrasonography allow incidental detection of previously unsuspected cysts and permit identification of their nature. The positive predictive value of TVS for the diagnosis of endometriomas and dermoid cysts is higher than 95% [8].

Dysgerminomas can be found in young patients presenting with subfertility as a result of abnormal gonads (insensitivity/dysgenesis) and have a 10–15% chance of being bilateral, but usually the contralateral side has only microscopic involvement not identifiable by ultrasound.

US appearance

Dermoids have variable appearance, and can present as (1) solid, hyperechoic, either homogeneous or heterogeneous masses; (2) fluid-filled areas with hyperechoic foci in their wall; and (3) a mixed pattern, with solid and liquid areas [9]. Germ cell tumors tend to be solid.

Diagnostic features

Cystic lesions with hazy hyperechoic content can be difficult to differentiate from endometriomas, but dermoids sometimes

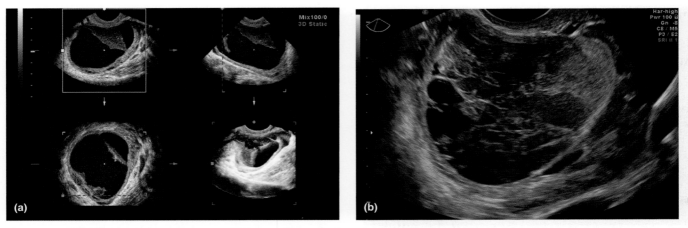

Figure 19.2. a) Fluid level with clot seen in transvaginal image of hemorrhagic ovarian cyst. (b) Transvaginal image of hemorrhagic ovarian cyst.

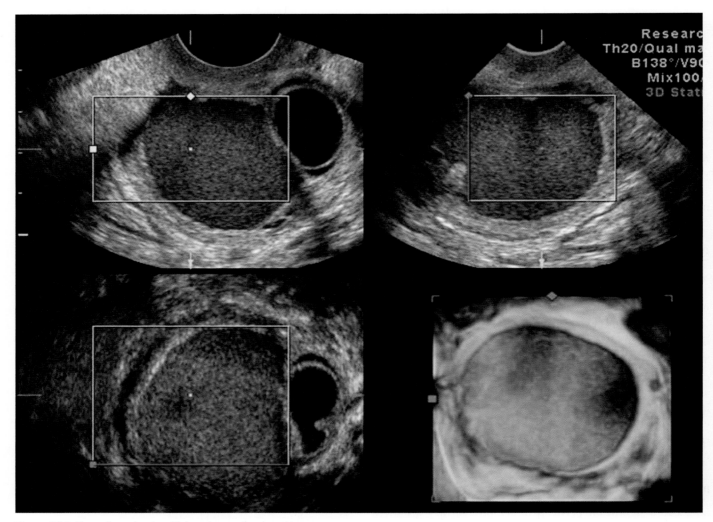

Figure 19.3. Three-dimensional multiplanar image of endometrioma.

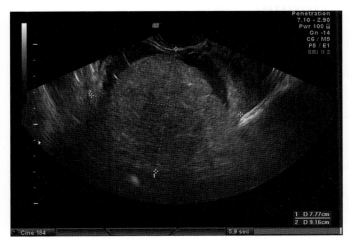

Figure 19.4. Transvaginal ultrasound image of dermoid cyst.

contain bright hyperechoic areas, fluid levels and/or calcifications (Figure 19.4). Moreover, posterior or edge acoustic shadowing is common and can be pronounced.

Fat is sometimes seen within dermoid cysts by CT, but for complex masses MRI may be indicated to exclude benign lesions (endometriomas, fibroids, dermoids) before any surgery is undertaken.

Reproductive significance

For malignant tumors, fertility-sparing surgery (unilateral salpingo-oophorectomy) is possible but should not compromise staging. Whether to undertake biopsy of the contralateral ovary is disputed as it may compromise ovarian function.

Sex cord tumors

Sex cord tumors include fibromas and granulosa cell tumors. The latter are hormonally active and may affect fertility, but are uncommon in this age group.

US appearance and diagnostic features

These tumors are usually solid but large ones may have cystic centers. Fibromas can be hypoechoic with sound attenuation, and may be associated with ascites, particularly when they are large. Less common is Meigs syndrome, which includes presence of fibroma, ascites, and right hydrothorax. In women with estrogen-secreting granulosa cell tumors, the endometrium is noted to be thickened and sometime heterogeneous.

Reproductive significance

Hormone-producing tumors are associated with anovulation and PCOS (polycystic ovary syndrome)-like phenotype if androgenic. Estrogen-secreting tumors on the other hand are often associated with menstrual disorders and possible breast enlargement [10]. Removal is often necessary, but fertility-sparing surgery is occasionally possible.

Cystadenomas and borderline ovarian tumors

These are the most common neoplastic tumors, but are more likely to be benign or borderline in the context of subfertility in women of reproductive age. In particular, prolonged use of clomiphene citrate for more than 12 cycles has been associated with increased risk of borderline ovarian tumor. A direct causal relationship has been disputed, though, and conflicting results and opinions seem to be a result of the interaction between nulliparity and infertility, the former being a very strong confounder and clearly associated with ovarian cancer [1].

US appearance

Mucinous tumors may be very large at presentation and are often multilocular with low-level echoes. Serous cystadenomas may contain calcifications also known as "psammoma" bodies.

Diagnostic approach

As with any complex mass, particularly when additional features suggestive of malignancy are present (septae, excrescences, ascites, bilaterality), it is important to scan the upper abdomen and liver as well as to check for hydronephrosis.

Doppler ultrasonography can provide additional information with regard to malignancy but is unreliable. Generally, absence of blood flow reduces the risk of malignancy, whereas the presence of low-resistance flow suggestive of neovascularization increases it.

MRI may be indicated to help distinguish a benign from a malignant lesion. CT is the imaging modality of choice for staging and determining operability but is not as good as ultrasound in demonstrating the degree of complexity of the primary tumor.

Reproductive significance

All complex ovarian cysts should be treated with caution, and liaison with a gynecologic oncologist is advisable. Ovarian or tubal malignancy may be uncommon in women of reproductive age, but it may occur, and stimulation of the ovaries should be avoided until complex lesions are managed, usually surgically, with conservative treatment reserved for certain cases where malignancy is considered very unlikely.

With regard to borderline tumors, studies have found pregnancy rates of 40–49% after conservative treatment [11,12]. A randomized controlled trial of 32 women affected by bilateral early-stage borderline tumors compared with bilateral cystectomy oophorectomy plus contralateral cystectomy, and found a significantly higher cumulative pregnancy rate in the bilateral cystectomy group after a follow-up period of 7 years, without detecting any difference in recurrence rate [13].

Hydrosalpinx or pyosalpinx

US appearance

These are usually complex cystic or tubular masses with echogenic walls (Figure 19.5a, b). Occasionally they can be difficult

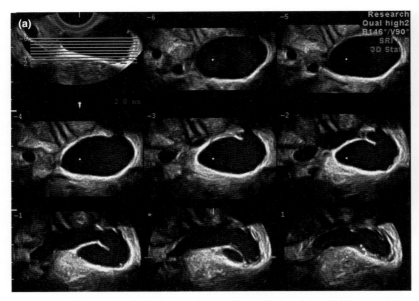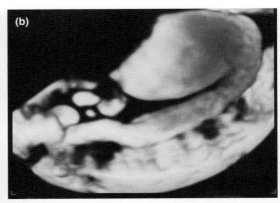

Figure 19.5. (a) Transvaginal 3D ultrasound image slices of hydrosalpinx; (b) 3D rendered image of hydrosalpinx.

to distinguish from fluid within pelvic adhesions or irregular ovarian cysts.

Diagnostic approach

Mucosal folds are characteristic and help differentiation from other cystic tumors. There is no peristalsis, they may appear convoluted, and the ovaries are seen separately. The presence of internal echoes and particulate matter suggests pyosalpinx.

Reproductive significance

It is now well recognized that hydrosalpinges have a detrimental effect on the outcome of IVF [14]. Transvaginal aspiration of hydrosalpinges [15] at the time of oocyte collection for IVF treatment has no benefit, whereas ultrasound-guided aspiration before commencement of ART leads to a greater ovarian response to stimulation, a greater number of embryos available for transfer, and a trend toward higher pregnancy rates.

Salpingostomy can be considered if the hydrosalpinx is thin walled, but the evidence to support this is lacking. On the other hand, guidance from NICE [1] states that women with hydrosalpinges should be offered salpingectomy, preferably laparoscopically, before IVF because this improves the chance of a live birth (grade A recommendation). Proximal tubal occlusion is another surgical option that may have less impact on ovarian performance and response to ovarian stimulation while maintaining satisfactory pregnancy rates [16].

Fimbrial and paraovarian cysts

Fimbrial and paraovarian cysts are a common finding in women of reproductive age and represent embryological remnants.

US appearance

These are small, round, unilocular, and thin walled (Figure 19.6). They represent müllerian and mesonephric duct remnants and carry no proven significance for fertility.

Diagnostic features

These should be separate from the ovaries. Gentle pressure with the transducer will displace the cyst(s) away from the homolateral ovary, unless there are adhesions.

Pedunculated subserosal and broad ligament leiomyomas

US appearance

Leiomyomas (fibroids) have a varied appearance but are usually hypoechoic, with poor through-transmission and concentric patterns (Figure 19.7). Calcification and cystic degeneration are possible. They may grow under the influence of estrogen in stimulated cycles.

Diagnostic approach

These should be seen separately from the ovaries and in continuation with the myometrium. Ultrasound alone is usually adequate, and the use of the transabdominal approach may be indicated. Occasionally, adhesions complicate diagnosis and MRI becomes helpful, but a bimanual examination may be informative before resorting to such diagnostic measures.

Reproductive significance

The main way these can affect reproductive potential varies and depends on their location. They can result in adhesions,

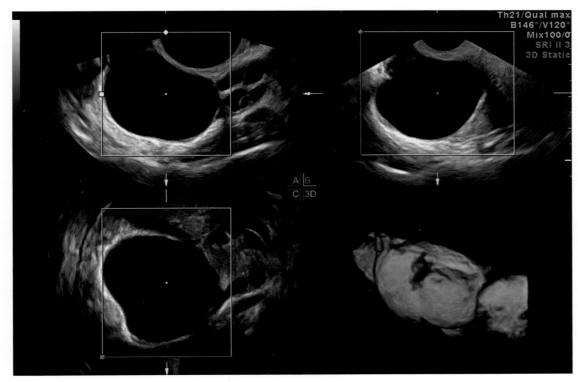

Figure 19.6. Transvaginal ultrasound image of paraovarian cyst.

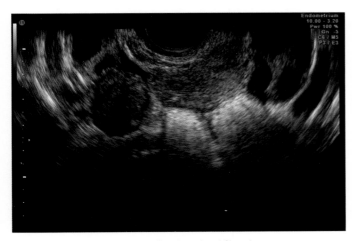

Figure 19.7. Ultrasound image of pedunculated fibroid.

compression, or stretching of fallopian tubes. Surgical intervention of subserous fibroids is not recommended for fertility reasons and may even be counterproductive by increasing scarring and adhesions; however, surgery may be considered for fibroids of considerable size and if they are causing symptoms.

The discussion of submucous and intramural fibroids and their potential impact on fertility is outside the scope of this chapter.

Peritoneal cysts

Peritoneal cysts can be the result of surgery, trauma, pelvic inflammatory disease, or endometriosis. The diagnostic approach may include a laparoscopy. The impact on fertility is dependent on the nature and extent of any coexisting adhesions involving the fallopian tubes.

New imaging techniques: three-dimensional ultrasonography

Recently three-dimensional (3D) or volume ultrasonography has been added to the gynecologic assessment armamentarium. There appear to be few differences in the diagnostic accuracy of standard 2D versus 3D images in detecting pelvic pathology [17], but 3D scanning can improve efficiency by reducing scanning time and therefore improving patient throughput [18]. Furthermore, 3D ultrasound is able to rapidly acquire and store ultrasonographic data that can later be retrospectively analyzed with little loss of information. It is therefore likely that the application of 3D ultrasound scanning will increase in the future for diagnostic purposes, particularly when the purchase cost of ultrasound equipment falls.

Concluding remarks

The availability of noninvasive ultrasonography has resulted in improved care for infertile women. The ability to diagnose and then decide on appropriate treatment is invaluable in helping women achieve better fertility outcomes where identified pathology is detrimental, but also in improving patient well-being where this may be more serious, such as malignancy, and is dealt with speedily. It is nevertheless imperative that appropriate measures are taken to reach the correct diagnosis to avoid unnecessary intervention or the failure to deal with a potentially serious condition. As such, there is no avoidance of the need for appropriate training, up-to-date, well-maintained equipment, and pathways to allow appropriate referral should further intervention or investigations be required when suspected pathology is identified.

Acknowledgments

The author are extremely grateful to Dr N. Raine-Fenning, Nottingham University, UK for kindly providing the images, some of which have been published (Raine-Fenning N, Jayaprakasan K, Deb S. Picture of the month. Three-dimensional ultrasonographic characteristics of endometriomata. *Ultrasound Obstet Gynecol* 2008; 31:718–24).

References

1. National Institute for Clinical Excellence. *Assessment and Treatment for People with Fertility Problems*. London: RCOG Press, 2004.

2. Jenkins JM, Anthony FW, Wood P, Rushen D, Masson GM, Thomas E. The development of functional ovarian cysts during pituitary down-regulation. *Hum Reprod* 1993; **8**(10): 1623–7.

3. Kupfer MC, Ralls PW, Fu YS. Transvaginal sonographic evaluation of multiple peripherally distributed echogenic foci of the ovary: prevalence and histologic correlation. *Am J Roentgenol* 1998; **171**(2): 483–6.

4. Nardo LG, Kroon ND, Reginald PW. Persistent unilocular ovarian cysts in a general population of postmenopausal women: is there a place for expectant management? *Obstet Gynecol* 2003; **102**(3): 589–93.

5. Kurjak A, Kupesic S. Ultrasonic assessment of ovarian endometriosis. In: Kupesic S, Kurjak A, de Ziegler D, eds. *Ultrasound and Infertility*. London: Informa Health Care, 1999.

6. Royal College of Obstetricians and Gynaecologists. The Investigation and Management of Endometriosis. *Green-top Guideline No. 24*. RCOG, London, 2006 [www.rcog.org.uk/index.asp?PageID=517].

7. Tsoumpou I, Kyrgiou M, Gelbaya TA, Nardo LG. The effect of surgical treatment for endometrioma on in vitro fertilization outcomes: a systematic review and meta-analysis. *Fertil Steril* 2009; **92**(1): 75–87.

8. Jermy K, Luise C, Bourne T. The characterization of common ovarian cysts in premenopausal women. *Ultrasound Obstet Gynecol* 2001; **17**(2): 140–4

9. Serafini G, Quadri PG, Gandolfo NG, Gandolfo N, Martinoli C, Derchi LE. Sonographic features of incidentally detected, small, nonpalpable ovarian dermoids. *J Clin Ultrasound* 1999; **27**(7): 369–73.

10. Van Holsbeke C, Domali E, Holland TK, et al. Imaging of gynecological disease (3): clinical and ultrasound characteristics of granulosa cell tumors of the ovary. *Ultrasound Obstet Gynecol* 2008; **31**(4): 450–6.

11. Tinelli FG, Tinelli R, La Grotta F, Tinelli A, Cicinelli E, Schonauer MM. Pregnancy outcome and recurrence after conservative laparoscopic surgery for borderline ovarian tumors. *Acta Obstet Gynecol Scand* 2007 **86**(1): 81–7.

12. Boran N, Cil AP, Tulunay G, et al. Fertility and recurrence results of conservative surgery for borderline ovarian tumors. *Gynecol Oncol* 2005; **97**(3): 845–51.

13. Palomba S, Zupi E, Russo T, et al. Comparison of two fertility-sparing approaches for bilateral borderline ovarian tumours: a randomized controlled study. *Hum Reprod* 2007; **22**(2): 578–85.

14. Siassakos D, Syed A, Wardle P. Tubal disease and assisted reproduction. *Obstet Gynecol* 2008; **10**: 80–7.

15. Sowter MC, Akande VA, Williams JA, Hull MG. Is the outcome of in-vitro fertilization and embryo transfer treatment improved by spontaneous or surgical drainage of a hydrosalpinx? *Hum Reprod* 1997; **12**(10): 2147–50.

16. Gelbaya TA, Kyrgiou M, Tsoumpou I, Nardo LG. The use of estradiol for luteal phase support in in vitro fertilization/ intracytoplasmic sperm injection cycles: A systematic review and meta-analysis. *Fertil Steril* 2008; **90**(6): 2116–25.

17. Benacerraf BR, Shipp TD, Bromley B. Improving the efficiency of gynecologic sonography with 3-dimensional volumes: a pilot study. *J Ultrasound Med* 2006; **25**(2): 165–71.

18. Hagel J, Bicknell SG. Impact of 3D sonography on workroom time efficiency. *Am J Roentgenol* 2007; **188**(4): 966–9.

Chapter 20

Scrotal ultrasonography in male infertility

Nabil Aziz and Iwan Lewis-Jones

Introduction

Male factor infertility is encountered in up to 60% of couples presenting with infertility. In half of these couples male impaired fertility is the only cause found, whereas in the other half both the male and female partners are contributing to the problem. The causes of male infertility are diverse, including congenital and acquired pathologies of the genital tract that ultimately affect spermatogenesis, sperm transport and storage, or sperm function. The effective and safe management of male infertility requires accurate etiological diagnosis. This is achievable by obtaining a thorough medical and surgical history, general and genital examination, and conducting appropriate investigative tests. These investigations include scrotal ultrasonography (US), which has proved valuable in confirming a clinical suspicion of genital pathology or unmasking unsuspected ones. Patients with fertility problems may be referred for scrotal US to evaluate testicular size, to assess testicular parenchyma, to examine epididymal integrity (partial or complete agenesis, obstruction), and to ascertain the presence of varicocele. Up to 50% of men referred for fertility assessment are found to have testicular abnormalities on scrotal ultrasonography (Table 20.1) [1,2,3]. Two-thirds of these abnormalities escape detection on physical examination [1,4]. Consequently, the role of ultrasonography is firmly established as a valuable tool in furnishing a reliable diagnosis of the cause of male infertility in modern clinical practice.

This chapter is concerned with detailing both the techniques and pathological findings of scrotal ultrasound scanning as pertinent to male infertility. The use of transrectal ultrasonography to assess the prostate and seminal vesicles is discussed elsewhere (Chapter 21).

Scrotal contents

The scrotum is composed of two mirror-image compartments (hemiscrota) with essentially identical contents separated by a median septum. Each compartment has a smooth, oval-shaped testis that measures approximately $50 \times 30 \times 20$ mm in the postpubertal male and is wrapped in a tightly adherent fibrous membrane termed the tunica albuginea. A remnant of the müllerian duct termed the appendix of the testis is found at the cephalic end of the testis in over 90% of men. This is detected on sonography when there is fluid in the tunica vaginalis (Figure 20.1). Along the posterior border of the testis the tunica albuginea extends inwardly, forming the mediastinum testis. Fibrous septa run from the mediastinum testis to the periphery, dividing the testicle into approximately 250 lobules. Each lobule contains 1 to 4 highly coiled seminiferous tubules that converge to form a single, straight tubule, which leads into the rete testis located in the mediastinum testis. Short efferent ducts (vasa efferentia) exit the testes, connecting the rete testis to the head of the epididymis. The epididymis is a tube approximately 6 m long that is tightly coiled to form a comma-shaped structure located along the superior and posterior margins of the testes. Anatomically, three regions of the epididymis are described: the head, which is the largest portion; the body, which is the longest portion and about 2–4 mm thick; and the tail. The tail ends by connecting to the vas deferens. Both the testis and epididymis are loosely enveloped by a double membrane called the tunica vaginalis. Developmentally, the tunica vaginalis is acquired from the peritoneal membrane as the testis migrates from the extraperitoneal space on the posterior abdominal wall to the scrotum. The vas deferens is a fibromuscular tube that turns sharply upward along the posterior margin of the testes. The vas deferens enters the pelvic cavity through the inguinal canal. Along the scrotal course of the vas deferens run arteries (testicular, deferential, and cremasteric), draining veins (pampiniform and cremasteric plexi), nerves, and lymphatics. These structures are tightly bound together by a fibrous sheath made up of three layers to form the spermatic cord. The testicular veins drain the posterior aspect of the testis into the pampiniform plexus situated anterior to the vas deferens. The drainage of the epididymis and the scrotal wall is via the cremasteric plexus situated behind the vas deferens, with multiple connections to the pampiniform plexus. The veins of the cremasteric plexus coalesce to form three or four vessels, which pass with the spermatic cord through the inguinal canal and eventually form a single testicular vein. The right testicular vein drains directly into the inferior vena cava but the left testicular vein drains into the left renal vein.

Ultrasonography in Reproductive Medicine and Infertility, ed. Botros R. M. B. Rizk. Published by Cambridge University Press. © Cambridge University Press 2010.

Ultrasonographic appearance of the normal scrotal contents

The normal scrotal wall thickness, on gray-scale ultrasound, is approximately 2–8 mm, depending on the state of contraction of the cremasteric muscle [5]. The normal testis is identified as an ovoid structure of moderate homogeneous echogenicity. Both testicles should be of the same echogenicity (Figure 20.2). If this is not the case, pathology should be suspected. Linear echogenic bands, coursing toward and coalescing at the mediastinum testis, correspond to the fibrous septa that are present and connect the tunica albuginea with the mediastinum testis. The mediastinum testis appears as an echogenic band situated peripherally in the testis parallel to the epididymis (Figure 20.3). The tunica albuginea is displayed as a hyperechoic line similar to the mediastinum testis

(Figure 20.2). The head of the epididymis should be approximately of the same echogenicity as the testicle. It should not exceed 12 mm in size. The body of the epididymis is less echogenic than the head and has a diameter of 2–5 mm (Figure 20.4). The tail is seen near the inferior pole of the testis with equal echogenicity to the body and measures <5 mm in length. The tunica vaginalis may contain a minimal amount of fluid. The appendix of the testis is seen when the amount of this fluid is increased (Figure 20.1). The appendix epididymis, which is a remnant of the wolffian duct, is detected as a cystic lesion on the top of the epididymal head (3–5 mm in diameter). On Doppler ultrasonography the flow in the testicular artery branches within the testis is of low resistance (RI 0.5–0.7). In general, there is no flow detectable in the epididymis. The draining veins in the spermatic cord are identifiable and measure no more than 2 mm in diameter.

Ultrasound technique

The scrotal ultrasound scan is carried out with the patient in the supine position, exposing the scrotum with the thighs and the

Table 20.1. The incidence of testicular abnormalities detected on scrotal ultrasonography in male patients referred for fertility assessment

	Nashan et al. (1990) [1]	Behre et al. (1995) [2]	Pierik et al. (1999) [3]	Sakamoto et al. (2006) [4]
Patients assessed (n)	658	1048	1372	545
Patients with abnormal scrotal scan (%)	40	50.4	38	65.3
Testicular tumors (%)	0.6	0.5	0.5	0.2
Testicular cyst (%)	1	1.1	0.7	0.6
Intratesticular hypo- or hyperechoic lesions (%)	4.5	12.6	–	–
Microlithiasis (%)	–	–	0.9	5.5
Spermatocele (%)	6	5.2	–	–
Epididymal cysts (%)	6		7.6	3.9
Hydrocele (%)	7	9.9	3.2	0.2
Varicocele (%)	21	18.5	29.7	57.4

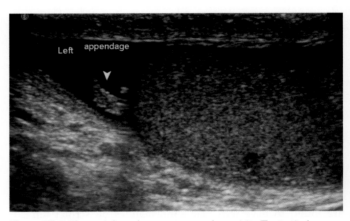

Figure 20.1. The testis has a homogeneous echogenicity. The testicular appendix may be visualized at the upper pole (arrowhead) when fluid accumulates in the tunica vaginalis.

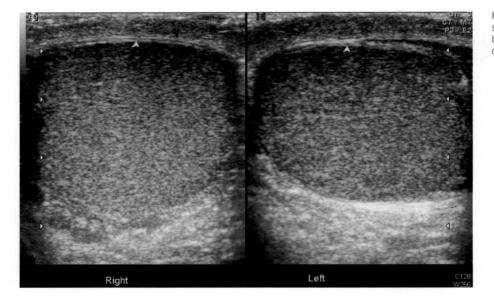

Figure 20.2. Both testicles are examined simultaneously in the transverse plane. They should be of the same echogenicity. The tunica albuginea is displayed as a hyperechoic line (arrowheads).

abdomen covered. The patient is asked to support the penis against the abdomen. With the thighs adducted, the scrotum and its contents are supported, but occasional further support may be required by a towel between the thighs. The testis, epididymal head, epididymal body, and epididymal tail are examined sequentially. Care must be taken not to compress the testis during measurement to avoid undersizing the antero-posterior diameter and oversizing the sagittal diameter. The contents of the spermatic cord are then examined and a Valsalva maneuver is used to assess the presence of reverse venous flow in the testicular veins. Some sonographers state that examination in the upright position may occasionally be needed for this maneuver.

A high-resolution, high-frequency (10–16 MHz) small-parts linear ray transducer is employed. When color Doppler is utilized it should be optimized to detect slow flow: the highest color gain setting allowing an acceptable signal-to-noise ratio, the lowest velocity scale, and the lowest wall filter. Pulsed

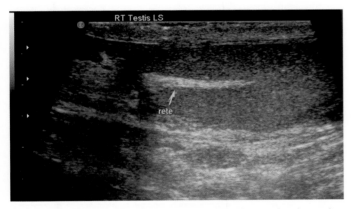

Figure 20.3. The mediastinum testis appears as an echogenic band extending from the posterior margin of the testis toward the center in the transverse plane view.

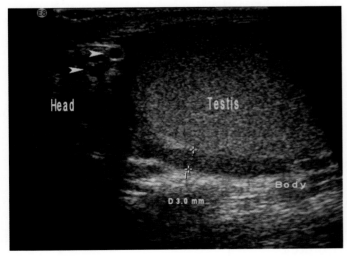

Figure 20.4. The head of the epididymis should be of approximately the same echogenicity as the testicle. The body of the epididymis is less echogenic than the head.

Doppler is also utilized to detect a subclinical varicocele by demonstrating the presence as well as the duration of reverse venous flow in the testicular veins.

Testicular abnormalities

Testicular size

The ultrasonographic testicular volumes are calculated as the length × width × depth × 0.71. The testicular volume estimated by the Prader orchiometer correlates closely with the measurements by ultrasonography except in small testes, where the orchiometer overestimates the testicular volume [6]. It is also reported that oligozoospermic patients are more likely to have a mean testicular volume below 10 ml, a mean length below 3.5 cm, a mean depth below 1.75 cm, and a mean width below 2.5 cm [7].

Testicular texture

Both testicles should be of the same echogenicity when compared (Figure 20.2). If this is not the case, pathology should be suspected. Hyperechogenic or hypoechogenic areas of the testicular tissue (Figure 20.5) are suggestive of testicular neoplasia and should be investigated further.

Intratesticular cysts

Intratesticular cysts are most commonly detected incidentally during ultrasound scanning. The incidence increases with age. Their appearance is similar to simple anechoic thin-walled cysts elsewhere (Figure 20.6). These should not be confused with cystic tumors of the testis, which appear as irregular with solid elements and are associated with abnormal vascularity. It is postulated that cysts result from obstruction of the spermatic ductal system. Cysts may be also found in the tunica albuginea and then may be palpated as a firm mass of pinhead size [8]. The origin of these cysts is unclear and could be congenital, or acquired as a result of infection or trauma (Figure 20.7).

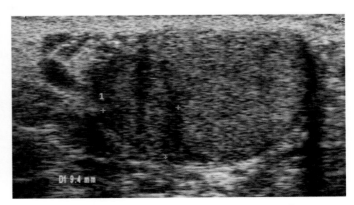

Figure 20.5. An ultrasound image of the testis depicts an area of hypoechogenicity suspicious for neoplasia.

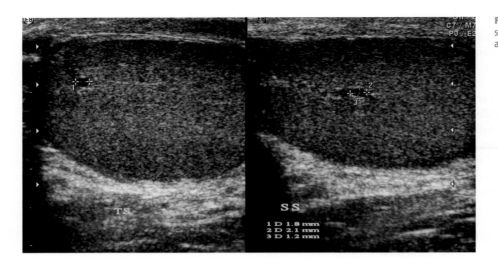

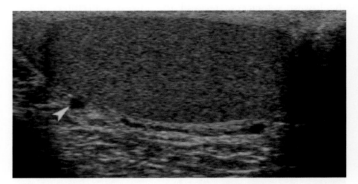

Figure 20.6. The intratesticular cyst has an average size of 2 mm and is similar in appearance to simple anechoic thin-walled cysts elsewhere.

Dilatation of the rete testis

Ectasia of the seminiferous tubules at the level of the mediastinum is a recognized benign condition of the testis and should not erroneously be interpreted as a tumor [9]. It is thought that tubular ectasia or cysts of the rete testis result from obstruction of the spermatic ductal system after infection or trauma. They are bilateral in approximately 45% of cases and are associated with an ipsilateral spermatocele in approximately 74% of cases [10].

Testicular microlithiasis

Testicular microlithiases are randomly distributed, 1–2 mm diameter, hyperechoic foci in one or both testes (Figure 20.8) [11]. They are detected in 0.6–6.7% of men undergoing testicular ultrasound scanning [12]. At one time it was thought to be associated with increased risk of germ cell tumors [13]. Because of the uncertainty as to what constitutes significant microlithiasis it was suggested that patients with severe microlithiasis (>5 microlithiases per field) should have annual follow-ups with repeat ultrasonographic examination of the testes and measurement of tumor markers [14]. However, recently available data suggest that men with incidental findings of testicular microlithiasis but who have otherwise normal testes have no increased risk of developing testicular cancer and for them no form of regular surveillance is required [15]. On the other hand, it is recommended that patients at high risk of developing testicular cancer, including infertile men with bilateral microlithiasis and men with a history of contralateral testicular tumor or history of cryptorchidism, require only regular testicular self-examination [12,15]. The role of surveillance with serial ultrasonographic examination of the testes and measurement of tumor markers in these individuals is prohibitively expensive and remains a matter of debate [12,15]. The need for clear guidelines for surveillance has been recently highlighted after demonstrating increased prevalence of testicular microlithiasis in men with familial testicular cancer and their relatives [16].

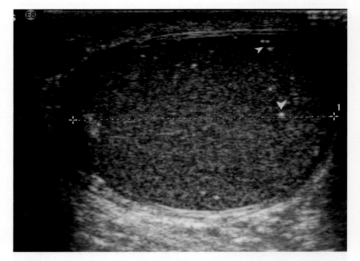

Figure 20.7. Cysts of the tunica albuginea (arrowhead) should not be confused with intratesticular cysts.

Figure 20.8. Testicular microlithiasis appears as 1–2 mm diameter hyperechoic foci (arrowheads) that are randomly distributed.

Hydrocele

A hydrocele is the accumulation of an abnormal amount of serous fluid between the two layers of the tunica vaginalis

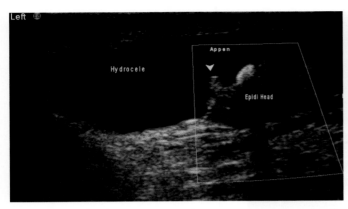

Figure 20.9. Hydrocele appears as a translucent space surrounding the testis.

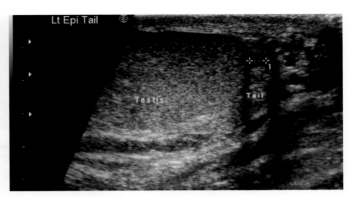

Figure 20.10. A cyst of the epididymal tail is demonstrated.

(Figure 20.9). A limited hydrocele is found in as many as 65% of men and is bilateral in 10% of cases. It may be primary (idiopathic) or secondary to virtually every underlying scrotal disease process. A hydrocele may communicate with the peritoneal cavity, when it can be demonstrated to be smaller in size on pressing on the testis or larger when the patient is asked to stand. It remains of the same size in any position if it is noncommunicating.

Cryptorchidism

In cryptorchidism one or both testes are not located in the scrotal sac but are located somewhere down the course of testicular descent, between the lower pole of the kidney and the external inguinal ring. In 75–80% of cases the testis is located in the inguinal canal between the internal and external inguinal rings. Ultrasound is needed to locate the testicle in the inguinal canal and to evaluate its size and to some extent the testicular parenchyma. Evaluation of the testicular parenchyma is important in view of fertility and the increased incidence of testicular malignancies (germ cell origin with hypoechoic areas) in cryptorchid testes. It is reported that 10% of all testicular neoplasms occur in undescended testes or in testis treated for cryptorchidism. This is because there is a 50-fold higher frequency of carcinomas in undescended testes compared with normally positioned testes [10]. Generally, the malignancy rate correlates with increasing distance of the testis from the scrotum; thus, malignant change is six times more common in the abdominal testis than in the inguinal testis [17].

Abnormalities of the epididymis

Epididymal cysts

Cysts of the epididymis are more commonly found in the head compared with the body and tail (Figures 20.4 and 20.10). They are reported in as many as 70% of men who undergo scrotal US. They are painless but may cause anxiety because of abnormal palpation. Epididymal cysts can be single or multiple, very tiny (1–2 mm), but occasionally larger.

Spermatocele

A spermatocele is a benign cyst arising from the epididymis and contains nonviable sperm, unlike the simple epididymal cysts that do not contain sperm. A spermatocele is most often incidentally noted by a patient or detected during a physical examination. Spermatoceles may vary in size between a few millimeters and several centimeters. Although occasionally found in other locations, most spermatoceles are located within the epididymal head and are thus palpated above the testicle and are usually asymptomatic. They can originate as diverticuli from the epididymis or rete testis [18]. Alternatively, they may be due to epididymal scarring and obstruction caused by infection or physical trauma to the testis. Ultrasonically, they appear as cysts with internal echoes (Figure 20.11). Recently, color Doppler sonography has been described in the evaluation of spermatoceles by demonstrating the "falling snow" sign [19]. It has been suggested that the "falling snow" sign can be used to enhance the diagnosis of a spermatocele as well as to evaluate a superficial cystic lesion with echogenic fluid and internal microdebris that is difficult to distinguish from a solid mass.

The epididymis in obstructive azoospermia

It has been shown that ultrasonographic abnormalities of the epididymis are significantly higher in obstructive azoospermia than in nonobstructive azoospermia [20]. An absent epididymis is self-evident on ultrasonography. Obstruction in the rete testis secondary to trauma or inflammation may lead to a tapering appearance of the whole of the epididymis. A tapering epididymal body with absent epididymal tail may also indicate proximal obstruction in the epididymis. Equally, absence or atrophy of the distal portion of the epididymis may also be demonstrated in azoospermic men diagnosed with combined bilateral absence of the vas deferens [21]. However, acquired obstruction of the vas deferens may be associated with dilated epididymis (Figure 20.12). Tubular ectasia secondary to obstruction may appear on epididymal ultrasonography as multiple anechoic tubular or round structures representing the dilated epididymal duct. This should

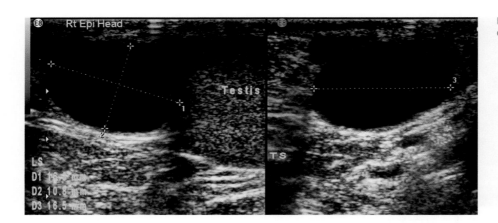

Figure 20.11. A spermatocele is seen in the region of the epididymal head.

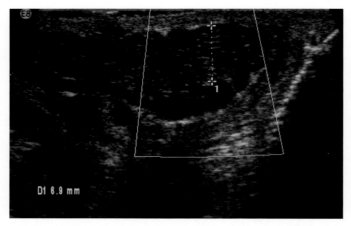

Figure 20.12. A dilated epididymal tail is suggestive of acquired distal (vas deferens) obstruction.

not be confused with a spermatocele or a simple epididymal cyst. Obstruction may also be explained by the presence of a masslike enlargement of any of the three epididymal regions caused by inflammation. In cases of inflammation-associated obstruction, cystic changes in the rete testis may be seen on ultrasound scanning, usually in association with epididymal obstruction [22].

Varicocele

The incidence of an idiopathic varicocele in the general male population is estimated at 15%, and in patients with subfertility at 37%. This implies that the majority of men with varicoceles are still fertile. Varicoceles are commonly found on the left side and are bilateral in 30% of patients. The varicocele is idiopathic when it is not related to the presence of a mechanical venous obstruction, e.g., renal masses.

Clinical varicoceles are diagnosed by physical examination and are graded on the basis of physical findings. Grade 1 varicoceles are small and palpable only with the Valsalva maneuver, owing to the engorgement and expansion of the pampiniform plexus (Figure 20.13); grade 2 varicoceles are moderate in size and are palpable without the Valsalva maneuver; and grade 3

varicoceles are large and visible through the scrotal skin, and are often termed a "bag of worms" [23]. While most large varicoceles are easily palpated, small varicoceles (subclinical) may only be detectable by ultrasonography. Several studies have shown that spermatic veins become clinically palpable when the diameter exceeds 2 mm on ultrasonography [24]. However, other studies have demonstrated that the upper diameter limit of spermatic veins in healthy normozoospermic men with normal scrotal palpation reaches 3.8 mm [4,25].

The size of the spermatic veins aside, for many clinicians the presence of reversed venous flow with Valsalva on color Doppler ultrasound is deemed essential to the diagnosis of a varicocele (Figure 20.14). However, few studies have demonstrated reversal of flow in varicoceles diagnosed in healthy men with normal sperm parameters [26]. Overall, color Doppler offers better diagnostic accuracy than physical examination in detecting venous reversed flow. One study reports that, compared with color Doppler ultrasonography, physical examination has a sensitivity in detecting left varicocele of 58.4%, a specificity of 79.3%, and an accuracy of 67.3% [4]. Another study has found that color Doppler has a sensitivity of 97% and specificity of 94% when compared with spermatic venography [27]. Moreover, 80% of patients with a normal examination but positive color Doppler (subclinical varicocele) have confirmatory venograms [28]. However, there is no current consensus on what flow parameters assessed with color Doppler and what cut-off values are to be used to make the diagnosis of a varicocele [29]. Moreover, the significant interobserver and intraobserver variability is another confounding factor when comparing different studies [25]. Accordingly, quantification of reversal of flow associated with varicoceles using color Doppler only may not be an adequate imaging modality, and pulsed-mode Doppler ultrasound is required to measure not only the presence but also the duration of reflux (Figure 20.15) [25,30,31,32]. Cornud et al. graded the degree of reflux into three different groups: grade1 (brief) reflux lasts less than 1 second and is considered physiological; grade 2 (intermediate) reflux lasts 1–2 seconds and decreases during the Valsalva maneuver, then disappears prior to the end of the maneuver; and grade 3 (permanent) reflux lasts more than 2 seconds and has a plateau aspect throughout the Valsalva

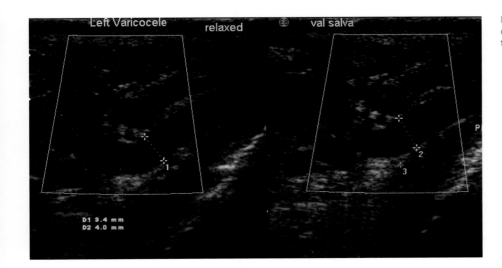

Figure 20.13. The assessment of varicocele demonstrates an increase in venous diameter during the Valsalva maneuver.

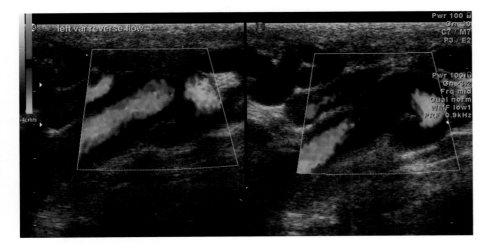

Figure 20.14. Doppler ultrasound of the testicular vein demonstrates flow reversal.

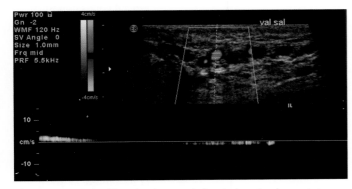

Figure 20.15. Pulsed Doppler ultrasound of testicular veins demonstrates reversal of venous flow on the Valsalva maneuver.

maneuver [30]. Although it did not correlate with the diameter of the spermatic vein, grade 3 reflux veins were found to be palpable in 60% of cases, whereas intermediate and brief reflux were never palpable.

From the above considerations it is recommended that the diameters of the veins are measured at rest and during a Valsalva maneuver (Figure 20.13), and the absence or presence of venous

reverse flow (reflux) is determined by color Doppler (Figure 20.14). It has been suggested that the velocity of the reflux using color Doppler may be recorded to standardize reporting of the condition [25]. Pulsed Doppler may be used to determine not only the presence but also the duration of reversed flow at rest and during Valsalva (Figure 20.15). A severe varicocele or right varicocele in an older man warrants further sonographic examination to exclude underlying disease processes causing secondary varicoceles (e.g., renal tumors, retroperitoneal masses).

From the current understanding of the available data, a guideline for the ultrasonographic criteria for the diagnosis of varicocele may be formulated as follows: (1) diameter of the veins >3 mm; (2) increase in size of the veins during Valsalva maneuver and/or in the upright position; and (3) retrograde flow during Valsalva and/or in the upright position. A combination of (1) and (2) is diagnostic of the condition and criterion (3) in itself is diagnostic as well. Varicoceles can be graded as follows: grade I, slight reflux (<2 s) during Valsalva; grade II, reflux (>2 s) during Valsalva, but no continuous reflux during the maneuver; and grade III, reflux at rest during normal respiration or continuously during the entire Valsalva maneuver.

Therapeutic application

The use of ultrasound-guided testicular sperm aspiration in azoospermic patients has been described [33]. A 21-gauge butterfly needle is directed into the testicular regions to be sampled under real-time gray-scale and power Doppler sonographic guidance, avoiding the echogenic mediastinum testis and the vascular plexus of the tunica albuginea, as well as the prominent testicular parenchymal vessels.

References

1. Nashan D, Behre HM, Grunert JH, Nieschlag E. Diagnostic value of scrotal sonography in infertile men: report on 658 cases. *Andrologia* 1990; **22**: 387–95.

2. Behre HM, Kliesch S, Schädel F, Nieschlag E. Clinical relevance of scrotal and transrectal ultrasonography in andrological patients. *Int J Androl* 1995; **18**(Suppl 2): 27–31.

3. Pierik FH, Dohle GR, van Muiswinkel JM, Vreeburg JT, Weber RF. Is routine scrotal ultrasound advantageous in infertile men? *J Urol* 1999; **162**: 1618–20

4. Sakamoto H, Saito K, Shichizyo T, Ishikawa K, Igarashi A, Yoshida H. Color Doppler ultrasonography as a routine clinical examination in male infertility. *Int J Urol* 2006; **13**: 1073–8.

5. Hricak H, Filly RA. Sonography of the scrotum. *Invest Radiol* 1983; **18**: 112–21.

6. Sakamoto H, Saito K, Ogawa Y, Yoshida H. Testicular volume measurements using Prader orchidometer versus ultrasonography in patients with infertility. *Urology* 2007; **69**: 158–62.

7. Sakamoto H, Yajima T, Nagata M, Okumura T, Suzuki K, Ogawa Y. Relationship between testicular size by ultrasonography and testicular function: measurement of testicular length, width, and depth in patients with infertility. *Int J Urol* 2008; **15**: 529–33.

8. Tammela TL, Karttunen TJ, Mattila SI, Makarainen HP, Hellstrom PA, Kontturi MJ. Cysts of the tunica albuginea – more common testicular masses than previously thought? *Br J Urol* 1991; **68**: 280–4

9. Rouvière O, Bouvier R, Pangaud C, Jeune C, Dawahra M, Lyonnet D. Tubular ectasia of the rete testis: a potential pitfall in scrotal imaging. *Eur Radiol* 1999; **9**: 1862–8.

10. Oyen RH. Scrotal ultrasound scan. *Eur Radiol* 2002, **12**: 19–34.

11. Janzen DL, Mathieson JR, Marsh JI, et al. Testicular microlithiasis: sonographic and clinical features. *Am J Roentgenol* 1992; **158**: 1057–60.

12. Costabile RA. How worrisome is testicular microlithiasis? *Curr Opin Urol.* 2007; **17**: 419–23.

13. Backus ML, Mack LA, Middleton WD, King BF, Winter TC 3rd, True LD. Testicular microlithiasis: imaging appearances and pathologic correlation. *Radiology* 1994; **192**: 781–5.

14. Laviopierre AM. Ultrasound of the prostate and testicles. *World J Surg.* 2000; **24**, 198–207.

15. Jaganathan K, Ahmed S, Henderson A, Rané A. Current management strategies for testicular microlithiasis. *Nat Clin Pract Urol.* 2007; **4**: 492–7.

16. Korde LA, Premkumar A, Mueller C, et al. Increased prevalence of testicular microlithiasis in men with familial testicular cancer and their relatives. *Br J Cancer* 2008; **99**: 1748–53.

17. Nguyen HT, Coakley F, Hricak H. Cryptorchidism: strategies in detection. *Eur Radiol* 1999, **9**: 336–43

18. Davis RS. Intratesticular spermatocele. *Urology* 1998; **51**(Suppl): 167–9.

19. Sista AK, Filly RA. Color Doppler sonography in evaluation of spermatoceles: the "falling snow" sign. *J Ultrasound Med* 2008; **27**: 141–3.

20. Moon MH, Kim SH, Cho JY, Seo JT, Chun YK. Scrotal US for evaluation of infertile men with azoospermia. *Radiology* 2006; **239**: 168–73.

21. Jequier AM, Ansell ID, Bullimore NJ. Congenital absence of the vasa deferentia presenting with infertility. *J Androl* 1985; **6**: 15–19.

22. Brown DL, Benson CB, Doherty FJ, et al. Cystic testicular mass caused by dilated rete testis: sonographic findings in 31 cases. *Am J Roentgenol* 1992; **158**(6): 1257–9

23. Dubin L, Amelar RD. Varicocele size and results of varicocelectomy in selected subfertile men with varicocele. *Fertil Steril* 1970; **21**: 606–9.

24. Chiou RK, Anderson JC, Wobig RK, et al. Color Doppler ultrasound criteria to diagnose varicoceles: correlation of a new scoring system with physical examination. *Urology* 1997; **50**: 953–6.

25. Cina A, Minnetti M, Pirronti T, et al. Sonographic quantitative evaluation of scrotal veins in healthy subjects: normative values and implications for the diagnosis of varicocele. *Eur Urol* 2006; **50**: 345–50.

26. Cvitanic OA, Cronan JJ, Sigman M, Landau ST. Varicoceles: postoperative prevalence–a prospective study with color Doppler US. *Radiology* 1993; **187**(3): 711–14.

27. Trum JW, Gubler FM, Laan R, van der Veen F. The value of palpation, varicoscreen contact thermography and color Doppler ultrasound in the diagnosis of varicocele. *Hum Reprod* 1996; **11**: 1232–5.

28. Petros JA, Andriole GL, Middleton WD, Picus DA. Correlation of testicular color Doppler ultrasonography, physical examination and venography in the detection of left varicoceles in men with infertility. *J Urol* 1991; **145**(4): 785–8.

29. Lee J, Binsaleh S, Lo K, Jarvi K. Varicoceles: the diagnostic dilemma. *J Androl* 2006; **29**: 143–6.

30. Cornud F, Belin X, Amar E, Delafontaine D, Helenon O, Moreau JF. Varicocele: strategies in diagnosis and treatment. *Eur Radiol* 1999; **9**: 536–45.

31. Meacham RB, Townsend RR, Rademacher D, Drose JA.. The incidence of varicoceles in the general population when evaluated by physical examination, gray scale sonography, and color Doppler sonography. *J Urol* 1994; **151**: 1535–8.

32. Kocakoc E, Kiris A, Orhan I, Bozgeyik Z, Kanbay M, Ogur E. Incidence and importance of reflux in testicular veins of healthy men evaluated with color duplex sonography. *J Clin Ultrasound* 2002; **30**: 282–7.

33. Belenky A, Avrech OM, Bachar GN, et al. Ultrasound-guided testicular sperm aspiration in azoospermic patients: a new sperm retrieval method for intracytoplasmic sperm injection. *J Clin Ultrasound* 2001; **29**: 339–43.

Transrectal ultrasonography in male infertility

Levent Gurkan, Andrew C. Harbin and Wayne J. G. Hellstrom

Male infertility: prevalence, clinical presentation, and diagnostic steps

Infertility is a clinical issue affecting approximately 15% of all couples. Male factor infertility is the sole cause in 30–40% of cases, while abnormalities involving both partners occur in approximately 20% of presentations. Despite the common misperception of the female partner as the major cause of conception difficulties, the male factor is present in at least half of the cases [1].

Standard evaluation of male infertility includes complete history, focused physical examination, laboratory testing (including semen analysis and determination of the hormone profile), and in certain situations, selective imaging. Male infertility may be caused by abnormalities in the normal development or fertilization capacity of spermatozoa (e.g., vascular, genetic, hormonal, or immunological) or interference in the transport of spermatozoa from the testis to the prostatic urethra (e.g., agenesis or obstruction).

Azoospermia, defined as the complete absence of spermatozoa in the ejaculate, can occur in either type of male infertility. Azoospermia is found in 5% of all infertile couples presenting to infertility clinics [2,3]. Obstructive infertility can be categorized into partial or complete. Complete obstruction, accounting for about 1% of cases of azoospermia, is localized to the epididymis in 30–67% of cases and to the testis in 15%. Distal ejaculatory duct obstruction occurs in only 1–3% of patients with obstructive azoospermia [4]. However, partial obstruction of the ejaculatory tract accounts for 5% of male factor infertility [5]. Functional obstruction of the distal seminal ducts, which is hypothesized to be related to local neuropathy, has also been reported [6].

Patients suffering from obstructive infertility may have a specific clinical history including hematospermia, postejaculatory pain, current or previous urethritis or prostatitis, obstructive or irritative urinary symptoms, previous scrotal swelling, infection or pain, prior scrotal surgery, previous inguinal herniorrhaphy, trauma, or chronic sinopulmonary infections [4]. Physical examination in such patients reveals at least one normal testis with a volume greater than 15 ml, although conceivably a smaller testis may be found in men with obstructive azoospermia and concomitant testicular failure. Other possible physical findings related to obstructive infertility are an enlarged or indurated epididymis, nodules in the epididymis or vas deferens, absence or partial atresia of the vas deferens, signs of urethritis, or prostatic abnormalities. While serum follicle-stimulating hormone (FSH) levels are usually normal in patients with obstructive infertility, normal FSH levels do not exclude azoospermia of testicular origin. In fact, serum FSH levels are normal in 40% of men with primary spermatogenic failure. Inhibin B, a negative feedback signal molecule produced by the Sertoli cells, may have a greater predictive value for the presence of normal spermatogenesis [7].

The importance of the history and physical examination in the majority of these patients cannot be overemphasized, as many physicians focus primarily on semen analysis and imaging. A physical examination should precede any type of radiologic or laboratory study. For example, congenital bilateral absence of the vas deferens (CBAVD) is easily detected by physical examination of the scrotal content and, in such circumstances, further radiologic examination of genital structures is not indicated (though an abdominal ultrasound may be required to rule out concurrent kidney abnormalities). In this subgroup of patients, the optimal therapy is assisted reproduction technologies (ART) involving open or percutaneous retrieval of gametes from the epididymis or testis. Hence a proper physical examination will circumvent the false hope of natural conception and the significant emotional and financial burden of unnecessary imaging studies.

Ultrasonographic evaluation of patients suspected of having obstructive infertility includes scrotal and transrectal ultrasound. Scrotal ultrasound is mainly used to evaluate the testis and epididymis, with special attention paid to anatomic structure and echogenicity. Transrectal ultrasound (TRUS) evaluates the distal components of the ejaculatory duct system including the ampullae of the vas deferens, the seminal vesicles, the ejaculatory ducts, and the prostate (Figure 21.1).

Candidates for TRUS imaging

The classic candidate for a TRUS evaluation has semen analysis findings consistent with complete distal ejaculatory obstruction, including low ejaculate volume (usually <1.5 ml),

Ultrasonography in Reproductive Medicine and Infertility, ed. Botros R. M. B. Rizk. Published by Cambridge University Press. © Cambridge University Press 2010.

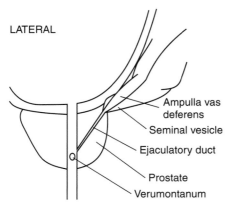

LATERAL

Ampulla vas deferens

Seminal vesicle

Ejaculatory duct

Prostate

Verumontanum

Figure 21.1. Schematic representation of the structures investigated in a typical TRUS study.

azoospermia, low pH (<7), and absence of fructose. Patients should have at least one palpable vas deferens and will usually have normal sex hormone profiles. Patients with partial distal obstruction may also be candidates for TRUS evaluation. These patients usually present with low volume of ejaculate, severe oligoasthenospermia (low count, low motility), and/or painful ejaculation. In contrast to complete obstruction, however, patients with partial obstruction will have borderline normal fructose levels in the ejaculate and no obvious physical or hormonal abnormalities [4].

Essentials of TRUS imaging

Transrectal ultrasound follows the same principles as other ultrasonographic evaluations. Sound waves are emitted by a transducer, and the reflected waves are converted into computer-generated images. The quality of the image depends mainly on the frequency of sound generated by the probe. Higher-frequency probes generate higher-quality images, but they have the disadvantage of the waves having a lower ability to penetrate tissue. The transrectal approach requires limited tissue depth, allowing the operator to use a higher-frequency biplane probe (7.0–7.5 MHz). Although the frequency used is lower than that for the superficial examination of the scrotum and penis (10 MHz), the close proximity of the probe to the prostate, ejaculatory ducts, and seminal vesicles provides adequate detailed anatomic information about these structures [1].

Technically, TRUS is minimally invasive and easy to perform. In most cases it can be performed as an outpatient procedure without the need for anesthesia. Prior to the procedure, rectal examination should be performed to exclude any structural abnormalities that could contraindicate or complicate TRUS examination. The examination can be performed with the patient in the lithotomy, knee–chest, or lateral decubitus position. Lateral decubitus position is the preferred position in our clinic as this provides easy access for the operator and less discomfort for the patient. The probe is inserted 8–9 cm above the anal verge, with adequate lubrication. The ampullae of the vas deferens, seminal vesicles, ejaculatory ducts, prostate, and surrounding structures are systematically examined in both transverse and sagittal planes. For medical and legal purposes, multiple images of these structures are captured and properly labeled with the patient's name, the name of the structure in the image, and the date. The operator is responsible for proper storage of these materials.

Embryological and anatomic considerations related to TRUS imaging

In order to understand the normal and pathological appearance of the ejaculatory structures on TRUS, it is important to appreciate their anatomic relationships and embryological origins.

As the vas deferens approaches the base of the prostate from a posterolateral direction, the distal end joins the seminal vesicle ducts to form the ejaculatory ducts. The ejaculatory ducts drain into the posterior urethra, lateral to the verumontanum. They are the common urethral entry pathway for both spermatozoa from the vas deferens and the seminal fluid from the seminal vesicles.

The ureters are derived embryonically from the wolffian (mesonephric) ducts. During the 7th week of embryological development, the wolffian ducts transform into the distal vas deferens and the ejaculatory ducts. This common origin is significant, as pathological findings in the vas deferens may predict more significant congenital abnormalities in the ureter and kidney (see below) [8]. The ejaculatory ducts on sagittal TRUS are tubular structures less than 2 mm in diameter, and run in a posterolateral to anteromedial direction. The sagittal plane is preferred, as identification of ejaculatory ducts on the transverse plane is difficult.

The prostatic utricle may seen at the verumontanum between the openings of the ejaculatory ducts. The embryonic origin of the prostatic utricle has been the subject of much debate, with some claiming it to be of endodermal origin [5] while others believe it to be a small remnant of the müllerian duct [8]. Others suggest it to be a combination of müllerian duct and urogenital sinus epithelium [9]. The true identity, as well as the clinical relevance, of the utricle's embryonic origin remains to be determined. While the size of the prostatic utricle varies, it is normally less than 6 mm on TRUS. However, in 10% of cases it is >10 mm.

The seminal vesicles are located behind the posterior wall of the bladder, superior to the prostate. Around the 13th week of embryological development, the seminal vesicles branch from the distal wolffian ducts, just proximal to their entry into the prostate. Abnormalities in other structures of wolffian origin, involving the vas deferens or ureters, are frequently associated with seminal vesicle malformations. On TRUS examination, the seminal vesicles appear as hypoechoic areas with fine septations. An anteroposterior diameter up to 15 mm is considered normal.

TRUS as a diagnostic tool

Traditionally, vasography after vasopuncture was used to evaluate the patency of the ejaculatory ducts. The procedure involves trans-scrotal cannulation of the vas deferens and injection of a solution containing a dye (e.g., methylene blue) or a radio-opaque substance, followed by cystoscopy or x-ray imaging, respectively [10]. Although vasography is still the gold standard, its use has been supplanted by TRUS. The primary concerns of vasography are its invasive nature, inherent costliness, high risk of iatrogenic stricture and vasal occlusion, and relative risks of anesthetic and radiation exposure [5]. Today, the major use of vasography is during definitive surgery for ejaculatory duct obstructions.

Magnetic resonance imaging (MRI) and computerized tomography (CT) have also been proposed for the evaluation of the ejaculatory system. Because of its low resolution, CT has been shown to have limited value in evaluating the ejaculatory ducts and surrounding structures. MRI with the use of an endorectal coil has proven to be valuable on T2 sequence imaging. Because of its multiplanar nature and high resolution, MRI is superior to TRUS in the diagnosis of small prostatic cysts, evaluation of cyst content, and inspection of the surrounding tissues. However, MRI has restricted use in these circumstances because of its high cost and low availability. Additionally, the low visibility of calcium on MRI makes the diagnosis of calcification problematic. Calcification and stone formation is recognized as one of the major causes of ejaculatory duct obstruction.

Because of its noninvasive nature, low cost, low rate of complications, and high diagnostic efficacy, TRUS is the preferred tool for the diagnosis of ejaculatory duct obstruction. It should be noted that in a recent study, TRUS findings correlated poorly with those obtained by definitive invasive studies [11]. Obstruction on TRUS was confirmed in only 52%, 48%, and 36% of vesiculography, seminal vesicle aspiration, and duct chromotubation studies, respectively. Relying only on the TRUS findings, 52% of patients in this study would have undergone unnecessary surgical intervention [11].

Pathological findings on a diagnostic TRUS procedure

The types of pathologies found on a TRUS evaluation include agenesis or hypoplasia of urogenital structures, cysts, dilatations, calcifications, and stones.

Agenesis of the vas deferens is seen in 1.0–2.5% of infertile men and 4.4–17.0% of azoospermic men, and is frequently accompanied by seminal vesicle agenesis. Ultrasonographic evaluation of the ipsilateral kidney should be performed in cases of unilateral vas deferens agenesis, as ipsilateral renal anomalies may be found in as many as 91% of cases [12]. This association exists, as already noted, because both the ureters and the vas deferens arise embryologically from the wolffian ducts. Genetic counseling is advised for infertile males with congenital agenesis of the vas deferens, as mutations in genes related to cystic fibrosis (CF) are found in 82% of these patients [13].

Seminal vesicle cysts are rare and can be either congenital or acquired. Congenital seminal vesicle cysts are frequently accompanied by ipsilateral renal agenesis or an ectopic ureter.

In the latter cases, the ureter is frequently attached to a dysplastic kidney and with entry into the seminal vesicle. Seminal vesicle cysts cause seminal vesicle duct obstruction only if they are medially located and reach sufficient size [14].

Prostatic cysts can be classified by location, sperm content, and embryological origin. Non-sperm-containing cysts are found in a midline location and are called either utricular cysts or müllerian duct cysts. The degree to which these two cysts differ, and the nature of that difference, remain to be determined. Some authors maintain that utricular cysts are of endodermal origin and are located near the verumontanum, while müllerian duct cysts are of mesodermal origin and are located closer to the prostatic base [5]. Other authorities argue that cysts of müllerian duct origin do not truly exist, and that all cysts of this nature derive from the prostatic utricle [9]. Whatever the embryonic origin, their appearance on TRUS is nearly identical. Sperm-containing cysts, called wolffian or ejaculatory duct cysts, are far less common than utricular/müllerian duct cysts [15]. They are usually found in a more paramedian location rather than strictly midline [16]. Sperm may be absent from wolffian cysts in the setting of concomitant epididymal obstruction or after long-term ejaculatory duct obstruction. This can make differentiation of wolffian cysts from utricular cysts difficult [17,18]. Other cystic formations that can be detected during a TRUS evaluation are congenital and retention prostatic cysts and local abscess formations. These cysts are less likely to cause obstruction because they are frequently located more laterally.

Fibrosis and calcification of the distal ejaculatory ducts, mainly secondary to inflammation or infection, are common causes of ejaculatory duct obstruction. These lesions appear on TRUS as hyperechoic regions. TRUS importantly can reveal the anatomic relationship between ejaculatory channels and calcifications. It can also detect proximal dilatation of the ejaculatory tract, which indirectly implies the presence of a distal obstruction. However, obstruction because of excessive fibrosis may occur without apparent dilatation of the ejaculatory duct. If there is no history of infection or surgical procedure, a subclinical infection is implicated in these situations [16].

Diagnostic criteria for distal ejaculatory duct obstruction

Distal ejaculatory duct obstruction (EDO) is strongly suspected in cases of azoospermia in which TRUS reveals dilated seminal vesicles with an anteroposterior length greater than 15 mm, or ejaculatory ducts with diameter greater than 2.3 mm (Figures 21.2 and 21.3) [19]. However, in cases of incomplete ejaculatory obstruction or without sufficient dilatation of the seminal vesicles or ejaculatory ducts, for example in cases of excessive fibrosis, it may be difficult to make a definitive clinical judgment based on the TRUS findings alone. In such cases of atypical presentation, verification of distal obstruction can be confirmed by transrectal aspiration of the seminal vesicles. Diagnosis of distal obstruction is supported by the presence of three or more motile spermatozoa per high-powered field in the

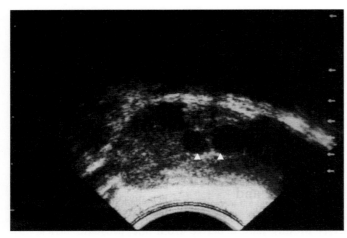

Figure 21.2. Transverse image of the prostate revealing dilated ejaculatory ducts (arrowheads).

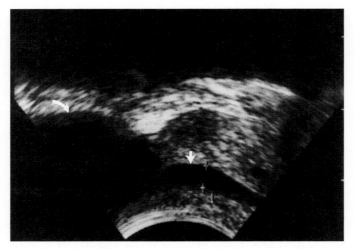

Figure 21.3. Longitudinal image of the junction of the seminal vesicle (curved arrow) and prostate revealing a dilated ejaculatory duct (straight arrow) that measured 3.6 mm.

aspirate. The sample is obtained 2 hours after ejaculation, since normal seminal vesicles will contain no motile spermatozoa at this time [20].

Therapeutic applications of TRUS

If TRUS evaluation reveals obstruction of the ejaculatory ducts secondary to fibrosis or calcification of the duct opening or compression by a superficial midline cyst, the preferred therapy is transurethral resection or unroofing of the ejaculatory ducts (TURED) [21]. The procedure varies depending on the pathological findings, but it may involve resection of the distal portion of the duct, unroofing of any cysts present, or a combination of both [22]. In TURED, because there are no guides to identify the ejaculatory ducts, the resection depth and the exact location of the obstructed lesion are not determined easily. Furthermore, complications such as rectal wall, external

sphincter, and bladder neck injury can theoretically occur more frequently, because of the small prostate volumes in these younger infertile men. Concurrent TRUS can be used to monitor resection depth during TURED in order to prevent complications and also to monitor the efficacy of the procedure. Dye (for direct visualization with cystoscopy) or a combination of dye and echo-enhancing contrast agent (for visualization with TRUS) is injected into the seminal vesicles, using TRUS to identify the ejaculatory ducts [23,24].

TRUS can also be used for therapeutic aspiration and reduction in the size of obstructive cysts. This method is preferred for deep cysts that are inaccessible by TURED. While this is a simple and noninvasive method of cyst reduction, it is not always curative and the cystic fluid often reaccumulates [15].

TRUS may also be used in azoospermic men with an obstruction distal to the seminal vesicles for sperm retrieval by seminal vesicle aspiration. The sperm retrieved by this method can be used for ART. Although described as successful in the literature, this is not a commonly performed procedure, as testicular sperm extraction (TESE) or epididymal aspiration (MESA) are the preferred methods for sperm retrieval. TRUS-guided aspiration of the seminal vesicles may be suitable for patients undergoing concurrent TRUS-guided aspiration of midline cysts [2,25].

Key points in clinical practice

- Infertility is a common problem affecting 15% of couples; male factor infertility accounts for about half of these cases.
- Obstructive infertility can present with a wide range of clinical scenarios including azoospermia, which is the absence of sperm in the ejaculate.
- Obstructive azoospermia is seen in 5% of infertile men; ejaculatory duct obstruction accounts for 1–3% of cases of obstructive azoospermia.
- The standard clinical evaluation of an infertile male includes history, physical examination, semen analysis, hormone profile, and selective imaging. Imaging should not be performed before the earlier steps are completed.
- Transrectal ultrasound is a useful tool for imaging of the distal structures of the ejaculatory system (including the ampulla of the vas deferens, the seminal vesicles, the ejaculatory ducts, and the prostate) and for diagnosis of ejaculatory duct obstruction (EDO).
- Although it has a low sensitivity, TRUS is currently preferred over MRI, CT, and vasography for diagnosis of EDO, because of its minimal risk, low cost, infrequent complications, and diagnostic efficacy.
- Pathological findings on TRUS include prostatic and seminal vesicle cysts, dilatations of the seminal vesicles and ejaculatory ducts, stones, and fibrosis or calcification of the ejaculatory ducts.
- TRUS findings suggestive of ejaculatory duct obstruction are dilated seminal vesicles with an anteroposterior length

greater than 15 mm, dilated ejaculatory ducts with a diameter greater than 2.3 mm, and the presence of spermatozoa in the seminal vesicle aspirate 2 hours after ejaculation.

- TRUS can be applied therapeutically for ART concurrently with TURED, aspiration and reduction of cyst size, and aspiration of seminal vesicle fluid.

References

1. Zahalsky M, Nagler H. Ultrasound and infertility: diagnostic and therapeutic uses. *Curr Urol Rep* 2001; **2**: 437–42.

2. Cerruto MA, Novella G, Antoniolli SZ, Zattoni F. Use of transperineal fine needle aspiration of seminal vesicles to retrieve sperm in a man with obstructive azoospermia. *Fertil Steril* 2006; **86**: 1764. e7–9.

3. Irvin DS. Epidemiology and etiology of male infertility. *Hum Reprod* 1998; **13**(Suppl 1): 33–44.

4. Dohle GR, Colpi GM, Hargreave TB, Papp GK, Jungwirth A, Weidner W. The EAU Working Group on Male Infertility. EAU guidelines on male infertility. *Eur Urol* 2005; **48**: 703–11.

5. Goluboff ET, Stifelman MD, Fisch H. Ejaculatory duct obstruction in the infertile male. *Urology* 1995; **45**: 925–31.

6. Colpi GM, Casella F, Zanollo A, et al. Functional voiding disturbances of the ampullo-vesicular seminal tract: a cause of male infertility. *Acta Eur Fertil* 1987; **18**: 165–79.

7. Pierik FH, Vreeburg JT, Stijnen T, De Jong FH, Weber RF. Serum inhibin B as a marker of spermatogenesis. *J Clin Endocrinol Metab* 1998; **83**: 3110–14.

8. Partin AW, Rodriquez R. The molecular biology, endocrinology, and physiology of the prostate and seminal vesicles. In: Walsh PC et al. *Campbell's Urology*, 8th edn. Philadelphia, PA: Saunders, 2002; 1238–84.

9. Kato H, Hayama M, Furuya S, Kobayashi S, Islam AM, Nishizawa O. Anatomical and histological studies of so-called Mullerian duct cyst. *Int J Urol* 2005; **12**: 465–8.

10. Weintraub MP, De Mouy E, Hellstrom WJ G. Newer modalities in the diagnosis and treatment of ejaculatory duct obstruction. *J Urol* 1993; **150**: 1150–4.

11. Purohit RS, Wu DS, Shinohara K, Turek PJ. A prospective comparison of 3 diagnostic methods to evaluate ejaculatory duct obstruction. *J Urol* 2004; **171**: 232–5.

12. Schlegel PN, Shin D, Goldstein M. Urogenital anomalies in men with congenital absence of the vas deferens. *J Urol* 1996; **155**: 1644–8.

13. Chillon M, Casals T, Mercier B, et al. Mutations in the cystic fibrosis gene in patients with congenital absence of the vas deferens. *N Engl J Med* 1995; **332**: 1475–80.

14. Shabsigh R, Lerner S, Fishman IJ, Kadmon D. The role of transrectal ultrasonography in the diagnosis and management of prostatic and seminal vesicle cysts. *J Urol* 1989; **141**: 1206–9.

15. Elder JS, Mostwin JL. Cyst of the ejaculatory duct/urogenital sinus. *J Urol* 1984; **132**: 768–71.

16. Kuligowska E, Fenlon HM. Transrectal US in male infertility: spectrum of findings and role in patient care. *Radiology* 1998; **207**: 173–81.

17. Silber SJ. Ejaculatory duct obstruction. *J Urol* 1980; **124**: 294–7.

18. Patterson L, Jarow JP. Transrectal ultrasonography in the evaluation of the infertile man: a report of three cases. *J Urol* 1990; **144**: 1469–71.

19. Nguyen HT, Etzell J, Turek PJ. Normal human ejaculatory duct anatomy: a study of cadaveric and surgical specimens. *J Urol* 1996; **155**: 1639–42.

20. Orhan I, Onur R, Cayan S, Koksal IT, Kadioglu A. Seminal vesicle sperm aspiration in the diagnosis of ejaculatory duct obstruction. *BJU Int* 1999; **84**: 1050–3.

21. Fisch H, Kang YM, Johnson CW, Goluboff ET. Ejaculatory duct obstruction. *Curr Opin Urol* 2002; **12**: 509–15.

22. Schroeder-Printzen I, Ludwig M, Kohn F, Weidner W. Surgical therapy in infertile men with ejaculatory duct obstruction: technique and outcome of a standardized surgical approach. *Hum Reprod* 2000; **15**: 1364–8.

23. Halpern EJ, Hirsch IH. Sonographically guided transurethral laser incision of a Mullerian duct cyst for treatment of ejaculatory duct obstruction. *Am J Roentgenol* 2000; **175**: 777–8.

24. Apaydin E, Killi RM, Turna B, Semerci B, Nazli O. Transrectal ultrasonography-guided echo-enhanced seminal vesiculography in combination with transurethral resection of the ejaculatory ducts. *BJU Int* 2004; **93**: 1110–12.

25. Boehlem D, Schmid HP. Novel use of fine needle aspiration of seminal vesicles for sperm retrieval in infertile men. *Urology* 2005; **66**: 880.

Chapter 22

Ultrasonographic evaluation of acute pelvic pain

Aimee Eyvazzadeh and Deborah Levine

Introduction

Acute pelvic pain is a common reason for women to seek urgent gynecologic evaluation. This challenging clinical condition requires immediate evaluation of the patient to reach the proper diagnosis. Women with acute pelvic pain are usually in their reproductive years and may be pregnant at the time of presentation. Proper diagnosis makes a substantial difference in the management of the patient, and, at times, preservation of reproductive function. Early in the work-up of acute pelvic pain it is important to establish whether the patient is pregnant since pregnancy (normal or abnormal) can cause pain. In addition, pregnant patients can have all the gynecologic and nongynecologic causes of pelvic pain that affect women of any age.

Acute pelvic pain generally lasts less than one month and does not recur. The source may be pregnancy-related, gynecologic, gastrointestinal, or urological (Table 22.1) and may range from the less alarming rupture of a follicular cyst to a life-threatening condition such as rupture of an ectopic pregnancy or a perforated appendix. Ruptured ectopic pregnancy, salpingitis, and hemorrhagic ovarian cysts are the three most commonly diagnosed gynecologic conditions presenting with acute pelvic pain.

Due to its noninvasive nature, safety, and reliability, ultrasound is the primary imaging modality for evaluation of women with acute pelvic pain and is a readily available tool in the fertility clinic. Many gynecologic disorders that cause acute pelvic pain demonstrate characteristic ultrasound findings, and familiarity with their sonographic appearances is essential for the clinician performing pelvic ultrasounds in the office as it will allow the physician to guide appropriate treatment of the affected patient and frequently will eliminate the need for further imaging evaluation. Real-time imaging allows the clinician to correlate the region of the patient's pain with the ultrasound findings, improving the specificity of diagnosis.

This chapter summarizes characteristic ultrasound findings of acute pelvic pain in women of reproductive age. Ultrasound findings seen in gynecologic, urological, gastrointestinal, and pregnancy-related conditions will be reviewed.

Pelvic pain in pregnant or nonpregnant patients

Ovarian cysts

The incidence of follicular cysts is increased in infertile patients taking drugs such as clomiphene citrate and gonadotropins for ovulation induction. Typically, ovarian cysts are functional, not disease-related, and disappear on their own. During ovulation, a follicle may grow but fail to rupture and release an oocyte. Instead of being reabsorbed, the fluid within the follicle persists and forms a follicular cyst. This cyst may cause pain. As patients come in frequently for ultrasound during infertility treatment, making them aware of the presence of this cyst is essential so that they may be informed about why they may experience acute pelvic pain in the future. Functional ovarian cysts usually disappear within 60 days without treatment. However, if the cyst is larger than 6 cm (Figure 22.1), or persists for longer than 6 weeks, then further testing may be needed.

The corpus luteum is a common site of pelvic pain, especially in patients who have undergone controlled ovarian hyperstimulation or ovulation induction resulting in multiple corpus luteum cysts. The corpus luteum cyst (Figure 22.2) is a normal finding in pregnancy and is the most common adnexal mass in pregnancy. Pain can be due to the size of the cyst, bleeding within the cyst, torsion, or rupture. If a hemorrhagic corpus luteum cyst is the cause of the patient's pain, it should be tender to direct pressure using the ultrasound probe (either transabdominal or transvaginal, depending on cyst position). If moving the cyst (or tissues around the cyst) with the ultrasound probe does not elicit the patient's pain, another source for the pelvic pain should be sought.

Corpus luteum cysts are typically less than 6 cm in diameter, but may be larger. Due to the cyst fluid, there is posterior through-transmission. The internal echotexture varies, depending on the stage of hemorrhage and the amount of fluid within the cyst. This is best appreciated with transvaginal scanning. The diagnosis of a hemorrhagic cyst can be made with the presence of fibrin strands, a retracting clot, septations, and wall irregularity [1,2]. The wall of the cyst may appear thick or thin, ranging from

Ultrasonography in Reproductive Medicine and Infertility, ed. Botros R. M. B. Rizk. Published by Cambridge University Press. © Cambridge University Press 2010.

Table 22.1. Causes of acute pelvic pain

Gynecologic	Adnexal torsion	
	Endometriosis	
	Infection	Pelvic inflammatory disease
		Tubo-ovarian abscess
	Ovarian	Corpus luteum cyst
		Ovarian hyperstimulation syndrome
		Endometrioma
		Mittelschmerz
		Ruptured cyst
		Neoplasm
	Uterine	Fibroids
		Dysmenorrhea
		Congenital obstructive müllerian anomaly
Pregnancy-related	Miscarriage	
	Ectopic pregnancy	
Gastrointestinal	Appendicitis	
	Constipation	
	Inflammatory bowel disease	
	Irritable bowel syndrome	
	Gastroenteritis	
	Diverticulitis	
Urological	Acute cystitis	
	Renal calculi	

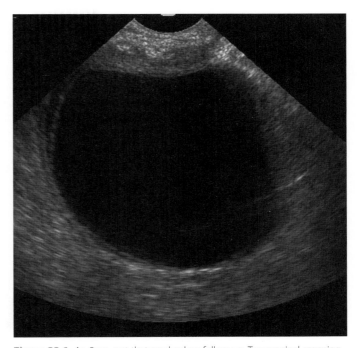

Figure 22.1. An 8 cm cyst that resolved on follow-up. Transvaginal scanning demonstrates an anechoic 8 cm cyst.

2 to 22 mm. The corpus luteum is a very vascular structure, and typically a ring of color flow can be demonstrated [3]. It is important to recognize that this flow is a normal finding, so as not to mistake a corpus luteum for an ectopic pregnancy.

Endometriosis

The prevalence of endometriosis in infertile women is 25–40%, while the prevalence in reproductive-age women is 3–10% [3]. Although the classic clinical presentation is dysmenorrhea with premenstrual intensification, dyspareunia, and chronic pelvic pain, some patients – who may or may not know they have the condition – experience acute pelvic pain. Ultrasound is helpful in the evaluation of women with an endometriotic cyst, since there is the classic appearance of a chocolate cyst with diffuse, low-level internal echoes (Figure 22.3) and at times scattered punctuate echogenicities in the cyst wall. Occasionally, endometriotic cysts may have septations, thickened walls, and wall nodularity. Blood flow in endometriomas is usually pericystic, especially noticeable in the hilar region, and usually visualized in regularly spaced vessels [4]. Dermoid cysts, hemorrhagic cysts, and cystic neoplasms may resemble endometriomas and must be considered in the differential diagnosis. Ultrasound has a limited role in the

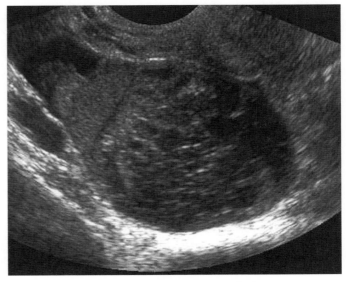

Figure 22.2. Hemorrhagic corpus luteum cyst. Note the heterogeneous cyst contents with strands of internal echoes and posterior increased through-transmission.

diagnosis of adhesions or superficial peritoneal implants. These are better assessed with MRI (if imaging diagnosis is desired) or laparoscopy (if direct visualization is desired).

Ovarian hyperstimulation

Ovarian hyperstimulation syndrome (OHSS) is an iatrogenic complication of superovulation induction therapy with a varied spectrum of clinical and laboratory manifestations,

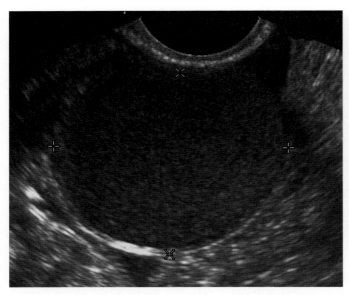

Figure 22.3. Endometrioma. Note 4 cm cyst (calipers) with diffuse homogeneous low-level internal echoes.

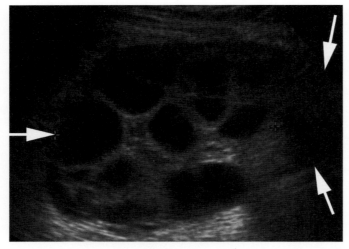

Figure 22.4. Ovarian hyperstimulation syndrome. Enlarged right ovary (arrows) measuring greater than 9 cm, with multiple cysts. Patient also had ascites and pleural effusions (not shown).

with abdominal pain as the most common first presenting symptom. Symptoms typically start 3–4 days after the hCG (human chorionic gonadotropin) trigger and peak 7 days after ovulation or oocyte retrieval unless a patient is pregnant, in which case symptoms may persist or worsen [5]. Ovarian hyperstimulation (Figure 22.4) is diagnosed by the presence of abdominal pain, enlargement of the ovary greater than 5 cm, and ascites [5]. Patients with OHSS may also have a hematocrit of 45% or more, elevated white blood cell count, oliguria, elevated liver enzymes, electrolyte abnormalities, dyspnea, anasarca, or acute renal failure. Patients with acute pain and ascites may benefit from sonographically guided drainage of ascites to relieve the abdominal pain and distension they experience. An

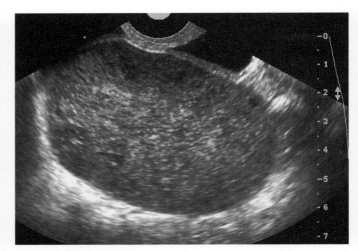

Figure 22.5. Torsion in a patient with acute right lower quadrant pain. Transvaginal view shows an enlarged edematous-appearing ovary.

indwelling "pig-tail" catheter should be considered for extended drainage, especially if the patient has severe pain, pulmonary compromise, or evidence of renal compromise unresponsive to fluid management. There are two potentially overlapping diagnoses in the evaluation of the patient with acute pelvic pain and ovarian hyperstimulation. The first is that if the patient is pregnant, ectopic pregnancy is still a possibility. The second is that ovarian torsion may coexist with hyperstimulation.

Ovarian torsion

Symptoms of ovarian torsion include severe lower abdominal pain, pelvic pain, and tenderness that are usually sudden in onset and localized to the torsed ovary, as well as nausea and vomiting. However, the signs and symptoms associated with torsion are variable and nonspecific. Confident and early diagnosis of ovarian torsion is imperative. Ultrasound demonstrates either an enlarged edematous-appearing ovary or an adnexal mass (Figure 22.5). The patient should have acute pain localized to the enlarged ovary There may be surrounding intraperitoneal fluid [6]. Doppler of ovarian torsion can be difficult because the ovaries have a dual blood supply, from the ovarian artery laterally and from the ovarian branch of the uterine artery medially, so that flow may appear normal even in a torsed ovary. Altered blood flow on Doppler studies may consist of absent arterial and venous flow (complete torsion), arterial flow present but with absent diastolic flow (partial torsion), or absent arterial but present venous flow (predictive of ovarian viability [7]. If no flow is visualized, it is often helpful to check the contralateral ovary to ensure that Doppler settings are appropriate to visualize ovarian flow. It should be emphasized that the presence of blood flow on Doppler studies should not dissuade one from making the diagnosis of torsion, as this finding may be present in incomplete torsion.

With isolated tubal torsion, the tube is usually distended and lacks flow or has reversed flow during diastole.

Leiomyomas

Leiomyomas undergoing degenerative changes are another cause of acute pelvic pain that may also complicate pregnancy. One in 500 pregnant women are admitted for fibroid-related complications [8]. The symptoms and signs are focal pain, with tenderness on palpation and sometimes low-grade fever. Color flow detects regularly separated vessels at the periphery of the leiomyoma, which exhibit moderate vascular resistance. Fibroids during pregnancy occasionally undergo red degeneration that is caused by hemorrhagic infarction (Figure 22.6). The sonographic diagnosis of a degenerating fibroid is made when the patient experiences pain localized to the region of the visualized fibroid. At times a lucent center will be visualized.

Pelvic inflammatory disease

Pelvic inflammatory disease (PID) may occur in many instances in the work-up of the infertile woman. It may be the cause of infertility. It may be exacerbated after hysterosalpingography, particularly in women with unexpected hydrosalpinx. It may occur following a pelvic procedure (Figure 22.7). Ultrasound findings of PID include thickening of the tubal wall (greater than or equal to 5 mm), incomplete septa within the dilated tube (as the tube folds back upon itself), enlarged ovaries associated with inflammation, and free fluid in the cul-de-sac [9]. If the distended tube is viewed in cross-section, it may demonstrate the "cog wheel" sign due to the thickened endosalpingeal folds. An enlarged ovary with increased numbers of small cysts, the so-called "polycystic ovary" appearance, appears to correlate with PID. A reasonable explanation for this reactive polycystic change is that the inflammation increases ovarian volume, by thickening the stroma and increasing the number and size of cysts [9]. The margins of the ovaries may also become indistinct in PID. When the ovary adheres to the tube, but is still visualized, this indicates a tubo-ovarian complex. A tubo-ovarian abscess is the result of a complete breakdown of ovarian and tubal architecture such that separate structures are no longer identified. Tubo-ovarian abscess may be treated by transvaginal drainage, allowing for improved response to antibiotics without an open procedure.

Chronic PID typically results in a hydrosalpinx from accumulation of fluid due to occlusion of the tube distally or at both ends. Several specific ultrasound findings can help distinguish a hydrosalpinx from other cystic adnexal lesions. A hydrosalpinx tends to be anechoic and more tubular, and often demonstrates the "incomplete septa" sign. The tubal wall is thin, less than 5 mm, and in cross-section demonstrates the "beads-on-a-string" sign. These beads are 2–3 mm hyperechoic nodules projecting from the wall, representing remnants of the endosalpingeal folds.

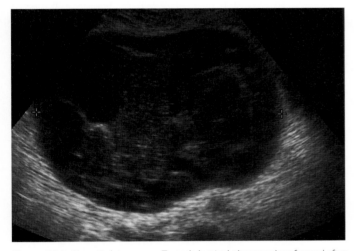

Figure 22.6. Necrotic leiomyoma. Transabdominal ultrasound performed after cesarean section in patient with pain shows a heterogeneous cystic and solid mass (calipers). Color Doppler (not shown) showed no flow. This was in the region of the patient's pain. Pathology was a necrotic leiomyoma.

Obstructed duplicated system

At times, acute pelvic pain can occur in the setting of a congenital obstructive müllerian anomaly, such as a didelphic uterus with an oblique vaginal septum obstructing one of the cervices, or an obstructed atrophic horn of a bicornuate uterus. At the time of presentation, a pelvic ultrasound can evaluate the

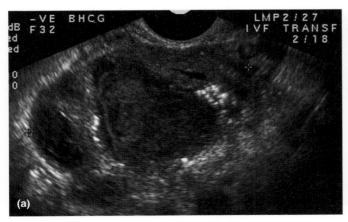

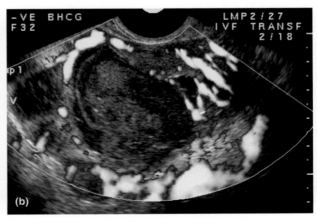

Figure 22.7. Pelvic inflammatory disease 3 weeks after IVF. (a) Transvaginal sagittal image of left adnexa shows heterogeneous fluid collections and bright echoes consistent with gas. (b) Power Doppler sonogram shows complex adnexal fluid collection with surrounding hyperemic tissue.

179

müllerian anomaly and collection of blood. Three-dimensional ultrasound can be helpful in showing the coronal view of the uterine horn(s). Vaginal ultrasound is helpful in delineating the number of cervices. Magnetic resonance imaging may be needed to better define the pelvic anatomy.

Gastrointestinal causes of acute pelvic pain

Appendicitis is the most common surgical emergency and should always be considered in differential diagnosis of acute right lower quadrant pain if the appendix has not been removed. Apart from clinical examination and laboratory tests, the combined ultrasound criteria of an appendix with a muscular wall thickness greater than or equal to 3.0 mm (6 mm transverse diameter) and visualization of a complex mass separate from the adnexa has proved most useful as a diagnostic test (sensitivity, 68%; specificity, 98%) [10]. Fluid around the appendix may be visualized, even if the appendix has not ruptured. An appendicolith can be seen as a shadowing mass, and is indicative of a ruptured (or soon to rupture) appendix. The method for visualizing the appendix is to scan the right lower quadrant, following the cecum to its end. The appendix should be visualized as a blind-ending tubular structure (Figure 22.8). The patient's pain may be increased by rapidly removing the ultrasound probe, stimulating rebound tenderness. In cases where the appendix is not visualized, but appendicitis is of concern, alternative imaging with CT (if the patient is not pregnant) or MRI (if it is available and the patient is pregnant) are helpful in diagnosing and excluding appendicitis.

Urinary tract

Dilatation of the renal pelvis and ureter are typical signs of obstructive uropathy and may be efficiently detected by ultrasound. Additional thinning of renal parenchyma suggests long-term obstructive uropathy. Stones can be seen at the ureteropelvic junction with transabdominal ultrasound and at the ureterovesical junction with either transabdominal or transvaginal ultrasound. If a stone is suspected but not visualized, assessment for ureteral jets (seeing Doppler flow in the bladder from the urine stream) may be helpful. For this study the bladder should be partially full with urine, and examination with color flow is performed in the region of the ureterovesicular junction. Absence of flow on the side of pain (with documented jets on the contralateral side) is an indication of an obstructing stone. However, jets may be present with partially obstructing stones, so visualization of jets does not exclude ureterolithiasis.

Pelvic pain in pregnancy

Normal pregnancy

Crampy pelvic pain due to hormonal changes, rapid growth of the uterus, and increased blood flow is a common sign of early pregnancy. This pain can be quite alarming and can cause anxiety in fertility patients, especially those experiencing pregnancy for the very first time. Showing the normal findings of intrauterine pregnancy can be helpful in these patients. The intradecidual sign (Figure 22.9), seen at 4.5–5 weeks of gestation, is visualized as a discrete hypoechoic fluid collection with an echogenic rim that is eccentrically located in the endometrial cavity, causing deviation of the endometrial stripe, and is the first sonographic demonstration of early pregnancy [11]. Because small endometrial fluid collections can simulate the intradecidual sign, care should be taken to ensure that the collection has a well-defined echogenic rim, is just beneath the central endometrial echo, and has an unchanging appearance [11]. Follow-up in patients at high risk for ectopic pregnancy or patients who have persistent symptoms is essential in order to ensure that an intrauterine pregnancy is present.

The double decidual sac sign is seen slightly later, when the decidua capsularis and decidua vera are seen as two distinct hyperechoic layers surrounding the early gestational sac [12]. At 5.5 weeks' gestation, the yolk sac appears as a small hyperechoic ring within the gestational sac. Later in pregnancy the embryo is visualized adjacent to the yolk sac. Cardiac activity should be seen by the time the embryonic pole is 5 mm [13].

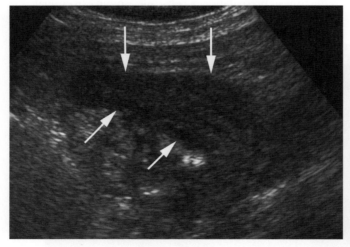

Figure 22.8. Appendicitis in a pregnant patient with acute right lower quadrant pain. Oblique transabdominal right lower quadrant image demonstrates the dilated appendix (arrows).

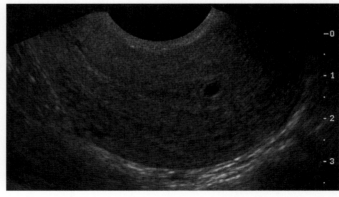

Figure 22.9. Intradecidual sign. Note the echogenic rim, eccentrically located in the endometrial cavity.

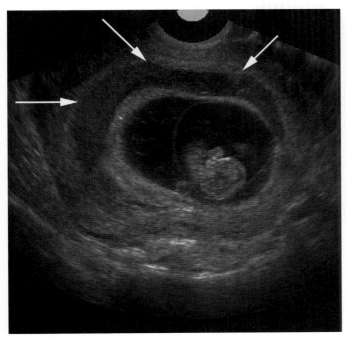

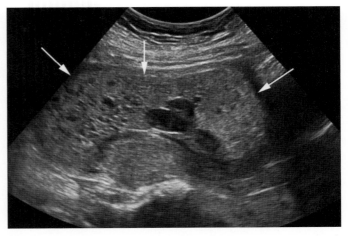

Figure 22.11. Molar pregnancy at 11 weeks' gestational age in a patient with pelvic pain. Sagittal transabdominal image shows the endometrial cavity (arrows) distended with echogenic material, with multiple small cysts compatible with a molar pregnancy. Human chorionic gonadotropin level was 550 000 mIU/ml.

Figure 22.10. Subchorionic hemorrhage at 10 weeks. Note the crescentic appearance of the blood products (arrows) as they conform to the uterine shape.

Subchorionic hemorrhage

If the patient also reports bleeding as well as acute-onset crampy pain, a subchorionic hemorrhage should be considered as part of the differential diagnosis. The presence of subchorionic hematoma is reportedly higher in the pregnant infertility population than in the general obstetric population [14]. It is caused by a partial detachment of the trophoblast from the uterine wall. The placental margin is displaced by anechoic or heterogeneous hypoechoic material. At times the blood products are of similar echogenicity to the placenta, and thus are difficult to visualize sonographically. Small collections have no clinical significance, whereas larger hematomas have a poorer prognosis. Seventy per cent of subchorionic hematomas resolve spontaneously by the end of the second trimester [15]. The hematoma can dissect in the potential space between the chorion and endometrial cavity and may be visualized as separate from the placenta. It usually has a falciform shape because it typically conforms to the shape of the uterus (Figure 22.10). As in all early pregnancy assessments, demonstration of cardiac activity is crucial in determining prognosis.

Spontaneous abortion

Whether pregnancies conceived through assisted reproductive technologies (ART) are at an increased risk of spontaneous abortion is inconclusive [16]. First-trimester spontaneous abortion occurs in 10–12% of clinically recognized pregnancies [17]. Most women with spontaneous abortion experience vaginal bleeding. Up to 25% of all pregnant women bleed some time during pregnancy, with about half of them eventually undergoing miscarriage. Pain may be constant or intermittent and crampy over the uterus or lower back.

Ultrasound thresholds (using transvaginal sonography) that ensure the highest specificity in the diagnosis of spontaneous abortion include the following: visualization of a yolk sac by the time the gestational sac has a mean sac diameter of 13 mm; visualization of an embryo by the time the mean sac diameter is 18 mm; and visualization of cardiac activity by the time the embryonic pole is 5 mm [18]. Between 6.5 and 10 weeks of gestation, the length of the amniotic cavity is similar to that of the embryo. At times a failed early pregnancy will present as an "empty amnion sign" [19]. Sonographic findings also include a thin decidual reaction (less than 2 mm), weak decidual amplitude, irregular contour of the sac, absent double decidual sac sign, and low position of the sac.

Molar pregnancy

Molar pregnancies are relatively uncommon, with geographic differences in the incidence of the complication. In the USA about 1 out of every 1000 pregnancies is a molar pregnancy. In Southeast Asia the incidence is 8 times higher [20]. Age over 40 is a risk factor for molar pregnancy, as is having a prior molar pregnancy (with a recurrence risk of 1 out of 100 [20]. Molar pregnancy can be associated with pelvic pain because of the rapid change in size of the uterus, the size of the associated theca lutein cysts, or torsion of the ovaries caused by the theca lutein cysts. The classic sonographic appearance of a complete mole has multiple cystic spaces representing hydropic villi; however, the size of the villi is directly proportional to gestational age, and early molar pregnancies frequently do not have the typical sonographic appearance (Figure 22.11) [21]. Other appearances that can be seen in the first trimester include an intrauterine anechoic fluid collection similar to a gestational sac, a fluid collection with a complex echogenic mass similar to an edematous placenta, a heterogeneously thickened endometrium, and echogenic fluid–fluid levels within the endometrium [21].

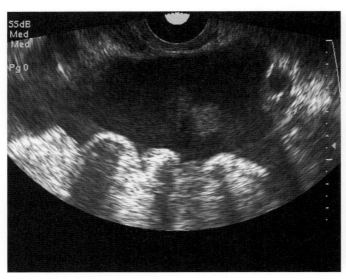

Figure 22.12. Hemoperitoneum in a patient with pelvic pain. Sagittal transvaginal sonogram shows fluid with debris in the cul-de-sac in a patient with a ruptured hemorrhagic cyst.

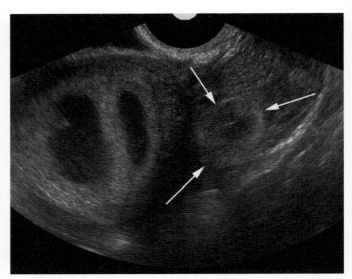

Figure 22.13. Heterotopic pregnancy in a pregnant patient with pelvic pain. Sagittal transvaginal sonogram shows diamniotic dichorionic intrauterine gestations and a third echogenic sac outside the uterus, due to a heterotopic gestation (arrows).

Hemoperitoneum

Hemoperitoneum is visualized sonographically as echogenic fluid in the cul-de-sac. Larger amounts of fluid will extend out of the pelvis and mimic ascites. When fluid with debris is visualized in the upper abdomen, a large of amount of hemoperitoneum should be suspected, even if the patient's hematocrit is normal, because a decrease in hematocrit may lag several hours behind the visualization of hemoperitoneum.

Hemoperitoneum in infertility patients after oocyte retrieval is reported in 0.03–0.50% of cases [22], in cases of ruptured ovarian cysts, and in cases of ectopic pregnancy. When echogenic fluid is visualized in a patient who has positive β-hCG results, this has a positive predictive value (86–93%) in the diagnosis of ectopic pregnancy and may be the only endovaginal sonographic finding [23]; however, a ruptured hemorrhagic corpus luteum cyst can also result in hemoperitoneum (Figure 22.12). If the patient is clinically unstable, differentiating between a ruptured ectopic and a ruptured hemorrhagic corpus luteum is unimportant, because in either case surgical management is indicated. In unstable patients who have demonstration of hemoperitoneum, the sonographic examination may not demonstrate an ectopic pregnancy. In the clinically stable patient it is more important to carefully examine the adnexa to determine whether an ectopic pregnancy is present. Imaging the kidneys is helpful in terms of assessing whether a large amount of hemoperitoneum is present.

Ectopic pregnancy

Up to 5% of IVF pregnancies are ectopic and 0.1–0.3% heterotopic, which is higher than the baseline ectopic rate of 1% [24,25] and heterotopic rate of 1/7000–30 000. With the higher incidence of heterotopic pregnancy in women undergoing ART, not only is visualization of an intrauterine gestational

sac important but careful attention to the adnexa is crucial (Figure 22.13). The most common signs and symptoms of an ectopic pregnancy include severe abdominal pain (90%), vaginal spotting (80%), and pelvic mass on examination (50%) [26]. The combination of ultrasound and hCG level is the best way to diagnose an ectopic pregnancy. A normal pregnancy shows a doubling time of the β-hCG value of 2 days (range 1.2–2.2 days) [27]. Patients typically present at about 5–6 weeks' gestational age, with 90% of ectopics having a β-hCG <6500 mIU/ml.

In general, an intrauterine gestational sac is expected to be visualized when β-hCG is 1000 mIU/ml (Second International Standard) or 2000 mIU/ml international reference preparation (IRP) [28,29]. It should be emphasized that the majority of studies of β-hCG in early pregnancy evaluated normal early pregnancy, and described an intrauterine gestational sac as any collection of fluid in the endometrial cavity. Small fluid collections of 2 mm without a decidual reaction were considered sufficient to describe an early gestational sac. It should be noted that this type of fluid collection can be caused by a decidual cyst or even a pseudosac, and therefore may not represent a normal intrauterine pregnancy; however, these values are helpful in triaging patients. When β-hCG is below the discriminatory zone (2000 mIU/ml, IRP) and no intrauterine gestation is present, the diagnosis could be an early intrauterine pregnancy, a miscarriage, or an ectopic pregnancy, and therefore close follow-up is indicated. When the β-hCG value is above the discriminatory zone, one can expect to see an intrauterine gestational sac; however, even without visualization of a sac there could still be a very early normal intrauterine pregnancy. Technical quality of the examination, presence of fibroids, intrauterine contraceptive devices, large hemorrhage, and multiple gestation may all contribute to nonvisualization of an early sac.

The most common location for ectopic pregnancy is in the fallopian tubes, occurring in up to 97% of cases. Of these, 80% are located in the ampullary region, 10% in the isthmic portion, 5% in the fimbrial portion, and 2–4% in the interstitial portion. Uncommon locations include the ovary, abdomen, cervix, and uterine scars [30]. Because most ectopic pregnancies are located within the tubes, it is important to scan above and below the ovaries and between the uterus and ovaries.

Sonographic diagnosis of ectopic pregnancy

Endometrial findings

When fluid is seen centrally in the endometrial cavity, this is termed a pseudosac. This fluid collection represents blood in the endometrial cavity, which can be present in both intra-uterine and ectopic pregnancies. The pseudosac has only one layer corresponding to the endometrial decidual reaction, compared with the double decidual sac sign seen in early intra-uterine pregnancy [12]. Decidual cysts, seen as small fluid collections without an echogenic rim located at the junction of the endometrium with the myometrium, were once thought to be highly specific for ectopic pregnancy [31], but are now known to be neither specific nor sensitive (Figure 22.14) [32].

Adnexal findings

The most specific finding for ectopic pregnancy is the presence of a live extrauterine pregnancy; however, this pathogno-monic sign is present only in only 8–26% of ectopic pregnancies on transvaginal sonography [33]. The next most specific sign is an extrauterine gestational sac containing a yolk sac, with or without an embryo [34]; care should be taken not to confuse a hemorrhagic cyst with debris mimicking a yolk sac or embryo.

An extraovarian tubal ring is 40–68% sensitive for ectopic pregnancy [35]. Slightly less specific but most common is a complex adnexal mass separate from the ovary [33,34]. These should be distinguished from a hemorrhagic corpus luteum cyst arising from the ovary. The transvaginal transducer can be used in "real-time" to determine whether the echogenic ring moves with, or is independent of, the ovary. Another sonographic finding that can help distinguish the corpus luteum from the adnexal ring of an ectopic pregnancy is the relative echogenicity of the wall of the corpus luteum compared with that of a tubal ectopic and of the endometrium. The wall of a corpus luteum is less echogenic than the wall of the tubal ring associated with an ectopic pregnancy, and is less echogenic than the endometrium [36]. If the diagnosis of an adherent ectopic pregnancy or an exophytic ovarian cyst cannot be confirmed and the patient is stable, a follow-up examination is reasonable, because an intrauterine pregnancy may be seen on follow-up, and a hemorrhagic cyst is expected to undergo evolution.

The least specific finding of ectopic pregnancy is the presence of any adnexal mass other than a simple cyst. Even a complex cyst in the ovary is more likely to be the corpus luteum than an ectopic pregnancy.

Use of color Doppler in diagnosis of ectopic pregnancy

Using color Doppler flow, uterine or extrauterine sites of vascular color can be identified in a characteristic placental shape, the so-called "ring-of-fire" pattern, and a high-velocity, low-impedance flow pattern may also be identified that is compatible with placental perfusion [37]. A ring of fire has been described as characterizing the appearance of flow around an ectopic pregnancy; however, the corpus luteum is also very vascular and can have a similar appearance [38]. Color Doppler is most helpful when an extra-ovarian mass has not yet been found, because use of Doppler may allow for detection of an ectopic surrounded by loops of bowel. Luteal flow can be helpful in identifying an ectopic pregnancy, because about 90% of ectopic pregnancies occur on the same side as luteal flow [39].

Interstitial pregnancy

Interstitial pregnancies represent 2–4% of ectopic pregnancies and are associated with higher morbidity and mortality than other tubal pregnancies [40]. The high morbidity from these pregnancies is caused by the interstitial portion of the tube dilating more freely and painlessly than the rest of the tube, and the implantation site location may be between the ovarian and uterine arteries. This leads to later clinical presentation, with rupture between 8 and 16 weeks and the potential for maternal mortality due to massive hemorrhage [40].

The diagnosis is suggested when what appears to be an intrauterine pregnancy is visualized high in the fundus and is not surrounded in all planes by 5 mm of myometrium [40]. This can be treated with laparotomy, systemic methotrexate [41], or transvaginal, sonographically guided injection of potassium chloride [42].

Cervical ectopic pregnancy

Cervical ectopic pregnancy occurs in fewer than 1% of ectopic pregnancies [43]. The sonographic diagnosis is made when a gestational sac with peritrophoblastic flow or a live embryo is identified within the cervix. When a gestational sac with a yolk sac or embryo is seen within the cervix without a heartbeat, the differential diagnosis includes spontaneous abortion and cervical ectopic pregnancy. Follow-up scanning allows for differentiation; in cases of ectopic pregnancy the sac does not change in position, whereas in spontaneous abortion the sac shape and position will change. Patients who have cervical ectopics tend to bleed profusely because the cervix does not have contractile tissue. Therefore, treatment by dilatation and curettage is more risky than treatment of an intrauterine pregnancy. Because of these risks, in the past, cervical ectopics were often treated with hysterectomy. Newer conservative therapies include sonographically guided local potassium chloride injection [42], systemic or local methotrexate [44], or preoperative uterine artery embolization before dilatation and evacuation [44].

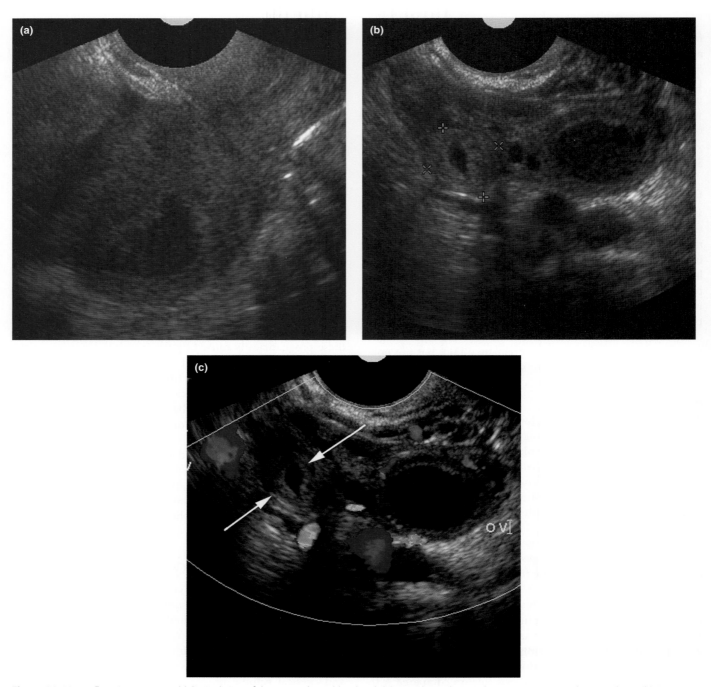

Figure 22.14a–c. Ectopic pregnancy. (a) Sagittal view of the uterus shows blood and debris in the endometrial cavity, consistent with a pseudosac. (b) Transverse view of the left adnexa shows the corpus luteum and adjacent ectopic pregnancy (calipers). Note how the echogenicity of the ectopic pregnancy is greater than that of the corpus luteum. (c) Color Doppler shows flow around the corpus luteum.

Scar pregnancy

Scars in the uterus can be sites for implantation of pregnancy. Cesarean section scar pregnancy is increasingly being reported [45]. Other procedures that scar the uterus put the patient at increased risk for scar pregnancy. For example, a pregnancy can implant in a myomectomy scar. On ultrasound, there is complete embedding of the gestational sac in the myometrium. In cesarean section scar ectopic pregnancy, the myometrium between the bladder and the sac becomes thinner or disappears because of distension of the sac. Only the thin, serosal layer is apparent. Criteria used for diagnosis are an empty uterus, empty cervical canal, and development of the sac in the anterior part of the lower uterine segment. Current noninvasive and minimally invasive treatments include sonographically guided methotrexate or potassium chloride injection [43,46], or intramuscular methotrexate [47]. Definitive treatment of a cesarean scar pregnancy is by laparotomy and hysterotomy, with repair of the accompanying uterine scar dehiscence.

Ovarian and abdominal ectopic pregnancy

Ovarian pregnancies usually appear as an ovarian cyst with a wide, echogenic outside ring. A yolk sac or embryo is less commonly seen, with the appearance of the contents lagging in comparison with the gestational age. Abdominal pain before 7 weeks' gestational age is typically present.

Abdominal pregnancies are rare. The pregnancy typically develops in the ligaments of the ovary, usually the broad ligament. It can then obtain blood supply from the omentum and abdominal organs. Sonographically, the pregnancy is seen separate from the uterus, adnexa, and ovaries. Treatment is by laparotomy or laparoscopy. Abdominal pregnancy can result in a life-threatening emergency. However, if it is diagnosed late in gestation, a viable pregnancy can result.

Pelvic pain after treatment with methotrexate

Within several days of the initiation of treatment, the majority of patients treated with systemic methotrexate for an ectopic pregnancy will experience some lower abdominal pain. Sonographic findings may include free fluid in the pelvis and an increase in the size of the adnexal mass. It may take up to 3 months for the adnexal mass to resolve after treatment [48]. Unless the patient is clinically unstable or has persistent symptoms, the increase in tubal size and vascularity should not cause concern as this is part of the healing process.

If a patient fails a single course of methotrexate or has pelvic pain that is increasing, ultrasound can be helpful. This may reveal a much larger mass and potentially a fetal pole with cardiac activity, which would prompt surgery rather than a second course of methotrexate. Otherwise, ultrasonography after methotrexate is indicated in cases where rupture is suspected due to worsening abdominal pain, hemodynamic instability, or failure of decline in β-hCG values by at least 15% between days 4 and 7, or increasing or plateauing β-hCG levels after the first week of treatment [49].

Key points in clinical practice

- Ultrasound is a rapid, noninvasive procedure, is usually not painful, requires no special dietary preparations, and is performed on an outpatient basis. The benefit of having the scans done by the infertility specialist is that immediate decisions regarding treatment based on ultrasound findings can be made. Real-time scanning allows correlation of imaging findings with clinical symptoms.

- Knowledge of the pregnancy status of the patient is helpful in assessing the potential etiology of pelvic pain, but it should be realized that patients who are pregnant can still have the many causes of pelvic pain seen in non-pregnant patients.

- The incidence of follicular cysts is increased in infertile patients taking drugs such as clomiphene citrate and gonadotropins for ovulation induction. When large or hemorrhagic, these cysts may cause pain. As patients come in frequently for ultrasound during infertility treatment, making them aware of the presence of this cyst is essential so that they may be knowledge about why they may experience acute pelvic pain in the future.

- If a patient continues to have pain after a presumed miscarriage, even if products of conception were confirmed cytologically, a heterotopic pregnancy should be a considered. If an adnexal mass suspicious of an ectopic pregnancy is not seen, a repeat quantitative β-hCG that continues to be high despite a presumed miscarriage would lead one to consider a heterotopic pregnancy.

References

1. Chiang G, Levine D. Imaging of adnexal masses in pregnancy. *J Ultrasound Med* 2004; **23**: 805–19.

2. Patel MD, Feldstein VA, Filly RA. The likelihood ratio of sonographic findings for the diagnosis of hemorrhagic ovarian cysts. *J Ultrasound Med* 2005; **24**: 607–15.

3. Ozkan S, Murk W, Arici A. Endometriosis and infertility: epidemiology and evidence-based treatments. *Ann N Y Acad Sci.* 2008; **1127**: 92–100.

4. Kurjak A, Kupesic S. Scoring system for prediction of ovarian endometriosis based on transvaginal color and pulsed Doppler sonography. *Fertil Steril* 1994; **62**: 81–8.

5. Golan A, Ron-El R, Herman A, et al. Ovarian hyperstimulation syndrome: an update review. *Obstet Gynecol Surv* 1989; **44**: 430–40.

6. Shadinger LL, Andreotti RF, Kurian RL. Preoperative sonographic and clinical characteristics as predictors of ovarian torsion. *J Ultrasound Med.* 2008 Jan; **27**(1): 7–13.

7. Fleischer AC, Stein SM, Cullinan JA, et al: Color Doppler sonography of adnexal torsion. *J Ultrasound Med* 1995; **14**: 523–8.

8. Katz VL, Dotters DJ, Droegemeuller W. Complications of uterine leiomyomas in pregnancy. *Obstet Gynecol* 1989; **73**: 593–6.

9. Horrow MM. Ultrasound of pelvic inflammatory disease. *Ultrasound Q* 2004; **20**: 171–9.

10. Worrell JA, Drolshagen LF, Kelly TC, Hunton DW, Durmon GR, Fleischer AC, Graded compression ultrasound in the diagnosis of appendicitis. A comparison of diagnostic criteria. *J Ultrasound Med* 1990; **9**(3): 145–50.

11. Chiang G, Levine D, Swire M, et al: The intradecidual sign: is it reliable for diagnosis of early intrauterine pregnancy?. *Am J Roentgenol* 2004; **183**: 725–31.

12. Bradley WG, Fiske CE, Filly RA. The double sac sign of early intrauterine pregnancy: use in exclusion of ectopic pregnancy. *Radiology* 1982; **143**: 223–6.

13. Levi CS, Lyons EA, Zheng XH, et al. Endovaginal US: demonstration of cardiac activity in embryos of less than 5.0mm in crown-rump length. 1990; *Radiology* **176**: 71–4.

14. Gago LA, Torres M, Diamond MP, Puscheck EE. Prognosis of subchorionic hemorrhage in early pregnancy. *Fertil Steril* 2005 Sep; **84**(Suppl 1): S115.

15. Nagy S, Bush M, Stone J, et al: Clinical significance of subchorionic and retroplacental hematomas detected in the first trimester of pregnancy. *Obstet Gynecol* 2003; **102**: 94–100.

16. Farr SL, Schieve LA, Jamieson DJ. Pregnancy loss among pregnancies conceived through assisted reproductive technology, United States, 1999–2002. *Am J Epidemiol.* 2007; **165** (12): 1380–8.

17. Simpson J, Carson S. Genetic and non-genetic casues of spontaneous abortions. In: Sciarra J, ed. *Gynecology and Obstetrics.* Philadelphia, PA: JB Lippincott, 1995; 20.

18. Filly RA. Ultrasound evaluation during the first trimester. In: Callen PW, ed. *Ultrasonography in Obstetrics and Gynecology.* Philadelphia, PA: WB Saunders, 1998; 63–85.

19. McKenna KM, Feldstein VA, Goldstein RB, et al. The empty amnion: a sign of early pregnancy failure. *J Ultrasound Med* 1995; **14**: 117–21.

20. Bracken MB, Brinton LA, Hayashi K. Epidemiology of hydatidiform mole and choriocarcinoma. *Epidemiol Rev* 1984; **6**: 52–75.

21. Lazarus E, Hulka C, Siewert B, et al: Sonographic appearance of early complete molar pregnancies. *J Ultrasound Med* 1999; **18**: 589–94.

22. Bergh T, Lundkvist Ö. Clinical complications during in-vitro fertilization treatment. *Hum Reprod* 1992; **7**: 625–6.

23. Nyberg DA, Hughes MP, Mack LA, et al. Extrauterine findings of ectopic pregnancy of transvaginal US: importance of echogenic fluid. *Radiology* 1991; **178**: 823–6.

24. Klemetti R, Sevón T, Gissler M, Hemminki E. Complications of IVF and ovulation induction. *Hum Reprod* 2005 Dec; **20**(12): 3293–300.

25. From the Centers for Disease Control and Prevention: Ectopic pregnancy–United States, 1990–1992. *JAMA* 1995; **273**: 533.

26. Pisarska MD, Carson SA, Buster JE. Ectopic pregnancy. *Lancet* 1998; **351** (9109): 1115–20.

27. Batzer R. Guidelines for choosing a pregnancy test. *Contemp Ob Gyn* 1985; **30**: 57.

28. Cacciatore B, Ulf-hakan S, Ylostalo P. Diagnosis of ectopic pregnancy by vaginal ultrasonography in combination with a discriminatory serum hCG level of 1000 IU/l (IRP). *Br J Obstet Gynaecol* 1990; **97**: 904–8.

29. Barnhart K, Mennuti MT, Benjamin I, et al. Prompt diagnosis of ectopic pregnancy in an emergency department setting. *Obstet Gynecol* 1994; **84**: 1010–15.

30. Dialani V, Levine D. Ectopic pregnancy: a review. *Ultrasound Q* 2004; **20**: 105–17.

31. Ackerman TE, Levi CS, Dashefsky SM, et al. Interstitial line: sonographic finding in interstitial (cornual) ectopic pregnancy. *Radiology* 1993; **189**: 83–7.

32. Yeh HC. Some misconceptions and pitfalls in ultrasonography. *Ultrasound Q* 2001; **17**: 129–55.

33. Nyberg DA, Mack LA, Jeffrey RB Jr, et al. Endovaginal sonographic evaluation of ectopic pregnancy: a prospective study. *Am J Roentgenol* 1987; **149**: 1181–6.

34. Russell SA, Filly RA, Damato N. Sonographic diagnosis of ectopic pregnancy with endovaginal probes: what really has changed?. *J Ultrasound Med* 1993; **12**: 145–51.

35. Atri M, de Stempel J, Bret PM. Accuracy of transvaginal ultrasonography for detection of hematosalpinx in ectopic pregnancy. *J Clin Ultrasound* 1992; **20**: 255–61.

36. Frates MC, Visweswaran A, Laing FC. Comparison of tubal ring and corpus luteum echogenicities: a useful differentiating characteristic. *J Ultrasound Med* 2001; **20**: 27–31.

37. Emerson DS, Cartier MS, Altieri LA, et al. Diagnostic efficacy of endovaginal color Doppler flow imaging in an ectopic pregnancy screening program. *Radiology* 1992; **183**: 413–20.

38. Levine D. Ectopic pregnancy. In: Callen PW, ed. *Ultrasonography in Obstetrics and Gynecology.* Philadelphia, PA: WB Saunders, 2000: 912–34.

39. Taylor KJ, Meyer WR. New techniques in the diagnosis of ectopic pregnancy. *Obstet Gynecol Clin North Am* 1991; **18**: 39–54.

40. Lee GS, Hur SY, Kown I, et al. Diagnosis of early intramural ectopic pregnancy. *J Clin Ultrasound* 2005; **33**: 190–2.

41. Fernandez H, Benifla JL, Lelaidier C, et al. Methotrexate treatment of ectopic pregnancy: 100 cases treated by primary transvaginal injection under sonographic control. *Fertil Steril* 1993; **59**: 773–7.

42. Doubilet PM, Benson CB, Frates MC, et al. Sonographically guided minimally invasive treatment of unusual ectopic pregnancies. *J Ultrasound Med* 2004; **23**: 359–70.

43. Celik C, Bala A, Acar A, et al. Methotrexate for cervical pregnancy. A case report. *J Reprod Med* 2003; **48**: 130–2.

44. Frates MC, Benson CB, Doubilet PM, et al. Cervical ectopic pregnancy: results of conservative treatment. *Radiology* 1994; **191**: 773–5.

45. Jurkovic D, Hillaby K, Woelfer B, et al. First-trimester diagnosis and management of pregnancies implanted into the lower uterine segment Cesarean section scar. *Ultrasound Obstet Gynecol* 2003; **21**: 220–7.

46. Seow KM, Huang LW, Lin YH, et al. Cesarean scar pregnancy: issues in management. *Ultrasound Obstet Gynecol* 2004; **23**: 247–53.

47. Haimov-Kochman R, Sciaky-Tamir Y, Yanai N, et al. Conservative management of two ectopic pregnancies implanted in previous uterine scars. *Ultrasound Obstet Gynecol* 2002; **19**: 616–19.

48. Atri M, Bret PM, Tulandi T, Senterman MK. Ectopic pregnancy: evolution after treatment with transvaginal methotrexate. *Radiology* 1992; **185**: 749–53.

49. American College of Obstetricians and Gynecologists. ACOG practice bulletin. Medical management of tubal pregnancy. Number 3, December 1998. *Int J Gynaecol Obstet* 1999; **65**(1): 97–103.

Chapter 23

Ultrasonographic evaluation of chronic pelvic pain

Nicole Brooks and Moshood Olatinwo

Introduction

Chronic pelvic pain (CPP) in women is defined as a "noncyclic pain of 6 or more months' duration that localizes to the anatomic pelvis, anterior abdominal wall at or below the umbilicus, the lumbosacral back, or the buttocks and is of sufficient severity to cause functional disability or lead to medical care" [1]. In the United States, the prevalence of chronic pelvic pain for women aged 18–50 years is reportedly as high as 15–20%, corresponding to about 9.2 million women per year [2]. This is comparable to the reported prevalence of 24% in Europe [3].

CPP is the most common indication for referral to women's health services and accounts for 20% of all gynecologic outpatient visits. This condition is a substantial burden on health care resources. Indeed, $881.5 million are spent per year on its outpatient management in the USA [3] and an estimated £158 million are spent annually on the management of this condition in the UK National Health Service [4]. However, despite the high prevalence and enormous cost, our current understanding of the etiology of chronic pelvic pain is limited. This is due to the fact that the specific cause(s) of chronic pelvic pain are often elusive, varied, and confusing. This lack of understanding of the pathophysiology of chronic pelvic pain has resulted in poor clinical management and, consequently, in significant dissatisfaction among women sufferers of chronic pelvic pain [5]. The traditional approach to diagnosis of chronic pelvic pain in female patients is based on the notion that the female reproductive system is the sole culprit in most cases. This traditional approach is faulty because most cases of chronic pelvic pain are caused by multiple pathologies [1]. How then can we improve our current approach to the management of this chronic disabling disease?

The answer is that we need to adopt a new paradigm for the management of this disease. An effective approach that is beneficial to women sufferers of chronic pelvic pain ought to integrate prompt pain management following initial consultation with a focused search for a specific diagnosis [5]. This assures that the initial concern of the patient is addressed by relieving the presenting symptom and improving their quality of life. Subsequently, ancillary investigations can then be offered to improve our ability to provide a comprehensive diagnosis and enable us to offer an integrated management approach based on identifiable pathology. A sensitive and readily available modality for pelvic imaging is ultrasonography.

Pelvic ultrasonography is a useful tool for the evaluation and management of chronic pelvic pain and may also provide an aid to counseling, as noted by a recent meta-analysis of published studies on chronic pelvic pain from the Cochrane Library [6]. Transvaginal ultrasonography is the preferred imaging method for evaluating the pelvis. However, when this modality fails to provide a reason for the patient's pain, other methods such as transrectal or transperineal modalities can provide essential information and improve diagnostic accuracy. Although laparoscopy is considered the gold standard in the diagnosis of several diseases that cause pelvic pain, it is invasive, expensive, and associated with significant risks [7]. Moreover, there is no evidence that it is superior in establishing the specific cause of chronic pelvic pain in the majority of patients [8]. In contrast, pelvic ultrasonography has been demonstrated to be a valuable diagnostic tool for the management and diagnosis of pelvic pain [9].

In this chapter we will describe how the use of pelvic ultrasonography can enhance our ability to diagnose the cause(s) of chronic pelvic pain and provide rationale for a targeted and effective treatment of this disease using specific examples.

Endometriosis

Endometriosis is a chronic condition characterized by growth of endometrial tissue in sites other than the uterine cavity, most commonly in the pelvic cavity, including the ovaries, the uterosacral ligaments, and the pouch of Douglas. It is the most commonly identifiable cause of chronic pelvic pain, occurring in up to 65% of sufferers. Traditionally, the diagnosis of endometriosis is established by visual inspection at the time of laparoscopy and confirmed when possible by histological examination. However, diagnostic laparoscopy often requires general anesthesia, and it is also associated with around a 3% risk of minor complications and a 0.5% risk of major complications [8].

A common gynecologic cause of chronic pelvic pain is an endometriotic cyst located within the ovary. Ovarian endometrioma appears on ultrasound as a round-shaped, homogeneous

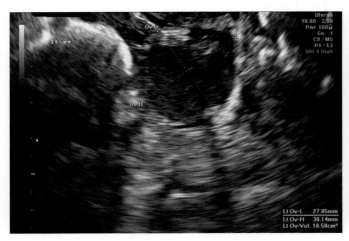

Figure 23.1. Endometrioma.

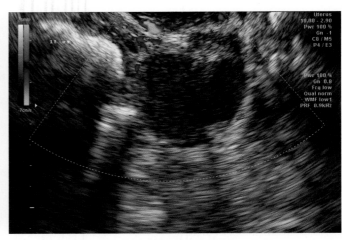

Figure 23.2. Endometrioma with Doppler imaging.

hypoechoic area of low-level echoes within the ovary [10] (Figures 23.1 and 23.2), and about 24% of all ovarian cysts are endometriomas. Several studies have shown that transvaginal ultrasonography (TVUS) is highly sensitive in differentiating between an endometrioma and other ovarian masses [11]. This is particularly important in the presurgical evaluation of patients because it allows the surgeon to discuss the extent of surgery and the possible complications that may occur at the time of surgery. Okaro et al. found near-perfect correlation between ovarian mobility during TVUS and during laparoscopy [7]. These authors noted that the association of ultrasound features of pelvic adhesions and peritoneal endometriotic implants (soft signs) in a patient with ovarian endometrioma is predictive of a poor response to medical therapy. Therefore, patients who have soft signs on TVUS may benefit from laparoscopic surgical management, while those patients without the soft or hard markers are ideally suited for medical therapy.

Noninvasive diagnostic modalities are essential for the evaluation of women with deeply infiltrating endometriosis involving the rectovaginal septum, the rectum, or the bladder. Rectovaginal endometriosis involves the connective tissue between the anterior rectal wall and the vagina and it often infiltrates both. The recommended treatment for rectovaginal endometriosis is complete surgical excision. Rectovaginal endometriosis is difficult to assess by clinical examination, and infiltration of the rectal wall can be suspected in only 40–68% of the cases. Therefore, imaging techniques are essential preoperatively to determine the extent of disease. They may also allow a more precise preoperative discussion with the patient about the requirement for bowel resection and possible colostomy formation [12].

Bowel endometriosis appears as an irregular hypoechoic mass, with or without hypoechoic or hyperechoic foci, penetrating into the intestinal wall on transvaginal ultrasonography. Using this imaging modality, Bazot et al. reported a sensitivity of 95%, a specificity of 100%, and an accuracy of 97% in

diagnosing colorectal involvement [13]. However, it is impossible to accurately determine the exact distance of rectal lesions from the anal margin or the depth of rectal wall involvement using this modality. In addition, locations above the rectosigmoid junction are beyond the field of view of a transvaginal approach. A sensitive modality for determining the extent of bowel endometriosis is preoperative transrectal ultrasonography (TRUS). TRUS for rectovaginal endometriosis is an extremely accurate modality that strongly predicts the need for extensive laparoscopic dissection and potential bowel resection [14]. Similarly, the addition of water-contrast in the rectum to transvaginal ultrasonography (RWC-TVUS) has also been shown to improve the diagnosis of rectal infiltration in women with rectovaginal endometriosis. RWC-TVUS was more accurate than TVUS in determining the presence of endometriotic infiltration, reaching at least the muscular layer of the rectal wall. The sensitivity of RWC-TVUS in identifying rectal lesions was 97%, the specificity 100%, the positive predictive value 100%, and the negative predictive value 91.3% [12].

Adenomyosis

Adenomyosis is a common disorder in the gynecologic population that consists of the presence of endometrial glands and stroma in the myometrium. Adenomyosis is associated with chronic pelvic pain, dysmenorrhea, dyspareunia, and feelings of pressure low in the pelvis due to uterine enlargement. Recently, ultrasound has emerged as a modality in the diagnosis of adenomyosis. As demonstrated by Kepkep et al. [15], the most valuable findings correlating with histopathological results are myometrial heterogeneity, a regularly enlarged uterus, myometrial cysts, and subendometrial echogenic linear striations in the myometrium (Figures 23.3 and 23.4). However, the diagnosis of adenomyosis by ultrasonography can be confounded by the frequent coexistence of adenomyosis with leiomyomata, endometrial hyperplasia, and endometrial polyps. In addition, the large size of the uterus may make transvaginal scanning

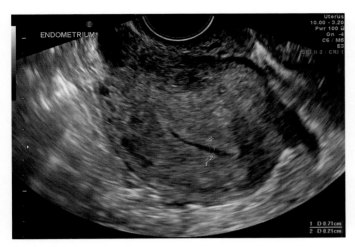

Figure 23.3. Adenomyosis.

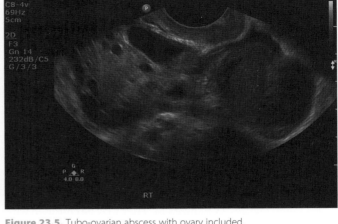

Figure 23.5. Tubo-ovarian abscess with ovary included.

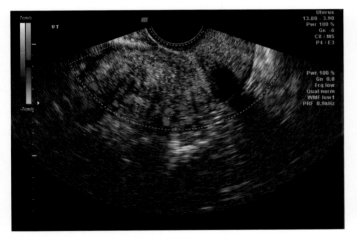

Figure 23.4. Adenomyosis with Doppler imaging.

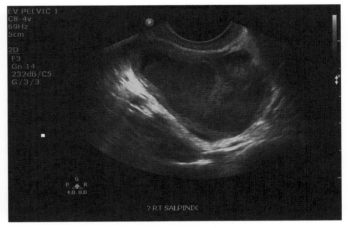

Figure 23.6. Tubo-ovarian abscess, cross-sectional view.

difficult as it may be impossible to visualize the entire uterus with the transvaginal probe.

Infection

Infection of the pelvis causes pain by several different mechanisms: pelvic inflammatory disease, puerperal infections, postoperative gynecologic surgery, and abortion-related infections. If the patient is suffering from chronic pelvic pain due to infection, the most likely cause is pelvic inflammatory disease and its sequelae. The fallopian tubes are rarely seen with ultrasonography because their normal diameter is less than 4 mm. When they become dilated with fluid secondary to inflammatory exudates the tubes become visible as elongated, tortuously dilated structures. These distended tubes may be visualized as anechoic or hyperechoic structures using transvaginal ultrasound. Ultrasonography is a validated diagnostic modality that can be used to distinguish pelvic vasculature from fallopian tubes [16].

The gold standard for diagnosis of pelvic inflammatory disease is laparoscopy. However, it is expensive and requires anesthesia, hospitalization, and surgical expertise for optimal outcome. Ultrasound can be very useful for initial diagnosis and treatment guidance [17]. Findings on ultrasound are subtle. Transvaginal scanning is generally preferred, with the exception of an enlarged uterus due to endometritis, which may be better visualized abdominally. Free fluid, when present, is generally clear or anechoic. As the infection progresses, there may be an increase in free fluid in the pelvis, and this free fluid may become echogenic due to the presence of pus, blood, and other inflammatory elements. Loculated areas or the presence of septa indicate encapsulated fluid. If the fluid noted is inhomogeneous and echoic, there is a correlation with infection. Also of note is the presence or absence of the sliding organ sign. If the organs are bound by adhesions, they are unable to move. This is not specific to pelvic inflammatory disease, but clinical suspicion can lead to diagnosis. Endometriosis and malignancy may also present with a lack of sliding organ sign.

The fallopian tubes may also have positive findings on ultrasound in the presence of pelvic inflammatory disease. Normally, the fallopian tubes are less than 4 mm in diameter [18]. They are rarely seen with ultrasonography unless fluid is surrounding or dilating them. With pelvic inflammatory disease the tubes become visible as elongated, tortuously dilated structures. Fluid distending the tubes may be anechoic or hyperechoic. The use of Doppler imaging is helpful to distinguish pelvic vasculature from fallopian tubes, and the presence of peristalsis helps differentiate bowel [19].

Due to the presence of septations in both hydrosalpinx and tubo-ovarian abscess, it can be difficult to distinguish between the two. With salpingitis Doppler flow is increased. Tubo-ovarian inflammatory masses are visualized as solid cystic or mixed mass (Figures 23.5 and 23.6). They may be confused with neoplasms due to septations and the presence of loops of bowel adhered to pelvic structures. In this case, Doppler of inflammatory masses tends to demonstrate decreased blood flow and a low pulsatile index, while malignant lesions usually demonstrate neovascularity and arteriovenous shunting. In general, the degree of pelvic distortion is proportionate to the severity of infection [20].

Pelvic congestion syndrome

Pelvic congestion syndrome (PCS) is a pelvic pain syndrome caused by retrograde flow in an incompetent ovarian vein. Symptoms associated with PCS include a shifting location of pain, deep dyspareunia, and postcoital pain, with exacerbation of symptoms after prolonged standing. The etiology of PCS is poorly understood and is believed to be an absence of ovarian vein valves or incompetence resulting from dilatation. This vascular incompetence leads to stasis, dilation, and retrograde blood flow. Dilated veins are seen more commonly in multiparous women. Other causes of venous stasis are pelvic vein kinking associated with malposition of the uterus, vascular compression, and the nutcracker syndrome [21].

Normal pelvic veins appear as tubular structures that are 4 mm or less in diameter. Diagnosis of PCS is a possibility when pelvic veins are greater than 5 mm in diameter and/or retrograde flow is present in the ovarian vein. Another finding that is consistent with this diagnosis is dilated arcuate veins crossing the myometrium. Additionally, women with pelvic congestion tend to have larger than normal uteri and ovaries due to cystic changes. The diagnostic sensitivity of pelvic ultrasonography may be enhanced by having the patient perform a Valsalva maneuver. This causes accentuation of the pelvic vasculature, enhancing the image of the ovarian veins.

The four main criteria for diagnosing PCS via ultrasound are:

1. Tortuous pelvic veins with a diameter greater than 6 mm. The mean diameter of the PCS group is about 8 mm.
2. Slow blood flow (about 3 cm/s) or reversed caudal flow.
3. Dilated arcuate veins in the myometrium that communicate between bilateral pelvic varicose veins.
4. Sonographic appearances of polycystic changes of the ovaries [21].

Conclusion

Ultrasound is a very useful tool for evaluating chronic pelvic pain sufferers. By performing an ultrasound as part of the initial evaluation for these patients, providers can provide treatment, counseling, and better direct pain management. When the diagnosis is less clear, other less common causes of pelvic pain can then be explored. These include pelvic neuromas and other myofascial causes of pain, irritable bowel syndrome, pelvic relaxation, and interstitial cystitis. With diagnosis of pelvic pathology, targeted and effective treatment can be prescribed. Patients have better satisfaction due to their understanding of their pain, with a goal of better productivity and return to normal function.

References

1. ACOG Committee on Practice Bulletins – Gynecology. Chronic Pelvic Pain: No. 51, March 2004. *Obstet Gynecol* 2004; **103**(3): 589–605.

2. Mathias SD, Kuppermann M, Leberman RF, Lipschutz RC, Steege JF. Chronic pelvic pain: prevalence, health-related quality of life, and economic correlates. *Obstet Gynecol* 1996; **87**: 321–7.

3. Zondervan KT, Yudkin PL, Vessey MP, et al. The community prevalence of chronic pelvic pain in women and associated illness behaviour: *Br J Gen Pract* 2001; **51**: 541–7.

4. Davies L, Gangar KF, Drummond M, Sounders D, Beard RW. The economic burden of intractable gynaecological pain. *J Obstet Gynaecol* 1992; **12**: S54–6.

5. Breivik H, Collett B, Ventafridda V, Cohen R, Gallacher D. Survey of chronic pain in Europe: prevalence, impact on daily life and treatment. *Eur J Pain* 2006; **10**: 177–83.

6. Stones W, Cheong YC, Howard FM. Interventions for treating chronic pelvic pain in women. *Cochrane Database Syst Rev* 2005; (**2**): CD000387.

7. Okaro E, Condous G, Khalid A, et al. The use of ultrasound based 'soft markers' for the prediction of pelvic pathology in women with chronic pelvic pain-can we reduce the need for laparoscopy? *BJOG* 2006; **113**: 251–6.

8. Kang SB, Chung HH, Lee HP, Lee JY, Chang YS. Impact of diagnostic laparoscopy on the management of chronic pelvic pain. *Surg Endosc* 2007; **21**: 916–19.

9. Okaro E, Valentin L. The role of ultrasound in the management of women with acute and chronic pelvic pain. *Best Pract Res Clin Obstet Gynecol* 2004; **18**(1): 105–23.

10. Mais V, Gueriero S, Afossa S, Angiolucci M, Paoletti AM, Melis GB, The efficiency of transvaginal ultrsonography in the diagnosis of endometriomas: *Fertil Steril* 1993; **60**(5): 776–80.

11. Guerriero S, Mais V, Ajossa S, et al. The role of endovaginal ultrasound in differentiating endometriomas from other

ovarian cysts. *Clin Exp Obstet Gynecol* 1995; **22**(1): 20–2.

12. Fedele L, Bianchi S, Portuese A, Borruto F, Dorta M. Transrectal ultrasonography in the assessment of rectovaginal endometriosis. *Obstet Gynecol* 1998; **91**(3): 444–8.

13. Bazot M, Malzy P, Cortez A, Roseau G, Amouyal P, Darai E. Accuracy of transvaginal sonography and rectal endoscopic sonography in the diagnosis of deep infiltrating endometriosis. *Ultrasound Obstet Gynecol* 2007; **30**: 994–1001.

14. Koninckx PR, Martin D. Treatment of deeply infiltrating endometriosis. *Curr Opin Obstet Gynecol* 1994; **6**: 231–41.

15. Kepkep K, Tuncay YA, Goynumer G, Tutal E. Transvaginal sonography in the diagnosis of adenomyosis: which findings are more accurate?. *Ultrasound Obstet Gynecol* 2007; **30**: 341–5.

16. Teissala K, Heinonon PK, Punnonen R. Transvaginal ultrasound in the diagnosis and treatment of tuboovarian abcess. *Br J Obstet Gynaecol* 1990; **97**(2): 178–80.

17. Bajo Arenas JM, Perez-Medina T, Troyano J. Sonography of pelvic infection. *Ultrasound Rev Obstetr Gynecol* 2005; **5**(1): 81–90.

18. Timor-Tritsch IE, Rottem S, Lewit N. The fallopian tubes. In: Timor-Tritsch, IE, Rottem S, eds. *Transvaginal Sonography*, 2nd ed. New York: Elsevier, 1991; 131–4.

19. Teissala K, Heinonon PK, Punnonen R. Transvaginal ultrasound in the diagnosis and treatment of tuboovarian abcess. *Br J Obstet Gynaecol* 1990; **97**(2): 178–80.

20. Ghiatas AA. The spectrum of pelvic inflammatory disease. *Eur Radiol Suppl* 2004; **14** (Suppl 3): E184–92.

21. Ganeshan A, Upponi S, Hon LQ, Uthappa MC, Warakaulle DR, Uberoi R. Chronic pelvic pain due to pelvic congestion syndrome: the role of diagnostic and Interventional radiology. *Cardiovascular Intervent Radiol* 2007; **30**: 1105–11.

Ultrasonography and IVF

Luciano G. Nardo and Tarek A. Gelbaya

Introduction

The availability of a good ultrasonography (US) service as part of clinical in-vitro fertilization (IVF) is of paramount importance. Over the last 25 years, progress in the field of assisted reproduction has paralleled that in ultrasonography. During the initial IVF attempts, follicular growth was monitored by measurement of urinary estrogen and plasma luteinizing hormone (LH) concentrations. The correlation between follicular size and urinary estrogen concentrations was poor, as many small follicles producing significant amount of estradiol (E_2) could not be measured by US. Hackelöer and Robinson [1] were the first to report successful monitoring of follicular size and number in patients undergoing ovulation induction using a transabdominal static B-scan. In 1982, O'Herlihy and co-workers published on the follicular size criteria and protocols for ovulation induction [2].

Oocyte retrieval started as a laparoscopic procedure until Lenz and colleagues described percutaneous transabdominal/transvesical aspiration of ovarian follicles in 1981. They demonstrated for the first time that oocyte retrieval could be performed as an ultrasound-guided outpatient procedure [3]. In 1983, transvaginal oocyte retrieval under transabdominal ultrasound (TAS) guidance was further described by Gleicher and collaborators [4]. The true impact on ovum pick-up came with the appearance of the mechanical transvaginal sector scanner, when Kemeter and Feichtinger described its use for transvaginal aspiration of ovarian follicles in IVF [5]. In the late 1980s, the greatest development of transvaginal imaging was in human assisted reproduction. In this field, both diagnostic and therapeutic approaches require the use of transvaginal ultrasonography (TVS), including the initial assessment of subfertile women for pelvic pathologies, surveillance of ovarian follicles and endometrial responses with or without medications, oocyte retrieval, embryo transfer, and diagnosis of clinical pregnancy.

Transvaginal and transabdominal approaches

The pelvic organs may be imaged using transabdominal or transvaginal ultrasonography. The transabdominal approach requires a full bladder in order to displace the bowel and provide an acoustic window through which pelvic organs can be visualized. Transvaginal ultrasound has become the method of choice for pelvic assessment and management of subfertile women. Nevertheless, TAS may be necessary for adequate visualization of pelvic-abdominal masses, enlarged uterus, or high (abdominal) ovaries. The elasticity of the vaginal wall and the close proximity of the vaginal probe to the pelvic structures allow the use of high-frequency ultrasound waves with short focal length, giving enhanced resolution compared with TAS. Care must be taken to minimize the risk of cross-infection by cleaning the probe thoroughly, changing the protective sheath after every examination, and using sterile sachets of gel. Current evidence does not suggest any adverse effects of ultrasound on the oocytes, embryos, or early pregnancy [6].

Initial investigations of the subfertile woman

Transvaginal ultrasound can be used to rule out pelvic pathology in subfertile women who suffer from other symptoms such as dysmenorrhea, chronic pelvic pain, deep dyspareunia, hirsutism, and/or menstrual disorders. In addition, TVS can be used in the evaluation and follow-up of women with known pelvic pathology, such as endometriosis, endometrial polyps, leiomyoma, uterine anomalies, and adnexal pathology. Although TVS is not a prerequisite for referring a couple for assisted conception, it enables accurate evaluation of pelvic anatomy and helps to reassure women, especially those with idiopathic subfertility.

Ultrasound of the uterus

The uterus is usually easily identifiable with its uniformly reflective myometrium and the midline endometrial echo. The appearance of the endometrium varies throughout the menstrual cycle, being very thin immediately after menstruation, thickening and becoming more prominent during the proliferative phase, assuming the trilaminar appearance before ovulation, and being thick and reflective in the secretory phase of the cycle. Figure 24.1 shows the typical appearance of the

Ultrasonography in Reproductive Medicine and Infertility, ed. Botros R. M. B. Rizk. Published by Cambridge University Press. © Cambridge University Press 2010.

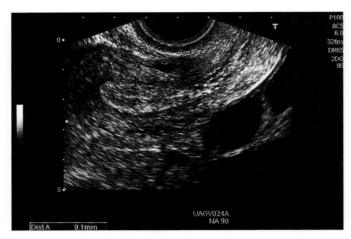

Figure 24.1. Trilaminar preovulatory endometrium.

preovulatory endometrium. A trace of endometrial fluid may normally be seen at the time of ovulation, leading to a slight separation of the endometrial layers, but this fluid usually disappears within 24 hours. The endometrial growth in stimulated cycles is very similar to that in the natural cycle, despite higher serum estradiol levels.

Leiomyoma

Fibroids may be identified by disruption of either the uniform myometrial reflectivity or the smooth uterine outline. They often contain highly reflective regions that will lead to acoustic shadowing. Very large fibroids are best seen with TAS as they often extend beyond the effective range of the transvaginal probe. The relationship of the fibroids to the uterine cavity is better examined by TVS. The effect of fibroids on fertility depends on the location and size of the fibroid, with large myomas indenting the endometrium having greater impact on fertility performance and pregnancy outcome [7].

Endometrial polyps

With the advent of TVS, saline sonohysterography, and improved Doppler technology the ultrasonographic diagnosis of endometrial polyps has become highly accurate [8]. Endometrial polyps are often seen on days 2–3 of the baseline TVS as a demarcated lesion with different echogenicity within the endometrial cavity. Many authors advise hysteroscopy and removal of the polyp before ovarian stimulation is commenced for IVF. This is particularly the case with polyps of 1 cm diameter or more. Stamatellos and co-authors reported no differences in pregnancy and miscarriage rates between women with small polyps (≤1 cm) and those with large or multiple polyps [9]. Saline infusion sonohysterograpy (SIS) can improve the diagnostic accuracy for detection of an endometrial polyp. The presence of thick endometrium on day 2 or 3 of the menstrual cycle should raise the possibility of a local endometrial lesion, and hysteroscopy should be considered in such cases.

Endometrial fluid

The ultrasound visualization of fluid in the endometrial cavity before embryo transfer in IVF cycles is associated with poor prognosis. The fluid may be cervical mucus that ascends into the endometrial cavity, but it may also be associated with fluid reflux from a hydrosalpinx [10] or subclinical uterine infection [11] or may be the result of abnormal endometrial development [12]. The identification of persistent fluid accumulation may prompt the clinician to freeze all embryos and postpone the embryo transfer.

Assessment of endometrial and uterine contour

Although there is a debate about the role of endometrial texture in implantation, endometrial contour is less disputed. Endometrial abnormalities such as fibroids and septa can cause implantation failure. The diagnosis of "double uterus" has traditionally been achieved through hysterosalpingography (HSG). However, this technique cannot differentiate between a unified corpus with a septum and a bicornuate uterus, nor between a complete septate and a didelphic uterus. Although some authors claim there are hysterographic criteria that can distinguish the various uterine malformations, it is currently accepted that accurate diagnosis requires knowledge of the morphology of the peritoneal surface of the uterine fundus. Hysteroscopy alone cannot provide an accurate diagnosis, and laparoscopy is required in order to assess the peritoneal configuration of the uterine fundus.

Accurate visualization of the fundus can be obtained by TVS with a sensitivity of 100% and a specificity of 80% [13]. A septate uterus on TVS is represented by a convex, flat and minimally indented (<1 cm) fundal contour with an echogenic structure dividing the cavity. Saline infusion sonohysterography may improve the information obtained by ultrasonography alone. Three-dimensional ultrasound seems to constitute a valid alternative to traditional ultrasound, showing a sensitivity and specificity close to 100% [14]. Uterine anomalies can be associated with congenital anomalies of the urinary tract; hence imaging of the urinary tract with appropriate techniques should be performed.

Ultrasound of the fallopian tubes

Normal fallopian tubes are not usually seen by ultrasound, though it is sometimes possible to visualize the fimbrial end within fluid in the pouch of Douglas.

Hydrosalpinx

Hydrosalpinges are easily identified by TVS (Figure 24.2). Typically the distended tube is coiled around the ovary in a sausage-shaped appearance. The presence of a hydrosalpinx adversely affects implantation and pregnancy rates. Two meta-analyses demonstrated a reduction by half in the probability of achieving a pregnancy in the presence of hydrosalpinx and a doubled rate of miscarriage [15,16]. TVS is useful in identifying the coexistence of periadnexal adhesions in

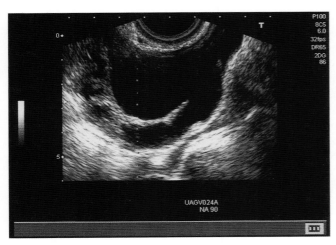

Figure 24.2. Hydrosalpinx.

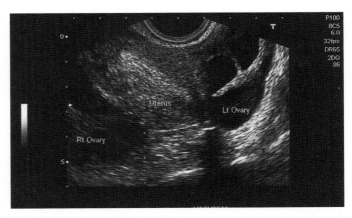

Figure 24.3. Uterus and ovaries.

women with hydrosalpinx. In these cases, the typical ultrasound appearance of a hydrosalpinx is associated with "loss of sliding signs" during the transvaginal examination. In subfertile women with dense pelvic adhesions, laparoscopic proximal division of the damaged fallopian tube(s) is an effective alternative to salpingectomy for hydrosalpinx prior to IVF [17].

Ultrasound for tubal patency

Different tests exist to investigate tubal patency in women seeking fertility. The most common diagnostics include laparoscopy and dye test, HSG, and hysterosalpingo-contrast sonography (HyCoSy). The advantage of HyCoSy is that it allows for concomitant ultrasound assessment of the ovaries and the uterus. In addition, it is well tolerated by women and provides an effective outpatient alternative to hysterosalpingography or laparoscopy and dye test [18].

Ultrasonography of the ovaries

The ovaries are usually seen lateral to the uterus (Figure 24.3), in close relationship to the internal iliac vessels. They can be identified by their echogenic stroma and sonolucent follicles. Occasionally, they may be located behind or above the uterus or under the anterior abdominal wall. A high ovary may be brought into the field of the view of the transvaginal probe by pressing firmly on the lower abdomen. The ovary tends to be of slightly lower reflectivity than the uterus, with low-level echoes surrounding the follicles. The ovarian volume can be estimated using the approximate formula: volume = length × width × depth × 0.5. The nonstimulated ovary in women with regular cycles has a mean volume of 9.8 ml [19].

Ultrasound and polycystic ovary

Ultrasound is important, but not essential, in the diagnosis of polycystic ovary syndrome (PCOS). The Rotterdam consensus meeting sponsored by the European Society for Human Reproduction and Embryology (ESHRE) and the American Society for Reproductive Medicine (ASRM) in 2003 stated that PCOS could be diagnosed by having two of the following three features, after the exclusion of related disorders: (1) oligo-ovulation or anovulation; (2) clinical and/or biochemical signs of hyperandrogenism; or (3) polycystic ovaries [20]. Ultrasound criteria for polycystic ovaries (PCO) were defined as the presence of 12 or more small follicles in each ovary measuring 2–9 mm in diameter and/or increased ovarian volume of more than 10 ml. The follicle distribution and stromal echogenicity and volume were omitted from the ultrasound features. Only one ovary fitting this definition is sufficient for the diagnosis of PCO. If there is a follicle more than 10 mm in diameter or a corpus luteum, the ultrasound should be repeated during the next cycle. The definition does not apply to women taking the oral contraceptive pill, since its use modifies the ultrasound morphology of the ovary [20].

Functional ovarian cysts

The normal follicle typically reaches a maximum diameter of 22–25 mm at ovulation, following which it shrinks or disappears gradually. Failure of the follicle to rupture may cause a follicular cyst. Luteal cysts result from failure of involution of the corpus luteum. Follicular and luteal cysts are characterized by echo-free contents, usually measuring less than 5 cm in diameter with a smooth outline. Most simple ovarian cysts in women of reproductive age are functional and will resolve spontaneously. If the cyst persists it may be aspirated transvaginally, and only if it recurs is cystectomy required. An irregular margin in a persistent cyst is an indication for cystectomy, though this is uncommon in young women seeking fertility treatment. Blood-filled ovarian cysts may be identified by internal echoes in the form of septa or gravity-dependent particulate debris.

Endometrioma

Endometrioma is an ovarian mass arising from growth of ectopic endometrial tissue in the ovary. Endometrioma may vary in size from 1 cm to a large, complex mass that occasionally may be difficult to differentiate from an ovarian neoplasm. Endometriomas contain thick, altered blood that typically

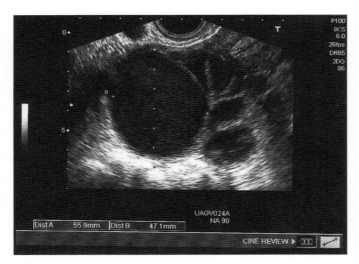

Figure 24.4. Endometrioma.

generates numerous low-level echoes (Figure 24.4). Of note, endometriomas that are not adjacent to clear fluid-containing cystic structures may be difficult to differentiate from ovarian stroma. However, by the use of pattern recognition, TVS can confidently diagnose 80% of endometriomas [21].

Dermoid cysts

Dermoid cysts may occasionally be identified in the ovaries of women of reproductive age. They can be cystic, solid, or complex depending on the components. The classic appearance is a well-circumscribed mass containing a fluid-debris level with a highly reflective internal echo, which produces acoustic shadow. Hair floating on sebum is strongly reflective and may cause shadow distally, obscuring the deeper tissues. In this case, only the anterior margin of the dermoid will be visualized, giving rise to the "tip of the iceberg" sign in which most of the volume of the mass is not seen.

Assessment of ovarian reserve

A variety of ovarian reserve tests are used in routine clinical practice to assess a woman's ovarian performance prior to controlled ovarian hyperstimulation (COH) for IVF. These include measurement of day 2 serum FSH, E_2, antimüllerian hormone (AMH), inhibin-B, and antral follicle count (AFC).

Follicular growth is a continuous process, independent of gonadotropin stimulation until the follicles reach 5 mm in diameter. Further growth of the follicles requires appropriate gonadotropin stimulation. Follicles measuring 2–5 mm (antral follicles) are seen by TVS in the early follicular phase of the menstrual cycle, and they normally develop under the influence of pituitary hormones as the cycle progresses. It has been reported that the number of antral follicles correlates well with the woman's age, ovarian reserve, and ovarian response to gonadotropin stimulation. There is a continuous and rapid loss of follicles due to apoptosis over the woman's reproductive life; and as the ovary ages, there is a noticeable reduction in the ovarian volume and the number of antral follicles. The AFC is regarded as a relatively good marker to predict poor ovarian response in assisted reproduction programs, providing better information than the patient's age alone or several endocrine markers [22]. The test can obviously be done at the time of the baseline ultrasound scan before commencing ovarian stimulation, thus avoiding repeat ultrasound scans. An AFC less than 6 correlates well with reduced ovarian reserve and poor response to ovarian stimulation, with a positive predictive value of 75% [23].

Monitoring ovarian response to gonadotropin stimulation

Ultrasound assessment of follicular growth was first introduced in 1978 when Hackelöer and Robinson [1] described a linear relationship between follicle size and circulating E_2 levels. Since then, TVS has been used to routinely monitor follicular growth in natural cycles, in ovulation induction programs, and during COH for assisted reproductive technology cycles.

During the natural cycle, a cohort of small antral follicles (2–5 mm in diameter) appears in the ovary very early in the proliferative phase. As FSH levels rise, further growth of the follicles occurs and the decline of FSH in the late follicular phase allows the selection of the single most sensitive follicle to continue to develop. Once the leading follicle reaches a diameter of approximately 14 mm, the daily growth rate is between 1.5 and 2.0 mm until reaching a diameter of 22–25 mm, when ovulation occurs. In natural cycles, serum E_2 levels correlate with follicle size, while the contribution of small atretic follicles to the steroidal milieu is negligible. Characteristic ultrasound appearance at the time of ovulation includes diminution in the follicle size, blurring of the follicle borders, and appearance of intrafollicular echoes and presence of a small amount of free fluid in the pouch of Douglas. Thereafter, an irregular, slightly cystic structure representing the corpus luteum shrinks throughout the luteal phase of the cycle until luteolysis occurs before menses.

Ultrasound scanning is useful in monitoring the response to clomiphene citrate in anovulatory women. TVS is usually performed 4–5 days after the last dose of clomiphene and every 2–3 days until a follicle of approximately 20 mm in diameter is seen.

Ovulation induction with gonadotropins overcomes the normal feedback mechanism that allows for physiological unifollicular ovulation causing growth of a cohort of follicles at various stages of development (Figure 24.5). To ensure safe clinical practice, a maximum of two leading follicles per cycle should be present. As the risk of ovarian hyperstimulation syndrome (OHSS) and multiple pregnancies is significant, it is important to monitor treatment response carefully by serial ultrasound scans and serum E_2 levels. In contrast to a natural cycle, the linear relationship between follicle size and E_2 measurements is lost due to the presence of many developing follicles that contribute to the circulating E_2. In ovulation induction cycles, a baseline ultrasound scan is performed to exclude

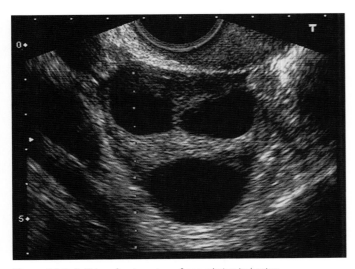

Figure 24.5. Follicles of various sizes after ovulation induction.

functional ovarian cysts, as well as other pelvic pathologies. Monitoring is usually carried out using TVS on day 8 of treatment. The dose of exogenous gonadotropins is adjusted according to the response. If more than two leading follicles (>17 mm) are seen, human chorionic gonadotropin (hCG) should be withheld and the cycle canceled to avoid the risk of multiple pregnancies.

Follicular size is best estimated by calculating the mean of the maximum follicular diameter in three planes. The interobserver variation in measurement is larger than the intraobserver variation, with the least interobserver variation being ±1.6 mm using TVS. This suggests that follicular tracking is more accurate when each scan is performed by the same operator [24]. In the presence of several follicles, the measurement of the largest four follicles in each ovary and a count of the remaining smaller follicles is considered as satisfactory. Follicular growth of approximately 2–3 mm per day is expected under normal circumstances.

Follicles can occasionally be confused with other pelvic structures, but they can be differentiated by rotating the transducer 90°. If the structure is a vessel, it will then elongate, acquiring a tubular shape. The internal iliac artery can easily be identified by its arterial pulsations, while a hydrosalpinx generally has a less regular shape (Figure 24.2).

Monitoring of the ovarian response in COH cycles can be carried out by TVS alone. Starting from day 8 of stimulation and then every other day, the dimensions of the growing follicles are plotted on a chart. Provided the TVS is performed by an experienced operator, daily measurements of serum E_2 concentrations may have limited value in predicting the success of the cycle or the risk of OHSS [25]. When FSH alone is used for ovarian stimulation in long protocols, the serum E_2 concentration is approximately half of the level found when human menopausal gonadotropins (hMG) is used. As serum E_2 concentrations appear to be proportional to the amount of LH in the gonadotropin preparation used in the stimulation regimen, the findings may be misleading.

Ultrasound assessment of the endometrium

The endometrium undergoes cyclic morphological as well as histological changes throughout the menstrual cycle. During menstruation, the endometrium appears as a thin echo that gradually thickens throughout the proliferative phase to reach the typical periovulatory trilaminar appearance (Figure 24.1). After ovulation, the rise in circulating progesterone induces stromal edema and growth of spiral arterioles, resulting in increased echogenicity of the thick secretory endometrium.

Ultrasound assessment of the endometrium has received a great deal of attention in the analysis of factors that affect embryo implantation. The literature has shown conflicting evidence about the predictive value of ultrasonography in the assessment of implantation failure and pregnancy potential.

Several investigators have reported no difference in endometrial thickness between pregnant and nonpregnant women [26,27], while others have observed a positive correlation between endometrial thickness and pregnancy outcome [28,29]. Zhang and co-authors found that increased endometrial thickness was associated with improved treatment outcome, but the association was dependent on patient age, duration of ovarian stimulation, and embryo quality [30]. Conversely, Richter and colleagues concluded that the higher clinical pregnancy and live-birth rates associated with increasing endometrial thickness were independent of the effects of patient age and embryo quality [31]. A meta-analysis of the literature demonstrated that endometrial thickness is a better negative than positive predictor of implantation [32]. Studies in the literature have proposed different endometrial thickness cut-off levels for successful implantation to occur: ≥6 mm [26], ≥10 mm [29], and ≥13 mm [33]. There have been no reports of adverse effects of a thickened endometrium on implantation, pregnancy, or miscarriage rates in IVF [34].

Endometrial echogenic patterns have also been studied. An association has been shown between the ultrasound endometrial texture and serum hormonal levels [33]. In IVF cycles, a preovulatory, multilayered appearance of the endometrial echo has been associated with a positive pregnancy outcome when compared with an incomplete, echogenic, and homogeneous pattern [26,33,35]. Synchronization between endometrial and embryo development is an essential prerequisite for successful implantation.

The endometrial thickness and pattern may provide useful information in cycles in which the endometrium is supplemented with estrogen and progesterone, such as in down-regulated frozen embryo transfer cycles as well as in recipients of donated oocytes or embryos. A minimal endometrial thickness of 6 mm is required before embryo replacement for pregnancy is achieved in oocyte recipients' cycles [36,37]. In a recent retrospective analysis of medicated frozen embryo replacement (FER) cycles, an endometrial thickness of 9–14 mm on the day of progesterone supplementation was found to be associated with higher implantation and pregnancy rates compared with an endometrial thickness of 7–8 mm [38]. In this study, the authors demonstrated that the lowest

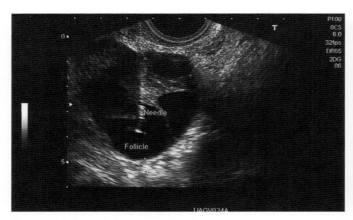

Figure 24.6. Ovary during oocyte retrieval.

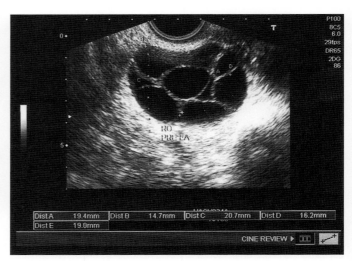

Figure 24.7. Ovary after stimulation, before oocyte retrieval.

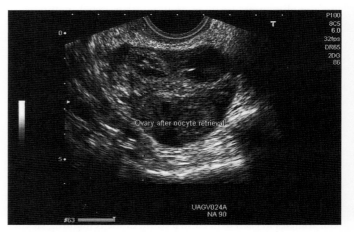

Figure 24.8. Ovary after oocyte retrieval.

pregnancy rates were associated with endometrial thickness <7 mm and >14 mm.

Uterine artery blood flow

There have been conflicting reports in the literature regarding the usefulness of the application of color Doppler ultrasound for monitoring and predicting pregnancy outcome of IVF cycles. Several studies used the pulsatility index (PI) as the measure of impedance and determined that a PI of <3.0 [39] or <3.34 [26] was more favorable for pregnancy. More recently, Steer and co-authors found similar results in women undergoing frozen embryo transfer in a down-regulated hormonally prepared cycle [40]. In contrast, other researchers found that uterine artery PI did not significantly change until the mid-luteal phase. No difference was found in uterine or ovarian artery PI between pregnant and nonpregnant women, but there was a nonsignificant increase in uterine receptivity when the uterine artery PI was in the range of 2.0–2.99 on the day of embryo transfer [41]. Other investigators used resistance index (RI) and found that it was significantly lower at the time of oocyte collection in women who achieved a pregnancy [35]. In a recent study, Ng and colleagues performed 3D ultrasound power Doppler one day after LH surge in women undergoing frozen embryo transfer in natural or clomiphene-induced cycles. The age of women was the only predictive factor for pregnancy. Endometrial thickness, endometrial volume, endometrial pattern, uterine PI, uterine resistance index (RI), and endometrial and subendometrial 3D power Doppler flow indices were similar between the nonpregnant and pregnant groups [42]. Currently, measurement of uterine artery blood flow should not be part of routine IVF practice.

Oocyte retrieval

Transvaginal ultrasound-guided aspiration of ovarian follicles provides a safe and effective means of oocyte retrieval. It is usually performed under sedation as a day-case procedure and requires minimal postoperative analgesia. The needle used for aspiration has a 17-gauge outer diameter and is approximately 11 inches (27 cm) long. The tip of the needle is

echogenic, enabling visualization by ultrasound at all times during the procedure (Figure 24.6). The needle is passed through a guide that is fixed to the transducer, allowing for proper alignment of the needle with the ultrasound beam. Care should be taken to avoid damage to internal iliac vessels or bowel by visualizing the needle tip at all times. Figures 24.7 and 24.8, respectively, show an ovary with three mature follicles before oocyte retrieval and an ovary immediately after the same procedure.

Ultrasound-guided embryo transfer

Embryo transfer is a crucial step of IVF treatment. It can be performed with or without ultrasound guidance. Embryo transfer entails the delivery of the embryo(s) into the uterine cavity, in a location where implantation is maximized. Embryo(s) contained in the soft Teflon catheter are placed about 1.5 cm from the fundus of the uterus.

The use of ultrasound guidance for embryo transfer was first described by Strickler and colleagues in 1985 [43]. TAS has been used to verify that the catheter has passed into the endometrial cavity and the embryo(s) has been transferred. Indeed, ultrasound guidance has many potential advantages. It facilitates the passage of the catheter through the sharp cervicouterine angle, avoids touching the fundus, confirms that the catheter is beyond the internal os in cases of elongated cervical canal, and minimizes endometrial disruption. Molding of the embryo transfer catheter according to the cervicouterine angle measured by TAS has been associated with increased clinical pregnancy and implantation rates [44]. Furthermore, in cases of impossible transcervical embryo transfer, TVS-guided transmyometrial transfer can be an option, especially in women with known tubal disease in whom intrafallopian transfer will not be possible [45]. Ultrasound guidance is useful for trainees as it enables them to master the technique of embryo transfer without compromising the success rate.

Whether ultrasound guidance improves clinical pregnancy per embryo transfer is debatable, however. Two meta-analyses reported higher pregnancy rates with ultrasound-guided embryo transfer compared with non-ultrasound-guided embryo transfer [46,47]. Conversely, a recent large random controlled trial concluded that TAS guidance during embryo transfer did not improve clinical pregnancy and implantation rates provided that the transfer was performed by an experienced operator [48]. Of interest, in this trial patients were not required to have a full bladder at the time of TVS-guided embryo transfer. Within our department, the use of ultrasound-guided embryo transfer has significantly improved implantation and clinical pregnancy rates [49].

Complications of IVF

Ultrasound is a cornerstone of prevention and diagnosis of potential IVF complications such as ovarian hyperstimulation syndrome (OHSS) and multiple pregnancies.

Ovarian hyperstimulation syndrome

Measures to prevent OHSS remain the most desirable approach. Management of OHSS is mostly expectant, with a small proportion of patients requiring hospitalization. The risk of OHSS is significantly increased in women with an ultrasound feature of PCO (odds ratio of 6.8, 95% confidence interval 4.9–9.6) [50]. The excessive ovarian response to stimulation with exogenous gonadotropin in women with PCO can be explained by the large pool of small antral follicles available for recruitment [51]. The initial dose of gonadotropins can be adjusted according to the appearance of the ovaries at the time of baseline ultrasound scan rather than to the diagnosis of PCOS.

Monitoring of follicular size and number during COH is essential for prevention of OHSS. A correlation between OHSS and the number of intermediate-sized follicles has been reported [52]. A combination of ultrasound monitoring of follicular growth/number and serial measurement of serum E_2 is used routinely in IVF to enhance the prediction rate of OHSS. Women who develop more than 20 follicles in both ovaries, with the majority being small (less than 14 mm in diameter), or

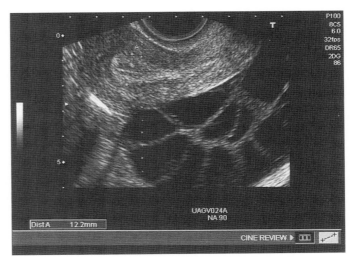

Figure 24.9. Ovary with signs of excessive response to ovarian stimulation.

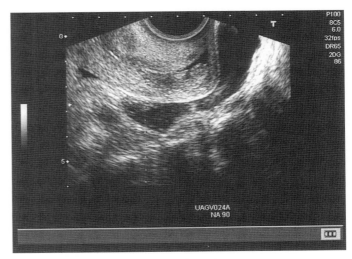

Figure 24.10. Free fluid in the pouch of Douglas

those who have high serum E_2 levels (>10 000 pmol/l) are at higher risk of OHSS. It is beyond the scope of this chapter to discuss strategies used to reduce the risk of OHSS.

Figure 24.9 shows an ovary with several follicles, which is in keeping with excessive response to stimulation. Figure 24.10 shows free fluid in the pouch of Douglas in a case of OHSS.

Early pregnancy complications and multiple pregnancies

Ultrasound is essential for the diagnosis of clinical pregnancy, confirmation of viability, dating of pregnancy, and diagnosis of ectopic and multiple pregnancies. In the UK, despite the policy of transferring no more than two embryos, the risk of multiple pregnancy remains high at approximately 20–25%. Information of a twin pregnancy in early gestation is important for counseling as well as management of potential complications and antenatal care.

References

1. Hackelöer BJ, Robinson HP. Ultrasound examination of the growing ovarian follicle and of the corpus luteum during the normal physiologie menstrual cycle. *Geburtshilfe Frauenheilkd* 1978; **38**: 163–8.

2. O'Herlihy C, Evans JH, Brown JB, de Crespigny LJ, Robinson HP. Use of ultrasound in monitoring ovulation induction with human pituitary gonadotropins. *Obstet Gynecol* 1982; **60**: 577–82.

3. Lenz S, Lauritsen JG, Kjellow M. Collection of human oocytes for in vitro fertilisation by ultrasonically guided follicular puncture. *Lancet* 1981; **23**: 1163.

4. Gleicher N, Friberg J, Fullan N, et al. EGG retrieval for in vitro fertilisation by sonographically controlled vaginal culdocentesis. *Lancet* 1983; **2**: 508–9.

5. Kemeter P, Feichtinger W. Trans-vaginal oocyte retrieval using a trans-vaginal sector scan probe combined with an automated puncture device. *Hum Reprod* 1986; **1**: 21–4.

6. Williams SR, Rothchild I, Wesolowski D, Austin C, Speroff L. Does exposure of preovulatory oocytes to ultrasonic radiation affect reproductive performance. *J In Vitro Fert Embryo Transf* 1988; **5**: 18–21.

7. Horne AW, Critchley HO. The effect of uterine fibroids on embryo implantation. *Semin Reprod Med* 2007; **25**: 483–9.

8. Brown SE, Coddington CC, Schnorr J, Toner JP, Gibbons W, Oehninger S. Evaluation of outpatient hysteroscopy, saline infusion hysterosonography, and hysterosalpingography in infertile women: a prospective, randomised study. *Fertil Steril* 2000; **74**: 1029–34.

9. Stamatellos I, Apostolides A, Stamatopoulos P, Bontis J. Pregnancy rates after hysteroscopic polypectomy depending on the size or number of the polyps. *Arch Gynecol Obstet* 2008; **277**: 395–9.

10. Sharara FI, McClamrock FI. Endometrial fluid collection in women with hydrosalpinx after human chorionic gonadotrophin administration: a report of two cases and implication for management. *Hum Reprod* 1997; **12**: 2816–19.

11. Drbohlav P, Halkova E, Masata J, et al. The effect of endometrial infection on embryo implantation in the IVF and ET program. *Ceska Gynekol* 1998; **63**: 181–5.

12. Sharara FI, Prough SG. Endometrial fluid collection in women with PCOS undergoing ovarian stimulation for IVF: A report of four cases. *J Reprod Med* 1999; **44**: 299–302.

13. Pellerito JS, McCarthy SM, Doyle MB, Glickman MG, DeCherney AH. Diagnosis of uterine anomalies: relative accuracy of MR imaging, endovaginal sonography, and hysterosalpingography. *Radiology*. 1992; **183**: 795–800.

14. Raga F, Bonilla-Musoles F, Blanes J, Osborne NG. Congenital Mullerian anomalies: diagnostic accuracy of three-dimensional ultrasound. *Fertil Steril* 1996; **65**: 523–8.

15. Zeyneloglu HB, Arici A, Olive DL. Adverse effects of hydrosalpinx on pregnancy rates after in vitro fertilization-embryo transfer. *Fertil Steril* 1998; **70**: 492–9.

16. Camus E, Poncelet C, Goffinet F, et al. Pregnancy rates after IVF in cases of tubal infertility with and without hydrosalpinx: meta-analysis of published comparative studies. *Hum Reprod* 1999; **14**: 1243–9.

17. Gelbaya TA, Nardo LG, Fitzgerald CT, Horne G, Brison DR, Lieberman BA. Ovarian response to gonadotropins after laparoscopic salpingectomy or the division of fallopian tubes for hydrosalpinges. *Fertil Steril* 2006; **85**: 1464–8.

18. Ayida G, Kennedy S, Barlow D, Chamberlain P. A comparison of patient tolerance of hysterosalpingo-contrast sonography (HyCoSy) with Echovist-200 and X-ray hysterosalpingography for outpatient investigation of infertile women. *Ultrasound Obstet Gynecol* 1996; **7**: 201–4.

19. Cohen HL, Tice HM, Mandel FS. Ovarian volumes measured by ultrasound: bigger than we think. *Radiology* 1990; **177**: 189–92.

20. Rotterdam ESHRE/ASRM-sponsored PCOS consensus workshop group. Revised 2003 consensus on diagnostic criteria and long-term health risks related to polycystic ovary syndrome (PCOS). *Hum Reprod* 2004; **19**: 41–7.

21. Calster BV, Timmerman D, Bourne T, et al. Discrimination between benign and malignant adnexal masses by specialist ultrasound examination versus serum CA-125. *J Natl Cancer Inst.* 2007; **99**: 1706–14.

22. Scheffer GJ, Broekmans FJM, Looman CWN, et al. The number of antral follicles in normal women with proven fertility is the best reflection of reproductive age. *Hum Reprod* 2003; **18**: 700–6.

23. Kwee J, Elting ME, Schats R, McDonnell J, Lambalk CB. Ovarian volume and antral follicle count for the prediction of low and hyper responders with in vitro fertilization. *Reprod Biol Endocrinol* 2007; **5**: 9.

24. Eissa MK, Hudson K, Docker MF, Sawers RS, Newton JR. Ultrasound follicle diameter measurement: an assessment of inter observer and intra observer variation. *Fertil Steril* 1985; **44**: 751–4.

25. Golan A, Herman A, Soffer Y, Bukovsky I, Ron-El R. Ultrasonic control without hormone determination for ovulation induction in in-vitro fertilization/embryo transfer with gonadotrophin-releasing hormone analogue and human menopausal gonadotropin. *Hum Reprod* 1994; **9**: 1631–3.

26. Coulam CB, Bustillo M, Soenksen DM, Britten S. Ultrasonographic predictors of implantation after assisted reproduction. *Fertil Steril* 1994; **62**: 1004–10.

27. Ayustawati, Shibahara H, Obara H, et al. Influence of endometrial thickness and pattern on pregnancy rates in in vitro fertilization-embryo transfer. *Reprod Med Biol* 2002; **1**: 17–21.

28. Gonen Y, Casper RF, Jacobson W, Blankier J. Endometrial thickness and growth during ovarian stimulation: a possible predictor of implantation in in-vitro fertilization. *Fertil Steril* 1989; **52**: 446–50.

29. Check JH, Nowroozi K, Choe J, Lurie D, Dietterich C. The effect of endometrial thickness and echo pattern on in vitro fertilization outcome in donor oocyte-embryo transfer cycle. *Fertil Steril* 1993; **59**: 72–5.

30. Zhang X, Chen CH, Confino E, Barnes R, Milad M, Kazer RR. Increased endometrial thickness is associated with improved treatment outcome for selected patients

undergoing in vitro fertilization-embryo transfer. *Fertil Steril* 2005; **83**: 336–40.

31. Richter KS, Bugge KR, Bromer JG, Levy MJ. Relationship between endometrial thickness and embryo implantation, based on 1,294 cycles of in vitro fertilization with transfer of two blastocyst-stage embryos. *Fertil Steril* 2007; **87**: 53–9.

32. Friedler S, Schenker JG, Herman A, Lewin A. The role of ultrasonography in the evaluation of endometrial receptivity following assisted reproductive treatments: A critical review. *Hum Reprod Update* 1996; **2**: 323–35.

33. Rabinowitz R, Laufer N, Lewin A, et al. The value of ultrasonographic endometrial measurement in the prediction of pregnancy following in vitro fertilization. *Fertil Steril* 1986; **45**: 824–8.

34. Dietterich C. Check JH. Choe JK. Nazari A. Lurie D. Increased endometrial thickness on the day of human chorionic gonadotropin injection does not adversely affect pregnancy or implantation rates following in vitro fertilization-embryo transfer. *Fertil Steril* 2002; **77**: 781–6.

35. Serafini P, Batzofin J, Nelson J, Olive D. Sonographic uterine predictors of pregnancy in women undergoing ovulation induction for assisted reproductive treatments. *Fertil Steril* 1994; **62**: 815–22.

36. Abdalla HI, Brooks AA, Johnson MR, Kirkland A, Thomas A, Studd JWW. Endometrial thickness: a predictor of implantation in ovum recipients. *Hum Reprod* 1994; **9**: 363–5.

37. Shapiro H, Cowell Casper RF. Use of vaginal ultrasound for monitoring endometrial preparation in a donor oocyte program. *Fertil Steril* 1993; **59**: 1055–8.

38. El-Toukhy T, Coomarasamy A, Khairy M, et al. The relationship between endometrial thickness and outcome of medicated frozen embryo replacement cycles. *Fertil Steril* 2008; **89**: 832–9.

39. Steer CV, Campbell S, Tan SL, et al. The use of transvaginal color flow imaging after in vitro fertilization to identify optimum uterine conditions before embryo transfer. *Feril Steril* 1992; **57**: 372–6.

40. Steer CV, Tan SL, Dillon D, Mason BA, Campbell S. Vaginal color Doppler assessment of uterine artery impedance correlates with immunohistochemical markers of endometrial receptivity required for the implantation of an embryo. *Fertil Steril* 1995; **63**: 101–8.

41. Tekay A, Martikainen H, Jouppila P. Blood flow changes in uterine and ovarian vasculature, and predictive value of transvaginal pulsed colour Doppler ultrasonography in an in-vitro fertilization programme. *Human Reprod* 1995; **10**: 688–93.

42. Ng EHU, Chan CCW, Tang OS, Yeung WSB, Ho PC. The role of endometrial and subendometrial vascularity measured by three-dimensional power Doppler ultrasound in the prediction of pregnancy during frozen-thawed embryo transfer cycles. *Hum Reprod* 2006; **21**: 1612–17.

43. Strickler RC, Christianson C, Crane JP. Curato A, Knight AB, Yang V. Ultrasound guidance for human embryo transfer. *Fertil Steril* 1985; **42**: 54–61.

44. Sallam HN, Agameya AF, Rahman AF, Ezzeldin F, Sallam AN. Ultrasound measurement of the uterocervical angle before embryo transfer: a prospective controlled study. *Hum Reprod* 2002; **17**: 1767–72.

45. Kato O, Takatsuka R, Asch RH. Transvaginal-transmyometrial embryo transfer: the Towako method; experiences of 104 cases. *Fertil Steril* 1993; **59**: 51–3.

46. Buckett WM. A meta-analysis of ultrasound-guided versus clinical touch embryo transfer. *Fertil Steril* 2003; **80**: 1037–41.

47. Sallam HN, Sadek SS. Ultrasound-guided embryo transfer: a meta-analysis of randomized controlled trials. *Fertil Steril* 2003; **80**: 1042–6.

48. Kosmas IP, Janssens R, De Munck L, et al. Ultrasound-guided embryo transfer does not offer any benefit in clinical outcome: a randomized controlled trial. *Hum Reprod* 2007; **22**: 1327–34.

49. Ali CR, Khashan AS, Horne G, Fitzgerald CT, Nardo LG. Implantation, clinical pregnancy and miscarriage rates after introduction of ultrasound-guided embryo transfer. *RBM Online* 2008; **17**: 88–93.

50. Tummon I, Gavrilova-Jordan L, Allemand MC, Session D. Polycystic ovaries and ovarian hyperstimulation syndrome: a systematic review. *Acta Obstet Gynecol Scand* 2005; **84**: 611–16.

51. Van Der Meer M, Hompes PG, De Boer JA, Schats R, Schoemaker J. Cohort size rather than follicle-stimulating hormone threshold level determines ovarian sensitivity in polycystic ovary syndrome. *J Clin Endocrinol Metab* 1998; **83**: 423–6.

52. Blankstein J, Shalev J, Saadon T, et al. Ovarian hyperstimulation syndrome: prediction by numbers and size of preovulatory ovarian follicles. *Fertil Steril* 1987; **47**: 597–602.

Chapter 25

Ultrasonography and hydrosalpinges in IVF

Annika Strandell and Seth Granberg

Background

In the beginning of the in-vitro fertilization (IVF) era, tubal factor infertility was the sole indication for the treatment. Today, other indications constitute the majority of treatments and tubal disease may account for as little as 20% in some IVF centers. It is notable that tubal factor infertility is often reported to yield worse results than other causes of infertility. Hydrosalpinx is a severe condition that has attracted special interest in research and clinical practice. Hydrosalpinx is a commonly used term to describe a heterogeneous spectrum of pathology of distal tubal occlusion. A strict definition is a collection of watery fluid in the uterine tube, occurring as the end stage of pyosalpinx. Historically, these patients have been treated with microsurgery through laparotomy and, in later times, through laparoscopy. The result, measured as intrauterine pregnancy, is dependent on the status of the tubal mucosa. As IVF has developed, the majority of patients have been referred to IVF, but this subgroup of patients with hydrosalpinx was found to have a poor prognosis. The impaired outcome has been demonstrated in several retrospective studies, summarized in meta-analyses showing a reduction by half in clinical pregnancy and delivery rates and a doubled rate of spontaneous abortion in women with hydrosalpinx [1]. It is not completely understood how the hydrosalpinx exerts its negative effects. The main theories have focused on the hydrosalpingeal fluid and its action through (1) possible embryotoxic properties; (2) mechanical leakage into the uterine cavity causing endometrial alterations hostile to embryo implantation and development; or (3) simply mechanical washout of embryos.

This chapter will focus on the reproductive problems associated with hydrosalpinx, including diagnosis, with particular focus on ultrasonography, and interventions to enhance outcome after IVF.

Diagnosis of tubal disease

The diagnosis of tubal disease is mainly based on the failure to detect tubal patency with laparoscopy, hysterosalpingography (HSG), or hysterosalpingo-contrast sonography (HyCoSy). Chlamydia antibody testing contributes to the evaluation of risk for tubal disease, although without giving any information on the structural appearance of the tubes.

Pelvic sonography is commonly performed in patients with a clinical diagnosis of pelvic inflammatory disease. Although the examination may be normal or sometimes nonspecific, there are a variety of findings that are characteristic of this process. Understanding of the sonographic features of pelvic inflammations, salpingitis, pyosalpinx, tubo-ovarian complex, and tubo-ovarian abscess will allow the interpreter to make more specific, clinically useful diagnoses. Furthermore, sonography can help to distinguish acute from chronic abnormalities in the fallopian tubes. This is of high importance in the assessment of the infertile couple.

In the following sections we will discuss the usefulness of ultrasound in diagnosing normal and abnormal fallopian tubes using two-dimensional (2D) and three-dimensional (3D) transvaginal ultrasonography (TVS) and hysterosalpingo-contrast sonography (HyCoSy).

2D Transvaginal ultrasonography

On standard TVS, normal fallopian tubes are commonly not visualized and dilated fallopian tubes have usually a nonspecific appearance and often are indistinguishable from other pelvic fluid collections and masses.

The most consistent sonographic feature of fallopian tube dilatation is a tubular "sausage"-shaped structure with a fold configuration. The wall of the structure is typically well defined and echogenic. The echogenic appearance has been described in patients with acute salpingitis [2,3]. Often linear echoes protruding into the lumen, a feature that may be related to the wrinkled nature of the fallopian tube epithelium, are seen [2,3].

Distended pelvic veins, a common finding on TVS, have a tubular appearance when imaged along their long axis. However, blood flow within them usually causes multiple low-level moving echoes on real-time sonography. Bowel loops can also resemble dilated fallopian tubes, but peristaltic motion is almost always evident in bowel loops, even if only transiently. The rectosigmoid colon is easily identified by administering a water enema, and the colon often has distinctive haustral markings.

Ultrasonography in Reproductive Medicine and Infertility, ed. Botros R. M. B. Rizk. Published by Cambridge University Press. © Cambridge University Press 2010.

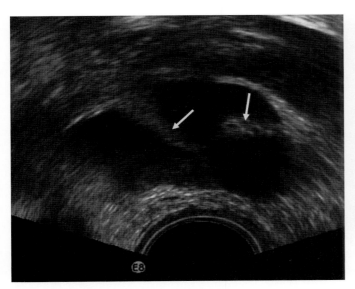

Figure 25.1. Illustration of a hydrosalpinx in 2D view.

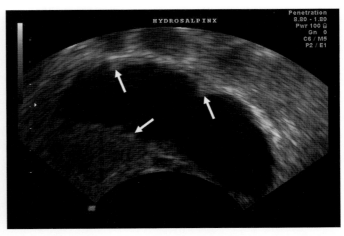

Figure 25.2. Illustration of the hydrosalpinx sign "beads on a string" (2D view), in a "sausage"-shaped cystic structure (arrows).

Adnexal masses may have some of the features of dilated fallopian tubes, but if an ovarian origin can be established, fallopian tube dilatation can be excluded. Moreover, in our experience, adnexal masses are rarely elongated and do not possess a well-defined echogenic wall.

It was concluded by Tessler et al. in 1989 that the findings of dilated fallopian tubes on TVS are sufficiently characteristic to allow the diagnosis to be made with this technique [2]. Distinguishing TVS characteristics of acute and chronic salpingitis were presented in an easily understandable way by Timor-Tritsch et al. (3), who identified chronic tubal inflammatory disease by the following TVS markers:

1. *Shape*: on the longitudinal section, a pear-shaped, ovoid, or retort-shaped structure containing sonolucent or sometimes low-level echoes.

2. *Wall structure*:
   a. Incomplete septa (Figure 25.1), defined as hyperechoic septa that originate as a triangular protrusion from one of the walls, but do not reach the opposite wall;
   b. "Beads-on-a-string" sign, defined as hyperechoic mural nodules measuring about 2–3 mm and seen on the cross-section of the fluid-filled distended structure (Figure 25.2).

3. *Wall thickness*: determined as "thick" if it is 5 mm or thicker (acute infection) and "thin" if it is less than 5 mm (chronic infection).

In a prospective study by Patel and co-workers, a hydrosalpinx was described by use of the criteria given by Timor-Tritsch and co-workers [3,4]. However, they also included in their definition "waist." The "waist" sign referred to diametrically opposed indentations along the wall of the cystic mass. The aim of the Patel study was to describe the "waist" sign as a feature of hydrosalpinx and to calculate the likelihood ratio of sonographic findings for predicting that a cystic adnexal mass is a hydrosalpinx. At least one incomplete septation was found in 65%, short linear projection in 77%, and small, round projection in 65%. Tubular shape ("sausage" shape)was found in 77% and waist sign in 50%. In this study they concluded that hydrosalpinx can be diagnosed with the highest likelihood when a tubular mass with the waist sign or a tubular mass with small, round projections is encountered. However, they also concluded that incomplete septations and short linear projections are less discriminating findings of hydrosalpinx. In another study, Guerriero and co-workers demonstrated the accuracy in identifying patients with hydrosalpinx using TVS, with a positive predictive value (PPV) of 93.3% [5]. Normal ultrasonography was also reliable because surgery generally confirmed the absence of hydrosalpinx. The false-negative rate was 2.6% and the negative predictive value (NPV) was 99.6%.

It has been proposed to establish cut-off values for the size of a hydrosalpinx, to decide when there is a need for intervention prior to IVF. However, the size of a hydrosalpinx, as measured by ultrasound, may vary during a cycle and it has not been possible to correlate IVF outcome with the precise size. Only two indexes of size have been established, "detection at ultrasonography" and "bilateral affection," and these are used to evaluate prognosis and choice of treatment [6].

3D Transvaginal ultrasonography

Conventional 2D ultrasound is a valuable diagnostic tool in the field of obstetrics and gynecology. Nevertheless, 3D ultrasound and rendering mode can illustrate even more sophisticated imaging with nearly real-time computerized reconstruction. 3D ultrasound can help in differentiating uterine malformations and intrauterine pathological lesions as well as adnexal pathology.

Images that may easily be overlooked or visualized incompletely on conventional 2D sonography can be clearly depicted on 3D ultrasound, once the volumes are scanned and stored digitally. In 3D ultrasound, three perpendicular planes displayed on the screen can be rotated and adjusted

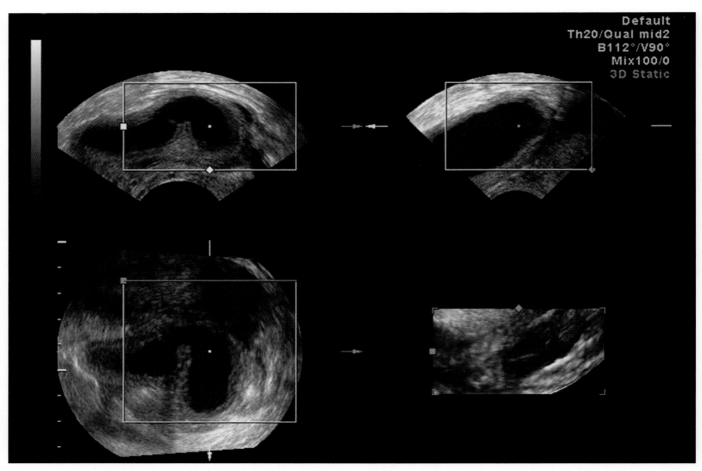

Figure 25.3. 3D ultrasound can be used to depict the hydrosalpinges in three orthogonal planes. The technique facilitates the discrimination between the tube and an ovarian cyst. Note the "sausage" shape (longitudinal plane) of the of the hydrosalpinges in the upper left box (see also Figure 25.4).

simultaneously into a more suitable anatomic orientation obtained from any arbitrary planes (Figure 25.3). Optimal display of stored volume data by rotation can also provide more detailed morphology for accurate diagnosis. Furthermore, the volumes acquired by 3D ultrasound can be digitally "manipulated" with the use of a variety of display modalities such as the multiplanar (orthogonal) views and various surface, transparency, and x-ray modes.

A new display modality was recently added to the existing ones: the 3D inversion mode, which has been described neatly by Timor-Tritsch and co-workers [7]. This new inversion rendering mode is available on the Voluson 730 Expert sonography machine (GE Medical Systems, Kretztechnik, Zipf, Austria) (Figures 25.4, 25.5, 25.6). Volumes obtained by this system can be analyzed on a laptop computer using 4DView 2000 version 2.1 computer software (GE Medical Systems). In this study, the inversion rendering mode proved useful in displaying the fluid-filled fallopian tubes. It clearly helped to differentiate between an ovarian and a tubal abnormality. The inversion mode in the case of hydrosalpinges provided further sonographic support of the 2D appearance of this condition.

They also concluded that they arrived at the diagnostic image faster than by scrolling through the original volume using only the orthogonal planes.

Hysterosalpingo-contrast sonography

In cases when hydrosalpinx is visualized by transvaginal ultrasound we do not recommend contrast instillation. There is an increased risk of infection and the information from the 2D sonography is sufficient to initiate a discussion on the need for laparoscopy.

Hysterosalpingo-contrast sonography (HyCoSy) involves the introduction of fluid into the uterine cavity and the fallopian tubes. It is an outpatient procedure that normally takes about 20 minutes. Sterile saline is used as an echo-free (negative) contrast medium for the assessment of the uterine cavity. For the examination of the fallopian tubes, a positive contrast medium is used, such as air, albumin with micro air bubbles, or galactose with micro air bubbles (Figures 25.7, 25.8). These positive contrast agents outline the fallopian tubes, giving a hyperechoic appearance.

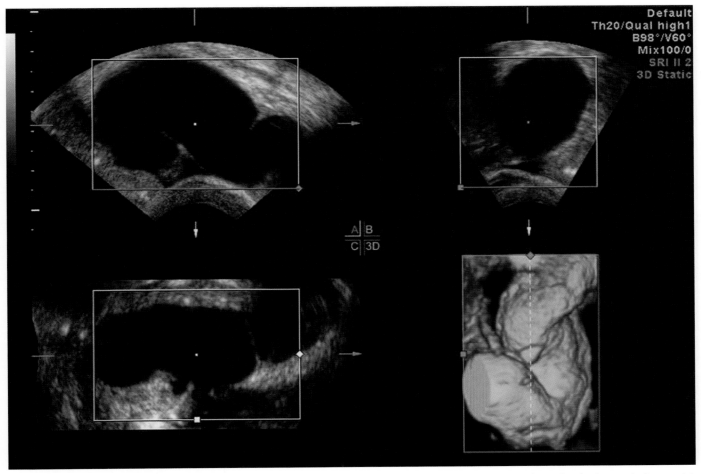

Figure 25.4. Steps in the 3D inversion rendering process of a hydrosalpinx. Acquisition in the three orthogonal planes and the rendered volume in the bottom right box. With activation of the "invert" button, the inverted volume appears in the bottom right box. Eliminating the surrounding nonpertinent structures with the electronic scalpel leaves the central structure of interest (bottom right box), the final inverted and rendered volume.

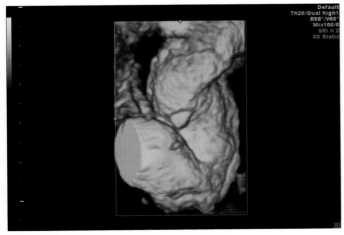

Figure 25.5. Rendered volume from the bottom right box in Figure 25.4. This figure can easily be shown as a loop.

Complete visualization of the entire fallopian tube using B-mode TVS and Echovist may not always be possible. Deichert and colleagues concluded that pulsed-wave Doppler in HyCoSy is recommended as a supplement to gray scale imaging in cases of suspected tubal occlusion or if there is intratubal flow demonstrable only over a short distance [8]. The additional use of color and pulsed-wave Doppler, when no flow of contrast medium is detected, has been shown to increase the diagnostic accuracy of HyCoSy [9]. The color Doppler gate is placed over the presumed mural portion of the tube and movement of contrast medium is registered. In this way a pulsed Doppler range gate can be used to obtain a flow velocity waveform. Such a pulsed Doppler waveform from the tube is diagnostic of tubal patency. The amplitude of the waveform will be proportional to the amount of pressure put on the syringe to instill the contrast medium. Characteristic Doppler spectra can be generated, representing patent, partially occluded, and completely occluded tubes [9].

Kupesic and Plavsic studied the diagnostic efficacy of 2D B-mode, color, and pulsed Doppler HyCoSy ($n = 152$) compared with 3D B-mode and power Doppler HyCoSy ($n = 152$). The sensitivity, specificity, PPV, and NPV of 2D hysterosonography compared with hysteroscopy for detection of uterine pathology were 93.6%, 97.3%, 98.2%, and 97.3%, respectively. The sensitivity, specificity, PPV, and NPV of 3D

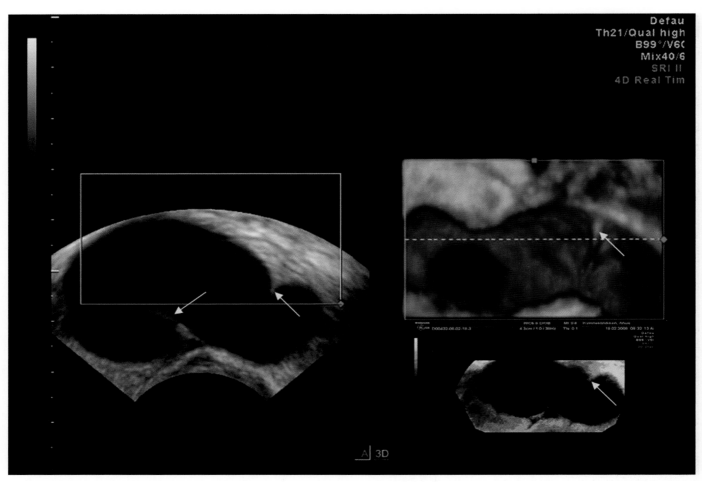

Figure 25.6. Figures of the same tube as in Figure 25.4 illustrating the pseudo septation, marked with arrows.

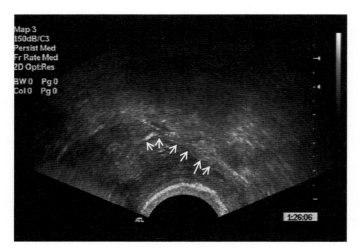

Figure 25.7. HyCoSy demonstrating the imaging of the left fallopian tube with positive contrast (marked with arrows).

hysterosonography compared with hysteroscopy were 97.9%, 100%, 97.9%, and 100%, respectively. Adding color and pulsed Doppler to 2D HyCoSy and power Doppler to 3D HyCoSy contributed to an increase in the diagnostic precision in detection of tubal patency. The sensitivity, specificity, PPV, and NPV of 3D power Doppler HyCoSy in detection of tubal patency compared with laparoscopy and dye intubation were 100%, 99.1%, 99.2%, and 100%, respectively. However, it was concluded that 2D and 3D HyCoSy are accurate methods for evaluation of uterine abnormalities and tubal patency in infertile patients and that 2D and 3D ultrasound do not differ statistically in diagnosing blocked or patent tubes [9].

Comparison of diagnostic methods

The role of HyCoSy as a first-line procedure for the assessment of tubal patency has been examined in several studies. In most of the studies the diagnostic capabilities of HyCoSy have been compared with the established reference methods of HSG or laparoscopy with dye insufflation, or both, and in the majority of the studies Echovist was used as the ultrasonographic contrast medium.

In a meta-analysis including more than 1000 women, a concordance of 83% in detecting tubal pathology was found when HyCoSy was compared with either HSG or laparoscopy with dye. Hysterosalpingo-contrast sonography showed "false"

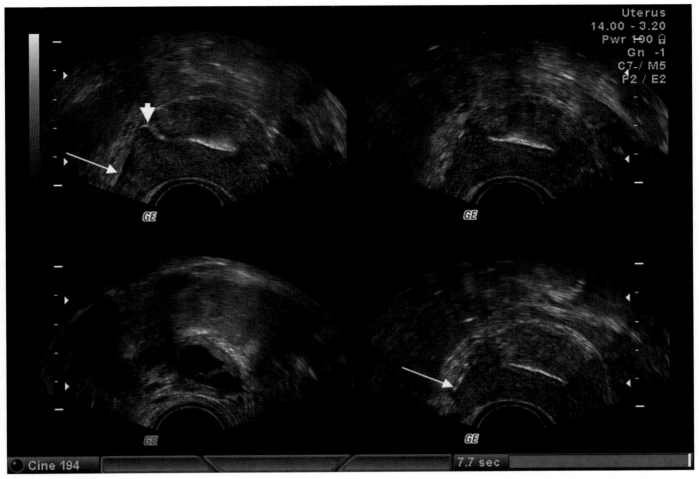

Figure 25.8. HyCoSy showing contrast passing through the right uterotubal junction (bold arrow), the middle part of the tube (arrow), the endometrium, and around the ovary.

occlusion of tubes in 10% when compared with laparoscopy with dye insufflation. When HyCoSy was compared with HSG, 13% "false" occlusions of tubes were found. "False" patency was found in 4% and 7% of tubes when HyCoSy was compared with HSG and laparoscopy, respectively. The concordance between HSG and laparoscopic findings for individual tubes was 76% [10].

In another study, Ayida and co-workers found 84% concordance at laparoscopy with the tubal patency findings at HyCoSy [11]. The percentage of women with a "normal pelvis" was 71%. Since the majority of the women had a normal pelvis, it was concluded that routine surgical procedures may not be necessary as part of first-line infertility investigations. Other studies, assessing the diagnostic capability of HyCoSy, have shown similar results. Hauge and co-workers found 90.9% concordance of tubal patency between HyCoSy and laparoscopy/hysteroscopy [12]. Compared with laparoscopy with dye, the sensitivity for diagnosis of occluded tubes using HyCoSy was 92.8%. The corresponding figures for specificity, PPV, and NPV were 96.2%, 92.8%, and 98.1%, respectively.

In a study by Strandell and co-workers, a simplified investigation protocol focusing on the use of HyCoSy – one blood test and semen analysis as an initial screening for infertility – was compared with a traditional infertility investigation protocol. The latter investigation included an HSG, postcoital test, and laparoscopy with dye. Agreement between the diagnosis based on the simplified protocol and the comprehensive protocol was found in 74% of the cases. In 13% there was partial agreement. In 36% the HyCoSy-based simplified protocol was considered sufficient to suggest treatment. It was concluded that a simplified approach could lead to a significant reduction in both the time and cost of first-line infertility investigations [13].

Although Echovist has been used as contrast agent in most of the studies assessing tubal patency, other noncommercial media have also been studied. One simple technique is to use "agitated saline," whereby 10 ml of saline and 10 ml of air are vigorously shaken and then injected into the uterine cavity. Using TVS, the bright, scintillating echoes reflecting micro bubbles are easily seen as they pass within the fallopian tubes. Comparing this technique with HSG, a concordance of 85% was found, with ultrasound being more sensitive in detecting uterine pathology [14].

Ultrasonography has the obvious advantage over HSG of being able to detect hydrosalpinx without the instillation of fluid, which carries a high risk of subsequent infection. Both methods, including instillation of contrast, can be used to diagnose a distally occluded tube without any fluid prior to instillation. Antibiotic prophylaxis is mandatory!

Chlamydia antibody testing (CAT) has been shown to be as accurate as HSG in diagnosing tubal disease [15]. The likelihood of tubal disease increases with the serum titer, but the method cannot reveal any structural damage of the tubes. CAT can be recommended as a tool to select patients for laparoscopy instead of HSG or HyCoSy if the suspicion of tubal disease is high.

Laparoscopy is obviously the ultimate method for diagnosis of hydrosalpinx and associated pathology of pelvic adhesions. However, the method is highly invasive and carries a risk of complications, and the opportunity should be taken to perform all diagnostic and therapeutic procedures at the same time if laparoscopy is indicated.

Benefits of an ultrasound-based approach

A woman's age is well known to be the most important factor affecting the outcome of fertility treatment, particularly IVF. In addition, the risk of miscarriage is dramatically increased in women in their late thirties or older, irrespective of reproductive history. Thus, prolonging the investigation of subfertile women of advanced reproductive age does not seem to be an optimal investigation strategy and may clinically delay treatment.

In publicly funded health services with limited resources, it is imperative to optimize cost–benefit ratios. Public health services usually have long waiting lists for infertility investigations. The capacity of operating theatres is limited, and the available funding may be severely restricted. In addition, factors such as the degree of available medical expertise and a high staff turnover may also turn the process of investigation into a lengthy and unnecessarily repetitive one. We thus see the suggested ultrasound-based approach as a logical development.

Ultrasonography in infertility investigations has proven to be as accurate and effective as the traditional alternatives, and in many cases even superior to HSG, hysteroscopy, and laparoscopy [8,9,10,11,12,13,14]. In addition, ultrasonography is a quick procedure that in the majority of cases causes little or no pain.

An ultrasound-based approach in basic infertility investigation has several additional benefits. Firstly, the approach is as streamlined as possible, since the results of various blood tests and semen analysis are already available at the time of the ultrasound scan. Based on the results of the tests and the ultrasound scan, further tests or even invasive procedures may be necessary. For instance, if poor sperm parameters are initially found and the gynecologic examination, including the ultrasonographic scan, has not shown any kind of pathology, no invasive procedures should be performed. If a second semen analysis shows similar poor sperm parameters to the first one, the couple should be directed to intracytoplasmic sperm injection (ICSI). For the female half of the couple, there is no need for tubal assessment. The uterus can be assessed by a 2D US and most pathology within the cavity will be detected by the infusion of sterile saline. The presence of submucosal fibroids is associated with decreased reproductive outcome, and hysteroscopic myomectomy should be considered. Thus, investigation can be tailored to the individual patient in an efficient way. Furthermore, since fewer laparoscopies are performed, the waiting list for operations is shortened for those women with proven pathology.

Secondly, the number of side-effects and complications secondary to the investigations themselves are also minimized. It is well known that side-effects and complications after HSG include exposure to radiation, uterine perforation, hemorrhage, hypersensitivity to iodine, and pain. When laparoscopy is performed there is always a risk of serious complications such as perforation of blood vessels and bowel injury. As previously mentioned, complications due to HyCoSy seem to be of a less serious character [8,9,10,11,12,13,14].

Finally, an ultrasound-based approach appears to be more cost-effective than traditional comprehensive infertility investigation protocols. Although the cost-effectiveness of various assisted reproduction technology strategies has been well documented [16,17], little is known about the costs of infertility investigations. However, the potentially largest cost savings in the assessment of infertility come from proper utilization of surgical procedures. Proper utilization of surgical procedures, usually endoscopic procedures, represents the single most significant factor in providing cost-effective infertility care [16,17]. Preliminary results suggest that an ultrasound-based fertility assessment not only reduces patient-related costs, but also is cost-effective in a public health service [16]. In conclusion, a huge body of evidence has shown that an ultrasound-based assessment of infertility provides diagnostic information that is comparable with the traditional invasive investigative methods. In our opinion ultrasonography, as we have described in this section, can be the routine standard for initial infertility investigations. In order to achieve this aim, units of reproductive medicine should invest in high-resolution ultrasound machines with sensitive Doppler equipment and ensure that their personnel are trained to use the equipment effectively.

Management of hydrosalpinx

The accumulating evidence on the negative influence of hydrosalpinx on IVF outcome started an intense debate about treatment options, most of which focused on surgical methods to dispose of the hydrosalpingeal fluid. Laparoscopic salpingectomy is the only method that has been properly evaluated in a sufficiently large randomized controlled trial, while all other methods need further evaluation. Reconstructive surgery may still be a treatment option when there is only mild to moderate tubal damage and the surgical competence, skill, and equipment are available.

Salpingectomy

A multicenter study in Scandinavia compared laparoscopic salpingectomy with no intervention prior to the first IVF cycle [6]. Of special interest were the groups with bilateral and/or ultrasound visible hydrosalpinges, which were previously shown to have a worse prognosis. The study demonstrated a significant improvement in pregnancy and birth rates after salpingectomy in patients with hydrosalpinges that were large enough to be visible on ultrasound. Clinical pregnancy rates were 46% vs. 22% ($P = 0.049$), and birth rates were 40% vs. 17% ($P = 0.040$) in salpingectomized patients vs. patients without any surgical intervention. The difference in outcome was not statistically significant in the total study population of 204 patients, which included patients with hydrosalpinges that were not visible on ultrasound, demonstrating that the benefit of salpingectomy is evident only if the hydrosalpinx is fluid-filled.

The psychological aspect of removing the tubes in an infertile patient is very important and has to be considered. Even if it is obvious that the patient would benefit from salpingectomy, it is crucial that she is psychologically prepared to undergo the procedure. In some cases, it takes one or several failed cycles before the patient is ready to give her consent.

This study constitutes the major part of a systematic review, including two additional smaller trials on salpingectomy showing a statistically significant increase in live birth rate, if salpingectomy precedes IVF (odds ratio 2.1, 95% CI 1.2–3.6) in all hydrosalpinx patients [18]. In a meta-analysis, including also the most recent published articles, the common risk ratio for ongoing pregnancy was 2.4 (95% CI 1.6–3.4), as depicted in Figure 25.9.

Also, the cumulative result from the Scandinavian study, including all subsequent cycles, demonstrated a doubled birth rate compared with patients with persistent hydrosalpinges (hazard ratio 2.1, 95% CI 1.6–3.6, $P = 0.014$) [19]. This result, as well as the compiled data from the Cochrane review, suggests that all patients with hydrosalpinx, regardless of size or fluid accumulation, should undergo salpingectomy. However, the cumulative data from the Scandinavian study revealed that the benefit of salpingectomy mainly affected patients with hydrosalpinges visible on ultrasound, and consequently, those are the only patients to be recommended prophylactic salpingectomy prior to IVF.

A cost-effectiveness analysis, based on the Scandinavian trial [20], showed that the strategy of performing salpingectomy prior to the first IVF cycle was more cost-effective than the strategy of suggesting surgery after one or two cycles had failed.

Author	Surgery Birth or ongoing pregnancy/ patients	No surgery Birth or ongoing pregnancy/ patients	Relative risk (95% CI)	Weight	Relative risk (95% CI)
Déchaud, 1998 [30]	13/30	6/30		13%	2.17 (0.95, 4.94)
Strandell, 1999 [6]	31/116	15/88		42%	1.57 (0.90, 2.72)
Goldstein, 1998 [31]	4/15	1/16		6%	4.27 (0.54, 33.98)
Kontoravdis, 2006 [22]	23/47	1/14		13%	6.85 (1.01, 46.32)
Moshin, 2006 [32]	23/60	8/66		26%	3.16 (1.53, 6,53)
Total	94/268	31/214		100%	2.37 (1.63, 3.44)

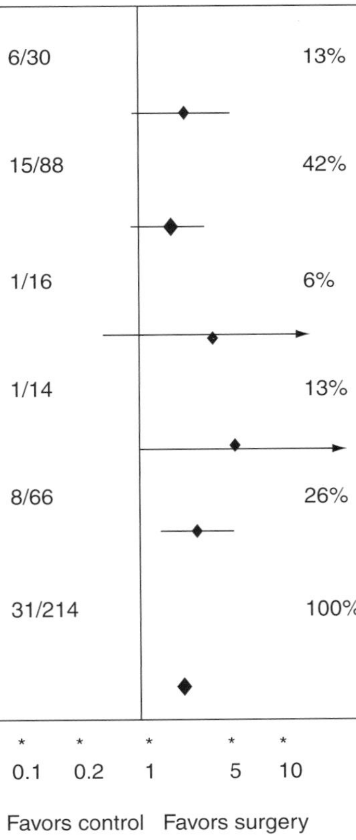

0.1   0.2   1   5   10

Favors control   Favors surgery

Figure 25.9. Meta-analysis comparing the effect of salpingectomy vs. no surgery in hydrosalpinx patients prior to IVF on birth or ongoing pregnancy rate. All published randomized controlled trials, including abstracts, are included.

The effect of salpingectomy on ovarian function has been debated because the close anatomic association of the vascular and nervous supply to the tube and ovary may increase the risk of damage if the surgery is too extensive or incautious. The results of hitherto published studies do not show any significant reduction in the overall number of oocytes retrieved at IVF after surgery. Of at least 10 publications, only one retrospective study reported impaired outcome from the ovary ipsilateral to the salpingectomy, compared with the contralateral ovary [21]. None of the randomized studies showed any difference, which is reassuring.

Tubal ligation

Proximal occlusion of the fallopian tube has been suggested as an alternative to salpingectomy prior to IVF, in particular when dense adhesions complicate an intended salpingectomy. Occlusion of the tube serves the purpose of interrupting the passage of fluid to the endometrial cavity, but leaves the hydrosalpinx in place, where it might interfere with the aspiration of oocytes. The procedure can be combined with distal fenestration of the hydrosalpinx, but the opening frequently re-occludes. In a randomized trial, 115 patients with hydrosalpinx were allocated to proximal tubal occlusion, salpingectomy, or no surgery prior to IVF [22]. Both surgical methods demonstrated significantly higher ongoing pregnancy rates (34% and 46%, respectively) compared with women having no surgery (6.6%), analyzed on an intention-to-treat basis ($P = 0.049$). Although this study was underpowered, the result supports the findings of previous retrospective studies, suggesting that proximal occlusion is effective.

The hysteroscopic route for tubal ligation has been tried in cases where laparosopy was contraindicated. The placement of microinserts, the Essure® device originally developed for tubal sterilization, and its favorable outcome have been reported in several publications. The hitherto largest case series reported on 10 women with unilateral hydrosalpinx and conditions that contraindicated laparoscopy [23]. Tubal occlusion was demonstrated by HSG in 9 patients before starting IVF.

Transvaginal aspiration

Ultrasound-guided transvaginal aspiration has been advocated as a treatment option to remove the hydrosalpingeal fluid. If the procedure is performed prior to stimulation, the fluid always reaccumulates. Even if it is done at the time of oocyte retrieval, the risk of reoccurrence is already high at the time of transfer. One recent randomized controlled trial investigated the effect of aspiration directly after oocyte retrieval compared with no aspiration [24]. Unfortunately, the study was stopped in advance and did not reach the required sample size. Clinical pregnancy rates for aspiration versus control groups were 31.3% (10/32) and 17.6% (6/34), respectively (RR = 1.8 [0.8, 4.3], $P = 0.20$). The result certainly suggests a benefit from aspiration, although additional studies are required to confirm that conclusion. Previous

studies were retrospective and inconclusive. The procedure should be combined with antibiotic cover. If a hydrosalpinx develops during stimulation, there is an alternative option to freeze all embryos and perform a salpingectomy prior to a freeze transfer.

Hydrosalpinx and spontaneous conception

After reconstructive surgery of the tubes, sufficient time should be allowed for spontaneous conception. Thus, only younger women would be suitable for salpingostomy. A large proportion of women undergoing surgery will not achieve an intrauterine pregnancy and will subsequently need IVF.

Women with a unilateral hydrosalpinx and a contralateral healthy tube can be recommended a unilateral salpingectomy and wait for spontaneous conception. They will not necessarily need IVF, as demonstrated by the Scandinavian trial on salpingectomy and case reports [13,19,25].

Follow-up of pregnancies

There are several reasons to examine patients with a history of hydrosalpinx with transvaginal sonography in early pregnancy. All patients with tubal disease carry an increased risk of ectopic pregnancy subsequent to both spontaneous and assisted conception. A transvaginal ultrasound examination in early gestation is important to rule out ectopic placentation. If more than one embryo has been transferred in IVF treatment, the risk of a heterotopic pregnancy should be remembered. The detection of an intrauterine pregnancy is not sufficient; the tubes and adnexae need to be carefully examined as well.

The risks of dehiscence in the uterine wall and cornual fistulae after salpingectomy have been described [26]. Rare ectopic placentations such as in the ovary and even in the retroperitoneal space have been described [27,28]. A recommendation of resection not too close to the uterus is appropriate, and close sonographic surveillance of the early pregnancy can be considered. Patients with a persistent hydrosalpinx have an increased risk of miscarriage. Counseling and additional ultrasound in early pregnancy are supportive for the patient. If miscarriage occurs, advice on salpingectomy can be proposed [29].

Key points in clinical practice

- Normal tubes cannot be visualized in most cases.
- Hydrosalpinx can be diagnosed with high accuracy by use of both 2D and 3D TVS.
- Contrast TVS should not be used in cases where a hydrosalpinx has been visualized by transvaginal ultrasound.
- Contrast TVS is an accurate and acceptable diagnostic tool in diagnosing blocked and patent tubes.
- In patients with hydrosalpinx on ultrasound and with a destroyed mucosa upon endoscopic inspection, IVF is the method of choice, but should be preceded by a discussion of

laparoscopic salpingectomy, which will double the patient's chances of a subsequent birth after IVF.

- In cases of severe adhesions to the hydrosalpinx, proximal occlusion of the tube can be performed.
- Salpingectomy for a unilateral hydrosalpinx increases the chance of spontaneous conception and live birth.
- If hydrosalpinx develops during stimulation, transvaginal aspiration before oocyte retrieval is an option.
- The risk of ectopic pregnancy is increased in patients with tubal disease after both spontaneous and assisted conception. These patients should be carefully examined with transvaginal ultrasound in early pregnancy.

References

1. Zeyneloglu HB, Arici A, Olive DL. Adverse effects of hydrosalpinx on pregnancy rates after in vitro fertilization-embryo transfer. *Fertil Steril* 1998; **70**: 492–9.

2. Tessler F, Perrella R, Fleischer A, Grant E. Endovaginal sonographic diagnosis of dilated fallopian tubes. *AJR* 1989; **153**: 523–5.

3. Timor-Tritsch IE, Lerner JP, Monteagudo A, Murphy KE, Helle DS. Transvaginal sonographic markers of tubal inflammatory disease. *Ultrasound Obstet Gynecol* 1998; **12**: 56–66.

4. Patel M, Acord D, Young S. Likelihood ratio of sonographic findings in discriminating hydrosalpinx from other adnexal masses. *Am J Roentgenol* 2006; **186**: 1033–8.

5. Guerriero S, Ajossa S, Lai MP, Mais V, Paoletti AM, Melis GB. Transvaginal ultrasonography associated with colour Doppler energy in the diagnosis of hydrosalpinx. *Hum Reprod* 2000; **15**: 1568–72.

6. Strandell A, Lindhard A, Waldeström U, et al. Hydrosalpinx and IVF outcome: A prospective, randomized multicentre trial in Scandinavia on salpingectomy prior to IVF. *Hum Reprod* 1999; **14**: 2762–9.

7. Timor-Tritsch IE, Monteagudo A, Tsymbal T, Strok I. Three-dimensional inversion rendering: a new sonographic technique and its use in gynecology. *J Ultrasound Med.* 2005; **24**: 681–8.

8. Deichert U, Schleif R, van de Sandt M. Transvaginal hystero-salpingo-contrast-sonography (HyCoSy) compared with conventional tubal diagnostics. *Hum Reprod* 1989; **4**: 418–24.

9. Kupesic S, Plavsic B. 2D and 3D hysterosalpingo-contrast-sonography in the assessment of uterine cavity and tubal patency. *Eur J Obstet Gynecol Reprod Biol.* 2007; **133**: 64–9.

10. Holz K, Becker R, Shurman R. Ultrasound in the assessment of tubal patency: a meta analysis of three comparative studies of Echovist 200 including 1007 women. *Zentralbl Gynacol* 1997; **119**: 266–373.

11. Ayida G, Chamberlain P, Barlow D, Kennedy S. Uterine cavity assessment prior to *in-vitro* fertilization: comparison of transvaginal scanning, saline contrast hysterosonography and hysteroscopy. *Ultrasound Obstet Gynecol* 1997; **10**: 59–62.

12. Hauge K, Flo K, Riedhart M, Granberg S. Can ultrasound-based investigations replace laparoscopy and hysteroscopy in infertility? *Eur J Obst Gynecol Biol Reprod.* 2000; **92**: 167–70.

13. Strandell A, Bourne T, Bergh C, Granberg S, Asztely M, Thorburn J. The assessment of endometrial pathology and tubal patency: a comparison between the use of ultrasonography and x-ray hysterosalpingography for the investigation of infertility patients. *Ultrasound Obstet Gynecol* 1999; **14**: 200–4.

14. Spalding H, Martikainen A, Tekay A, Jouppila P. A randomized study comparing air to Echovist as a contrast medium in the assessment of tubal patency in infertile women using transvaginal sonography. *Hum Reprod* 1997; **12**: 2461–4.

15. Land JA, Evers JL, Goossens VJ. How to use Chlamydia antibody testing in subfertility patients. *Hum Reprod* 1999; **14**: 268–70.

16. Nargund G. Time for an ultrasound revolution in reproductive medicine. *Ultrasound Obstet Gynecol* 2002; **20**: 107–11.

17. Mol BW, Bonsel GJ, Collins JA, et al. Cost-effectiveness of in vitro fertilization and embryo transfer. *Fertil Steril* 2000; **74**: 748–54.

18. Johnson NP, Mak W, Sowter MC. Surgical treatment for tubal disease in women due to undergo in vitro fertilisation. *Cochrane Database Syst Rev* 2004 (3): CD002125. DOI: 10.1002/14651858. CD002125.pub2.

19. Strandell A, Lindhard A, Waldenstrom U, Thorburn J. Hydrosalpinx and IVF outcome: cumulative results after salpingectomy in a randomized controlled trial.

20. Strandell A, Lindhard, A., Eckerlund I. Cost-effectiveness analysis of salpingectomy prior to IVF-based on randomized controlled trial. *Hum Reprod* 2005; **20**: 3284–92.

21. Lass A, Ellenbogen A, Croucher C, et al. Effect of salpingectomy on ovarian response to superovulation in an in vitro fertilization-embryo transfer program. *Fertil Steril* 1998; **70**: 1035–8.

22. Kontoravdis A, Makrakis E, Pantos K, et al. Proximal tubal occlusion and salpingectomy results in similar improvement in in vitro fertilization outcome in patients with hydrosalpinx. *Fertil Steril* 2006; **86**: 1642–9.

23. Mijatovic V, Veersma S, Emanuel MH, Schats R, Hompes PGA. Essure® hysteroscopic tubal occlusion device for the treatment of hydrosalpinx prior to in vitro fertilization–embryo transfer in patients with a contraindication for laparoscopy. *Fertil Steril* 2009; Jan 13 [Epub ahead of print].

24. Hammadieh N, Coomarasamy A, Ola B, Papaioannou S, Afnan M, Sharif K. Ultrasound-guided hydrosalpinx aspiration during oocyte collection improves pregnancy outcome in IVF: a randomized controlled trial. *Hum Reprod* 2008; **23**: 1113–17.

25. Aboulghar MA, Mansour RT, Serour GI. Spontaneous intrauterine pregnancy following salpingectomy for a unilateral hydrosalpinx. *Hum Reprod* 2002; **17**: 1099–100.

26. Inovay J, Marton T, Urbancsek J, et al. Spontaneous bilateral

Hum Reprod 2001; **16**: 2403–10.

cornual uterine dehiscence early in the second trimester after bilateral laparoscopic salpingectomy and in-vitro fertilization. *Hum Reprod* 1999; **14**: 2471–3.

27. Hsu CC, Yang TT, Hsu CT. Ovarian pregnancy resulting from cornual fistulae in a woman who had undergone bilateral salpingectomy. *Fertil Steril* 2005; **83**: 205–7.

28. Iwama H, Tsutsumi S, Igarashi H, Takahashi K, Nakahara K, Kurachi H. A case of retroperitoneal ectopic pregnancy following IVF-ET in a patient with previous bilateral salpingectomy. *Am J Perinatol.* 2008; **25**: 33–6.

29. Zolghadri J, Momtahan M, Alborzi S, Mohammadinejad A, Khosravi D. Pregnancy outcome in patients with early recurrent abortion following laparoscopic tubal corneal interruption of a fallopian tube with hydrosalpinx. *Fertil Steril* 2006; **86**: 149–51.

30. Déchaud H, Daurès JP, Arnal F, Humeau C, Hédon B. Does previous salpingectomy improve implantation and pregnancy rates in patients with severe tubal factor infertility who are undergoing in vitro fertilization? A pilot prospective randomized study. *Fertil Steril* 1998; **69**: 1020–5.

31. Goldstein DB, Sasaran LH, Stadtmauer L, Popa R. Selective salpingostomy-salpingectomy (SSS) and medical treatment prior to IVF in patients with hydrosalpinx. *Fertil Steril* 1998; **70 [Suppl 1]**: S320.

32. Moshin V, Hotineanu A. Reproductive outcome of the proximal tubal occlusion prior to IVF in patients with hydrosalpinx [Abstracts of the 22nd Annual Meeting of ESHRE, Prague. Czech republic, 18–21 June, 2006 edition.] *Hum Reprod Suppl 1* 2006; **21**: i193–i194.

Chapter 26

Ultrasonographic evaluation of ovarian reserve

Timur Gurgan, Aygul Demirol and Suleyman Guven

Introduction

Ovarian reserve, a term that has evolved in the era of assisted reproductive technologies (ART), refers to the residual oocyte–granulosa cell repertoire that, at any given age, is available for procreation. Both quantitative and qualitative deteriorations in the oocyte complement, and therefore a waning ovarian reserve, are recognized phenomena associated with advancing age. As a woman ages, thousands and thousands of follicles per year are lost due to atresia. At the same time, after a period of optimal fertility in her twenties, a woman's fertility decreases in her thirties, and comes to an end at the beginning of her forties [1,2].

A spectrum of markers prognostic of ovarian reserve are validated to varying degrees in the infertile population. These include biochemical markers (follicle-stimulating hormone [FSH], estradiol [E2], inhibin B, antimüllerian hormone, FSH/LH [luteinizing hormone] ratio), and ovarian ultrasonographic morphometric markers that are assessed in the early follicular phase (basal) of the menstrual cycle [1].

Four morphological markers have been commonly used: (1) ultrasonographic assessment of antral follicle count; (2) measurement of ovarian volume; (3) measurement of mean ovarian diameter and size; (4) assessment of ovarian blood flow of the stroma [3].

Antral follicle count

On cycle day 1, menstruation arrives and a new cycle begins. During the follicular phase an orderly sequence of events takes place that ensures that the proper number of follicles are ready for ovulation. Folliculogenesis is a process that is initiated well prior to the arrival of menstruation. Once a primary follicle leaves the resting state it will take 85 days, or three complete menstrual cycles, to reach the point of ovulation. The follicle destined to ovulate is recruited in the first few days of the third cycle. It will measure 1–2 mm on cycle day 1. The first morphological evidence of maturation is differentiation of the granulosa cell layer and enlargement of the oocyte [4].

Folliculogenesis is continuous throughout life. Each day a cohort of follicles reaches 2–5 mm size and either is available to be further recruited by FSH or will undergo atresia. Thus, a cohort is always ready and continuously available for a response to FSH [4].

Folliculogenesis is thought to occur in four phases: recruitment, selection, dominance, and ovulation. Recruitment takes place during cycle days 2, 3, and 4. The term recruitment indicates that a cohort of quasi-synchronous follicles has entered a gonadotropin-dependent rapid growth phase. By cycle day 5, both menstrual flow and follicular recruitment end. Selection refers to the reduction of the cohort size down to the species-specific ovulatory quota. Fluid accumulates amid the granulosa cell mass. The antrum is formed as the oocyte is displaced to one side by this process. Follicles at this stage measure 4–6 mm. By day 6, the follicle destined to become dominant secretes the greatest amount of estradiol, which, in turn, increases the density of FSH receptors on the granulosa cell membrane. The nondominant follicles cease development and then become atretic [4].

The pool of primordial follicles in the ovary is related to the number of growing antral follicles. Antral follicles are responsive to gonadotropin stimulation and the measure of ovarian reserve can be defined as the total number of follicles that can be stimulated to grow under maximal stimulation. There is a gradual decline in the number of primordial follicles with increasing age. The antral follicle count (AFC) is defined as the number of follicles smaller than 10 mm in diameter detected by transvaginal ultrasound in the early follicular phase. Ultrasound measurement of the ovarian AFC is a reproducible test with low interobserver variability at clinically important levels (low AFC) and can predict response to gonadotropin stimulation [5].

Transvaginal sonography (TVS) is the best means for assessment of total AFC. To determine the diameter of the follicle, the mean of measurements in two perpendicular directions should be taken (Figure 26.1). The numbers of follicles in both ovaries should be added for the total antral follicle count. The follicles visualized and counted by TVS in the early follicular phase should be 2–10 mm in size. Normal AFC in one ovary ranges from 5 to 10 (Figures 26.2 and 26.3) [6].

AFC is an ultrasound marker of ovarian aging. In the ART literature, a lower AFC has been associated with poor ovarian response. Various cut-off points for a low AFC, most often less than 4 or 6, have been described in predicting poor ovarian response (Figures 26.4 and 26.5) [7].

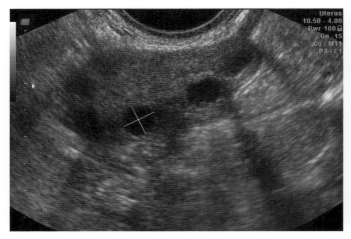

Figure 26.1. Measurement of the diameter of the follicle (4.2 mm); the mean of measurements in two perpendicular directions should be taken.

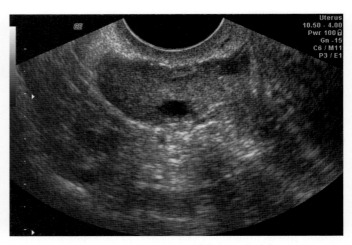

Figure 26.4. In the axial section, two antral follicles in the left ovary suggest poor ovarian reserve.

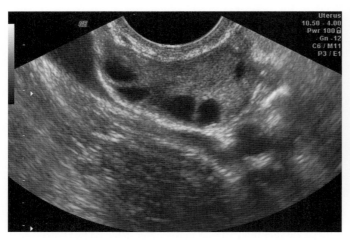

Figure 26.2. Five antral follicles in the left ovary suggest normal ovarian reserve.

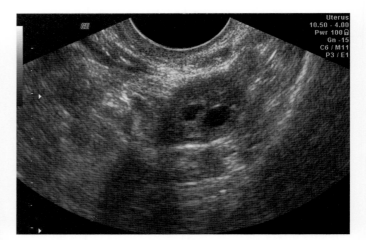

Figure 26.5. In the transverse section, two antral follicles in the left ovary suggest poor ovarian reserve.

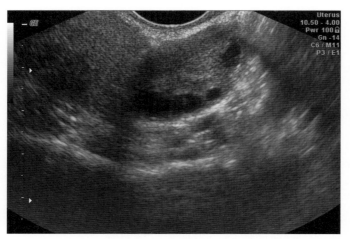

Figure 26.3. Six antral follicles in the left ovary suggest normal ovarian reserve.

Frattarelli and co-workers studied the predictive value of AFC in a period of desensitization with respect to ovarian response in 256 patients undergoing IVF. The correlation of AFC was positive with the number of mature follicles ($r = 0.52$), the number of oocytes ($r = 0.38$), and the number of embryos. They also determined the threshold number of antral follicles that could predict the ovarian response. A total number <4 was associated with a high risk of cancellation (41.0 vs. 6.4%) and with a poor rate of pregnancy (23.5 vs. 57.6%) [8].

From a prospective study including 327 consecutive IVF patients who had a basal ultrasound scan of their ovarian reserve during the early follicular phase and had a first IVF cycle between 1 and 3 months later, AFC correlates negatively with age and positively with the total number of follicles and E2 on hCG day and with the number of oocytes. The AFC has predictive value for ovarian response in an IVF cycle, with a cut-off value of seven follicles, above which there are more chances of normal response. Its predictive value is higher than that of basal FSH (bFSH). The number of antral follicles is shown as an independent marker of poor response, with an importance comparable with basal FSH and age. The value of AFC in predicting pregnancy is lower. However, patients with eight or more follicles may achieve statistically significantly higher pregnancy rates [3].

A great advantage of AFC over any other test is its potential usefulness in its ability to concomitantly predict low and high responders. The cut-off level of >14 antral follicles gave the highest combination of sensitivity and specificity and also gave the highest accuracy. This result had a sensitivity of 82% and a specificity of 89%. AFC >14 could lead to the decision to adjust the gonadotropin dose in trying to prevent a hyper-response leading to OHSS. Of course, the choice of the cut-off level depends on the appreciation of false-positive and false-negative results and on the consequences drawn by the clinician from an abnormal test [6].

The cut-off level of <6 antral follicles had a sensitivity of 41% and a specificity of 95%. The accuracy was 89% (which means that 89% of the patients had a correctly predicted test). In case of a result of <6 antral follicles, the test correctly predicted poor response to stimulation in an IVF treatment in 75% (positive predictive value) [6]. Recently, Hendriks et al. published a meta-analysis on the AFC as a predictor for poor ovarian response and concluded that AFC is an adequate test for the prediction of poor ovarian response, comparing to bFSH [9].

The way an AFC is performed differs between centers. Most often follicles of 2–5 mm or 2–10 mm are counted. The number of smaller antral follicles up to 6 mm reflects ovarian reserve better than the total AFC if follicles of 2–10 mm are counted. The larger antral follicles up to 13 mm may also be an important reflection of the remaining follicle pool. In a recent study, it was reported that the numbers of follicles measuring 2, 3, 4, 5, and 6 mm all declined with age, whereas the number of follicles measuring 7 mm or more did not. The number of small antral follicles (2–6 mm) is significantly correlated with all endocrine ovarian reserve tests. Independently of age, the number of small antral follicles measuring 2–6 mm represents the functional quantitative ovarian reserve. Therefore, if an AFC is performed, only follicles sized 2–6 mm could be counted and used for the interpretation of the outcome [10].

A recent study [7] investigated whether AFC differed between obese and normal-weight women in late reproductive age. They found that AFC was slightly lower in obese women compared with normal-weight women, although the differences were not statistically significant. There may be two possible explanations for the observed negative effect of body mass index. First, lower number of AFC in overweight and obese women may reflect a decrease in ovarian reserve. This first explanation is supported by the observation that obese women are less fertile (even in the presence of ovulatory menstrual cycles) and more prone to miscarriage than normal-weight women. In addition, obese women exhibit decreased ovarian response to gonadotropin stimulation during super-ovulation. Second, obesity may affect ovarian hormonal production, sequestration, or clearance.

AFC may be a useful tool for predicting pregnancy loss in IVF pregnancies. Women with an AFC of <7.5 on day 3 of stimulation were 4.2 times more likely to have an abortion and 5.5 times more likely to have a biochemical pregnancy loss following an IVF pregnancy, compared with those who had more than 7.5 antral follicles. This may be explained with the hypothesis that women with diminished ovarian reserve (OR) have significantly higher rates of pregnancy loss than do patients with normal OR [11].

In conclusion, AFC performs well as a test for ovarian response, being superior to or at least similar to complex, expensive, and time-consuming endocrine tests, and probably most applicable in general practice.

Ovarian volume

Ovarian volume decreases significantly in each 10-year period of a woman's fertile life. Andolf et al. [12] showed that ovarian size decreases in women >40 years old and that this trend is not related to parity. Higgins et al. [13] found a dramatic drop in ovarian volume at the menopause, with the average upper limit of normal falling from $18 \, cm^3$ in premenopausal women to $8 \, cm^3$ in postmenopausal women. Transvaginal sonography is a reasonably accurate tool for measuring ovarian volume.

The volume of each ovary is calculated by measuring in three perpendicular directions and applying the formula for an ellipsoid: $(D_1 \times D_2 \times D_3 \times \pi/6)$ (Figure 26.6). The volumes of both ovaries are added for the total basal ovarian volume (BOV). The ovaries should be visualized and measured in the early follicular phase [6]. Only measurement of ovaries not containing cysts or large follicles will achieve an accurate net ovarian volume. Therefore in most of these studies, only ovaries with follicles of <10–15 mm were included. However, the maximum follicular size eligible for ovarian volume measurement without skewing the net results is not clear [14].

With a sample of 140 IVF cycles, Lass and associates [15] proved that a mean volume of $<3 \, cm^3$ is associated with an increased risk of cancellation and of poor response to IVF. Assuming that ovarian volume in healthy women aged 25–51 years is associated with the pool of primordial follicles, ovarian volume predicts reproductive age and the age of menopause [16]. Furthermore, Syrop et al. also reported that, like maternal age and smoking status, ovarian volume may be a clinically important predictor of reproductive success, being superior to cycle day 3 FSH or estradiol concentrations as an assessment of ovarian reserve [17]. However, use of this parameter presents problems in cases with a history of ovarian surgery with reduction of ovarian tissue, in the presence of a polycystic ovary (the volume of which increases at the expense of the stroma), follicular persistence, or ovarian tumor pathology. For these reasons, ovarian volume is a poor predictor of the number of oocytes obtained in an IVF cycle [6].

Total volume of the ovaries detected by transvaginal ultrasound is correlated with the outcome parameters but not better than the count of antral follicles. Its performance was slightly to moderately less than that of AFC, both for poor and high response [6].

The results of a recent meta-analysis show that ovarian volume as a test for the occurrence of poor ovarian response after

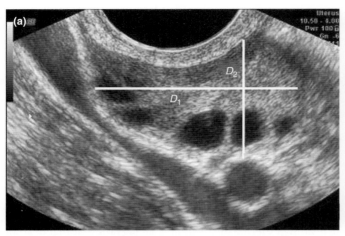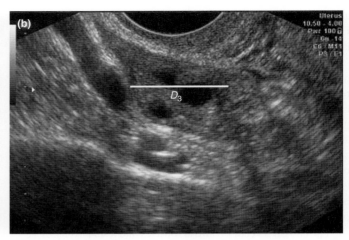

Figure 26.6. The volume of each ovary is calculated by measuring in three perpendicular directions and applying the formula for an ellipsoid: $D_1 \times D_2 \times D_3 \times \pi/6$. The measurements D_1 and D_2 are shown in (a) in an axial section of one ovary. The measurement D_3 is shown in (b) in a transverse section of one ovary.

IVF is only modestly accurate. Evidence for the accuracy of ovarian volume in predicting nonpregnancy clearly is lacking. Measuring ovarian volume in the early follicular phase therefore does not appear to be a test of choice for ovarian reserve assessment in IVF-indicated patients. Ovarian volume will remain rather stable across the third and fourth decades of female life but starts to decline after the age of 36 years. As such, the test potentially bears the same relation to reproductive status as applies for basal FSH. The test becomes abnormal only at the edge of a woman's entrance to the naturally infertile period of life (i.e., the age range 38–42 years), while she is still having regular cycles. In screening of IVF populations using ovarian volume, only a very limited number of cases will be identified as poor responders or as low-prognosis patients, because of the choice to use a very low cut-off to prevent false-positive cases. The performance of ovarian volume in the prediction of poor ovarian response after IVF is clearly lower than that of AFC. In the prediction of nonpregnancy, the performance of ovarian volume and the AFC is equally poor. Therefore, AFC may be considered to be the test of first choice in the assessment of diminished ovarian reserve [18].

Mean ovarian diameter/size

Using the largest cross-sectional sagittal view of the ovary, the mean ovarian diameter could be calculated from measurement of two perpendicular diameters [19]. The formula $(D_1 + D_2)/2$ should be used to calculate mean ovarian size [20] (Figure 26.7).

Frattarelli et al. reported that a mean ovarian diameter of <20 mm on cycle day 3 predicts higher cancellation rates during ART cycles. However, in patients who continued and underwent oocyte retrieval, no difference in the pregnancy or delivery rates was apparent. Likewise, they demonstrated that ovarian diameter correlates well with ovarian reserve and stimulation parameters [19].

In one prospective observational study it was confirmed that mean ovarian diameter correlates significantly with mean ovarian volume. The mean ovarian diameter significantly correlated

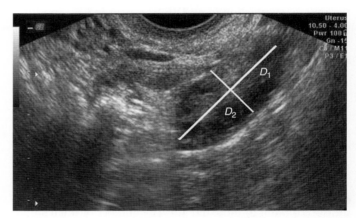

Figure 26.7. The measurements D_1 and D_2 are shown in an axial section of the left ovary. The formula $(D_1 + D_2)/2$ should be used to calculate mean ovarian size.

with age, day 3 FSH, day 3 LH, and day 3 estradiol. By using a simplified method to determine ovarian size, the physician can more effectively assess ovarian reserve during baseline ultrasound examination and thus change the patient's stimulation protocol to optimize results [20].

A recent study [1] investigated the association between individual ovarian dimensions (ovarian length [{right ovarian length + left ovarian length}/2], width ({right ovarian width + left ovarian width}/2), and overall diameter ({mean length + mean width}/2), advancing age, and declining OR in an infertile population. It was demonstrated that although all three of the individual ovarian dimensions are reliable prognosticators of OR, as reflected by the FSH levels, the mean ovarian width exhibits a more robust relationship with OR status compared with the ovarian length or the average of the two dimensions [1].

Ovarian stromal blood flow

The combination of transvaginal ultrasound and pulsed color Doppler is increasingly used in gynecology to assess the

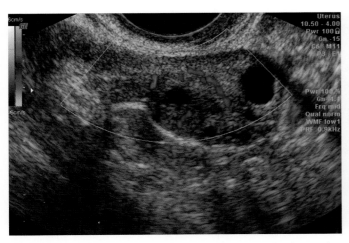

Figure 26.8. In this transverse section of a transvaginal Doppler ultrasound scan, the presence of stromal blood flow suggests normal ovarian reserve.

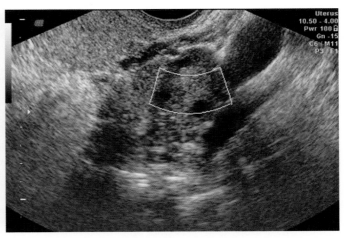

Figure 26.9. In this transverse section of a transvaginal Doppler ultrasound scan, the absence of stromal blood flow suggests poor ovarian reserve.

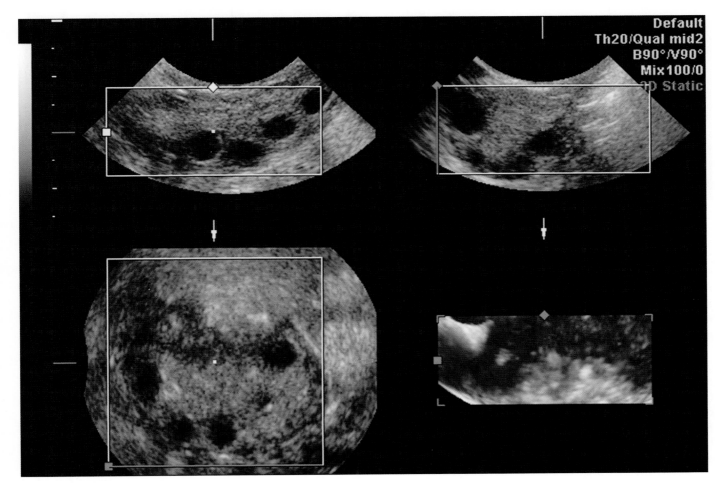

Figure 26.10. Measurement of AFC using 3D ultrasound in a woman with normal AFC.

hemodynamic changes in various physiological and pathological situations of the pelvic organs. The physiological significance of basal ovarian stromal blood flow was investigated for the assessment of ovarian reserve (Figures 26.8 and 26.9). In this study it was concluded that undetectable basal ovarian stromal blood flow in at least one ovary is related to low ovarian reserve in infertile women undergoing IVF-ET. It seems that undetectable basal stromal blood flow is not solely a technical issue, but rather is linked to the pathophysiology of ovarian aging [21].

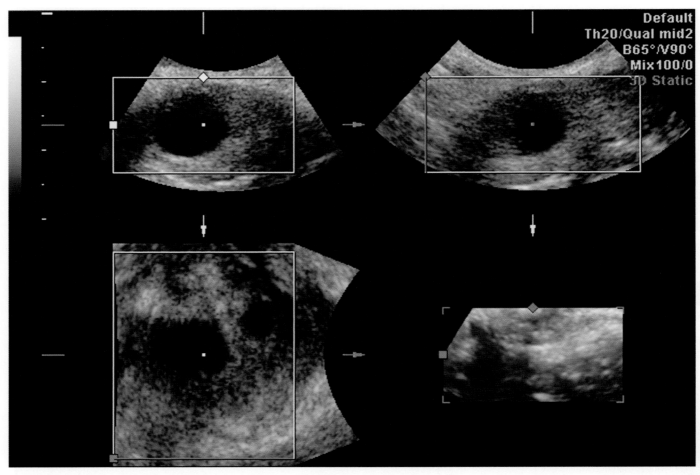

Figure 26.11. Measurement of AFC using 3D ultrasound in a woman with low AFC.

In 60% of women with low reserve, as compared with only 6% of women with good ovarian reserve, basal stromal blood flow was undetectable in at least one of the ovaries. The fact that the pregnancy rate was significantly higher in the "good ovarian reserve" group than in the "absence of basal stromal blood flow" group reinforces these findings [21].

Poor responders have ovarian arterial flow that is altered in the early follicular phase, in spontaneous cycles, and after pituitary inhibition. Ovarian stromal peak systolic velocity (PSV) was the most important single independent predictor of ovarian response in patients with a normal basal serum FSH level. Patients with high PSV ($\geq$10 cm/s) had a significantly higher median number of mature oocytes retrieved and a higher clinical pregnancy rate (35.3% versus 11.3%) than patients with low PSV (<10 cm/s), even after controlling for age [22].

Using 3D ultrasonography

Only one study has compared the predictive value of AFC measurement made using both 2D and 3D ultrasound in determining the outcome of response to ovarian stimulation as measured by the number of follicles that develop, the number of oocytes retrieved, and the pregnancy rate following ART (Figures 26.10 and 26.11). The authors indicated that a pretreatment AFC measured using methods specific to 3D ultrasound offers minimal additional information over that derived from conventional 2D ultrasound in the prediction of the number of follicles measuring 10 mm or more that will be evident on the day of hCG, the actual number of oocytes that will be retrieved thereafter, and the incidence of nonconception. Furthermore, measurements made with the inversion mode take significantly longer than those made with the 2D equivalent and 3D multiplanar view techniques [23].

References

1. Bowen S, Norian J, Santoro N, Pal L. Simple tools for assessment of ovarian reserve (OR): individual ovarian dimensions are reliable predictors of OR. *Fertil Steril* 2007; **88**(2): 390–5.

2. Broekmans FJ, Scheffer GJ, Bancsi LF, Dorland M, Blankenstein MA, te Velde ER. Ovarian reserve tests in infertility practice and normal fertile women. *Maturitas* 1998; **30**(2): 205–14.

3. Soldevila PN, Carreras O, Tur R, Coroleu B, Barri PN. Sonographic assessment of ovarian reserve. Its correlation with outcome of in vitro fertilization cycles. *Gynecol Endocrinol* 2007; **23**(4): 206–12.

4. Queenan J. The menstrual cycle. In: Lewis V, ed.

Reproductive Endocrinology and Infertility. Austin, TX: Landes Bioscience, 2007; 3–10.

5. Bukulmez O, Arici A. Assessment of ovarian reserve. *Curr Opin Obstet Gynecol* 2004; **16**(3): 231–7.

6. Kwee J, Elting ME, Schats R, McDonnell J, Lambalk CB. Ovarian volume and antral follicle count for the prediction of low and hyper responders with in vitro fertilization. *Reprod Biol Endocrinol* 2007; **5**: 9.

7. Su HI, Sammel MD, Freeman EW, Lin H, DeBlasis T, Gracia CR. Body size affects measures of ovarian reserve in late reproductive age women. *Menopause* 2008; **15**(5): 857–61.

8. Frattarelli JL, Levi AJ, Miller BT, Segars JH. A prospective assessment of the predictive value of basal antral follicles in in vitro fertilization cycles. *Fertil Steril* 2003; **80**(2): 350–5.

9. Hendriks DJ, Mol BW, Bancsi LF, Te Velde ER, Broekmans FJ. Antral follicle count in the prediction of poor ovarian response and pregnancy after in vitro fertilization: a meta-analysis and comparison with basal follicle-stimulating hormone level. *Fertil Steril* 2005; **83**(2): 291–301.

10. Haadsma ML, Bukman A, Groen H, et al. The number of small antral follicles (2–6 mm) determines the outcome of endocrine ovarian reserve tests in a subfertile population. *Hum Reprod* 2007; **22**(7): 1925–31.

11. Elter K, Kavak ZN, Gokaslan H, Pekin T, et al. Antral follicle assessment after down-regulation may be a useful tool for predicting pregnancy loss in in vitro fertilization pregnancies. *Gynecol Endocrinol* 2005; **21**(1): 33–7.

12. Andolf E, Jörgensen C, Svalenius E, Sundén B, et al. Ultrasound measurement of the ovarian volume. *Acta Obstet Gynecol Scand* 1987; **66**(5): 387–9.

13. Higgins RV, van Nagell JR Jr, Donaldson ES, et al. Transvaginal sonography as a screening method for ovarian cancer. *Gynecol Oncol* 1989; **34**(3): 402–6.

14. Lass A, Brinsden P. The role of ovarian volume in reproductive medicine. *Hum Reprod Update* 1999; **5**(3): 256–66.

15. Lass A, Skull J, McVeigh E, Margara R, Winston RM. Measurement of ovarian volume by transvaginal sonography before ovulation induction with human menopausal gonadotrophin for in-vitro fertilization can predict poor response. *Hum Reprod* 1997; **12**(2): 294–7.

16. Van Der Meer M, Hompes PG, De Boer JA, Schats R, Schoemaker J. Cohort size rather than follicle-stimulating hormone threshold level determines ovarian sensitivity in polycystic ovary syndrome. *J Clin Endocrinol Metab* 1998; **83**(2): 423–6.

17. Syrop CH, Dawson JD, Husman KJ, Sparks AE, Van Voorhis BJ. Ovarian volume may predict assisted reproductive outcomes better than follicle stimulating hormone concentration on day 3. *Hum Reprod* 1999; **14** (7): 1752–6.

18. Hendriks DJ, Kwee J, Mol BW, te Velde ER, Broekmans FJ. Ultrasonography as a tool for the prediction of outcome in IVF patients: a comparative meta-analysis of ovarian volume and antral follicle count. *Fertil Steril* 2007; **87**(4): 764–75.

19. Frattarelli JL, Lauria-Costab DF, Miller BT, Bergh PA, Scott RT. Basal antral follicle number and mean ovarian diameter predict cycle cancellation and ovarian responsiveness in assisted reproductive technology cycles. *Fertil Steril* 2000; **74**(3): 512–17.

20. Frattarelli JL, Levi AJ, Miller BT. A prospective novel method of determining ovarian size during in vitro fertilization cycles. *J Assist Reprod Genet* 2002; **19**(1): 39–41.

21. Younis JS, Haddad S, Matilsky M, Radin O, Ben-Ami M. Undetectable basal ovarian stromal blood flow in infertile women is related to low ovarian reserve. *Gynecol Endocrinol* 2007; **23**(5): 284–9.

22. Engmann L, Sladkevicius P, Agrawal R, Bekir JS, Campbell S, Tan SL. Value of ovarian stromal blood flow velocity measurement after pituitary suppression in the prediction of ovarian responsiveness and outcome of in vitro fertilization treatment. *Fertil Steril* 1999; **71**(1): 22–9.

23. Jayaprakasan K, Hilwah N, Kendall NR. Does 3D ultrasound offer any advantage in the pretreatment assessment of ovarian reserve and prediction of outcome after assisted reproduction treatment? *Hum Reprod* 2007; **22**(7): 1932–41.

Ultrasonography in oocyte retrieval for IVF

Matts Wikland and Lars Hamberger

Introduction

During the preclinical development of in-vitro fertilization (IVF) in the human, oocytes were frequently obtained at laparotomies for various indications and the time for the operative procedure was generally not scheduled close to ovulation. In 1968 Dr. Robert Edwards, a physiologist in Cambridge, UK, and pioneer in human IVF, contacted the British gynecologist Patrick Steptoe, a clinician who had helped to develop and utilize the laparoscopic technique for oocyte retrieval. This new technique played a key role in the collaboration and it was agreed that Steptoe would aspirate follicles through the laparoscope. Edwards would then fertilize the eggs in vitro and culture them for an appropriate time, and Steptoe would, if indicated, replace them in the uterine cavity through the cervical canal. Subsequently, laparoscopy became the technique of choice for oocyte aspiration during the 10 first years of the IVF era. Compared with laparotomy, laparoscopy was a relatively simple technique with a high oocyte recovery rate. General anesthesia and intubation of the patient was the standard procedure even if a few groups gradually came to use only local anesthesia combined with conscious sedation in selected patients [1]. There was also discussion in this connection whether the gas insufflated in the abdominal cavity could influence the maturing oocyte negatively. The use of pure carbon dioxide was changed by some groups to a gas mixture with 90% N_2, 5% O_2, and 5% CO_2 [2]. Postoperatively the patient frequently stayed overnight in the hospital. In summary the whole procedure was relatively laborious and expensive, requiring special instruments, and for practical reasons many IVF groups at that time could not manage more than one or two patients per day.

With the introduction of ultrasound for monitoring follicular growth and maturation as the sole instrument instead of repeated hormonal determinations (estradiol and luteinizing hormone [LH]), the knowledge that ultrasound also could be used for follicular aspiration meant that an interesting alternative technique had been born.

Ultrasonography

At the time of the worldwide clinical introduction of IVF around 1980, the technical ability to visualize pelvic organs by use of ultrasound also developed rapidly in parallel. This technique was first used in connection with IVF for diagnostic purposes, and the possibility of utilizing the technique for monitoring of follicular maturation was demonstrated [3,4]. However, even earlier a Danish group had described a technique for ultrasound-guided percutaneous punctures of cystic as well as solid tumors in different organs [5]. Another Danish group was the first to report successful oocyte collection under the guidance of abdominal ultrasound. However, no pregnancies were reported in this first publication [6].

Parallel with Lenz and Lauritsen [6], our own group started at the beginning of the 1980s to use a similar technique for ultrasound-guided follicular aspirations [2,7] We could also at that time report the first clinical pregnancy in the world resulting in a healthy child by use of this new application. The techniques utilized at this time were abdominal ultrasound scanning and abdominal, transvesicle puncture of mature follicles. The puncture was most often performed under light general anesthesia. The urinary bladder was first emptied and thereafter filled with 200–400 ml of isotonic saline colored with methylene blue; this made the ovaries more easily visible and the filled bladder also made the ovaries more firmly attached to the abdominal wall. The abdominal sector scanner transducer was placed in a sterile plastic bag and the sterilized needle was mounted to the short side of the transducer by use of a needle guide (Figure 27.1). The aspiration needle (inner diameter 1 mm) was connected via Teflon tubing to a sampling flask, which in turn was connected to a vacuum pump. A negative pressure of 90–100 mmHg was applied. Thereafter, the puncturing line (seen on the monitor) was adjusted to the middle of the follicle to be punctured. The echo from the tip of the needle could easily be followed on the monitor since shallow, circular tracks had been made on the needle tip.

In 1983 our group started to work on vaginal ultrasound scanning [8,9].

At that time only mechanical sector transducers were available, not ideal for follicular punctures transvaginally. We approached the Danish ultrasound company Bruel and Kjaer because it came to our knowledge that they had developed a small probe for cranial scanning during neurosurgical operative procedures. With minor modifications, this probe could also be

Ultrasonography in Reproductive Medicine and Infertility, ed. Botros R. M. B. Rizk. Published by Cambridge University Press. © Cambridge University Press 2010.

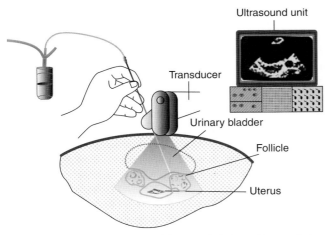

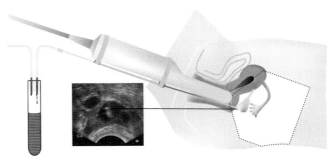

Figure 27.3. Illustration of the principle for TVOR. Note the ultrasound image with the bright echo from the needle tip induced by the shallow grooves on the needle tip.

Figure 27.1. Schematic drawing of the original abdominal/transvesical puncturing technique.

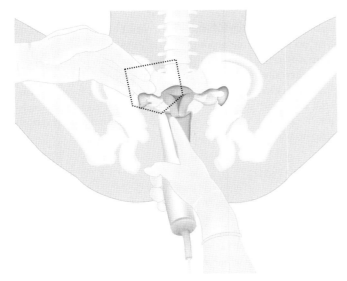

Figure 27.2. Principle of scanning with the vaginal transducer from Bryel and Kjaer, Denmark.

used as a vaginal transducer (Figure 27.2). The ovaries could now easily be scanned without using the full-bladder technique, and transvaginal ultrasound-guided oocyte retrieval (TVOR) could generally be performed with only use of some sedative in combination with local anesthesia (Figure 27.3). Even if we initially had major problems convincing other ultrasound manufacturers of the advantages of vaginal probes for both diagnostic and operative procedures, it was not long before they started to copy Bruel and Kjaer's idea with a vaginal ultrasound transducer. Other IVF groups also promptly started to apply the new technique clinically in their IVF programs [10,11].

TVOR very soon replaced the more complicated and expensive laparoscopic procedure and today only few centers in the world apply other approaches for oocyte retrieval.

Over the years the technique has been improved in many ways, partly as result of the ultrasound equipment becoming more sophisticated. The technical development has resulted in extremely refined images compared with those from the equipment used 20 years ago. In the following we will point in more detail to various aspects of this development.

Today most commercial ultrasound machines are supplied with a vaginal transducer that can be used for puncture of follicular and other ovarian or paraovarian structures via the vaginal route. It is important, however, to choose a fairly long transducer that facilitates both the scanning and puncture procedures. In our experience a frequency of 5–7 MHz gives both a sufficient penetration depth and enough resolution for scanning of the lower pelvis. The shape of the transducer should allow attachment of a sterile cover (e.g., one finger of a sterile glove) in an easy manner. The needle guide should be easy to attach to the transducer when it has been placed in the sterile cover.

Needles

Many manufacturers such as Cook Ltd., Wallace Ltd., and the former producer Swemed – now owned by Vitrolife – sell needles that are specially designed for oocyte aspiration. Certain differences in length, diameter, and shape of the tip exist and each of these may have specific advantages. In our opinion, after more than 20 years' experience of TVOR and having also tested and developed many of the available needles on the market, is that the sharpness of the needle tip is the most important property. A sharp needle also leads to less pain and discomfort for the patient, which is of crucial importance if the puncture is performed under local anesthesia. It is furthermore important that the needle is provided with grooves of some kind that will strengthen the ultrasound echo, making it easier to identify the exact position of the tip. Today, most needles used for ultrasound-guided puncture do have such preparations.

The diameter of the needle is of importance for a number of reasons. An 18–20-gauge (outer diameter) needle is in our experience optimal. Since it is rather thin it causes less pain but is thick enough to avoid the needle deviating from the puncturing line, a problem that is especially obvious if the ovaries are located high up in the pelvis. The inner diameter is also of pronounced importance since too narrow a diameter may harm the oocyte–cumulus complex [12]. In our experience, an inner diameter of 0.8–1.0 mm does not seem to negatively affect the oocyte–cumulus complex provided the negative aspiration pressure does not exceed 120 mmHg. A fingertip handle at the distal part of the needle facilitates the puncture procedure.

Needle connections and aspiration pressure

In order to increase the oocyte recovery rate it was found that Teflon tubing between needle and sampling tube was optimal. Today there are various sampling sets commercially available, including needle, tubing, and sampling tubes. The sterility and nontoxicity should be guaranteed by testing on mouse embryos (MEA; mouse embryo assay). Each set must be used only once. At follicular puncture the negative pressure in the system can be established either by use of a syringe or with a vacuum pump (see below). In our initial experiments many years ago we found that a negative pressure varying between 90 and 120 mmHg appeared optimal for both oocyte recovery in preovulatory follicles and avoiding any damage to the oocyte–cumulus complex. However, when applying the in-vitro maturation (IVM) technique in which much smaller follicles are punctured (around 5–8 mm in diameter), thinner needles and a reduced negative pressure(40–60 mmHg) have been found optimal [13]. The negative pressure is preferably created by use of a suction pump whereby the pressure can be safely controlled in a standardized manner. Today a variety of such pumps are commercially available. In the early days of IVF a syringe was frequently connected to the needle. This turned out to be a risky alternative since it was easy to apply a short-lasting excessive negative pressure, which could permanently damage the oocyte–cumulus complex [14].

Flushing of follicles and the use of double-channel or single-channel needles has been debated ever since the start of TVOR. The rationale behind this argument is that flushing of follicles gives a higher yield in terms of oocytes, a higher number of embryos for transfer, and thus a higher pregnancy rate. However, when more careful randomized comparisons were performed, for example, by Kingsland and co-workers [15], no significant differences were found between the two procedures apart from a shorter operating time in the nonflushing group. In a more recent study by Bagtharia and Haloob [16], though, it was demonstrated that only 40% of the oocytes were retrieved in the first aspirate, while 82% were retrieved after two flushes and 97% were retrieved when up to four flushes were performed. On the basis of this study they concluded that up to four was the optimal number of flushing. These two examples point to the fact that slight but important differences in equipment, as well as experience and handling, can lead to big differences in the clinical results.

In our own program we do not routinely flush follicles and have had 70% oocyte recovery rate during the past 15 years. In natural-cycle IVF or in minimally invasive IVF programs, and also in IVM programs, other routines must of course be worked out in order to optimize the results in each center.

General or local anesthesia

Right from the beginning 25 years ago our group started to perform TVOR under local anesthesia with conscious sedation. Our experience convinced us fairly quickly that most patients (more than 95%) found it acceptable or preferable to undergo the procedure with local anesthesia, which was also accompanied by much lower cost and much shorter postoperative surveillance. However, certain IVF groups prefer general anesthesia, at least in some more-sensitive patients. Furthermore, randomized control trials have concluded that the pain relief is superior when a paracervical block (PCB) in combination with sedation is used compared with sedation alone [17,18]. The PCB is generally applied at four locations around the cervix in the vaginal mucosa. Our own group has long used only 100 mg of lidocaine injected at four points in combination with conscious sedation (0.25 mg Alfentanil) administered once or twice during the procedure. In a separate study we tested the concentration of lidocaine that could be reached in the follicular fluid at aspiration and compared fertilization, cleavage rates, and pregnancies in oocytes aspirated from follicles with high lidocaine concentrations with those using low or no measurable amounts of the local anesthetic. No significant differences were found in the 40 patients tested [19].

Another alternative technique for pain relief during oocyte aspiration is electro-acupuncture. We and others have demonstrated that, with good knowledge and experience of the technique, it can be a valid alternative to other analgesic methods during oocyte retrieval [20].

Complications

Bleeding

Despite all the advantages of TVOR that have been described in the preceding sections, it should be kept in mind that the sharp aspiration needle may injure pelvic organs and structures, resulting in serious complications. The most common problem is postoperative hemorrhage. Bleeding from the vaginal wall has been reported with frequencies varying between 1.4% and 18.4% [21]. However, such bleeds generally cease spontaneously or on application of a sponge in the vagina.

Injury to intraperitoneal and/or retroperitoneal pelvic blood vessels has also been reported to occur (~1%) [22].

A severe intra-abdominal bleed should be suspected if the patient shortly after the puncture experience symptoms such as weakness, dizziness, dyspneic complaints over abdominal pain, and tachycardia. Careful hemodynamic monitoring and repeated measurements of the hemoglobin concentration should be performed. The patient will naturally not leave the hospital until convincing data confirm that any suspected bleeding has stopped.

Infection

Pelvic infections in connection with TVOR have been reported by various investigators at a low frequency. Sustained lower abdominal pain, dysuria, and fever are symptoms that may be related to the operative procedure and indicate an infection. Owing to the small risk of pelvic infections after oocyte pick-up there has been discussion whether prophylactic antibiotics should be given in all cases. However, even if use of prophylactic antibiotics is controversial it should be considered in the presence of risk factors, for example, if endometrioma or cystic structures such as hydrosalpinx have been punctured. Our own group does not use prophylactic antibiotics routinely and only four cases of pelvic infections have been diagnosed out of a total of 12 500 TVOR. Cleaning of the vagina prior to puncture can be performed by use of iodine solutions, for example (although our group has only used sterile saline solution). Awareness of even mild potential infection is of great importance for the outcome and in such a case embryo transfer should not be performed. The embryo could instead be frozen and transferred one or two months after the infection has been treated.

Negative effects on the oocyte

The possible adverse effects of ultrasound on an oocyte are theoretically probably more important during the retrieval procedure than during scanning for monitoring of follicular development. The oocyte is probably most vulnerable to damage during the final resumption of the first meiotic division, which in the IVF-ET programs is achieved with human chorionic gonadotropin (hCG) 36–38 hours before oocyte retrieval. Randomized studies comparing ultrasonographically versus laparoscopically guided follicle aspiration, however, have not been interpreted to suggest any differences with regard to pregnancy and take-home baby rates [23]. In conclusion, available data regarding possible adverse effects of ultrasonography on oocytes have been interpreted to indicate that the technique, in this respect, is as safe as laparoscopy.

Concluding remarks

The TVOR procedure has now been used for 25 years in millions of ovum pick-ups (OPUs) all over the world. The technique has been shown to be both simple and safe and is well accepted by the patients, even when performed under local anesthesia with conscious sedation. It can thus be performed as an outpatient procedure. Since it was first introduced the technique has been refined in many ways and can today be regarded as the gold standard for OPU. The low cost compared with the laparoscopic procedure has probably meant that more infertile patients have been given access to ART.

References

1. Belaish-Allart JC, Hazout A, Guilett Rosso F, Glissant M, Testart J, Frydman R. Various techniques for oocyte recovery in an in vitro fertilization and embryo transfer program. *J In Vitro Fert Embryo Transf* 1985; **2**: 99–104.

2. Hamberger L, Wikland M, Nilsson L, Janson PO, Sjögren A, Hillensjö T. Methods for aspiration of human oocytes by various techniques. *Acta Med Rom* 1982; **20**: 370–8.

3. Hackeloer BJ, Flemming R, Robinson HP, Adam AH, Couts JRT. Correlation of ultrasonic and endocrinologic assessment of human follicular development. *Am J Obstet Gynecol* 1979; **135**: 122–8.

4. Wikland M, Nilsson L, Hamberger L. The use of ultrasound in a human in vitro fertilization program. *Ultrasound Med Biol* 1983; **8**(Suppl 2): 609–13.

5. Holm HH, Kvist-Kristensen J, Rasmusen SN, Northeved A, Bardebo H. Ultrasound as a guide in percutaneous puncture technique. *Ultrasonics* 1972; **10**: 83–6.

6. Lenz S, Lauritsen JG. Ultrasonically guided percutaneous aspiration of human follicles under local anaesthesia: a new method of collecting oocytes for in vitro fertilization. *Fertil Steril* 1982; **38**: 673–7.

7. Wikland M, Nilsson L, Hansson R, Hamberger L, Janson PO. Collection of human oocytes by use of sonography. *Fertil Steril* 1983; **39**: 603–8.

8. Wikland M, Fishel SB, Hamberger L. Oocyte recovery by sonographic techniques. *International Conference on Human In-Vitro Fertilization. Serono Symposium* Montreal, Canada, 1984, 79–84.

9. Wikland M, Enk L, Hamberger L. Transvesical and transvaginal approaches for the aspiration of follicles by use of ultrasound. *Ann NY Acad Sci* 1985; **442**: 683–9.

10. Dellenbach P, Nissand I, Moreau L, Feger B, Plumere C, Gerlinger P. Transvaginal sonographically controlled ovarian follicle puncture for egg retrieval. *Lancet* 1984; **1**: 1467.

11. Feichtinger W, Kemeter P. Transvaginal sector scan sonography for needle guided transvaginal follicle aspiration and other applications in gynaecologic routine and research. *Fertil Steril* 1986; **45**: 722–5.

12. Awonuga A, Waterstone J, Oyesanya O, Curson R, Nargund G, Parsons J. A prospective randomized study comparing needles of different diameters for transvaginal ultrasound-directed follicle aspiration. *Fertil Steril* 1996; **65**: 109–13.

13. Mikkelsen AL, Smith S, Lindenberg S. Possible factors affecting the development of oocytes in in-vitro maturation. *Hum Reprod* 2000; **15**(Suppl. 5): 11–17.

14. Choen J, Avery S, Campbell S. Follicular aspiration using a syringe suction system may damage zona pellucida. *J In Vitro Fert Embryo Transf* 1986; **4**: 224–6.

15. Kingsland CR, Taylor CT, Aziz N, Bickeston N. Is follicular flushing necessary for oocyte retrieval? A randomized trial. *Hum Reprod* 1991; **6**: 382–3.

16. Bagtharia, S., Haloob, AR. Is there a benefit from routine follicular flushing for oocyte retrieval? *J Obstet Gynecol* 2005; **25**: 374–6.

17. Ng EH, Tang OS, Chui DK, Ho PC. A prospective randomized double blind and placebo-controlled study to assess the efficacy of paracervical block in the pain relief during egg collection in IVF. *Hum Reprod* 1999; **14**: 2783–7.

18. Ng EH, Chui DK, Tang OS, Ho PC. Paracervical block with and without conscious sedation: a comparison of the pain levels during egg collection and the postoperative side effects. *Fertil Steril* 2001; **75**: 707–11.

19. Wikland M, Enk L, Evers H, Hamberger L, Jakobsson AH, Nilsson L. Lidocaine does not influence the in vitro fertilization and embryo

cleavage in a human IVF/ET program. *Abstract ESHRE Annual Meeting* Copenhagen, 1989.

20. Stener-Victorin E. The pain-relieving effect of electro-acupuncture and conventional analgesic methods during oocyte retrieval: a systematic review of randomized control trials. *Hum Reprod* 2005; **20**: 339–49.

21. Tureck RW, García CR, Blasco L, Mastroianni L. Perioperative complications following transvaginal oocyte retrieval for in vitro fertilization. *Obstet Gynecol* 1993; Apr; **81**(4): 590–3.

22. Serour GI, Aboulghar M, et al. Complications of medically assisted conception in 3,500 cycles. *Fertil Steril* 1998; **70**: 638–42.

23. Flood J, Mausher S, Simonetti S, Kreiner D, Acosta A, Rosenwaks ZJ. Comparison between laparoscopically and ultrasonographically guided transvaginal follicular aspiration methods in an in vitro fertilization program in the same patients using the same stimulation protocol. *J In Vitro Fert Embryo Transf* 1989; **6**: 180–5.

Chapter 28

Ultrasonography-guided embryo transfer: evidence-based practice

Gautam N. Allahbadia

Summary

Thirty years from the first report of a successful in vitro fertilization–embryo transfer (IVF-ET) procedure in 1978, the field of assisted reproductive technology (ART) now enjoys a remarkable increase in success rates, primarily due to improvements in stimulation protocols, laboratory techniques, culture media, technical expertise, and instrumentation. However, the persistently low ART success rates despite what appears as a satisfying treatment protocol have befuddled the scientific fraternity, led to the analytical assessment of every aspect of the technique, and proved the previously held notion of embryo transfer (ET) as being a mere mechanical art wrong. It has now been established beyond doubt that embryo transfer, though imaginatively simple, is one of the most scientifically sophisticated techniques and a significant determinant of success in the long series of cumbersome clinical and laboratory protocols involved in ART that can either dilute or optimize the outcome of treatment.

Although unobvious, yet, inherent defects in the genetic constitution of oocytes and embryos cannot be overcome by an efficient embryo transfer technique, and morphologically good embryos are not necessarily the "best" embryos, a judgmental, methodical, and atraumatic transfer technique under visual ultrasound guidance has, in our hands, proven to impact positively on ART outcomes. Research evaluating the causes of failure following embryo transfer, advances in ultrasound technology, catheter design, and function, identification of the site of maximum implantation potential, and fresh evaluation of the influence of transferred matter and intrauterine forces on embryo implantation, have all contributed to an almost unanimous concept that there is more to the technique of embryo transfer than a blind and mindless ejection of the embryo through the catheter and have taken the science of embryo transfer a leap ahead. Embryo transfer is a true blend of art and science!

Recent publications have stressed that despite its apparent simplicity, the technique of embryo transfer is of utmost importance in maximizing the chances of pregnancy. There is now a general agreement in the IVF community that a smooth and atraumatic embryo transfer is critical for achieving high success rates, and the choice of technique and the choice of embryo replacement catheter may both play a crucial role in uterine embryo replacement.

Rationale

Ultrasound-guided embryo transfer (USG-ET) is widely suggested as a standard clinical practice that improves overall embryo implantation and pregnancy rates. Although a majority of studies in the past have concluded that USG-ET holds a clear advantage over the "clinical touch" method or blind embryo transfer, various studies on this issue suffer from methodological pitfalls [1]. Recent evidence from single-operator, randomized controlled trials testifies to the contrary and has re-addressed the absolute necessity of USG-ET. Is USG-ET an indispensable constituent of the ET technique? Does the catheter choice under USG-ET impact the outcome? If USG-ET must be used, does transvaginal USG-ET score over the transabdominal technique? While attempting to answer these questions in the sections below, we will also discuss how recent advances in ultrasound technology and catheter design have influenced the practice of ET.

Introduction

Many women undergoing an assisted reproductive technology (ART) cycle will not achieve a live birth. Failure at the embryo transfer stage may be due to poor embryo quality, lack of uterine receptivity, or the transfer technique itself. The success of the ET is dependent upon multiple factors including embryo quality, proper endometrial receptivity, and the embryo transfer technique. Uterine contractions, expulsion of embryos, blood or mucus on the catheter tip, bacterial contamination of the catheter, and retained embryos have all been associated with problematic and unsuccessful embryo transfers. Variables affecting pregnancy and recognized as important for successful embryo implantation include the ease of ET [2], the presence of blood or mucus on the transfer catheter [3,4,5], the type of catheter used [6], catheter loading [7,8,9], and the technique used to perform the transfer [10,11,12], uterine depth and the precise depth of embryo replacement in the uterine cavity [13], avoidance of uterine junctional zone contractions [14,15], and

Ultrasonography in Reproductive Medicine and Infertility, ed. Botros R. M. B. Rizk. Published by Cambridge University Press. © Cambridge University Press 2010.

Table 28.1. Advantages of ultrasound-guided embryo transfer

1. Facilitates placement of soft catheters.

2. Avoids touching the fundus.

3. Confirms that the catheter is beyond the internal os in cases of an elongated cervical canal.

4. Allows direction of the catheter along the contour of the endometrial cavity, thereby avoiding disruption of the endometrium, plugging of the catheter tip with endometrium, and instigation of bleeding.

5. Full bladder required to perform transabdominal ultrasonographic guidance is in itself helpful in straightening the cervical uterine access and improving pregnancy rates [24].

6. May facilitate an uncomplicated access through the cervix to access the uterine cavity, thus overcoming cervical stenosis [25].

7. Facilitates tracking of the site of embryo deposition

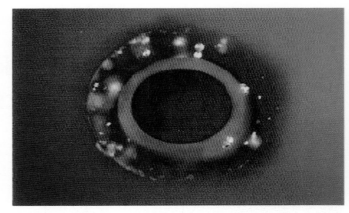

Figure 28.1. Cross-section of the SureView catheter.

the experience of the physician [16,17]. It has been suggested that the clinician's perception of transfer difficulty was the most important variable of all [18]. Initially, intrauterine ETs were performed blindly, but transabdominal ultrasound [12] and, more recently, vaginal ultrasound guidance [19] have added more consistency to the procedure.

Optimizing the technique of ET would, therefore, provide the best chance for pregnancy. It is imperative that all efforts be made to avoid difficult embryo transfers provoking bleeding, remove cervical mucus, and to deposit embryos as gently as possible during IVF, avoiding maneuvers that might trigger uterine contractions, which could adversely affect the results of this treatment. Evaluation before IVF treatment must include a trial transfer and uterine ultrasonography to evaluate the transfer step, anticipate problems, and thus improve treatment. The use of soft catheters and ultrasound guidance facilitate embryo transfer [20].

The embryo transfer catheter may be inserted in one of two ways: blindly by "clinical touch" or with ultrasonographic guidance. Ultrasound-guided embryo transfer during an IVF cycle was initially reported during the mid 1980s [12,21], and has gradually become an integral part of the embryo transfer technique for many IVF clinics. The use of ultrasound guidance for proper catheter placement in the endometrial cavity has been suggested as a means of improving the technique of embryo transfer [22]. No standard evidence-based protocol exists, but ET with ultrasound guidance has been shown to significantly increase the chance of embryo implantation, an ongoing pregnancy, and a live birth and to improve the ease of transfer [23]. The advantages of ultrasonographic guidance are summarized in Table 28.1 [24,25].

Ancillary advantages include the assessment of the ovaries and the presence of excessive peritoneal fluid volume to confirm that the risk for the ovarian hyperstimulation syndrome is not so great as to preclude embryo transfer. Fluid in the endometrial cavity can also be ruled out. The benefit of USG-ET may be due to the reduction in the incidence of difficult transfers [26,27], endometrial trauma [26,28], and bleeding [5,29] that can cause strong fundo-uterine contractions. Ultrasound can ensure catheter placement into the endometrial cavity, [30] or

decrease the chance of improper embryo placement [31,32]. It allows an examination of the relationship between the site of embryo placement and the possible outcome [33]. Two recent studies demonstrated that cavity depth, as noted by ultrasound at the time of embryo transfer, differed from the cavity depth via office trial transfer by >1.0 cm in >30% of cases [30,34]. However, the main disadvantages of using ultrasound guidance during embryo transfer may be the additional time and personnel required as well as patient discomfort due to a full bladder and the urge to urinate [35].

It is suggested that the decrease in cervical and uterine trauma can play a role in increasing the pregnancy rates associated with USG-ET [36]. Over the past two years, we have been performing transabdominal sonography (TAS)-guided embryo transfers using the SureView catheter (Wallace, UK) for all ETs in our program. For acutely anteverted uteri, we routinely mold the catheter according to the uterocervical angle seen on TAS. Molding of the embryo transfer catheter according to the uterocervical angle, measured by sonography, has been shown to increase the clinical pregnancy and implantation rates and diminish the incidence of difficult and bloody transfers. Use of the stylet under sonographic guidance to negotiate difficult cervical passage makes the ET technique very easy and less traumatic and bloody [37].

Several transfer catheters with stronger ultrasound reflection have been developed [38]. The use of the echogenic SureView and the Cook echo-dense catheters simplify ultrasound-guided embryo transfer as compared with the widely used standard soft Wallace catheter. The echodense tip [Cook Echo-Tip catheter (Cook Ob/Gyn, Australia)] is a modification of the soft-tip Wallace catheter in that the catheter has an echogenic stainless steel band at the tip of the inner sheath or echogenicity extending along the whole length of the catheter (SureView Wallace embryo replacement catheter). The echogenicity is brought about by small air bubbles contained within the polyurethane of the catheter itself and present along the whole length of the catheter (Figure 28.1). Limiting the time of embryo manipulation during the transfer technique may increase pregnancy rates after ART. The Sure-Pro and the Sure-Pro Ultra embryo transfer catheter sets, that include the echogenic properties of the SureView

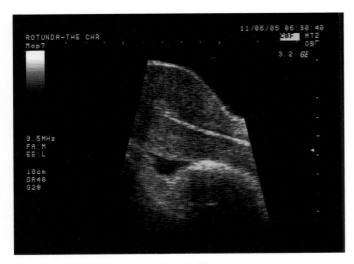

Figure 28.2. SureView catheter with air bubble.

catheters along with an obturator and stylet, respectively, have also been introduced for difficult embryo transfers. The catheter picture under ultrasound is likened to a "candle or torch in the uterus" (Figure 28.2). The exact basis on which USG-ET improves clinical pregnancy rates and embryo implantation is unclear, although confirming the position of the tip of the embryo transfer catheter actually within the uterine cavity is, obviously, a major benefit.

Clinical discussion

Does ultrasound guidance during embryo transfer really make a difference?

Several studies [22,35,36,39,40,41,42] have demonstrated a significantly higher pregnancy outcome following transabdominal USG-ET, while few [43,44,45] have reported the contrary. Recent studies from single-operator, randomized controlled trials [1,46] have demonstrated no significant impact of USG-ET over the clinical touch method.

Matorras et al. [36] conducted a prospective randomized (computer-generated random table) trial to compare embryo transfer under abdominal US guidance ($n = 255$ women) with clinical touch embryo transfer ($n = 260$), and concluded that USG-ET is associated with a significant increase in the clinical pregnancy rate (26.3% vs 18.1%; $P < 0.05$) and implantation rate (11.1% vs. 7.5%; $P < 0.05$) and a significant decrease in the difficulty of transfers (3% vs. 19%; $P < 0.05$) compared with the clinical touch group. They attributed the increase in pregnancy rates associated with USG-ET to a decrease in cervical and uterine trauma. Sallam and Sadek [39], in a meta-analysis of four randomized controlled studies comprising a total of 2051 patients (1024 ultrasound-guided embryo transfers; 1027 clinical touch method transfers), also concluded that USG-ET increases the clinical pregnancy and ongoing pregnancy rates significantly compared with the clinical touch method, while there were no differences in the incidence of ectopic pregnancy,

multiple pregnanies, or miscarriage rate. Similar results have been obtained by Buckett [35] in his systematic review and meta-analysis of eight randomized, controlled trials (four non-randomized or quasi-randomized and four genuinely randomized) to determine the relative efficacy of USG-ET and embryo transfer by clinical touch alone; these were further confirmed by Li et al. [40] in their prospective randomized trial, who recommended that embryo transfer should be performed under ultrasound guidance. However, a contemporary study from Brazil by de Camargo Martins et al. [43] reported no significant difference in pregnancy and implantation rates following embryo transfer with and without ultrasound guidance, and concluded that, as long as previous mock transfers are routinely performed during a cycle preceding assisted reproduction and the clinician considers transfer to be easy, ultrasound does not benefit the process of embryo transfer. This study was, nevertheless, very small to arrive at a concrete conclusion.

In an exhaustive Cochrane Database Systematic Review that included 13/15 randomized controlled trials only, Brown et al. [22] reported significantly higher live birth/ongoing pregnancies per woman randomized associated with USG-ET (452/1376 compared with 353/1338 for clinical touch; odds ratio [OR] 1.40; 95% confidence interval [CI] 1.18–1.66; $P < 0.0001$) in six studies. They suggested that for a population of women with a 25% chance of pregnancy using clinical touch, this would be increased to 32% (28–46%) by using USG-ET. There were no statistically significant differences in the incidence of adverse events between the two comparison groups, with the exception of blood on the catheter. Although they concluded that ultrasound guidance does appear to improve the chances of live/ongoing and clinical pregnancies compared with clinical touch methods, the authors recognized that this study was limited in quality, with only one of the 13 studies reporting details of both computerized randomization techniques and adequate allocation concealment [22].

Abou-Setta et al. [41] further buttressed the observations of Brown et al. [22] in the largest ever meta-analysis conducted to date, comprising of a systematic review of prospective, randomized, controlled trials comparing ultrasound with clinical touch methods of embryo catheter guidance. They reported a significantly increased chance of a live birth (OR 1.78; 95% CI 1.19–2.67), ongoing pregnancy (OR 1.51; 95% CI 1.31–1.74), clinical pregnancy (OR 1.50; 95% CI 1.34–1.67), embryo implantation (OR 1.35; 95% CI 1.22–1.50), and easy transfer rates after ultrasound guidance (OR 0.68; 95% CI 0.58–0.81). Twenty studies comprising 5968 ET cycles in women were analyzed. There was no difference in multiple pregnancy, ectopic pregnancy, or miscarriage rates. They concluded that USG-ET significantly increases the chance of live birth and ongoing and clinical pregnancy rates compared with the clinical touch method [41].

García-Velasco et al. [44] contested the observations in these extensively researched studies in their prospective, randomized, controlled trial on 374 patients and concluded no significant benefit of ultrasound guidance over clinical touch transfers with regard to pregnancy, implantation, miscarriage or multiple pregnancy rates. Although ectopic pregnancies were only observed in the clinical touch group (0% vs. 2.7%), there was no significant difference. However, it must be noted that this study, in contrast to the previous studies, was performed on oocyte recipients, where the oocyte quality and endometrial receptivity were, perhaps, largely controlled [44].

In yet another attempt to compare pregnancy rates after USG-ET and embryo transfer based on ultrasonographic length measurement, ultrasonographic guidance was not shown to significantly influence the pregnancy compared with previous ultrasonographic length measurement [45]. However, this study could possibly be biased in that, while the intervention group was prospective, the control group was retrospective, overlooking any changes in techniques or protocols that may have taken place besides the comparison in question. Additionally, patients undergoing both IVF and intracytoplasmic sperm injection were included in the study, which may further confound the results.

Flisser et al. [46] analyzed the influence of USG-ET on the clinical outcome of IVF in comparison with the "clinical touch" method of transcervical embryo transfer by one physician, to determine whether transabdominal ultrasound should be routinely applied to all cases of embryo transfer in this practice in a retrospective study. Demographic and cycle characteristics and the difficulty of ET were controlled. They concluded that USG-ET does not confer any additional advantage and, in experienced hands, the "clinical touch" method of embryo transfer yields equivalent results to transabdominal ultrasound-guided embryo placement. However, in patients with a prior history of difficult uterine sounding or embryo transfer, transabdominal ultrasound guidance may still play a role.

In a further effort to determine whether the implementation of ultrasound guidance will improve the clinical outcomes of ET compared with the standard clinical touch method of embryo catheter placement, Eskandar et al. [42] performed a prospective, single-operator, randomized, controlled trial in which 373 women underwent transcervical, intrauterine ET with or without ultrasound guidance. They reported significantly higher live-birth/ongoing pregnancy rates (40.98% vs. 28.42%; OR 1.66; 95% CI 1.07–2.57) and clinical pregnancies (40.98% vs. 28.42%; OR 1.75; 95% CI 1.14–2.69) in the USG-ET group compared with the clinical touch ET group. Demographics and cycle characteristics were not different between the two groups.

Owing to methodological biases inherent in combining numerous studies with varying stimulation protocols, different laboratory techniques, different operators, and different interpretations, evident in previous studies, Kosmas et al. [1] recently conducted a randomized, double-blind controlled trial by a single experienced operator to verify the superiority of USG-ET. Three hundred women aged <40 underwent fresh USG-ET with the K-J-SPPE echo tip soft catheter, or with the traditional K-Soft catheter if ultrasound was not used. The authors reported no difference in the pregnancy outcome or difficulty in cervical negotiation between the two groups and concluded that in

patients undergoing ET by an experienced operator, ultrasound guidance did not provide any benefit in terms of overall clinical pregnancy and embryo implantation rates.

Transvaginal ultrasound-guided embryo transfer enables the visualization of (1) the guiding cannula and transfer catheter placement in relation to the endometrial surface and uterine fundus during embryo transfer, (2) the position and movement of a transfer-associated air bubble, and (3) the impact of subendometrial myometrial contraction leading to endometrial movement. The tactile assessment of embryo transfer catheter placement is unreliable and the outer guiding catheter has been shown to either inadvertently abut the fundal endometrium (17.4% transfers), indent the endometrium (24.8% transfers), or embed in the endometrium (33.1% transfers). While unavoidable subendometrial transfers occurred in 22.3% of transfers, ultrasound-guided transfer avoided accidental tubal transfer in 7.4% of the transfers. Endometrial movement due to subendometrial myometrial contraction was obvious in 36.4% of cases, with active motion of the transfer-associated air bubble occurring in 28.1% [26].

Transvaginal vs. transabdominal ultrasound-guided embryo transfer

Transvaginal sonography gives a much better view of the uterine cavity than transabdominal sonography. We attempted to evaluate whether transabdominal sonographic guidance (TAS) or transvaginal sonographic guidance (TVS) during embryo transfer is a better tool for increasing pregnancy rates in patients undergoing oocyte donation [47]. Two hundred and eighty-six infertile patients undergoing oocyte donation were included in this study. Transabdominal ($n = 169$) and transvaginal ($n = 117$) USG-ET, performed by the same physician, was documented on video. The main outcome measures studied were the ease of passage of the catheter, ease of visualization of the ET catheter, and the pregnancy and implantation rates after transabdominal versus transvaginal USG-ET. The age groups, laboratory techniques, number and grade of embryos transferred, and the embryo transfer catheter (SureView, Wallace, UK) in both the groups were comparable. A clinical pregnancy was defined by the presence of an intrauterine gestational sac at 7 weeks. Superior visualization on sonography during ET was achieved in all the patients who had a transvaginal USG-ET. A similar number of easy transfers were performed in both the TAS-guided ($n = 160$) and TVS-guided ($n = 110$) groups (94.6% vs. 94%, respectively). The pregnancy rate was comparable between the groups (52.07% TAS vs. 52.13% TVS) as was the implantation rate (28.6% TAS vs. 26.3% TVS). No differences were found in the miscarriage rate (9.7% TAS vs. 9.1% TVS) or in the multiple pregnancy rates (26.62% TAS vs. 27.35% TVS). We could not show any benefit in terms of pregnancy rate in oocyte recipients for whom ET was performed under transvaginal sonographic visualization of the endometrial cavity [26]. This technique gave us superior visualization of the ET catheter tip and the air bubble

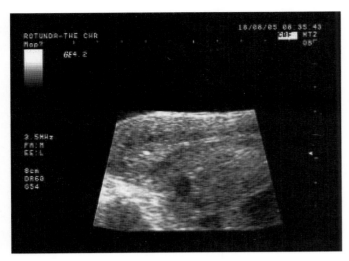

Figure 28.3. Placement of air bubble with the SureView catheter.

containing the culture media and embryos and was also better tolerated by the majority of patients because of the comfort of an empty bladder. However, it was technically more cumbersome and demanding on the physician's skills since the ET technique had to be controlled with one hand only. We recommend TAS-guided ET for all patients without compromising success rates in an oocyte donation program [47].

Kojima et al. [48] have confirmed that the use of transvaginal USG-ET, although technically difficult, shows the ability to maximize the chances of achieving a successful pregnancy outcome compared with the clinical touch method.

Does the catheter choice in USG-ET really make a difference?

Previous investigations have not conclusively shown improved pregnancy rates with ultrasonographic guidance, possibly because of the need for catheter movement for identification of the tip and resultant disruption of the endometrium. The immediate identification of the catheter may provide a method for precise, atraumatic ET [28]. The combination of a modern catheter and ultrasound allows visual monitoring of the entire ET process while navigating embryo placement within the uterine cavity with high precision. A recent development is the availability of the soft Wallace echogenic catheter (SureView Wallace Embryo Transfer Catheter; Smiths Medical, Kent, UK), which utilizes new technology specifically designed to visually enhance the catheter's appearance under ultrasound. The Wallace SureView Embryo Transfer Catheter (Figure 28.1) combines the advantages of the traditional ultrasoft Wallace catheter and the echogenic properties that make the entire length of the catheter visible to the physician doing the embryo transfer under ultrasonographic guidance. The attending physician can be more accurate regarding the embryo deposition site when using the SureView catheter (Figure 28.3).

It has been postulated that new echodense catheters that are more readily detectable by ultrasound may refine transfer

techniques in addition to USG-ET, thus improving the IVF outcome [49]. The echo-dense tip of the Cook Echo-Tip catheter is seen consistently with ultrasound guidance, minimizing the need for catheter movement to identify the tip [50]. The use of the echodense catheter facilitates catheter identification under ultrasound and, thus, reduces the duration of the embryo transfer procedure. The time elapsed from when the loaded catheter was handed to the physician up to embryo discharge was significantly shorter in the echogenic catheter group than in the standard catheter group [49].

Karande et al. [50] compared the performance of a new coaxial catheter system with an echo-dense tip (Cook Echo-Tip catheter) with a Wallace catheter during ultrasound-guided ET in a prospective, randomized study on 251 patients undergoing USG-ET by a single physician with a standardized technique. They reported no significant difference in the implantation rate (30% vs. 35%), clinical pregnancy rate (57% vs. 55%), or the ongoing pregnancy rate (49% vs. 47%) between the two catheters and concluded that the Cook Echo-Tip catheter, with its echogenic tip, simplifies USG-ET. However, it does not significantly impact pregnancy success rates in comparison with the use of a Wallace catheter.

Coroleu et al. [49] conducted a prospective, randomized, controlled trial to compare the IVF outcome in women undergoing embryo transfer with either the standard soft Wallace catheter (standard catheter group, $n = 95$) or the new echogenic soft Wallace catheter (echogenic catheter group, $n = 98$) under ultrasound guidance by a single healthcare provider. Women were randomly assigned to either of the groups, according to a computer-generated randomization table. There were no significant differences in the clinical pregnancy rates between the standard catheter and echogenic catheter groups (41.0% vs. 54.1%, respectively; $P < 0.08$). However, the authors interpreted the significantly high twin pregnancy rate ($P < 0.01$) in the echogenic catheter group as the underlying source for obtaining a significant increase in implantation rate in this group (37.1%) as compared with the standard catheter group (23.2%). In accordance with Karande et al. [50], they also concluded that although the use of the echogenic Wallace catheter simplifies ultrasound-guided embryo transfer, no definite benefit in terms of pregnancy rates was obtained. However, an association with a significant increase in the number of twin pregnancies was observed.

Wood et al. [51] evaluated two different embryo transfer techniques of potential clinical importance, performed in 518 cycles over two contiguous time periods in order to observe any corresponding change in clinical pregnancy rate (CPR) per transfer: (1) embryo transfer catheter; (2) ultrasound guidance. Ultrasound visualization was considered to be excellent/good when the catheter could be followed from the cervix to the fundus by TAS with retention of the embryo-containing fluid droplet; and fair/poor if visualization could not document the sequence of events. The CPR was significantly higher with the use of the soft (Frydman or Wallace) catheters compared with the use of the hard (Tefcat, Tom Cat, or Norfolk) catheters

(36% vs. 17% respectively; $P < 0.000$). The clinical pregnancy rate per transfer was significantly higher in the ultrasound guidance group (38% vs. 25%; $P < 0.002$), and in all excellent/good ultrasound-guided transfers (41.5% vs.16.7%, $P < 0.038$) compared with fair/poor transfers. They concluded that embryo transfer performed with a soft catheter under ultrasound guidance with good visualization resulted in a significant increase in clinical pregnancy rates [51].

We conducted a prospective, randomized study to compare the standard Wallace catheters versus SureView catheters used for ET under ultrasound guidance All the transfers were performed by a single physician at a fixed distance (15 ± 2 mm from the uterine fundus) and the same transfer technique was scrupulously maintained with all the patients. Ultrasound visualization of the catheter to obtain the pre-selected position for embryo transfer was assessed as excellent/good when the catheter could be easily tracked during the first pass with minimal transducer movement in the transverse plane. Fair/poor visualization during the procedure was recorded if marked transducer or catheter movements were necessary for the appropriate catheter. The ease of each transfer procedure was assessed according to the following criteria: *very easy*, when the catheter passed smoothly through the cervix; *easy*, when the rigid outer Teflon sheath was required; and *difficult*, when the use of a tenaculum was necessary in addition to the above. We observed better ease of transfer and excellent visualization with the SureView catheters [52].

However, in contrast to the previously published evidence, Aboulfotouh et al. [53] maintain that, under ultrasound guidance, individual catheter choice does not significantly affect the statistical clinical pregnancy rate in a modern clinical IVF practice, possibly as a result of a decreasing incidence of difficult transfers and endometrial injury at ET under ultrasound guidance.

Recent advances

Two-dimensional vs. three-dimensional ultrasound guidance

From the studies discussed above, it is evident that two-dimensional ultrasound guidance is an integral part of embryo transfer techniques that facilitates the visualization of catheter passage through the cervix into the endometrial cavity, minimizes trauma and, thus, improves clinical pregnancy rates. However, catheter three-dimensional ultrasound guidance may be a better tool for monitoring catheter placement and assessing the relationship of the catheter tip to the uterine cavity.

To compare the precision of catheter placement and position by two- and three-dimensional ultrasound, Letterie [54] pre-screened the cervix, uterus, and endometrial cavity of 24 patients in two dimensions, at the midline in the longitudinal plane of the uterus. Embryo transfers were then performed under two-dimensional guidance. Following satisfactory embryo transfer catheter placement, the catheter was held in

place for 60–120 seconds and net volume acquisition was attained during this interval. All images were stored and retrospectively reviewed. Embryo transfer catheter placement with two-dimensional ultrasound guidance was then compared with the images obtained simultaneously in three planes. The two-dimensional ultrasound images suggested that the catheter was 2 cm from the uterine fundus and in the midline. Out of the 21/24 satisfactory three-dimensional images that were available for review and comparison, the three-dimensional ultrasound images confirmed placement and agreed with the findings of two-dimensional ultrasound images in 17 of 21 patients. In 4 patients, the catheter tip on three-dimensional ultrasound was observed to be displaced either anteriorly or laterally from the ideal region, as suggested by two-dimensional ultrasound. In one case, the catheter tip on three-dimensional ultrasound was observed to be far laterally in the region of the uterine cornua. The authors concluded that although two-dimensional ultrasound-guided embryo transfer continues to be the standard for image-guided transfers, enabling convenient visualization of the catheter tip, the precision of catheter tip placement and, consequently, embryo transfer may be improved with three-dimensional imaging. Four of 21 patients studied had catheter tip placement in a different and less-than-ideal area when studied with three-dimensional ultrasound. Three-dimensional imaging may provide an improvement in embryo transfer technique and have a positive impact on overall pregnancy rates [54].

Maximal implantation potential

Gergely et al. [55] attempted to evaluate the use of the maximal implantation potential (MIP) point in conjunction with a 3D/4D ultrasound in order to facilitate embryo transfers and potentially improve pregnancy rate in a retrospective, observational study on 1222 patients who underwent 3D/4D-ultrasound-guided embryo transfers. They reported improved visualization, a greater accuracy in the placement of embryos within the uterine cavity, and a pregnancy rate of 36.66% (average patient age, 37.6 years) following embryo transfers at the MIP point and concluded that embryo transfers at the MIP, which can be identified and individualized for each patient, are associated with good implantation and pregnancy rates [55].

Conclusion

The goal of transcervical embryo transfer is to deliver embryos to the uterine fundus in a gentle, atraumatic manner at the presumed site of maximum implantation potential. Studies evaluating the role of ultrasound-guided ET have had mixed results, and although the meta-analyses of prospective randomized controlled trials suggest an improvement in pregnancy outcome, most of these studies suffer from methodological pitfalls [1], varying in stimulation protocols, the indications for ART, the technique of ET, the experience of the operator, laboratory techniques, and culture media and conditions. Evidence from recent single-operator, prospective randomized trials, addressing the utility of ultrasound-guided ET, has shown no clear advantage compared with the "clinical touch" method in the hands of an experienced operator. While ultrasound-guided ET is clearly advantageous in visualizing the course of the catheter in the uterine cavity and avoiding endometrial trauma, it is not indispensable to the technique if details of uterine measurement have been obtained at a mock transfer and may be reserved for patients with a prior history of difficult uterine sounding or embryo transfer.

With regard to the technique of ultrasound-guided ET, although transvaginal USG-ET has been shown to be better tolerated by patients because of the comfort of an empty bladder, and to yield superior visualization of the ET catheter tip compared with transabdominal ultrasound-guided ET, it is technically more cumbersome and demanding on the physician's skills. Therefore, unless technically equipped personnel are available to perform transvaginal USG-ET, it may be more appropriate to use transabdominal ultrasound-guided ET.

The evolution of the new echogenic catheters, such as SureView Wallace Embryo Transfer Catheter and Cook Echodense catheters, which employ new technology specifically designed to visually enhance the catheter's appearance under ultrasound, enables visual monitoring of the entire ET process while navigating embryo placement within the uterine cavity with high precision. However, research in this direction suggests that although the echogenic catheters simplify USG-ET by improving visualization and refining the ET technique, they do not significantly impact pregnancy success rates in comparison with the use of a Wallace catheter. Hence, under ultrasound guidance, individual catheter choice does not significantly affect the statistical clinical pregnancy rate in a modern clinical IVF practice, owing to the advantages conferred by ultrasound guidance in itself.

Although the essential features of embryo transfer in humans remain unchanged since its first description by Edwards et al. [56] nearly 20 years ago, the only constant in life is change. Hence, today, the fertility physician must make a conscious effort to keep up with the technology to optimize results. The application of technology such as 3D and 4D sonography, as well as focused research on the point of deposition of embryos, will probably lead the way forward. However, the lack of prospective, randomized trials in this area precludes making too many assumptions. Identification of appropriate ultrasound-guided simulation training techniques in ET would ensure adequate fellowship training without affecting the outcome of ART cycles [23].

Since no large trial has so far demonstrated an adverse effect, and because those patients who may benefit from its use can often not be predicted reliably, the routine application of ultrasonography can be justified. The routine use of echogenic catheters will add to the refinement of the technique for all ultrasonography-guided embryo transfers. A large-scale single operator, prospective, randomized controlled trial that incorporates all the features of modern IVF technology and the advances in ET techniques known to date would be beneficial in assessing the true prognostic value of these developments. The learning curve involved in overcoming the advantages conferred by ultrasound guidance during ET and relying solely on tactile feedback without compromising the ART outcome would be worth examining.

References

1. Kosmas IP, Janssens R, De Munck L, et al. Ultrasound-guided embryo transfer does not offer any benefit in clinical outcome: a randomized controlled trial. *Hum Reprod* 2007; **22**(5): 1327–34.

2. Mansour RT, Aboulghar MA. Optimizing the embryo transfer technique. *Hum Reprod* 2002; **17**, 1149–53.

3. Alvero R, Hearns-Stokes RM, Catherino WH, Leondires MP, Segars JH. The presence of blood in the transfer catheter negatively influences outcome at embryo transfer. *Hum Reprod* 2003; **18**: 1848–52.

4. Glass KB, Green CA, Fluker MR, Schoolcraft WB, McNamee PI, Meldrum D. Multicenter randomized trial of cervical irrigation at the time of embryo transfer (Abstract). *Fertil Steril* 2000; **74** (Suppl 1): S31.

5. Goudas VT, Hammitt DG, Damario MA, Session DR, Singh AP, Dumesic DA. Blood on the embryo transfer catheter is associated with decreased rates of embryo implantation and clinical pregnancy with the use of *in vitro* fertilization-embryo transfer. *Fertil Steril* 1998; **70**: 878–82.

6. van Weering H, Schats R, McDonnell J, Vink JM, Vermeiden J, Hompes P. The impact of the embryo transfer catheter on the pregnancy rate in IVF. *Hum Reprod* 2002; **17**: 666–70.

7. Meldrum DR, Chetkowski R, Steingold KA, de Ziegler D, Cedars MI, Hamilton M. Evolution of a highly successful *in vitro* fertilization embryo transfer program. *Fertil Steril* 1987; **48**: 86–93.

8. Correa-Perez JR, Fernandez-Pelegrina R. Air transfer in the catheter–good or bad? *Fertil Steril* 2004; **83**: 520–1.

9. Allahbadia GN, Gandhi GN, Kadam KS. A prospective randomized comparison of two different embryo transfer catheter loading techniques. *Fertil Steril* 2005; **84**(Suppl. 1), S114–15.

10. van de Pas MMC, Weima S, Looman CWN, Broekmans FJM. The use of fixed distance embryo transfer after IVF/ICSI equalizes the success rates among physicians. *Hum Reprod* 2003; **18**: 774–80.

11. Coroleu B, Carreras O, Veija A, et al. Embryo transfer under ultrasound guidance improves pregnancy rates after *in vitro* fertilization. *Hum Reprod* 2000; **15**: 616–20.

12. Leong M, Leung C, Tucker M, Wong C, Chan H. Ultrasound-assisted embryo transfer. *J In Vitro Fert Embryo Transf* 1986; **3**: 383–5.

13. Coroleu B, Barri PN, Carreras O, et al. The influence of the depth of embryo replacement into the uterine cavity on implantation rates after IVF: a controlled, ultrasound-guided study. *Hum Reprod* 2002; **17**: 341–6.

14. Fanchin R, Righini C, Olivennes F, Taylor S, de Ziegler D, Frydman R. Uterine contractions at the time of embryo transfer alter pregnancy rates after *in vitro* fertilization. *Hum Reprod* 1998; **13**: 1968–74.

15. Lesny P, Killick SR, Tetlow RL, Robinson J, Maguiness SD. Embryo transfer and uterine junctional zone

contractions. *Hum Reprod Update* 1999; **5**: 87–8.

16. Papageorgiou T, Hearns-Stokes RM, Leondires MP, et al. Training of providers in embryo transfer: what is the minimum number of transfers required for proficiency? *Hum Reprod* 2001; **16**: 1415–19.

17. Karande VC, Morris R, Chapman C, Rinehart J, Gleicher N. Impact of the "physician factor" on pregnancy rates in a large assisted reproductive technology program: do too many cooks spoil the broth? *Fertil Steril* 1999; **71**: 1001–9.

18. Lass A, Abusheikha N, Brinsden P, Kovacs GT. The effect of a difficult embryo transfer on the outcome of IVF. *Hum Reprod* 1999; **14**: 2417.

19. Anderson RE, Nugent NL, Gregg AT, Nunn SL, Behr BR. Transvaginal ultrasoundguided embryo transfer improves outcome in patients with previous failed *in vitro* fertilization cycles. *Fertil Steril* 2002; **77**: 769–75.

20. Frydman R. [Impact of embryo transfer techniques on implantation rates] [Article in French]. *J Gynecol Obstet Biol Reprod (Paris)* 2004; **33**(1 pt 2): S36–9.

21. Strickler RC, Christianson C, Crane JP, Curato A, Knight AB, Yang V. Ultrasound guidance for human embryo transfer. *Fertil Steril* 1985; **43**(1): 54–61.

22. Brown JA, Buckingham K, Abou-Setta A, Buckett W. Ultrasound versus 'clinical touch' for catheter guidance during embryo transfer in women. *Cochrane Database Syst Rev* 2007; **(1)**:CD006107.

23. Porter MB. Ultrasound in assisted reproductive technology. *Semin Reprod Med* 2008; **26**(3): 266–76.

24. Lewin A, Schenker JG, Avrech O, Shapira S, Safran A, Friedler S. The role of uterine straightening by passive bladder distention before embryo transfer in IVF cycles. *J Assist Reprod Genet* 1997; **14**: 32–4.

25. Christianson MS, Barker MA, Lindheim SR. Overcoming the challenging cervix: techniques to access the uterine cavity. *J Low Genit Tract Dis* 2008; **12**(1): 24–31.

26. Woolcott R, Stanger J. Potentially important variables identified by transvaginal ultrasound-guided embryo transfer. *Hum Reprod* 1997; **12**(5): 963–6.

27. Mirkin S, Jones EL, Mayer JF, Stadtmauer L, Gibbons WE, Oehninger S. Impact of transabdominal ultrasound guidance on performance and outcome of transcervical uterine embryo transfer. *J Assist Reprod Genet* 2003: **20**; 318–22.

28. Letterie GS, Marshall L, Angle M. A new coaxial catheter system with an echodense tip for ultrasonographically guided embryo transfer. *Fertil Steril* 1999 Aug; **72**(2): 266–8.

29. Sallam HN. Embryo transfer: Factors involved in optimizing the success. *Curr Opin Obstet Gynecol* 2005; **17**: 289–98.

30. Pope CS, Cook EK D, Arny M, Novak A, Grow DR. Influence of embryo transfer depth on *in vitro* fertilization and embryo transfer outcomes. *Fertil Steril* 2004; **81**: 51–8.

31. Schoolcraft WB, Surrey ES, Gardner DK. Embryo transfer: Techniques and variables affecting success. *Fertil Steril* 2001; **76**: 863–70.

32. Pasqualini RS, Quintans S. Clinical practice of embryo transfer. *Reprod Biomed Online* 2002; **4**: 83–92.

33. Cavagna M, Contart P, Petersen CG, et al. Implantation sites after embryo transfer into the central area of the uterine cavity. *Reprod Biomed Online* 2006; **13**(4): 541–6.

34. Shamonki MI, Spandorfer SD, Rosenwaks Z. Ultrasound-guided embryo transfer and the accuracy of trial embryo transfer. *Hum Reprod* 2005; **20**(3): 709–16.

35. Buckett WM. A meta-analysis of ultrasound-guided versus clinical touch embryo transfer. *Fertil Steril* 2003; **80**: 1037–41.

36. Matorras R, Urquijo E, Mendoza R, Corcóstegui B, Expósito A, Rodríguez-Escudero FJ. Ultrasound-guided embryo transfer improves pregnancy rates and increases the frequency of easy transfers. *Hum Reprod* 2002; **17**(7): 1762–6.

37. Allahbadia GN, Kadam KS, Gandhi GN, Arora S, Mhatre YP, Virk S. The stilette for a SureView. *Fertil Steril* 2006; **86**(Suppl 3): S252.

38. Coroleu B, Barri PN, Carreras O, et al. Effect of using an echogenic catheter for ultrasound-guided embryo transfer in an IVF programme: a prospective, randomized, controlled study. *Hum Reprod* 2006; **21**(7): 1809–15.

39. Sallam HN, Sadek SS. Ultrasound-guided embryo transfer: a meta-analysis of randomized controlled trials. *Fertil Steril* 2003; **80**(4): 1042–6.

40. Li R, Zhuang GL, Cai ZM, Wang H, Zhong K, Zhou WY. [Clinical analysis of ultrasound-guided embryo transfer after in-vitro fertilization] [Article in Chinese] *Zhonghua Fu Chan Ke Za Zhi* 2004; **39**(3): 180–3.

41. Abou-Setta AM, Mansour RT, Al-Inany HG, Aboulghar MM, Aboulghar MA, Serour GI. Among women undergoing embryo transfer, is the probability of pregnancy and live birth improved with ultrasound guidance over clinical touch alone? A systemic review and meta-analysis of prospective randomized trials. *Fertil Steril* 2007; **88**(2): 333–41.

42. Eskandar M, Abou-Setta AM, Almushait MA, El-Amin M, Mohmad SE. Ultrasound guidance during embryo transfer: a prospective, single-operator, randomized, controlled trial. *Fertil Steril* 2008; **90**(4):1187–90.

43. de Camargo Martins AM, Baruffi RL, Mauri AL, et al. Ultrasound guidance is not necessary during easy embryo transfers. *J Assist Reprod Genet*. 2004; **21**(12): 421–5.

44. García-Velasco JA, Isaza V, Martinez-Salazar J, Landazábal A, et al. Transabdominal ultrasound-guided embryo transfer does not increase pregnancy rates in oocyte recipients. *Fertil Steril* 2002; **78**(3): 534–9.

45. Lambers MJ, Dogan E, Kostelijk H, Lens JW, Schats R, Hompes PG. Ultrasonographic-guided embryo transfer does not enhance pregnancy rates compared with embryo transfer based on previous uterine length measurement. *Fertil Steril* 2006; **86**(4): 867–72.

46. Flisser E, Grifo JA, Krey LC, Noyes N. Transabdominal ultrasound-assisted embryo transfer and pregnancy outcome. *Fertil Steril* 2006; **85**(2): 353–7.

47. Allahbadia GN, Kadam KS, Gandhi GN, Mhatre YP, Virk S, Kaur K. TAS or TVS – that is the question? *Fertil Steril* 2006; **86**(Suppl 3): S53.

48. Kojima K, Nomiyama M, Kumamoto T, Matsumoto Y, Iwasaka T. Transvaginal ultrasound-guided embryo transfer improves pregnancy and implantation rates after IVF. *Hum Reprod* 2001; **16**(12): 2578–82.

49. Coroleu B, Barri PN, Carreras O, et al. Effect of using an echogenic catheter for ultrasound-guided embryo transfer in an IVF programme: a prospective, randomized, controlled study. *Hum Reprod* 2006; **21**(7): 1809–15.

50. Karande V, Hazlett D, Vietzke M, Gleicher N.

A prospective randomized comparison of the Wallace catheter and the Cook Echo-Tip catheter for ultrasound-guided embryo transfer. *Fertil Steril* 2002; **77**(4): 826–30.

51. Wood EG, Batzer FR, Go KJ, Gutmann JN, Corson SL. Ultrasound-guided soft catheter embryo transfers will improve pregnancy rates in in-vitro fertilization. *Hum Reprod* 2000; **15**(1): 107–12

52. Allahbadia GN, Athavale UR, Kadam KS, Gandhi GN, Digra GS, Kaur K. A prospective randomized

comparison of the Wallace catheter and the SureView catheter for ultrasound-guided embryo transfer (ET). *Fertil Steril* 2005; **84**(1): S117.

53. Aboulfotouh I, Abou-Setta AM, Khattab S, Mohsen IA, Askalani A, el-Din RE. Firm versus soft embryo transfer catheters under ultrasound guidance: does catheter choice really influence the pregnancy rates? *Fertil Steril* 2008; **89**(5): 1261–2.

54. Letterie GS. Three-dimensional ultrasound-guided embryo transfer: a

preliminary study. *Am J Obstet Gynecol* 2005; **192**(6): 1983–7.

55. Gergely RZ, DeUgarte CM, Danzer H, Surrey M, Hill D, DeCherney AH. Three dimensional/four dimensional ultrasound-guided embryo transfer using the maximal implantation potential point. *Fertil Steril* 2005; **84**(2): 500–3.

56. Edwards RG, Fishel SB, Cohen J, et al. Factors influencing the success of in vitro fertilization for alleviating human infertility. *J In Vitro Fert Embryo Transf* 1984; **1**: 3–23.

Chapter 29

Ultrasonography-guided embryo transfer: clinical experience

Mostafa Abuzeid and Botros Rizk

Introduction

Successful outcome after in-vitro fertilization-embryo transfer (IVF-ET) depends on embryo quality, endometrial receptivity, and the technique of embryo transfer. Meticulous and atraumatic transfer procedure is essential for successful outcome [1,2,3,4]. Rizk (2008) noted a strong correlation between the ease of embryo transfer and the pregnancy rate [4,5,6,7,8,9]. Unfortunately, there is a reluctance to adopt new techniques of embryo transfer (ET) among clinicians [8]. In addition, there is little attention in the literature to this procedure compared with other steps of in-vitro fertilization treatment [3]. In this chapter we briefly review the principles for optimizing chances of successful ET and the role of ultrasound scan in ET. There will be emphasis on some practical points regarding ET techniques.

Effect of cervical mucus and blood

The presence of cervical mucus has been thought to increase rates of embryo retention and embryo expulsion [10]. It may also be a source of embryo contamination [11,12]. In addition, it may be present in the endometrial cavity as an extension from the cervical canal (Figure 29.1).

Furthermore, fluid may inadvertently enter the endometrial cavity during cervical lavage prior to ET [13,14]. Every effort should be made to carefully remove cervical mucus prior to ET. This requires gentle and through technique of suction and gentle irrigation using flushing media. The mere presence of blood is suggestive of difficult transfer. The presence of blood is associated with poor pregnancy rate due to difficult transfer rate and its sequelae and also due to the increased chance of embryo retention [8].

Uterine contraction

Uterocervical contraction could lead to embryo expulsion. One should therefore strive to avoid initiation of uterine contractions during ET. Stimulation of the cervix by grasping of the cervix with a tenaculum can cause uterine contractions through release of oxytocin [15]. In addition, passage of the outer rigid sheath of the ET catheter through the internal os may lead to

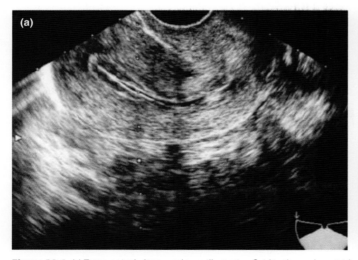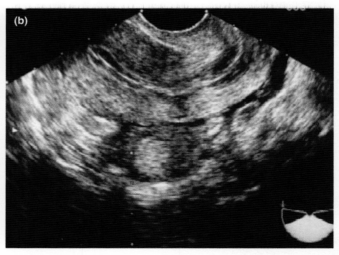

Figure 29.1. (a) Transvaginal ultrasound scan illustrating fluid in the endometrial cavity as the result of cervical mucus reaching into the lower area of the endometrial cavity. (b) Transvaginal ultrasound scan illustrating no fluid in the endometrial cavity after cervical mucus has been aspirated.

prostaglandin release. Furthermore, touching the uterine fundus, especially with a rigid catheter, can initiate uterine contractions [16].

Proper delivery of embryos inside the uterine cavity

Meticulous ET should ensure proper delivery of embryos inside the uterine cavity (Figure 29.2). This depends on several factors, including uterocervical angle, length of cervical canal, and how far the ET catheter is advanced. The so-called problematic cervix that leads to difficult ET procedure and perhaps inadequate transfer of embryos into the uterine cavity is most commonly secondary to distortion in the cervical canal or uterocervical angle. Figure 29.3 illustrates different types of uterocervical angles [17].

Figure 29.4 depicts transvaginal ultrasound pictures of difficult uterocervical angles that may complicate ET procedures. Such distortions are usually congenital in nature, sometimes as

a result of cervical fibroid (Figure 29.5) and/or rarely as a result of a large nabothian follicle (Figure 29.6), or multiple nabothian follicles (Figure 29.7).

In our experience, we rarely come across a true cervical stenosis, although theoretically this could be present as a result of previous surgery on the cervix, e.g., cone biopsy. Cervical polyp may also interfere with ET procedure and should be removed prior to IVF-ET.

An unusual angle can be seen in patients with acutely anteverted/anteflexed uterus or with retroverted uterus, especially if it is retroverted and fixed secondary to pelvic adhesions. It is also found in patients with extensive pelvic adhesions, leading to tilting of the uterus to one side, i.e., laterally. The uterus may also be tilted to one side – leading to an unusual lateral angulation in patients with unicornuate uterus – especially in association with endometriosis and pelvic adhesions. In rare cases, the uterocervical angle may have the shape of almost a half-circle appearance for no obvious reason (Figure 29.8).

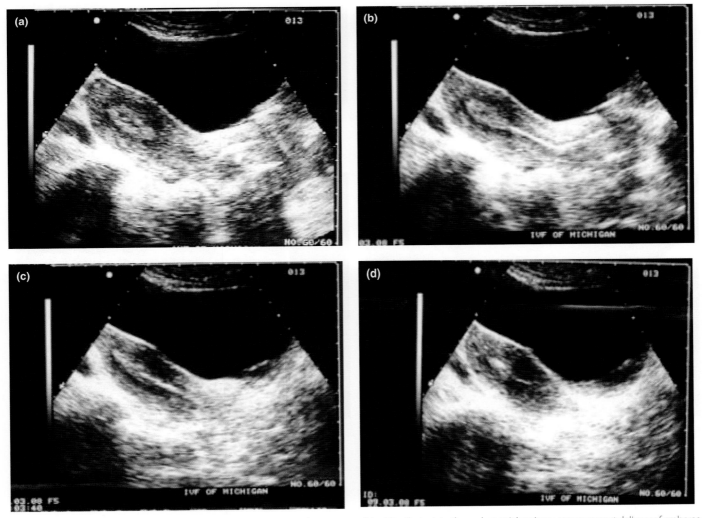

Figure 29.2 (a–d). Transvaginal ultrasound scans illustrating proper advancement of the ET catheter into the endometrial cavity to ensure correct delivery of embryos inside the endometrial cavity.

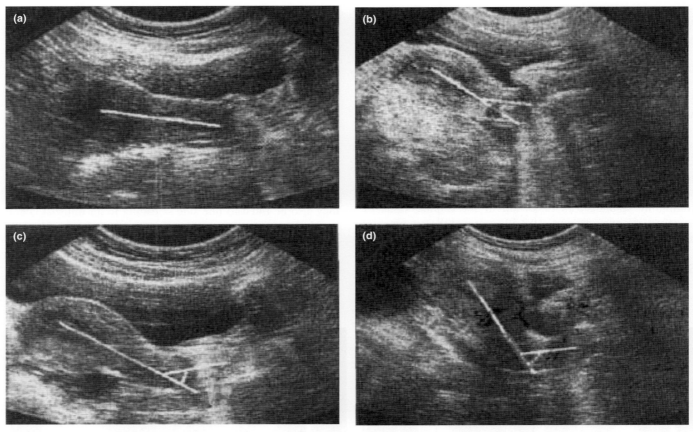

Figure 29.3. Transvaginal ultrasound scan of uterocervical angle. (a) No angle; (b) small angle (<30°); (c) moderate angle (30–60°); (d) large angle (>60°).

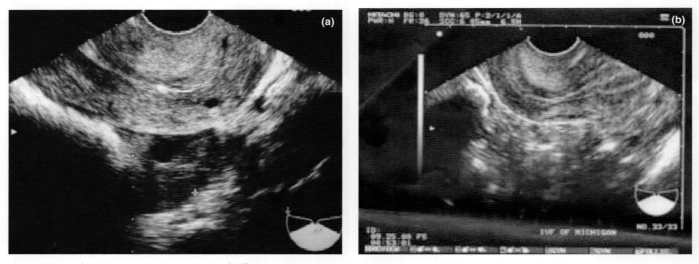

Figure 29.4 (a, b). Transvaginal ultrasound scan of difficult uterocervical angles: almost 90°.

Sometimes the difficulty is due to a narrowed external os, when it is difficult to advance the outer catheter. Sometimes the cervix is very short, and flush with the lateral fornix.

Some patients who underwent cesarean section may have an acute angle between the cervical canal and the lower uterine segment. This may be secondary to a healed cesarean scar pulling on and distorting this area. Others may occasionally have a distorted angle as a result of adhesions between the uterus and the anterior abdominal wall. In addition, the cervix may also be high in position after

Table 29.1. Principles that optimize the chances of successful ET

Proper evaluation of the uterine cavity and cervical canal

Thorough and gentle removal of cervical mucus and avoidance of cervical bleeding

Avoidance of initiation of uterine contractions

Proper delivery of the embryos inside the uterine cavity

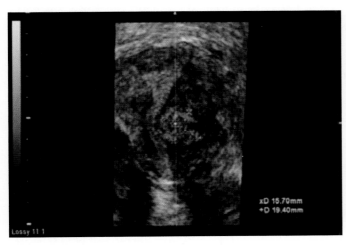

Figure 29.5. Cervical fibroid distorting uterocervical angle.

cesarean section, which can make it difficult to visualize the cervix.

Optimizing embryo transfer procedure

Certain steps need to be adopted to optimize ET procedure and, in turn, the chances of pregnancy (Table 29.1). Most of these steps are done on the day of ET, but some of them should be done well ahead of the ET procedure, i.e., prior to starting ovulation induction and certainly prior to retrieval procedure. Certain pathologies that may influence treatment or interfere with implantation or with ET procedures need to be identified and dealt with. History, physical examination, transvaginal ultrasound scan, saline sonogram, and mock ET trial are mandatory steps. The use of 3D ultrasound to detect subtle abnormalities, especially arcuate uterus and short uterine septum, is gaining momentum. Table 29.2 illustrates ovarian, fallopian tube, cervical, uterine, and endometrial cavity issues that need evaluation. Any significant pathology, e.g., submucous fibroid (Figure 29.9), or uterine septum (Figures 29.10, 29.11, 29.12, 29.13, 29.14), needs to be corrected surgically prior to IVF treatment.

When a problematic cervix is identified, a plan of action needs to be formulated. Currently most practitioners perform ET under ultrasound guidance. This helps in making the ET procedure easy and atraumatic and, in turn, optimizes the chances of a successful transfer. In some patients the problem can be solved by bladder distension and ultrasound guidance. In others, a cervical suture needs to be placed on the day of retrieval, to be used for traction and straightening of the uterocervical angle.

Figure 29.15 illustrates an ET catheter tip in a false passage. In some patients, modified general anesthesia may be needed,

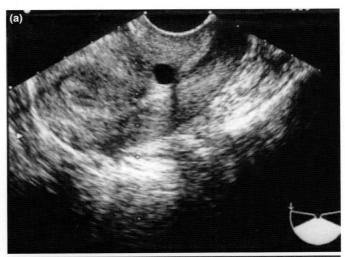

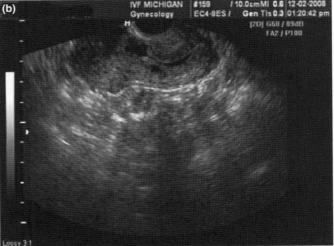

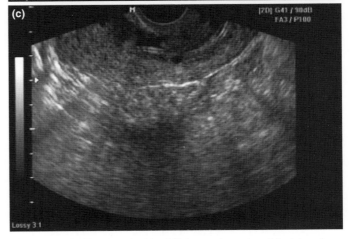

Figure 29.6. (a, b) Large nabothian follicle near the region of the internal os. (c) A large nabothian follicle near the region of the internal os interfering with advancement of the ET catheter tip into the endometrial cavity.

and in others transvaginal ultrasound-guided ET may be required. In a few patients, cervical dilatation and even hysteroscopy and resection of a ridge may be required [18,19]. In this case, some investigators suggest leaving a Foley catheter

Table 29.2. Transvaginal gynecologic ultrasound evaluation prior to IVF-ET treatment

1. Ovary	Position of ovary – accessible or not	
	PCO changes	
	Ovarian cysts, e.g., endometriomas	
	Dermoids	
2. Fallopian tube	Hydrosalpinx	
	Large paratubal cyst	
3. Cervical canal	Length	
	Nabothian follicles	
	Polyps	
	Fibroids	
	Fibroid tissue	
	Curve	
	Assessment of utero cervical angle	
4. Uterus	Size	
	Position	Anteverted
		Retroverted
		Axial
		Lateral tilt (2° to adhesions)
	Adhesions to abdominal wall, e.g., after cesarean section	
	Fibroids	
	Adenomyosis	
	Distortion of endometrial cavity	Polyps
		Submucous fibroids
		Adenomyosis
		Scar tissue
	Type of endometrial lining	
	Effect of previous cesarean section	

in utero for one week after such procedures [19]. If a mock trial is impossible and in the presence of at least one patent and healthy fallopian tube, tubal transfer, e.g., gamete intrafallopian transfer or tubal embryo transfer, should be planned (Figure 29.16).

On the day of oocyte retrieval, transvaginal ultrasound evaluation for a variety of issues should be performed, as summarized in Table 29.3.

On the day of ET, transabdominal ultrasound scan-guided ET should be planned. Table 29.4 summarizes some important points during this procedure. At the time of ET, bladder filling should be optimum (Figures 29.17, 29.18, 29.19). It should not be underdistended or overdistended (Figure 29.20).

Figure 29.21a illustrates fluid in the endometrial cavity, while Figure 29.21b illustrates the endometrial cavity after fluid has been aspirated before the ET procedure. Table 29.5 summarizes some important practical points that need to be adopted to optimize ET procedure. Patients who have undergone cesarean

section require adequate evaluation to determine whether they have some of the factors that may make the ET procedure difficult. In some instances, the uterus may be adherent to the anterior abdominal wall (Figure 29.22) and, in turn, the cervix may be high in position.

In these cases, one cannot use a short catheter (18 mm). A suture on the anterior lip of the cervix on the day of retrieval may be helpful. In addition, the bladder should not be very full as it will never be in front of the uterus and it may potentially create a curve between the cervical canal and endometrial cavity (Figure 29.23). In some patients the C-section scar in the lower uterine segment may lead to an unfavorable angle between the cervix and the endometrial cavity (Figure 29.24).

In turn, a false passage can be created as one is passing the catheter through the cervical canal. Application of cervical traction by pulling on a suture placed in the anterior lip of the cervix may help in straightening that angle, reduce the likelihood of false passage, and facilitate the process of ET [20]. Alternatively, advancing the outer sheath more than usual after fashioning its curve may help in overcoming the problem. When it is impossible to perform a mock trial, it is better to consider tubal embryo transfer (TET) [21] or gamete intrafallopian transfer (GIFT) [22], providing one fallopian tube is patent and healthy (Figure 29.16). Otherwise, if both tubes are damaged, one may utilize the technique of transmyometrial surgical ET proposed by Kato et al. [23].

Embryo transfer under ultrasound guidance

Woolcott and Stanger have demonstrated suboptimal placement of the catheter tip in approximately 50% of patients when transvaginal ultrasound-guided ET was performed [24]. In fact, they showed subendometrial placement of the tip of the catheter in 24.8% (Figures 29.25, 29.26); the catheter tip was abutting the fundus in 17.4% and near the opening of the fallopian tube in 7.4% [24]. Strickler et al. [25] were the first to use transvaginal ultrasound to ensure proper positioning of the ET catheter. The technique has been adopted by several investigators [26,27,28,29].

Transabdominal ultrasound-guided ET has been shown not only to improve the ease with which the procedure of ET is done [30], but also to improve the pregnancy rate [31] and delivery rate [32]. This is logical because, during ultrasound-guided ET, one can see the tip of the catheter as it advances through the cervical canal. One is able to determine how far the tip of the catheter has advanced into the endometrial cavity (Figure 29.27) and one can ensure that the catheter is along the endometrial cavity and not in a false passage.

One of the challenges is the relationship between the cervical canal and the endometrial cavity. In some cases, owing to retroversion and less commonly to acute anteversion, there may be a bad angle that makes it difficult to negotiate the cavity. This angle can also be due to a curved cervical canal. Sometimes there is a curve in the endometrial cavity, giving it a banana shape (Figure 29.28). This could be secondary to

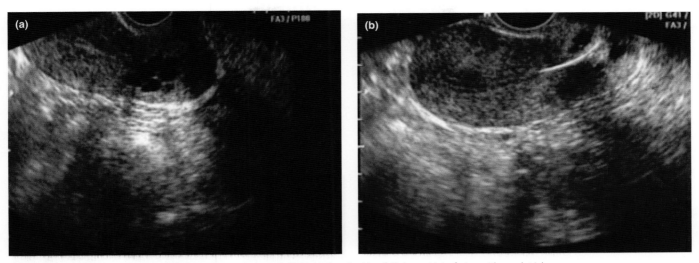

Figure 29.7. (a) Multiple nabothian follicles in the cervical canal. (b) Multiple nabothian follicles not interfering with mock trial.

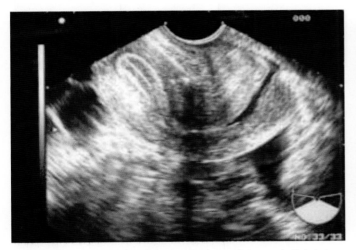

Figure 29.8. Uterocervical angle having the shape of almost a half-circle in appearance.

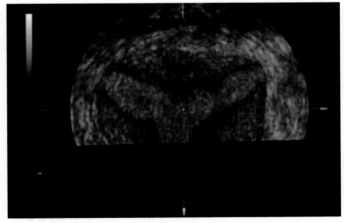

Figure 29.10. 3D ultrasound illustrating a short, incomplete uterine septum.

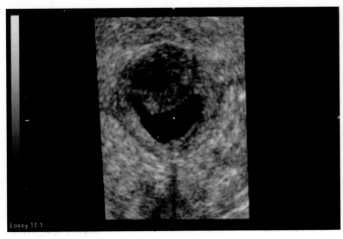

Figure 29.9. 3D saline sonogram illustrating type 2 fundal submucous fibroid.

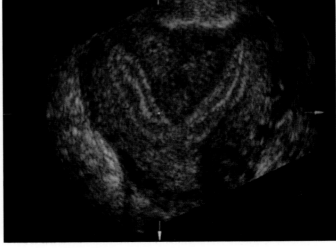

Figure 29.11. 3D ultrasound illustrating a long, complete uterine septum.

Table 29.3. Transvaginal gynecologic ultrasound evaluation on day of oocyte retrieval

Size of ovaries
Number of follicles
Position of ovaries
Aspiration of hydrosalpinx
Aspiration of cervical mucus
Aspiration of endometrial fluid
Aspiration of a large cervical cyst
Fluid in peritoneal cavity

Table 29.4. Transabdominal gynecologic ultrasound scan on day of ET

Bladder size should be optimal	Not overdistended
	Not underdistended
Aspirate cervical canal under direct vision	
Trial catheter under direct vision	
Transfer catheter only when situation under control	
Transfer catheter in complete view all the time	

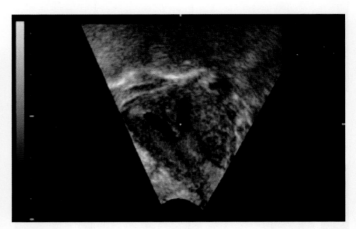

Figure 29.14. 3D saline sonogram illustrating a long, complete uterine septum.

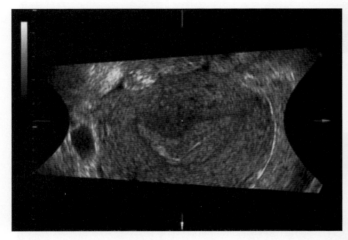

Figure 29.12. 3D ultrasound illustrating asymmetric cornual regions as a result of the short, incomplete uterine septum with its apex deviated to one side.

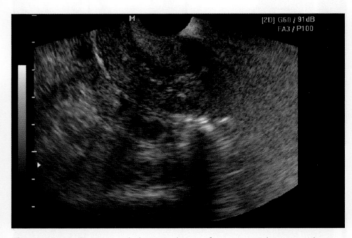

Figure 29.15. Transvaginal ultrasound scan of a retroverted uterus with embryo transfer catheter tip in a false passage in the myometrium.

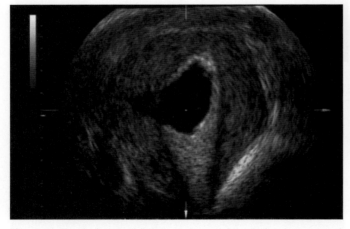

Figure 29.13. 3D ultrasound illustrating asymmetric cornual regions as a result of the short, incomplete uterine septum with its apex deviated to one side.

adenomyosis in the posterior wall of the myometrium, or to an intramural fibroid.

Ultrasound guidance allows the clinician to visualize the tip of the catheter as it is advanced along the cervical canal into the endometrial cavity (Figure 29.27). It therefore confirms that the catheter is advanced beyond an angle along the course of the cervical canal instead of the tip going into a false passage. In addition, it ensures that the tip of the catheter is beyond the internal os in cases of elongated cervix and, thus, avoids transfer of embryos into the cervical canal. Furthermore, ultrasound guidance facilitates placement of soft catheters; it avoids touching the anterior or posterior fundus walls; and it allows the direction the catheter along the course of the endometrial cavity, in turn avoiding shearing of the endometrium causing bleeding, or plugging of the catheter tip, which may lead to retention of the embryos. It enables the clinician to deposit the embryos in the desired area near the uterine fundus and, more importantly, the clinician is able to visualize the ease with which

Table 29.5. Practical points that optimize the ET procedure

Medication	Motrin
	Valium
	Sedation
Size of speculum	
Position of speculum	
Lateral retractor	
Suture in the:	Anterior lip
	Posterior lip
Type of catheter:	Soft catheter
	Echogenic catheter
	Stylet catheter
Curve of catheter	
Need to advance rigid outer sheath through internal os	

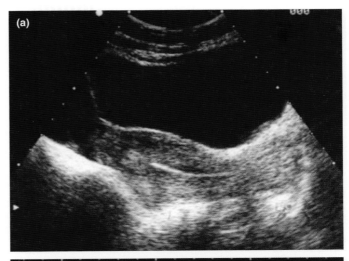

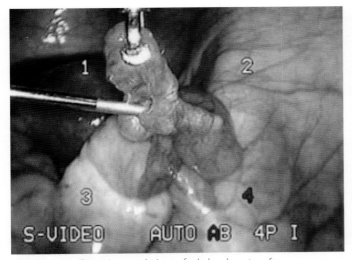

Figure 29.16. Illustrating a technique of tubal embryo transfer.

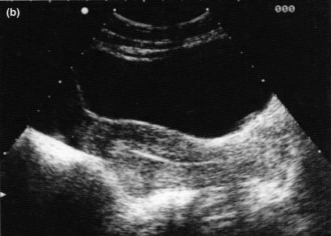

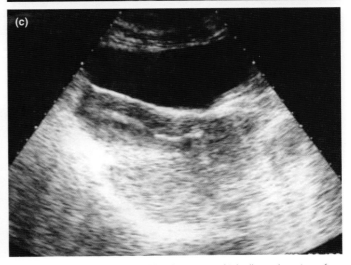

Figure 29.18 (a–c). Perfect bladder distension, which allows clear view of endometrial lining and, in turn, perfect advancement of ET catheter along the endometrial cavity and proper delivery of embryos in the desired area.

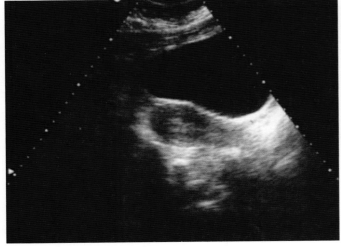

Figure 29.17. Perfect bladder distension.

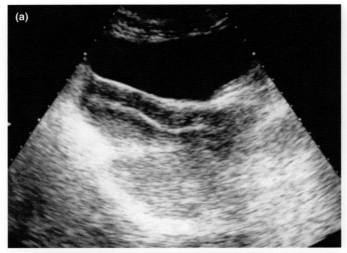

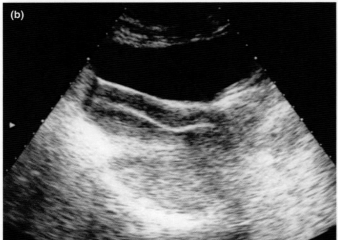

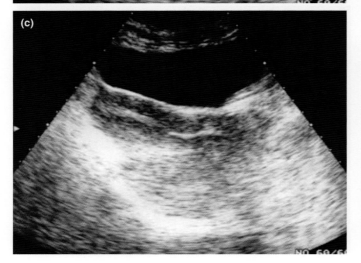

Figure 29.19 (a–c). Perfect bladder distension, which allows clear view of endometrial lining and, in turn, perfect advancement of ET catheter along the endometrial cavity and proper delivery of embryos in the desired area.

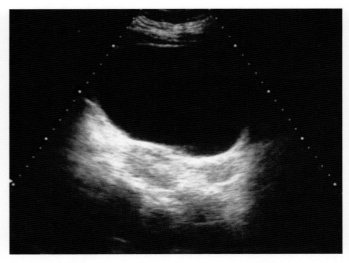

Figure 29.20. Overdistended bladder. Note: the endometrial lining is not clear.

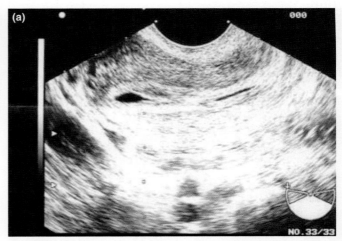

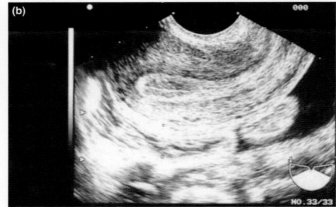

Figure 29.21. (a) Fluid in the endometrial cavity. (b) Same patient after aspiration of endometrial fluid using a Wallace embryo transfer catheter on the day of oocyte retrieval.

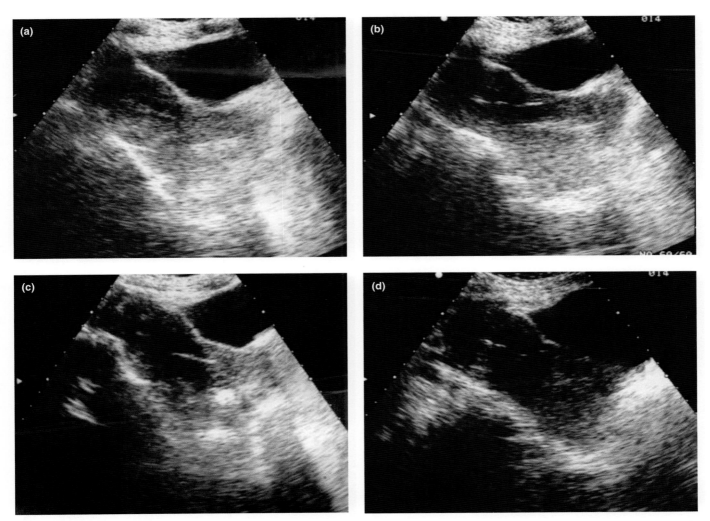

Figure 29.22 (a–d). The uterus is adherent to the anterior abdominal wall as a result of previous cesarean section. The ET catheter tip is being advanced into the endometrial cavity.

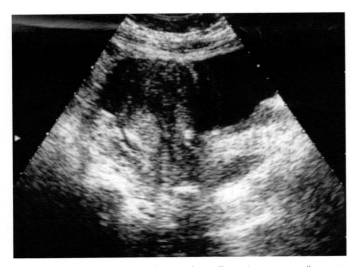

Figure 29.23. Transabdominal ultrasound scan illustrating a uterus adherent to the anterior abdominal wall as a result of previous cesarean section. This picture shows that the more the bladder is filled, the greater the likelihood of creating a curve at the uterocervical angle.

the drop of culture medium containing the embryos (as indicated by the drop of air seen on ultrasound) comes out of the catheter tip (bullet appearance). This is compared with the situation in which the drop of culture medium stays near the tip of the catheter (no bullet appearance), which may suggest that the catheter tip is touching the fundus or part of the anterior/posterior or lateral walls or that the tip is surrounded by mucus or blood.

This technique requires a full bladder, which, by itself, may simplify embryo transfer by straightening the cervical uterine access [33,34,35]. However, the degree of bladder filling should be optimal. If it is minimally filled, the view of the endometrium is not clear and its straightening effect is not present. On the other hand, a markedly distended bladder has several disadvantages, including patient discomfort, a suboptimal view of the endometrial lining, and a change in cervical position as a result of pushing on the vaginal speculum. In addition, a very full bladder may push a retroverted uterus still further backward, which compromises the view of the endometrial lining. Furthermore, if the uterus is adherent to the abdominal wall,

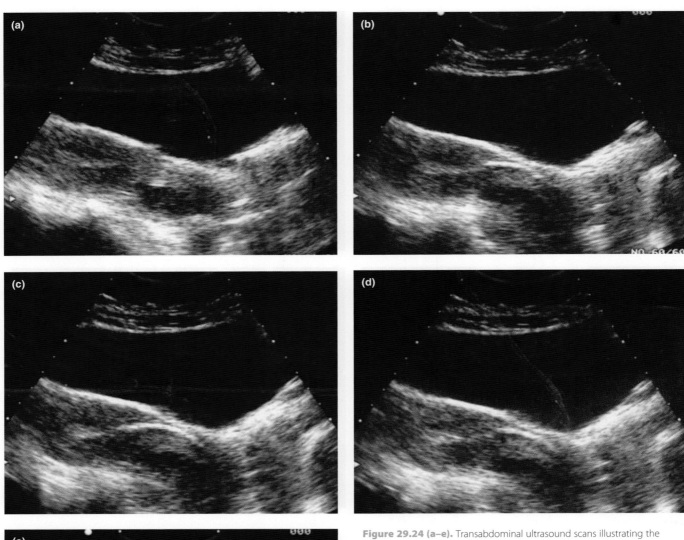

Figure 29.24 (a–e). Transabdominal ultrasound scans illustrating the angle at the uterocervical junction as a result of previous cesarean section. The pictures illustrate the ET catheter tip being advanced clearly, then withdrawn after completion of the procedure.

overfilling of the bladder will not only have no effect on the view of the endometrial lining, but also may further distort the relationship between the cervical canal and the uterine cavity. Therefore, care should be taken to ensure optimal filling, but not underfilling or overfilling, of the bladder.

Ultrasonographic guidance of ET may also have other potential advantages. Cervical lavage before ET should be done under ultrasound guidance, which ensures complete removal of cervical mucus and avoidance of pushing of washing medium into the endometrial cavity. The latter is accomplished by avoiding

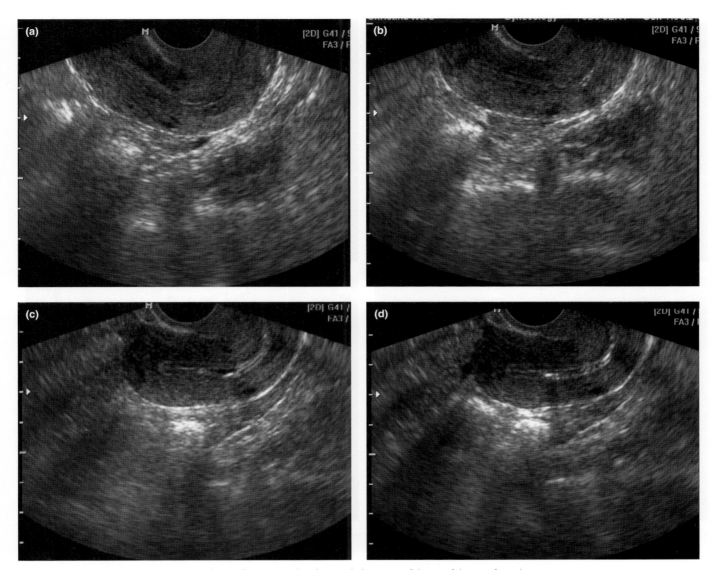

Figure 29.25 (a–d). Transvaginal ultrasound scans illustrating subendometrial placement of the tip of the transfer catheter.

advancing the tip of the catheter more than 50% of the length of the cervical canal. In the presence of a pinpoint nulliparous os, suction of the cervical mucus should be performed, but one should not perform cervical lavage as fluid may enter the endometrial cavity. Failure to monitor cervical cleansing and lavage by ultrasound may potentially have harmful effects, e.g., trauma to the region of internal os or even the endometrial cavity and the possibility of pushing fluid into the endometrial cavity. New technology from General Electric (GE, New York) allows ultrasonography-guided ET using a 4D mode, with significant advantage in the transfer process.

Key points in clinical practice

- Transvaginal ultrasound is mandatory for evaluation of the uterus and endocervical canal prior to and on the day of oocyte retrieval.

- Transabdominal ultrasound guidance is essential for meticulous and atraumatic ET.
- Cervical suture should be considered in patients with a history of:
  - Difficult mock trial
  - Problematic cervix
  - Pelvic adhesions (previous cesarean section)
  - Obesity
- If severe difficulty is expected, consider:
  - Transvaginal ultrasound
  - Tubal embryo transfer
  - 4D ultrasound is a very useful tool and may eventually replace 2D ultrasound for embryo transfer.

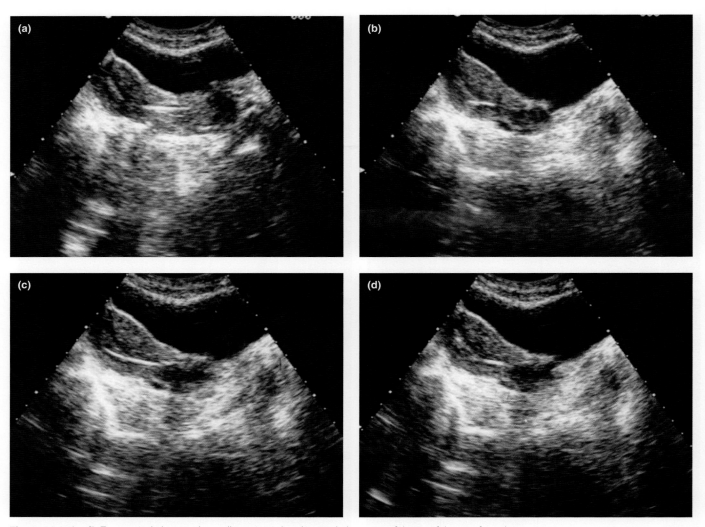

Figure 29.26(a–d). Transvaginal ultrasound scan illustrating subendometrial placement of the tip of the transfer catheter.

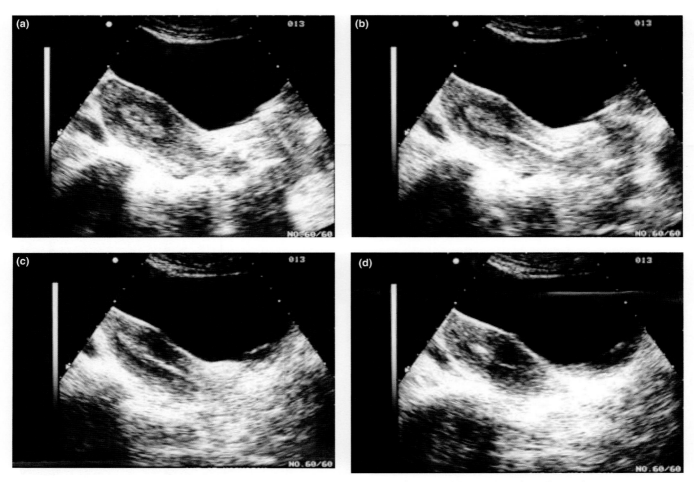

Figure 29.27 (a–d). Transabdominal ultrasound scan illustrating controlled advancement of the ET catheter tip along the endometrial cavity to ensure proper placement of embryos.

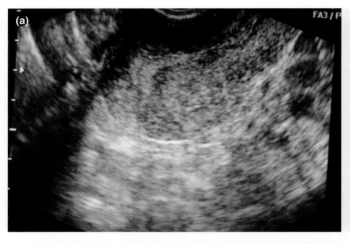

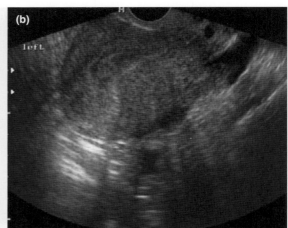

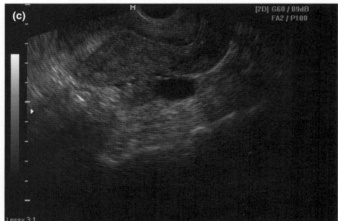

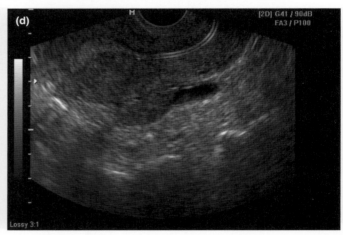

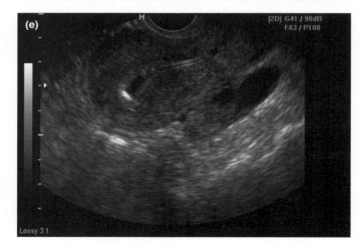

Figure 29.28. (a–c) A curve in the endometrial cavity, giving it a banana shape. (d) Mock trial catheter in a patient with a banana-shaped cavity. (e) Saline sonogram in a patient with a banana-shaped cavity. Note the tip of the catheter touching the anterior wall of the uterus.

References

1. Meldrum DR, Chetkowski R, Steingold KA, de Ziegler D, Cedars MI, Hamilton M. Evolution of a highly successful in vitro fertilization-embryo transfer program. *Fertil Steril* 1987; **48**: 86–93.

2. Schoolcraft WB, Surrey ES, Gardner DK. Embryo transfer: techniques and variable affecting success. *Fertil Steril* 2001; **76** (5): 863–870.

3. Mansour RT, Aboulghar MA. Optimizing the embryo transfer technique.

Hum Reprod 2002; **17**(5): 1149–53.

4. Rizk B. The Infuence of a difficult embryo transfer on the result. In: Allahbadia GN, ed. *Embryo Transfer*, chapter 39. New Delhi: Jaypee Brothers Medical Publishers, 2008: 391–6.

5. Englert Y, Puissant F, Camus M, Van Hoeck J, Leroy F. Clinical study on embryo transfer after human in vitro fertilization. *J In Vitro Fert Embryo Transf* 1986; **3**: 243–6.

6. Mansour R, Aboulghar M, Serour G. Dummy embryo transfer: a technique that

minimizes the problems of embryo transfer and improves the pregnancy rate in human in vitro fertilization. *Fertil Steril* 1990; **54**: 678–81.

7. Wood EG, Batzer FR, Go KJ, Gutmann JN, Corson SL. Ultrasound-guided soft catheter embryo transfers will improve pregnancy rates in in-vitro fertilization. *Hum Reprod* 2000; **15**: 107–12.

8. Visser DS, Fourie FL, Kruger HF. Multiple attempts at embryo transfer: effects on pregnancy outcomes in an in vitro fertilization and embryo transfer program. *J Assist Reprod Genet* 1993; **10**: 37–43.

9. Tomas C, Tapanainen J, Martikainen H. The difficulty of embryo transfer is an independent variable for predicting pregnancy in in-vitro fertilization treatments [Abstract]. *Fertil Steril* 1998; **70**(Suppl 1): S433.

10. Mansour RT, Aboulghar MA, Serour GI, Amin YM. Dummy embryo transfer using methylene blue dye. *Hum Reprod* 1994; **9**: 1257–9.

11. Fanchin R, Harmas A, Benaoudia F, Lundkvist U, Olivennes F, Frydman R. Microbial flora of the cervix assessed at the time of embryo transfer adversely affects in vitro fertilization outcome. *Fertil Steril* 1998; **70**: 866–70.

12. Egbase PE, al-Sharhan M, al-Othman S, al-Mutawa M, Udo EE, Grudzinskas JG. Incidence of microbial growth from the tip of the embryo transfer catheter after embryo transfer in relation to clinical pregnancy rate following in vitro fertilization and embryo transfer. *Hum Reprod* 1996; **11**: 1687–9.

13. McNamee P, Huang T, Carwile A. Significant increase in pregnancy rates achieved by vigorous

irrigation of endocervical mucus prior to embryo transfer with a Wallace catheter in an IVF-ET program [Abstract]. *Fertil Steril* 1998; **70** (Suppl 1): S228.

14. Glass KB, Green CA, Fluker MR, Schoolcraft WB, McNamee PI, Meldrum D. Multicenter randomized trial of cervical irrigation at the time of embryo transfer [Abstract]. *Fertil Steril* 2000; **74**: (Suppl 1): S31.

15. Dorn C, Reinsberg J, Schlebusch H, Prietl G, Van der Ven H, Krebs D. Serum oxytocin concentration during embryo transfer procedure. *J Obstet Gynecol Reprod Biol* 1999; **87**: 77–80.

16. Lesney P, Killick SR, Tetlow RL, Robinson J, Maguiness SD. Embryo transfer–can we learn anything new from the observation of junctional zone contractions? *Hum Reprod* 1998; **13**(6): 1540–6.

17. Sallam HN. Embryo transfer: Factors involved in optimizing the success. *Curr Opin Obstet Gynecol* 2005; **17**: 289–98.

18. Abusheikha N, Lass A, Akagbosu F, Brinsden P. How useful is cervical dilation in patients with cervical stenosis who are participating in an in vitro fertilization-embryo transfer program? The Bourn Hall experience. *Fertil Steril* 1999; **72**: 610–12.

19. Yanushpolsky EH, Ginsburg ES, Fox JH, Stewart EA. Transcervical placement of a Malecot catheter after hysteroscopic evaluation provides for easier entry into the endometrial cavity for women with histories of difficult intrauterine inseminations and/or embryo transfers: a prospective case series. *Fertil Steril* 2000; **73**: 402–5.

20. Johnson N, Bromham DR. Effect of cervical traction

with a tenaculum on the uterocervical angle. *Br J Obstet Gynaecol* 1991; **98**(3): 309–12.

21. Sasy M, Abdel Fattah A, Abozaid T, et al. Comparison between ultrasound-guided embryo transfer and tubal embryo transfer after intracytoplasmic sperm injection. *Middle East Fertil Soc J* 2003; **8**(3): 223–8.

22. Lodi S, Abdel Fattah A, Aboziad T, et al. Gamete intra-fallopian transfer or intrauterine insemination after controlled ovarian hyperstimulation for treatment of infertility due to endometriosis. *Gynecol Endocrinol* 2004; **19**: 152–9.

23. Kato, O, Takatsuka R, Asch R. Transvaginal-transmyometrial embryo transfer: The Towako Method. *Fert Steril* 1993; **59** (1): 51–3.

24. Woolcott R, Stanger J. Potentially important variables identified by transvaginal ultrasound-guided embryo transfer. *Hum Reprod* 1997; **12**: 963–6.

25. Strickler RC, Christianson C, Crane JP, Curato A, Knight AB, Yang V. Ultrasound guidance for human embryo transfer. *Fertil Steril* 1985; **43**: 54–61.

26. Hurley VA, Osborn JC, Leoni MA, Leeton J. Ultrasound-guided embryo transfer: a controlled trial. *Fertil Steril* 1991; **55**: 559–62.

27. Lindheim SR, Cohen MA, Sauer MV. Ultrasound guided embryo transfer significantly improves pregnancy rates in women undergoing oocyte donation. *Int J Gynecol Obstet* 1999; **66**: 281–4.

28. Kojima K, Nomiyama M, Kumamoto T, Matsumoto Y, Iwasaka T. Transvaginal ultrasound-guided embryo transfer improves pregnancy

and implantation rates after IVF. *Hum Reprod* 2002; **16**: 2578–82.

29. Anderson RE, Nugent NL, Gregg AT, Nunn SL, Behr BR. Transvaginal ultrasound-guided embryo transfer improves outcome in patients with previous failed in vitro fertilization cycles. *Fertil Steril* 2002; **77**: 769–75.

30. Kan AKS, Abdalla HI, Gafar A, et al. Embryo transfer: ultrasound-guided versus clinical touch. *Hum Reprod* 1999; **14**(9): 1259–61.

31. Coreleu B, Carreras O, Veiga A, et al. Embryo transfer under ultrasound guidance improves pregnancy rates after in vitro fertilization. *Hum Reprod* 2000; **15**(3): 616–20.

32. Abou-Setta AM, Mansour RT, Al-Inany H, Aboulghar MM, Aboulghar MA, Serour GI. Among women undergoing embryo transfer, is the probability of pregnancy and live birth improved with ultrasound guidance over clinical touch alone? A systemic review and meta-analysis of prospective randomized trials. *Fertil Steril* 2007; **88** (2): 333–40.

33. Sundstrom P, Wramsby H, Persson PH, Liedholm P. Filled bladder simplifies human embryo transfer. *Br J Obstet Gynecol* 1984; **91**: 506–7.

34. Lewin A, Schenker JG, Avrech O, Shapira S, Safran A, Friedler S. The role of uterine straightening by passive bladder distention before embryo transfer in IVF cycles. *J Assist Reprod Genet* 1997; **14**: 32–4.

35. Abou-Setta AM. Effect of passive uterine straightening during embryo transfer: a systematic review and meta-analysis. *Acta Obstet Gynecol* 2007; **86**: 516–22.

30 First-trimester pregnancy failure

William W. Brown, III

Introduction

Transvaginal sonography (TVS) has revolutionized the medical care available to women in early pregnancy by essentially replacing the historical approach of clinical assessment alone. Today's machine and software improvements and high-resolution probe capabilities allow providers a remarkable real-time window with which to observe many aspects of embryological development. By their doing so, this standard-of-care technology is now widely used to detect fetal structural defects in the first trimester and to screen for chromosomal anomalies.

Unfortunately, not all pregnancies are normal and many fail. Approximately 25% of women will risk losing their pregnancy by presenting with bleeding, and one-half of those will miscarry, although actual rates of spontaneous abortion (SAB) may vary and depend upon many factors, including maternal age and previous obstetric history. The vast majority of these losses occur during the embryonic period of development and are due to chromosomal abnormalities. Ultrasound is often the primary modality used to diagnose, and sometimes predict, miscarriage, and it is essential to recognize the altered images that deviate from normal and imply or threaten adverse outcome. The application of ultrasound in the management of early pregnancy failure is highlighted in this chapter.

Many clinical presentations in early pregnancy warrant TVS, including an unknown last menstrual period (LMP) with a positive pregnancy test, threatened abortion with bleeding, confirmation of viability in the infertility patient, and acute onset of pelvic pain. The focus of the examination is to determine the location of the pregnancy, to document viability when possible, and to confirm or establish gestational age. A complete pelvic study should evaluate the uterus, cervix, endometrial cavity, cul-de-sac, bilateral adnexa, and, when appropriate, the abdomen for signs of hemoperitoneum. While the pregnancy status may be the primary reason for investigation, it is important not to overlook other incidental findings which can sometimes substantially complicate an otherwise normal pregnancy, such as a coexistent intrauterine device, uterine or adnexal masses, or congenital uterine anomalies.

First-trimester sonography in normal and failed early pregnancy

Gestational sac

In a normally developing pregnancy, the early embryonic blastocyst implants into the uterine endometrium by 23 days of menstrual age. The gestational sac (GS) is an ultrasound term that signifies the conceptus; it is seen as a spherical, fluid-filled cavity within the endometrium that is surrounded by an echogenic rim (Figure 30.1). It may be visible with high-frequency endovaginal transducers as early as the end of the second week after fertilization, and it is the earliest ultrasound sign of an intrauterine pregnancy. The specific ultrasound appearance of the fluid collection within the endometrial cavity, as well as its size and its correlation with serum human chorionic gonadotropin (hCG) levels, are all very important since the differential diagnosis includes a normal pregnancy, simple fluid, embryonic demise, blood, decidual cyst, and the pseudosac of an ectopic pregnancy. Unfortunately, the mere presence of even a true GS does not guarantee viability, as the loss rate at this stage of pregnancy is still as high as 11.5% [1].

The anechoic space that represents the earliest GS is the exocoelomic fluid of the blastocyst, and it is surrounded by an echogenic ring of trophoblastic tissue comprised of chorionic villi. A measured thickness of the sac rim of 2 mm or more can help identify the fluid collection as an intrauterine pregnancy, and this chorionic membrane should also have an echodensity that exceeds that of the myometrium [2]. The earliest visible GS is more likely to be located eccentrically buried within the endometrium, and it is small enough not to distort the endometrial lining interface (Figure 30.2).

One ultrasound finding that can reliably signal a pregnancy within the uterus is the double decidual sac sign (DDS) (Figure 30.3). Here there are two echogenic rings surrounding the sonolucent sac [3]; the inner is the decidua capsularis, the outer is the decidua parietalis or decidua vera, and the two rings are separated by a thin layer of fluid. Unfortunately, this finding is not always present until the gestational sac mean sac diameter (MSD) is approximately 10 mm. By then, on endovaginal

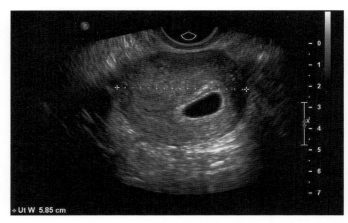

Figure 30. 1. Transverse view of the uterus revealing an early gestational sac. The sonographic hallmarks are a fluid-filled, sonolucent chorionic cavity surrounded by an echogenic rim of trophoblastic-decidual tissue.

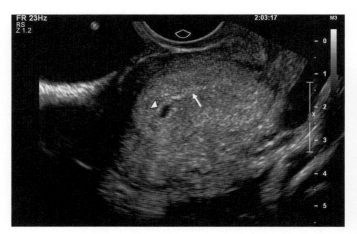

Figure 30.2. Despite very early menstrual dating, features that help distinguish the sonolucent structure shown as a likely gestational sac (arrowhead) are its echogenic rim and its eccentric location in relation to the endometrial interface (arrow). Once a true yolk sac becomes visible within the gestational sac, the intrauterine location of the pregnancy is confirmed.

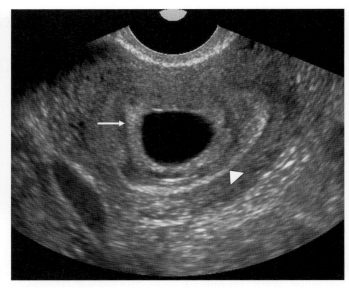

Figure 30.3. Double decidual sac sign, consisting of the inner decidua capsularis (arrow) and the outer decidua parietalis (or vera, arrowhead).

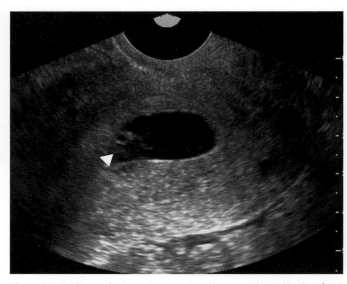

Figure 30.4. Abnormal intrauterine gestational sac as evidenced by ill-defined, irregular debris (arrowhead) in close proximity to the yolk sac.

ultrasound, it is easier and typically more predictable to locate the yolk sac as a definitive means of confirming pregnancy location within the uterus, thereby diminishing the clinical usefulness of the DDS sign.

Because both hCG levels and GS growth are directly related to trophoblastic function, there is a correlation between sac size, hCG level, and gestational age. The discriminatory level for hCG at which the GS should always be seen on transvaginal ultrasound is commonly cited to be between 1000 and 2000 mIU/ml, and the value in a viable pregnancy of less than 10 weeks' gestation should rise by at least 53% in two days [4]. This information is of critical importance to the care provider who is faced with the clinical possibility of ectopic pregnancy or, more commonly, the nonviable intrauterine pregnancy or spontaneous miscarriage. In addition, once the GS is firmly visualized, the MSD can be expected to grow at a rate of about 1.1 mm per day [5], and no less than 0.6 mm per day. Such a MSD is obtained by averaging the cephalocaudad, anteroposterior,

and transverse sac dimensions as measured from the chorionic fluid interface.

The GS, unfortunately, cannot serve as an accurate or precise measurement of gestational age due to its wide confidence limits, but it can and should be used to monitor the sequential sonographic milestones of the early, normal intrauterine pregnancy. GS growth rate, location, appearance (Figure 30.4), and size can all be used as helpful indicators when assessing pregnancy viability and the likelihood of continued normal growth. A poor or weak choriodecidual reaction of the surrounding sac rim, irregular sac contour (Figure 30.5), and low-set position of the sac within the lower uterine segment are all strong indicators of a nonviable pregnancy, and serial ultrasound follow-up examination is warranted. Bromley et al. [6] describe a small GS

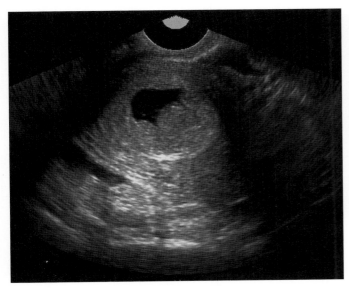

Figure 30.5. Abnormal gestational sac. Note the poorly defined chorionic rim and the distinctly nonspherical, irregular sac shape. Such combined abnormal findings increase the risk of first-trimester pregnancy failure.

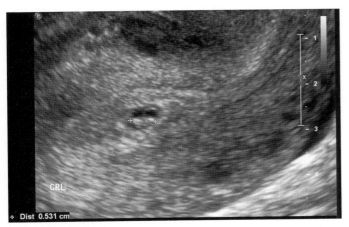

Figure 30.6. Abnormally small gestational sac surrounding a 5.3 mm embryo (calipers). This finding is confirmed when the mean diameter of the sac is less than 5 mm greater than the crown-rump length, or long axis measurement, of the embryo.

where the MSD is less than 5 mm greater than the crown–rump length, or embryonic size (Figure 30.6). This finding carries with it a high risk of embryonic demise, and in those pregnancies that do survive there is the risk of preterm labor and low birth weight [7], as well as triploid or trisomy chromosomal abnormalities [8]. Finally, although these ultrasound signs do not singularly denote a pregnancy absolutely destined to fail, the risk of demise does increase when these findings occur in combination with one another (Figure 30.5).

Yolk sac

The first structure to be identified inside the GS, before visualization of the embryo or its cardiac pulsation, is the yolk sac (YS). This spherical, echogenic, ringlike formation has a sonolucent center (Figure 30.7) and is most commonly seen at the periphery of the chorionic cavity; its presence confirms a true

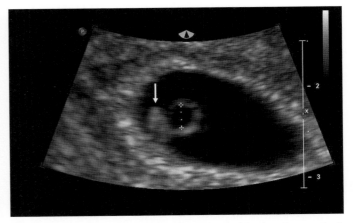

Figure 30.7. Very early embryo (arrow) located at the left edge of a normal yolk sac (calipers).

GS and an intrauterine pregnancy with 100% positive predictive value (PPV) [9]. Although the amniotic membrane and the YS differentiate at the same early time in pregnancy, the YS is much more readily visible due to its echogenicity. What is actually being seen is the embryological secondary yolk sac, and, as the pregnancy progresses, it assumes a clearly obvious extra-amniotic location. The YS should be detectable by 37–40 menstrual days or when the MSD ranges from 5 to 13 mm [10] on endovaginal ultrasound and by 6 gestational weeks, or 20 mm MSD on transabdominal ultrasound. Before placental function is established, this tiny and important structure is responsible for all of the nutritional and physiological support of the developing embryo. Early on, the YS represents the sole metabolic transport system between mother and offspring, managing necessary secretory, endocrine, immunologic, and hematopoietic functions. As well, it is the site for formation of primordial germ cells. Thus, its clinical relevance is not surprising. Yolk sac growth is steady during the embryonic period up to 11 weeks of gestation, when it attains a maximum size of around 6 mm and then naturally regresses to disappear typically by the end of the first trimester.

It should be noted that studies attempting to address an association between YS abnormalities and poor pregnancy outcome have differed in design and study populations. It is unknown whether YS abnormalities are due to primary deficiencies of the structure itself, which may then go on to cause pregnancy failure, or whether the YS changes are secondary to embryonic maldevelopment and death. What does tend to be repeated in the majority of the literature, however, even when the study population may or may not be presenting with signs of first-trimester bleeding, is that various abnormalities of the YS can forebode pregnancy failure. The YS should be visible by the time the GS reaches the discriminatory MSD value previously noted; in fact, Mara and Foster [11] emphasized that a YS should indeed be present in all normal-outcome pregnancies. In addition, once it is visualized, its premature regression can be associated with embryonic death. Other predictors of poor pregnancy outcome include absence of the YS in the presence of an embryo and nonspecific abnormalities of appearance,

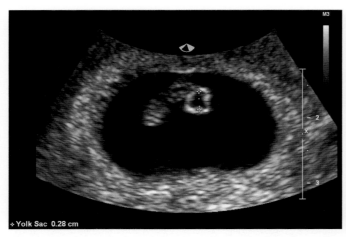

Figure 30.8. Abnormal yolk sac (calipers) seen lying to the right of an early embryo. The bright surrounding rim of this structure is irregular in shape.

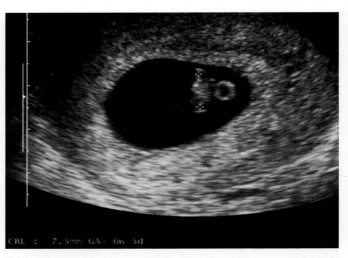

Figure 30.10. The embryonic complex seen within the exocoelomic fluid of the gestational sac. Displayed from left-to-right are the amnion, embryo (calipers), and yolk sac. Courtesy of Dr. Dolores Pretorius.

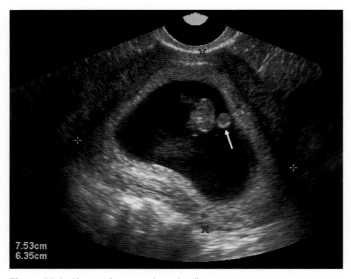

Figure 30.9. Abnormal, opaque (arrow) yolk sac.

such as shape (Figure 30.8) or contour, opacification (Figure 30.9), calcification, and floating central location within the GS [12]. Findings regarding YS shape can be notoriously transient, so follow-up ultrasound should be ordered. Finally, YS size matters because significant variations above or below the reported mean for a given gestational age can be highly predictive for pregnancy loss [13]. Interestingly, however, some pregnancies with this same finding actually progress normally, and in those that are lost in miscarriage the karyotype of the abortus may either be normal or abnormal.

Yolk sac findings that vary from normal deserve close clinical attention because such findings may herald impending pregnancy loss and, possibly, an increased risk of karyotypic abnormality in surviving gestations. This observation has caused several authors to recommend that attention by ultrasound be paid to the size and shape of the YS in all pregnancies up to 10 weeks. In those cases that are complicated by abnormal YS findings and where viability is maintained into the second trimester, ultrasound anatomic survey or genetic evaluation should be offered.

Embryo

The next structure to become visible inside the chorionic sac, after the yolk sac, is the early embryo. As a part of what will comprise the embryonic complex along with the amnion and yolk sac (Figure 30.10), the embryo has been present since 9 days post conception, and it begins to become recognizable around 40 menstrual days when it is seen as a linear echodensity measuring 2–3 mm immediately alongside the secondary YS (Figure 30.7). The consistency of this anatomic and ultrasound relationship between the very early embryo and the YS is helpful to the clinician who is seeking to ascertain normal progressive growth and, ultimately, viability of the pregnancy. During gestational weeks 5 through 9, which represent the embryonic period of development and organogenesis, the embryo or "fetal pole" is measured along its long axis. Although such a determination has long been called a "crown–rump length" (CRL), true anatomic structures are not really identifiable as such until the measurement reaches at least 17–18 mm and the fetal period has begun at 10 weeks of gestation or 70 days from the last menstrual period.

The first embryonic system to develop and function is the cardiovascular system; the new heart is very prominent at this stage and starts to beat as early as 35 menstrual days. It follows that sometimes the examiner may actually appreciate cardiac pulsations even before an embryonic size is clear enough to measure, even with magnification. Despite such an interesting occurrence, however, with most standard transvaginal instrumentation it is still the exception to document heart activity when the embryo is seen and ≤3 mm. What is clinically most relevant is to know the embryonic size by which the heartbeat should always be visible, for such a foolproof "discriminatory" value would give 100% positive predictability for embryonic demise. With such information in hand, the provider can comfortably offer the patient medical or surgical options for

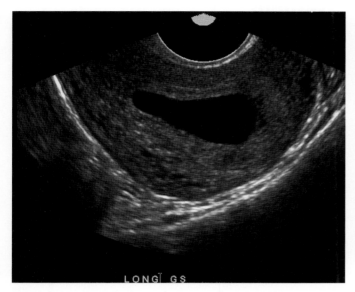

Figure 30.11. Longitudinal view of a retroverted uterus showing an empty gestational sac. When no yolk sac or embryo is present, the discriminatory mean sac diameter can be used to help confirm the diagnosis of embryonic demise and a failed pregnancy.

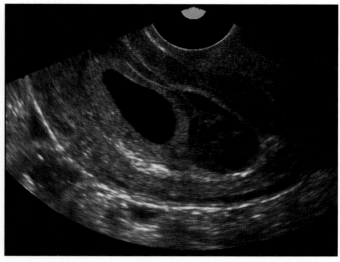

Figure 30.12. A moderate-sized subchorionic hemorrhage is seen to the right of the gestational sac. The mixed, complex echoes, representing blood and varying stages of clot, separate the chorionic membrane and the decidua.

uterine evacuation, if that is her wish, without concerns for inadvertently terminating a desired, viable pregnancy.

Studies dating back almost twenty years suggest that an embryo measuring 5 mm or more should have visible heart motion, and the absence thereof implies pregnancy failure [14]. However, as will be discussed later in this chapter, there are many influencing factors that can affect the meaning and interpretation of this result. Accordingly, when the embryo is of borderline size and no heartbeat is seen, a follow-up ultrasound is recommended, and the CRL should be seen increasing in size over time at the average rate of 1 mm/day [5]. Once cardiac motion is detected, the rate of pregnancy loss is low at approximately 5%, but it increases with confounding issues such as advanced maternal age, a history of recurrent pregnancy loss, and signs of threatened miscarriage. A slow embryonic heart rate in the early first trimester, especially when found to be ≤90 beats/minute, raises the chance of spontaneous abortion [15], as well as a higher anomaly rate in surviving pregnancies. In this situation, also, a repeat follow-up ultrasound examination is warranted.

The ability to sonographically visualize the early embryo depends upon the gestational age, as well as on several technical ultrasound factors. In a high-volume infertility practice, the timing of conception is known with exactness. Quite often, however, the timing of ovulation is imprecise, so it is helpful to have some objective criteria that will assist in determining the normal progress of pregnancy, embryonic viability, and dating. The most commonly quoted discriminatory range for MSD by which a "fetal pole" should be seen within the chorionic sac is 16–18 mm, although Rowling et al. [16] showed that some sacs of this size can appear empty even up to 19 mm MSD and still ultimately yield live embryos that go on to normal delivery. If a large GS is truly void of both embryo and YS, this is most likely due to embryonic demise, rather than representing an "anembryonic" pregnancy (Figure 30.11).

Before the embryo is seen, the GS itself can be a means of estimating gestational age through the simple formula: MSD (mm) + 30 = menstrual age (days). In the absence of a known ovulation date, though, the length of the embryo is the most accurate way to assess dating and assign a predicted due date. Especially in very early pregnancies, use of the following Goldstein formula [17] may be preferable to the older nomograms that are pre-packaged on most ultrasound machines: embryonic length (mm) + 42 = menstrual age (days). Lastly, in addition to gestational age assessment, early pregnancy CRL growth delay may signal pregnancies that carry a risk for spontaneous miscarriage, intrauterine growth restriction [18], and triploidy.

Subchorionic bleeding

Subchorionic hemorrhage (SCH), also called subchorionic hematoma, represents a situation when there is a crescent-shaped fluid collection between the chorionic membrane and the decidua. The fluid collection, felt to be blood and serum, is presumably due to a type of placental abruption where the bleeding detaches the trophoblastic tissue from the decidua of the uterine wall. The ultrasound images of acute bleeding are hyperechoic and isoechoic to the surrounding rim of the GS and are heterogeneous; however, after 1–2 weeks the SCH typically appears isoechoic to the chorionic fluid (Figures 30.12, 30.13). The prevalence of this condition may be as low as 1.3% in a general obstetric population [19] or as high as 39.5% in patients who present with signs and symptoms of threatened abortion [20]. The natural history of this problem is such that 70% of the time SCH resolves by the end of the second trimester.

The various reports in the literature over the past fifteen years are conflicting regarding the sonographic finding of SCH and its clinical significance, especially its relationship to either

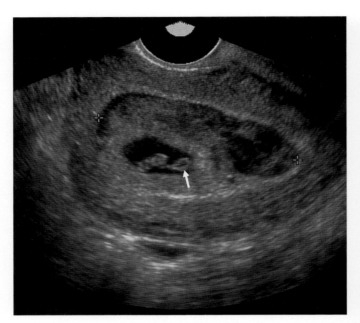

Figure 30.13. A large subchorionic hemorrhage (calipers) covering more than 50% of the gestational sac surface area is seen, along with an abnormally shaped yolk sac (arrow).

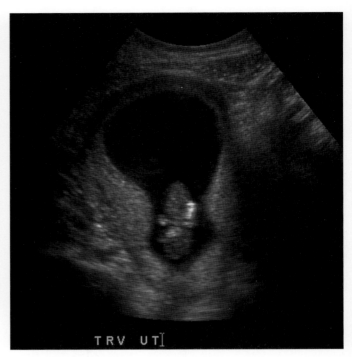

Figure 30.14. Inevitable miscarriage. The patient presented to the emergency department with severe pelvic cramping and bleeding, and a coronal view of the uterus reveals that rhythmic uterine contractions are forcing the gestational sac and embryo well into the cervix.

pregnancy failure or adverse pregnancy outcomes in the latter part of pregnancy. There are many reasons for such discrepant findings, and they include differing study designs, differing mean gestational ages at diagnosis, small case numbers, absence of appropriate control groups, technical variations such as the route of ultrasound, unlike definitions for hematoma size and location, and varying patient populations. Although clinical bleeding alone in the first trimester increases the risk of spontaneous abortion [8,20], two authors [21,22] do still confirm that the finding of SCH in a patient presenting with signs of threatened abortion only further exacerbates the chance of miscarriage, with loss rates approaching 18–20%. Interestingly, however, these results seem most applicable when the hematoma is large and the gestational age at diagnosis is less than 9 weeks. Even in an unselected population, similar results have been reported. The sonographic size of a SCH may not tell the whole story of its effect, however, because it does not take into consideration the amount of outflow from the cervix or the amount of blood reabsorbed from the uterus.

What might the finding of SCH imply regarding pregnancy outcome? In a low-risk group of women [23], an intrauterine hematoma found on routine prenatal scans between 5 and 12 weeks of gestation identified patients who are at increased risk of pre-eclampsia, pregnancy-induced hypertension, abruptio placenta, fetal growth restriction, and cesarean section due to fetal distress. These findings were independent of whether or not the pregnancy was complicated by vaginal bleeding at the time of SCH detection. Other reports also have confirmed similar results [19]. Vaginal bleeding in early pregnancy and SCH may both simply be signs of abnormal placentation. Given the potential for third-trimester pregnancy complications, it makes sense to closely follow such patients clinically, but

there are no clear guidelines about what forms such heightened observation and management should take.

Retained products of conception

Once an empty sac or embryonic demise is definitively diagnosed, the spontaneous completion rates with expectant management for such pregnancies are relatively low at around 50–60%. Although on rare occasions an ultrasound may actually reveal a patient in the very act of miscarriage (Figure 30.14), sonography is more commonly used in the clinical setting of spontaneous abortion. The diagnostic dilemma for the physician in this situation, where pregnancies have been complicated by bleeding and cramping and passing tissue, is when and whether to intervene for retained products of conception (POC) in an effort to avoid further bleeding and infection. Fortunately, the completion rate for incomplete miscarriage is high, at 80–96% [8], for ultrasound predictors of endometrial histology are vague. Many authors who have looked at endometrial thickness alone have used arbitrary cut-off values for curettage, and even an endometrium measuring <2 mm does not exclude POC. It appears that most women with a stripe thickness <10 mm do well without active management, and if it is >10 mm then these other findings may heighten the risk of complication: endometrial heterogeneity, irregular endometrial–myometrial interface [24], and the presence of a focal endometrial mass (Figure 30.15). Ultimately, in many situations of this kind, it is more likely the patient's

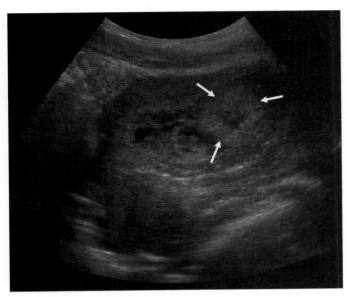

Figure 30.15. Retained products of conception from an incomplete miscarriage are shown in this longitudinal transvaginal image by the complex, thickened, and heteroechoic endometrial stripe and the suggestion of an intracavitary mass (arrows).

clinical condition, and not specific ultrasound findings, that dictates clinical decisions about active intervention to empty the uterus.

Using discriminatory values with caution

It seems intuitive to expect certain ultrasound developmental landmarks to be visible within well-defined gestational time periods. A discriminatory level, then, is the measured point at which absence of a specific sonographic finding can reliably predict a nonviable pregnancy. Such values are used routinely in clinical practice, especially to confirm early pregnancy viability in previously infertile women and in those patients who present with signs of threatened miscarriage.

It is noteworthy that discriminatory values used in this chapter appear as a range, rather than as a single specific cut-off number. That is because a review of the literature reveals conflicting data on the absolute parameters that can be consistently used to diagnose an abnormal or failing pregnancy at a single visit. This should come as no surprise, as any of the following conditions can certainly impact the measurement and reporting of a defined discriminatory value:

- **Operator skill at ultrasound performance and interpretation.** The imaging results of transvaginal sonography are operator-dependent, and the scanning planes are limited. It can be difficult to visualize such things as a very early embryo that is peripherally located up against the wall of the gestational sac.
- **Operator visual acuity.** This confounder is minimized with appropriate image magnification.
- **Measuring error or mathematical miscalculation.**

- **Inadequate image optimization.** Image quality can be negatively affected by such things as improper focal zone placement at or just below the area of interest.
- **Timing of hCG testing and ultrasound.** Given that both laboratory and ultrasound parameters in early pregnancy are changing daily, it becomes important to know the exact timing of these tests. If the hCG is measured even 24 hours later than the ultrasound, its value could have increased by as much as 1.7 times by then.
- **Myometrial heterogeneity, fibroids, or an intrauterine device.** Ultrasound imaging posterior to any of these structures can inhibit the ability to adequately visualize small, early-pregnancy structures.
- **Maternal obesity.** High-frequency ultrasound transducers do not penetrate well, so imaging resolution at a distance from the transvaginal probe is impeded.
- **Uterine position.** This is especially significant when the position is midplane and the endometrial cavity contents are parallel to the ultrasound beam.
- **Transducer frequency.** In studies where higher-frequency probes are used, discriminatory values are consistently lower [10], and the ability to visualize structures such as the GS, YS, and embryonic fetal heart can be transducer-dependent.
- **Equipment age, maintenance status and variability.**
- **Exact ultrasound criteria definitions.** There are differing definitions in the cited literature even for what, exactly, constitute criteria for an early pregnancy. Whereas some authors describe a GS as a fluid collection specifically surrounded by an echogenic rim, others emphasize the eccentric location of the fluid sac with or without mentioning the quality of the peripheral choriodecidual reaction.
- **Multiple gestation or small GS size.** Twin pregnancies, not uncommon in an infertility practice, may affect interpretation of either the visible sac size or the measured hCG level.
- **Unusually large GS size or a growth-restricted embryo.**
- **Variations or imprecision in hCG measurement.** hCG assays may be different from one laboratory to another due to each test and its coefficient of variation (standard deviation/mean). In addition, the analyzers for these tests at different sites may or may not require a sample dilution to interpret and record a result greater than 500 mIU/ml.

When applied to an unselected patient population, therefore, caution must be exercised when using any single value or result to definitively diagnose a failed pregnancy. Discriminatory values used to characterize pregnancies as normal or abnormal should be used as a conservative clinical guideline only. A desired pregnancy may warrant repeat serial ultrasound, and possibly hCG measurement, as necessary to finally confirm a failed pregnancy prior to surgical intervention. In fact, in some countries such repetitive ultrasounds are part of the recommended care policy when embryonic death is suspected [25].

Key points in clinical practice

- It is imperative for the physician to be fully knowledgeable regarding the sonographic hallmarks of early, normal pregnancy.

- The presence of the YS confirms the diagnosis and location of the GS, and detectable fetal heart motion documents viability.

- Pregnancy failure should be suspected when the GS, the YS, or embryo, and then embryonic heart motion are not present despite adequate discriminatory values for hCG, MSD, and embryonic length, respectively. In addition, lack of normal growth of the GS or embryo over time implies the same.

- Published discriminatory values may not be applicable in every clinical setting, and their use should be applied very carefully. Especially when measured values are borderline, liberal use of follow-up studies is encouraged.

- Several minor ultrasound deviations from normal involving the GS, YS, and embryo can also represent early warning signs of adverse pregnancy outcome.

References

1. Goldstein SR. Embryonic death in early pregnancy: a new look at the first trimester. *Obstet Gynecol* 1994; **84**(2): 294–7.

2. Yeh HC. Efficacy of the intradecidual sign and fallacy of the double decidual sac sign in the diagnosis of early intrauterine pregnancy. *Radiology* 1999; **210**(2): 579–82.

3. Bree RL, Edwards M, Bohm-Velez M, Beyler S, Roberts J, Mendelson EB. Transvaginal sonography in the evaluation of normal early pregnancy: correlation with HCG level. *Am J Roentgenol* 1989; **153**(1): 75–9.

4. Barnhart KT, Sammel MD, Rinaudo PF, Zhou L, Hummel AC, Guo W. Symptomatic patients with an early viable intrauterine pregnancy: HCG curves redefined. *Obstet Gynecol* 2004; **104**(1): 50–5.

5. Nyberg DA, Mack LA, Laing FC, Patten RM. Distinguishing normal from abnormal gestational sac growth in early pregnancy. *J Ultrasound Med* 1987; **6**(1): 23–7.

6. Bromley B, Harlow BL, Laboda LA, Benacerraf BR. Small sac size in the first trimester: a predictor of poor fetal outcome. *Radiology* 1991; **178**(2): 375–7.

7. Smith GC, Smith MF, McNay MB, Fleming JE. First-trimester growth and the risk of low birth weight. *N Engl J Med* 1998; **339**(25): 1817–22.

8. Jauniaux E, Johns J, Burton GJ. The role of ultrasound imaging in diagnosing and investigating early pregnancy failure. *Ultrasound Obstet Gynecol* 2005; **25**(6): 613–24.

9. Nyberg DA, Mack LA, Harvey D, Wang K. Value of the yolk sac in evaluating early pregnancies. *J Ultrasound Med* 1988; **7**(3): 129–35.

10. Rowling SE, Langer JE, Coleman BG, Nisenbaum HL, Horii SC, Arger PH. Sonography during early pregnancy: dependence of threshold and discriminatory values on transvaginal transducer frequency. *Am J Roentgenol* 1999; **172**(4): 983–8.

11. Mara E, Foster GS. Spontaneous regression of a yolk sac associated with embryonic death. *J Ultrasound Med* 2000; **19**(9): 655–6.

12. Harris RD, Vincent LM, Askin FB. Yolk sac calcification: a sonographic finding associated with intrauterine embryonic demise in the first trimester. *Radiology* 1988; **166**(1 pt 1): 109–10.

13. Chama CM, Marupa JY, Obed JY. The value of the secondary yolk sac in predicting pregnancy outcome. *J Obstet Gynaecol* 2005; **25**(3): 245–7.

14. Brown DL, Emerson DS, Felker RE, Cartier MS, Smith WC. Diagnosis of early embryonic demise by endovaginal sonography. *J Ultrasound Med* 1990; **9**(11): 631–6.

15. Chittacharoen A, Herabutya Y. Slow fetal heart rate may predict pregnancy outcome in first-trimester threatened abortion. *Fertil Steril* 2004; **82**(1): 227–9.

16. Rowling SE, Coleman BG, Langer JE, Arger PH, Nisenbaum HL, Horii SC. First-trimester US parameters of failed pregnancy. *Radiology* 1997; **203**(1): 211–17.

17. Goldstein SR, Wolfson R. Endovaginal ultrasonographic measurement of early embryonic size as a means of assessing gestational age. *J Ultrasound Med* 1994; **13**(1): 27–31.

18. Reljic M. The significance of crown-rump length measurement for predicting adverse pregnancy outcome of threatened abortion. *Ultrasound Obstet Gynecol* 2001; **17**(6): 510–12.

19. Ball RH, Ade CM, Schoenborn JA, Crane JP. The clinical significance of ultrasonographically detected subchorionic hemorrhages. *Am J Obstet Gynecol* 1996; **174**(3): 996–1002.

20. Johns J, Hyett J, Jauniaux E. Obstetric outcome after threatened miscarriage with and without a hematoma on ultrasound. *Obstet Gynecol* 2003; **102**(3): 483–7.

21. Bennett GL, Bromley B, Lieberman E, Benacerraf BR. Subchorionic hemorrhage in first-trimester pregnancies: prediction of pregnancy outcome with sonography. *Radiology* 1996; **200**(3): 803–6.

22. Maso G, D'Ottavio G, De Seta F, Sartore A, Piccoli M, Mandruzzato G. First-trimester intrauterine hematoma and outcome of pregnancy. *Obstet Gynecol* 2005; **105**(2): 339–44.

23. Nagy S, Bush M, Stone J, Lapinski RH, Gardo S. Clinical significance of subchorionic and retroplacental hematomas detected in the first trimester of pregnancy. *Obstet Gynecol* 2003; **102**(1): 94–100.

24. Alcazar JL, Baldonado C, Laparte C. The reliability of transvaginal ultrasonography to detect retained tissue after spontaneous first-trimester abortion, clinically thought to be complete. *Ultrasound Obstet Gynecol* 1995; **6**(2): 126–9.

25. Hately W, Case J, Campbell S. Establishing the death of an embryo by ultrasound: report of a public inquiry with recommendations. *Ultrasound Obstet Gynecol* 1995; **5**(5): 353–7.

Chapter 31

Ectopic pregnancy

Botros Rizk, Mostafa Abuzeid, Christine B. Rizk, Sheri Owens, John C. LaFleur and Youssef Simaika

An ectopic pregnancy is defined as any pregnancy in which implantation occurs at a location other than the endometrium [1]. The Arabian writer Abulcasis is credited with the first description of ectopic pregnancy in AD 963 [2]. Ectopic pregnancies account for 1.4% of all reported pregnancies and result in 11.5–17.6% of all maternal deaths annually [3,4,5]. Although the mortality from ectopic pregnancy is less than 1 per 1000, ectopic pregnancy has a risk of death 10 times greater than that of childbirth and 50 times greater than that of legally induced abortion [6]. In 1987, 30 women in the United States died from ectopic pregnancy [2]. Although the death rate from ectopic pregnancy has declined by more than tenfold as a result of early diagnosis by ultrasonography, it is still a leading cause of mortality in the first trimester of pregnancy. The risk of death is greater in black and unmarried women [2].

The incidence of ectopic pregnancy continues to rise in the United States [1,2,3,4,5,6,7,8]. Since 1970, the first year for which statistics were compiled by the Centers for Disease Control (CDC), the incidence of ectopic pregnancy in the United States has steadily increased from 4.5/1000 to 19.7/1000 [4]. It is estimated that more than 100 000 ectopic pregnancies occur in the United states. Factors that have contributed to the increased incidence of ectopic pregnancy over the last three decades include an increase in pelvic inflammatory disease, improved therapy for salpingitis that results in patent but scarred fallopian tubes, microsurgical tubal surgery, and assisted reproductive technologies [6,7,8,9,10,11,12,13,14,15,16]. Previous ectopic pregnancy, endometriosis, and pregnancy with an intrauterine device in place also increase the risk of an ectopic gestation.

The majority of ectopic pregnancies, 90–95%, are located in the fallopian tubes. The majority of these tubal pregnancies are located in the ampullary region of the fallopian tube and less commonly in the isthmical region. In 2–4%, the pregnancy implants in the intramural portion of the fallopian tube, termed interstitial or cornual pregnancy. Cervical pregnancy, when the gestational sac implants in the cervix, is rare. Abdominal ectopic pregnancy is a very rare form of ectopic pregnancy in which the gestational sac implants in the peritoneal cavity. Heterotopic pregnancy refers to the coexistence of intrauterine and extrauterine pregnancies at the same time [9,10,11,12,13,14,15,16,17,18].

Tubal ectopic pregnancy

The increased prevalence of pelvic inflammatory disease and the use of assisted reproductive technologies (ART) have increased the incidence of ectopic pregnancy over the past three decades [12]. Rare forms of ectopic pregnancy have been reported following the widespread use of ART. Rizk et al. have reported four bilateral tubal pregnancies and one unilateral tubal twin pregnancy [10].

Clinical presentation of ectopic tubal pregnancy

The classic presentation of ectopic pregnancy includes the triad of pelvic pain, abnormal vaginal bleeding, and an adnexal mass. This classic triad is less commonly seen today. More commonly, abnormal vaginal bleeding or pelvic tenderness is encountered as the leading presenting symptom. Abdominal pain has been reported in 90–100% of ectopic pregnancy and frequently begins far in advance of tubal rupture. Abnormal vaginal bleeding or amenorrhea is associated with 75% of cases. The possibility of ectopic pregnancy should be considered in all women with lower abdominal pain and a positive pregnancy test.

The most common clinical finding on physical examination is adnexal tenderness, which has been reported to occur in 75–90% of ectopic pregnancies. Internal hemorrhage may be severe enough to cause hypovolemic shock, particularly if there has been a delay in diagnosis.

The differential diagnosis includes threatened or incomplete abortion, pelvic inflammatory disease, adnexal torsion, degeneration of a uterine leiomyoma, endometriosis, or appendicitis, as discussed in Chapter 22.

Ultrasonographic appearance of tubal ectopic pregnancy

Ultrasonography is the primary diagnostic modality for the diagnosis of ectopic pregnancy (Figures 31.1, 31.2, 31.3, 31.4, 31.5, 31.6, 31.7). Transvaginal ultrasonography has revolutionized female pelvic imaging [19,20,21,22,23,24,25]. If a woman of reproductive age presents with pelvic pain, vaginal bleeding, and a positive pregnancy test, ultrasonography should be performed as an emergency. The optimal approach for the

Ultrasonography in Reproductive Medicine and Infertility, ed. Botros R. M. B. Rizk. Published by Cambridge University Press. © Cambridge University Press 2010.

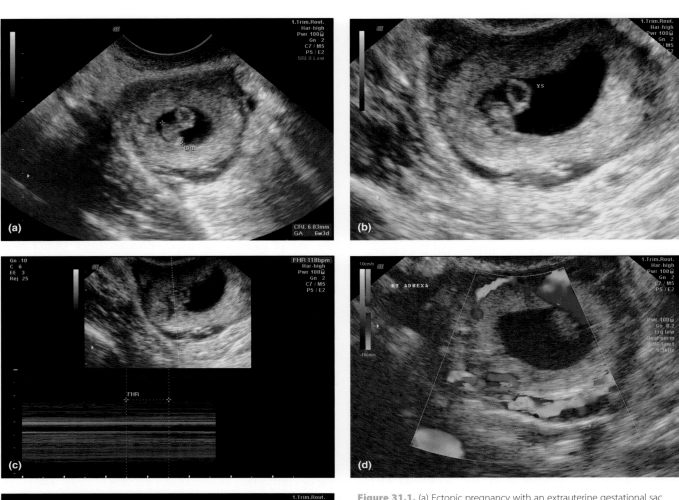

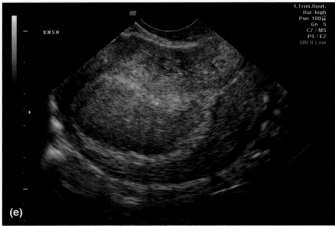

Figure 31.1. (a) Ectopic pregnancy with an extrauterine gestational sac containing a live embryo. The figure shows the measurement of the crown–rump length (calipers) and the echogenic ring of the ectopic pregnancy. (b) Ectopic pregnancy with an extrauterine gestational sac containing a yolk sac and fetal pole. (c) Ectopic pregnancy with an extrauterine gestational sac; the embryo has cardiac activity documented by M-mode (dotted line on image). Calipers measure a single heartbeat. (d) Ectopic pregnancy with an extrauterine gestational sac, with color Doppler demonstrating considerable blood flow. (e) Transvaginal ultrasound of the uterus showing no intrauterine gestational sac.

evaluation of suspected ectopic pregnancy is to focus on the uterus in an effort to detect an intrauterine pregnancy [7]. Approximately 90% of women with a positive pregnancy test referred for ruling out of an ectopic pregnancy are ultimately shown to have an intrauterine pregnancy. This frequency, combined with the knowledge that coexistent intrauterine and extrauterine pregnancies are rare, makes it initially logical to search for an intrauterine pregnancy [6,7,8].

The visualization of a fluid-filled sac outside the uterine cavity that contains an embryo with or without cardiac activity or a yolk sac is definitive for ectopic pregnancy (Figures 31.1, 31.2, 31.3). Stiller et al. [19] and Fleicher et al. [20] observed that approximately one-sixth to one-third of ectopic pregnancies develop to yolk sac formation or cardiac activity. This strict criterion has the highest specificity (100%) but the lowest sensitivity (20%) in identifying ectopic pregnancy. A more common

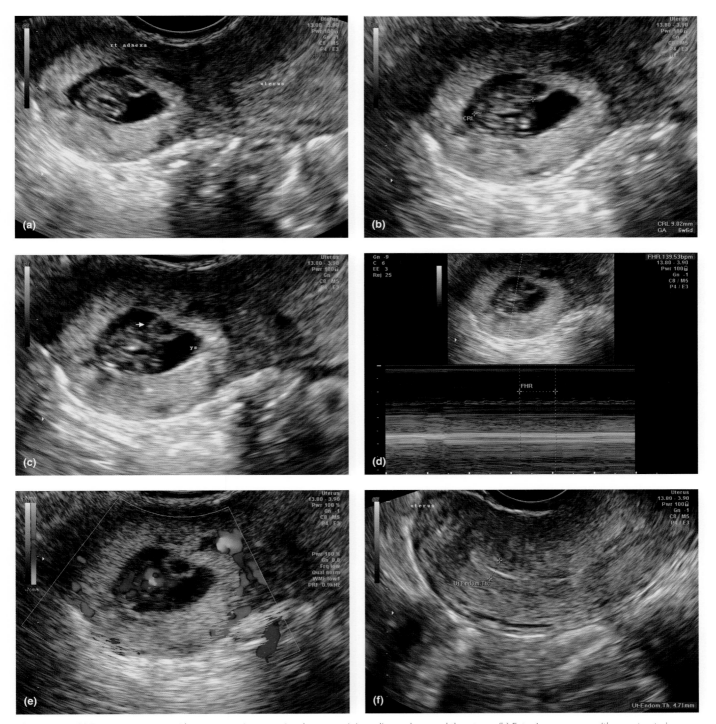

Figure 31.2. (a) Ectopic pregnancy with an extrauterine gestational sac containing a live embryo and the uterus. (b) Ectopic pregnancy with an extrauterine gestational sac showing the crown–rump length of the embryo (calipers). (c) Ectopic pregnancy with an extrauterine gestational sac showing the embryo and yolk sac (arrow). (d) Ectopic pregnancy with an extrauterine gestational sac; the embryo has cardiac activity documented by M-mode (dotted line). Calipers measure a single heartbeat. (e) Color Doppler imaging demonstrating blood flow in the embryo and surrounding gestational sac. (f) Transvaginal ultrasonography of the uterus; sagittal view of uterus reveals no evidence of an intrauterine gestational sac.

ultrasonographic finding in a woman with ectopic pregnancy is a complex adnexal mass [6,7,8]. The presence of this finding has a sensitivity of 20–80% and a specificity of 93–99%.

On the basis of the results of 10 studies, Brown and Doubilet concluded that the most useful criterion was the presence of any noncystic adnexal ovarian mass [24]. This criterion, which includes living ectopics, tubal rings, and common solid or cystic masses, had a high specificity (99%), positive predictive value (96%), sensitivity (84%), and negative predictive value (95%). Therefore, in the absence of an intrauterine pregnancy, the

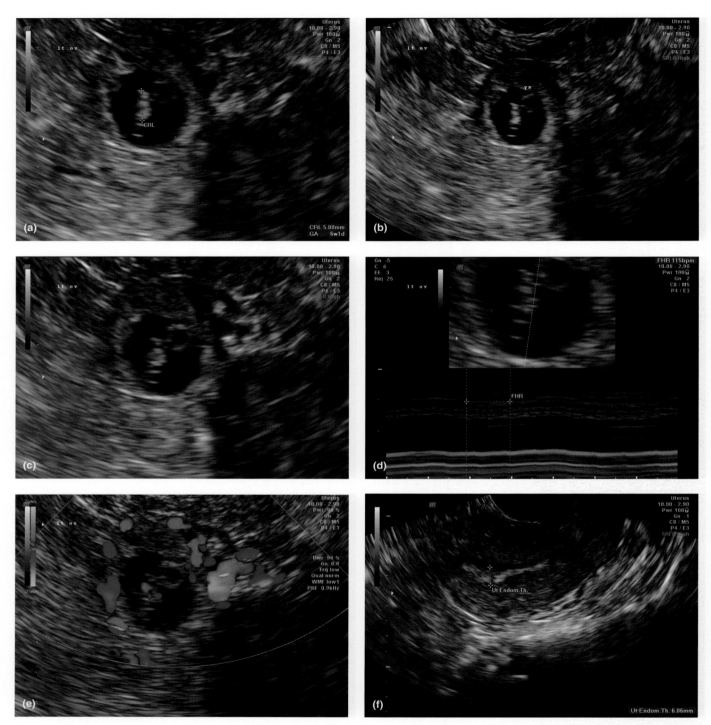

Figure 31.3 (a) Ectopic pregnancy with an extrauterine gestational sac, demonstrating crown–rump length and coronal view of the left ovary. (b) Ectopic pregnancy with an extrauterine gestational sac, revealing yolk sac and a coronal view of the left ovary. (c) Ectopic pregnancy with an extrauterine gestational sac, revealing the embryo and the yolk sac and a coronal section of the left ovary. (d) Ectopic pregnancy with an extrauterine gestational sac; the embryo has cardiac activity documented by M-mode (dotted line). Caliper reveals single heartbeat. (e) Transvaginal color Doppler of an ectopic pregnancy demonstrating blood flow within the embryo and considerable blood flow surrounding the gestational sac. (f) Transvaginal sagittal view of the uterus, revealing a thin endometrium (6 mm) and no gestational sac. (g) Transvaginal view of the uterus, revealing no gestational sac.

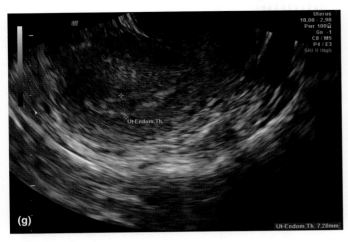

Figure 31.3. (cont.)

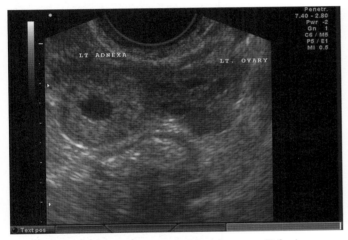

Figure 31.4. Transvaginal coronal view of the left ovary and left adnexa, demonstrating an extrauterine gestational sac with an echogenic ring but no fetal pole or fetal heart.

ultrasonographic visualization of a complex adnexal mass that is separate from the ovary can be used to diagnose an ectopic pregnancy (Figure 31.4). However, in 15–35% of patients with ectopic pregnancy, no adnexal masses will be identified despite meticulous ultrasonographic technique [24].

Ultrasonography of the uterus in ectopic pregnancy

The endometrium varies in appearance and thickness in tubal pregnancy (Figures 31.1e, 31.2f, 31.3f). There is no specific endometrial pattern or thickness that can be used to suggest an ectopic pregnancy, or to differentiate the endometrial appearance in women subsequently shown to have an ectopic pregnancy versus a normal or abnormal intrauterine pregnancy.

Pseudogestational sac

The uterine cavity may contain secretions or blood and what is often termed a pseudogestational sac, because it can be mistaken for a true gestational sac. However, a pseudogestational sac does not have the true characteristics of a true gestational sac. It lacks the double echogenic ring around it and has no embryo or yolk sac within it [6,7,8]. The double decidual sac sign has been suggested as a finding that characterizes an early intrauterine pregnancy and reliably discriminates an intrauterine gestational sac from the pseudogestational sac of an ectopic pregnancy before the ability to visualize either the yolk sac or the embryo [6]. The double sac that consists of two concentric rings surrounding a portion of the gestational sac was thought to represent the decidua parietalis (vera) adjacent to the decidua capsularis. Filly (1996) [6] observed by endovaginal sonography that the inner ring is composed of the chorionic villi proliferating around the developing gestation, while the outer ring is the deeper and more echogenic layer of the decidua vera

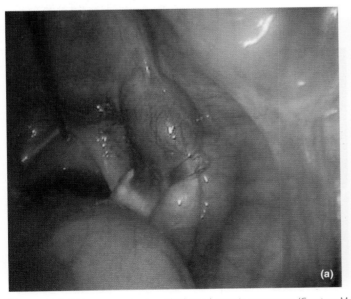

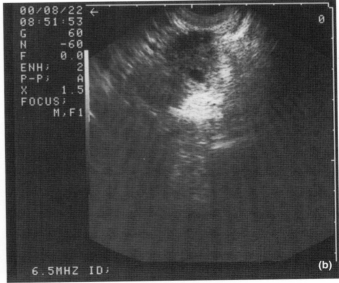

Figure 31.5. (a) Laparoscopic view of isthmical ectopic pregnancy. (Courtesy M. I. Abuzeid.) (b) Ultrasonographic view of isthmical ectopic pregnancy. (Courtesy M. I. Abuzeid.)

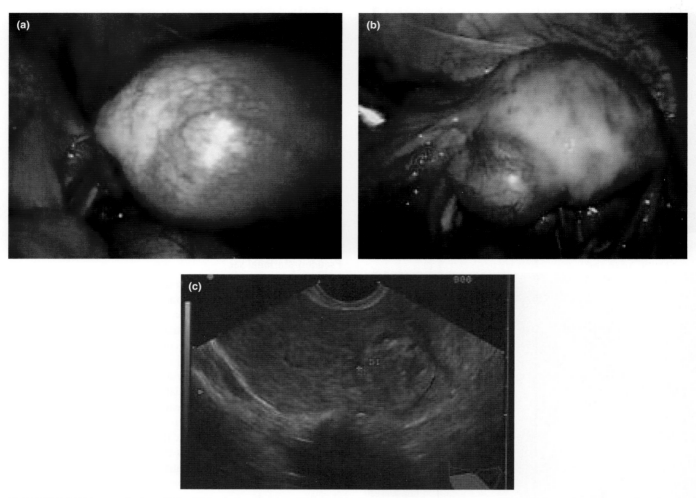

Figure 31.6 (a) Laparoscopic view of interstitial ectopic pregnancy. (Courtesy M. I. Abuzeid.) (b) Laparoscopic view of interstitial ectopic pregnancy after pitressin injection. (Courtesy M. I. Abuzeid.) (c) Ultrasonographic view of interstitial ectopic pregnancy. (Courtesy M. I. Abuzeid.)

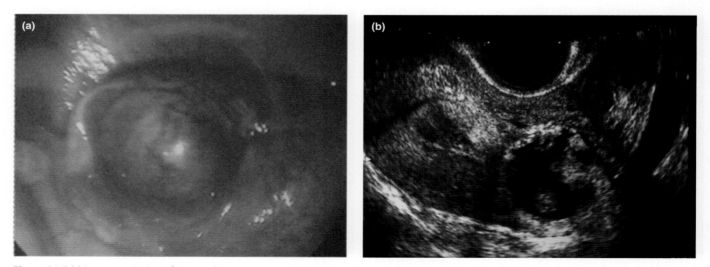

Figure 31.7 (a) Laparoscopic view of interstitial ectopic pregnancy. (Courtesy S. Marcus.) (b) Ultrasonographic view of interstitial ectopic pregnancy. (Courtesy S. Marcus.)

(Figure 30.3, Chapter 30). When the decidua vera is uniformly echogenic throughout its entire thickness, a true double decidual sac sign cannot be demonstrated [6]. In contrast, the pseudogestational sac is composed of an echogenic ring surrounding an intraendometrial fluid collection. However, Filly cautioned that the double decidual sac sign does not absolutely exclude a pseudogestational sac, nor does its presence confirm that a intrauterine pregnancy is normal [6].

Evaluation of intrauterine contents beyond exclusion of an intrauterine pregnancy does not improve diagnostic pregnancy. A pseudogestational sac may be present in 5–35% of ectopic pregnancies.

Doppler ultrasonography in the diagnosis of adnexal masses and ectopic pregnancy

The use of color and pulsed Doppler could improve the sensitivity of making the diagnosis of ectopic pregnancy. The rationale for using Doppler is to detect a high-velocity, low-resistance arterial flow patterns within the trophoblastic tissue in the ectopic pregnancy (Figures 31.1c, 31.1d, 31.2d, 31.2e, 31.3d, 31.3e). Once color flow identifies a possible ectopic pregnancy, the use of pulsed Doppler and determining the resistance index could differentiate an ectopic pregnancy from a corpus luteum [25]. There is an overlap in the resistance index of the ectopic pregnancy and corpus luteum. The blood flow around the ectopic is sometimes referred to as the "ring of fire." In contrast, the lack of flow cannot be used to exclude an ectopic pregnancy.

Pellerito et al. performed endovaginal sonography and endovaginal imaging in 155 patients with clinical suspicion of ectopic pregnancy [3]. Sixty-five patients (42%), had surgically confirmed ectopic pregnancies. They diagnosed 36 of the ectopic pregnancies with endovaginal sonography alone, the criteria being an extrauterine gestational sac or an ectopic fetus (sensitivity 54%). Endovaginal color flow imaging diagnosed 62 ectopic pregnancies when an ectopic fetus or sac was visualized or placental was flow identified in an adnexal mass separate from the uterus, with a sensitivity of 95%. The authors concluded that the use of color Doppler flow imaging, in addition to vaginal sonography, increased the sensitivity in the detection of ectopic pregnancy. They utilized a low-impedance pattern separate from the ovary to suggest or diagnose placental flow. Several of the early or dead ectopic pregnancies demonstrated no evidence of placental flow. All the avascular ectopic pregnancies demonstrated serum hCG levels less than 6000 mIU/ml. Only one of the 65 ectopic pregnancies (1.5%) was a solid avascular mass. Doppler may provide additional information about some adnexal masses [3]. However, the actual diagnosis depends on the gray scale features, and Doppler should not be considered mandatory during the evaluation of an ectopic pregnancy [6,7,8].

Endometrial Doppler in the diagnosis of ectopic pregnancy

The application of color and duplex Doppler to the endometrium has been used to differentiate a true gestational sac from a pseudogestational sac. The rationale for using Doppler with an early intrauterine pregnancy is to identify a high-velocity, low-resistance arterial flow associated with developing chorionic villi [6,7,8]. The resistance index should be <0.6. The specificity of this application remains to be determined, because a failed intrauterine pregnancy may or may not demonstrate blood flow in the developing trophoblast.

Free fluid in ectopic pregnancy

Free intraperitoneal fluid is not diagnostic for ectopic pregnancy. Isolated free fluid has been observed in 15% of patients with ectopic pregnancy. The fluid may result from active bleeding from the fimbriated end of the tube or rupture of the fallopian tube. A ruptured corpus luteum or hemorrhagic ovarian cyst could also be the source of the intraperitoneal fluid. The echogenicity of the intraperitoneal fluid may also help to suggest the absence or presence of hemoperitoneum.

Ultrasonography and human chorionic gonadotropin levels in the diagnosis and management of ectopic pregnancy

If an ectopic pregnancy cannot be clearly visualized by transvaginal sonography, and in the absence of an intrauterine gestational sac, it is imperative to determine the quantitative serum level of β-hCG. In normal pregnancy, hCG levels double every 48 hours during the first 6 weeks and, using sensitive radioimmunoassay, the serum level can be determined 23 days after the last normal menstrual period, which is approximately 8 days after ovulation. If the result of the hCG test is negative, a developing pregnancy is excluded. A chronic, nonliving ectopic pregnancy is a rare exception to this rule. If the pregnancy test is positive, the serum β-hCG level should be determined and correlated with the findings of transvaginal ultrasonography.

Human chorionic gonadotropin discriminatory zone

A normal intrauterine gestational sac should be visualized by ultrasonography when the level is 1000 mIU/ml or greater [26]. Failure to identify a normal intrauterine gestational sac when this discriminatory zone is reached suggests either an abnormal intrauterine pregnancy with a spontaneous abortion or an ectopic pregnancy [26]. If the β-hCG level is increasing on further evaluation and still no intrauterine gestational sac is identified, an ectopic pregnancy is suggested unless the patient has experienced a spontaneous abortion. The history is often crucial for suggesting the correct diagnosis. Rizk et al. [14] cautioned that in multiple pregnancy, where the β-hCG level would be greater than for the expected gestational age, hCG levels should be interpreted taking into consideration the multiplicity as determined by the ultrasonographic appearance.

Management of ectopic pregnancy

Ultrasonography has revolutionized the management of tubal ectopic pregnancy [21,22,23,24,25,26]. Early diagnosis allows medical treatment to be the first-line choice in appropriate cases. Prior to ultrasonography, most cases were treated surgically by laparoscopy (Figures 31.5, 31.6, 31.7) or laparotomy. The management of ectopic pregnancy was revolutionized by Lawson et al., who reported the successful treatment of four women in England and Wales by salpingectomy. Conservative management has been considered for more than a century. One of the earliest reports of conservative treatment, vaginal puncture to treat ectopic pregnancy instead of laparotomy, was reported by Kelly in 1896 in the Johns Hopkins Hospital bulletin [27]. Encouraged by his success, he treated 10 other cases using vaginal puncture. Mahfouz in 1938 presented a comprehensive and elegant management of a series of ectopic pregnancy in Cairo, Egypt, where he debated the role of salpingostomy versus salpingectomy [28].

Many modalities of ultrasonographically guided treatment have been reported, including injection of potassium chloride in the fetal heart of the ectopic gestation or methotrexate in the ectopic gestational sac. Feichtinger and Kemeter treated unruptured ectopic pregnancies by needling and injection of methotrexate or prostaglandin (PGE_2) under transvaginal sonographic control [29]. Timor-Tritsch et al. used transvaginal salpingocentesis for treatment of ectopic pregnancy [30]. Rizk et al. utilized potassium chloride for the treatment of extrauterine pregnancy for selected cases of heterotopic pregnancies after in-vitro fertilization at Bourn Hall Clinic [11].

Interstitial (cornual) ectopic pregnancy

Interstitial or cornual ectopic pregnancy is a pregnancy that implants in the interstitial or intramural portion of the fallopian tube (Figures 31.6 and 31.7). Interstitial pregnancies account for 2–4% of ectopic pregnancies. The term cornual pregnancy is frequently used interchangeably with interstitial pregnancy, although strictly it should be reserved for pregnancies that develop in a rudimentary uterine horn. It has been suggested that the interchangeable use of these terms in clinical practice can create problems for clinicians interpreting ultrasound reports, as the clinical course and management differ markedly between intrauterine cornual gestations and ectopic interstitial gestations [31]. In contrast to a tubal ectopic pregnancy which may rupture at 6–8 weeks of gestation, an interstitial ectopic pregnancy may progress without symptoms until rupture occurs at 12–16 weeks, although the study by the Society for Reproductive Surgeons (SRS) has questioned this statement [32]. The SRS study analyzed 32 cases of interstitial pregnancy reported to the Registry between 1999 and 2002. Fourteen of 32 patients experienced rupture at less than 12 weeks of gestation. Their conclusion is that interstitial pregnancies could rupture earlier than assumed [32].

Ultrasonography of interstitial pregnancy

The diagnosis of interstitial pregnancy should be suspected when ultrasonography demonstrates eccentric implantation of the gestational sac at the superior fundal level of the uterus (Figures 31.6 and 31.7). Ultrasonographic diagnosis of interstitial pregnancy is possible at an early stage before rupture. Timor-Tritsch et al. used three sonographic criteria for diagnosis of interstitial pregnancy: (1) an empty uterine cavity; (2) a chorionic sac seen separately 1 cm from the most lateral edge of the uterine cavity; and (3) a thin myometrial layer surrounding the chorionic sac [33].

The interstitial line sign is another useful ultrasound diagnostic criterion [34]. It is an echogenic line that extends into the upper regions of the uterine horn and borders the margins of the intrauterine gestational sac. Ackerman et al. suggested that the thin echogenic line likely represents the interstitial portion of the fallopian tube. This sign had 80% sensitivity and 98% specificity for the ultrasonographic diagnosis of interstitial pregnancy [35].

Distinguishing between interstitial ectopic pregnancy and an eccentrically located intrauterine pregnancy can present a diagnostic dilemma [5]. The appearance of myometrium around the sac appears to be the most useful ultrasonographic feature in making the distinction. 3D ultrasonography could also be very useful in differentiating a questionable ectopic from an eccentrically located intrauterine pregnancy [35]. In a subseptate uterus, the eccentric location of the pregnancy might make it difficult to distinguish it from a cornual pregnancy.

Management of interstitial pregnancy

The conventional management of interstitial pregnancy is hysterectomy or cornual wedge resection with or without ipsilateral salpingectomy through laparotomy [6]. Although hysterectomy or cornual resection is a perfect method for terminating the pregnancy, these are not desirable in patients who wish to preserve their fertility.

Conservative management has been used with laparoscopy, hysteroscopy, or medical treatment (Figure 31.6b).Tanaka et al. introduced medical treatment with methotrexate in 1982 [36], Reich et al. reported the first case of laparoscopic management in 1988 [37], and Meyer and Mitchell utilized hysteroscopic management in 1989 [38]. Various hemostatic techniques have been used laparoscopically, including diluted intramyometrial pitressin (Figure 31.6b). electrocauterization [39], fibrin glue [40], ultrasonic cutting and coagulating surgical devices (harmonic scalpel), and tourniquet suture [41]. Timor-Tritsch et al. treated cornual pregnancy using methotrexate and, in a case of heterotopic pregnancy, potassium chloride [33].

Cervical ectopic pregnancy

Cervical ectopic pregnancy is very rare in naturally conceived pregnancies [42]. Its incidence represents 0.15–0.20% of all ectopic pregnancies [6,7,8]. Its actual incidence has been estimated to vary between 1 per 1000 and 1 per 20 000 pregnancies. Rizk and Brinsden observed that cervical pregnancy is still very rare following assisted reproduction [13]. Patients are at high risk of potential life-threatening hemorrhage, which may lead to hysterectomy or to a loss of future reproductive potential. Transvaginal ultrasonography has revolutionized the diagnosis of cervical pregnancy, allowing the utilization of conservative options. Uncontrollable hemorrhage remains the most serious aspect of medical care and its management has included a variety of innovative options, including angiographic uterine artery embolization, curettage and local prostaglandin injection, hysteroscopic resection, uterine artery ligation and cervicotomy, intracervical injections of vasoconstrictive agents, and Shirodkar-type cervical cerclage [43,44,45].

Ovarian pregnancy

Primary ovarian pregnancy is a rare form of ectopic pregnancy. In 1614, Mercier was the first to suggest that pregnancy might occur within the ovary [46], but it was not until 1899 that Catherine Van Tussenbroek of Amsterdam convinced a skeptical medical establishment of the occurrence of this condition by presenting the first accurate clinical and histological description of the abnormality [47]. The classic anatomic and histological criteria for the diagnosis of an authentic case of ovarian pregnancy were suggested by Spiegelberg in 1878. The conceptus occupied the anatomic location of the ovary, which was connected to the uterus by the utero-ovarian ligament; ovarian tissue was histologically distinguishable about the wall of the conceptus, and the ipsilateral tube was intact [48,49,50].

Incidence of ovarian pregnancy

The incidence of ovarian pregnancy has been reported to range from as low as 1 in 60 000 to as high as 1 in 7000. Its occurrence remains rare despite the different forms of ectopic pregnancy seen following assisted conception [51,52].

Mechanism of ovarian pregnancy

The likely mechanism of this occurrence is the reverse migration of one of the embryos through the fallopian tube with subsequent implantation in the ovary, although other possibilities cannot be excluded.

Clinical picture of ovarian pregnancy

The clinical pictures of ovarian pregnancy and tubal pregnancy are indistinguishable during early gestation. Most ovarian pregnancies (75–90%) rupture in the first trimester, with two-thirds rupturing during the first 8 weeks. Indeed, among the sites in which pregnancy may develop ectopically, the ovary may have the greatest ability to accommodate a pregnancy and offer the highest chance of development to term and survival of the infant. As many as 4–12% of ovarian pregnancies have been reported to be maintained into the third trimester.

Management of ovarian pregnancy

Early diagnosis by ultrasonography allows the conservation of the ovary. Rizk et al. reported successful surgical removal of an ovarian ectopic pregnancy with ovarian preservation followed by a successful IVF attempt with a subsequent intrauterine pregnancy [52].

Abdominal pregnancy

Abdominal pregnancy is a rare form of ectopic pregnancy in which the gestational sac implants in the peritoneal cavity of the abdomen or pelvis. Abdominal pregnancy may be primary or secondary. In primary abdominal pregnancy, the pregnancy implants directly in the peritoneal cavity of the abdomen or the pelvis. In secondary abdominal pregnancy, the pregnancy begins as a tubal pregnancy and then reimplants in the peritoneal cavity after the expulsion of the gestational sac from the end of the tube or after the rupture of the fallopian tube.

Maternal mortality in abdominal pregnancy

Maternal mortality is significantly increased in abdominal pregnancy due to the high incidence of internal hemorrhage or sepsis. In many abdominal pregnancies, the fetus dies early in pregnancy. However, the pregnancy can remain alive to the second or even third trimester.

Ultrasonography of abdominal pregnancy

In the early part of the first trimester, abdominal pregnancy is very difficult to distinguish from tubal pregnancy by ultrasonography. In the late first trimester, demonstration of a live fetus outside the uterus is highly suggestive of abdominal pregnancy, because the fallopian tube cannot contain a pregnancy as large as 12 weeks [8]. It is important to delineate the margin of the uterus carefully in order to demonstrate that the gestational sac lies outside the uterus. Other important ultrasonographic features of abdominal pregnancy include oligohydramnios and abnormal fetal lie, usually above the maternal pelvis and extra-uterine placental tissue. A live fetus is born in 10–20% of advanced abdominal pregnancies, but neonatal mortality is very high because of pulmonary hyperplasia and oligohydramnios. Advanced abdominal pregnancy should be managed by prompt delivery of the fetus and removal of the placenta if it appears that the blood supply can be effectively controlled. If the placenta cannot be removed, and there are large vessels involved, the cord should be ligated and the placenta left in situ. Methotrexate treatment of abdominal pregnancy has been associated with several deaths and should not be considered.

Lithopedion

Lithopedion is a rare form of calcified and mummified abdominal pregnancy. Rizk et al. reported a lithopedion that had been present for the longest period, almost 50 years after its occurrence in the patient. In that situation, the patient presented with signs of colon cancer, and during radiography and CT scan a lithopedion was diagnosed that was 6 months in size [53].

Heterotopic pregnancy

The incidence of heterotopic pregnancy in spontaneously conceived pregnancies is 1/4000 to 1/30 000. Among pregnancies achieved by assisted reproduction, that incidence can increase to as high as 1–4% [9,11,15]. The diagnosis of heterotopic pregnancy is usually delayed because of the presence of an intrauterine pregnancy, which could be hazardous. Because of the importance of this entity in reproductive medicine, we have dedicated the next chapter to heterotopic pregnancy.

Key points in clinical practice

- Ectopic pregnancy represents 0.14% of pregnancies but contributes to 11.6% of maternal mortality.

- Tubal pregnancy represents 90–95% of all ectopic pregnancy. The majority of tubal pregnancies are located in the ampullary region of the fallopian tube.

- Transvaginal ultrasonography has revolutionized the diagnosis and management of ectopic pregnancy.

- A combination of transvaginal sonography and hCG determination is the best approach for the early diagnosis of ectopic pregnancy.

- The visualization of a fluid-filled sac outside the uterine cavity that contains an embryo with or without cardiac activity or a yolk sac is definitive for ectopic pregnancy.

- This strict criterion has the highest specificity (100%) but the lowest sensitivity (20%) in identifying an ectopic pregnancy.

- A more common ultrasonographic finding in a woman with an ectopic pregnancy is an adnexal mass.

- Despite meticulous ultrasonography, no adnexal mass will be identified in 15–35% of patients with ectopic pregnancy.

- A pseudogestational sac may be present in 5–35% of ectopic pregnancies and, if mistaken for a true uterine gestational, the diagnosis could be delayed.

- Doppler ultrasound may provide useful information about adnexal masses; however, the final diagnosis depends on the grayscale features.

- If an ectopic pregnancy is diagnosed by transvaginal sonography, systemic methotrexate is the first line of treatment.

- Conservative management of ectopic pregnancy could be achieved by transvaginal salpingocentesis, injection of methotrexate into the sac, or injection of potassium chloride into the fetal heart.

- Interstitial pregnancies represent 2–4% of ectopic pregnancies. However, they may be catastrophic because of rupture.

- Rupture of interstitial pregnancy has been thought to occur between 12 and 16 weeks. However, at least one-third could rupture between 8 and 12 weeks.

- 3D ultrasonography is very helpful in distinguishing interstitial pregnancy and eccentrically located intrauterine pregnancy.

- Conservative management of interstitial pregnancy has been achieved successfully by laparoscopy, hysteroscopy, or methotrexate injection.

- Laparoscopic management of interstitial pregnancy requires careful hemostatic measures such as electrocoagulation or laparoscopic suturing and pitressin injection.

- Abdominal pregnancy is a rare form of ectopic pregnancy in which the gestational sac implants in the peritoneal cavity.

- Maternal mortality is significantly increased in abdominal pregnancy due to the high incidence of internal hemorrhage or sepsis.

References

1. Lipscomb GH. Ectopic pregnancy. In: Copeland J, ed. *Textbook of Gynecology*, 2nd edn. Philadelphia and London: WB Saunders, 2000; 273–86.

2. Ory SV. Surgery for ectopic pregnancy. In: Gershensen DM, DeCherney AH, Curry SL, Brubaker L, eds. *Operative Gynecology*, 2nd edn. Philadelphia and London: WB Saunders, 2001; 665–81.

3. Pellerito JS, Taylor KJ, Quedens-Case C, et al. Ectopic pregnancy: evaluation with endovaginal color flow imaging. *Radiology* 1992; **183**: 407–11.

4. Centers for Disease Control and Prevention. Ectopic pregnancy: United States 1990–92. *Morb Mortal Wkly Rep* 1995; **44**: 46–8.

5. Dorfman SF, Grimes DA, Cates W Jr, et al. Ectopic pregnancy United States clinical aspects: 1979–1980 *Obstet Gynecol* 1984; **64**: 386.

6. Filly RA. Ectopic pregnancy. In: Callen P, ed. *Ultrasonography in Obstetrics and Gynecology*, 3rd edn. Philadelphia and London: WB Saunders, 1994; 641–59.

7. Laing FC. Ectopic pregnancy. In: Timor-Tritsch IE, Goldstein SR, eds. *Ultrasound in Gynecology*, 2nd edn. Philadelphia: Churchill Livingstone Elsevier, 2007; 161–75.

8. Doubilet PM, Benson CB. Ectopic Pregnancy. In: Doubilet PM, Benson CB, eds. *Atlas of Ultrasound in Obstetrics and Gynecology: A Multimedia Reference*. Philadelphia: Lippincott Williams and Wilkins, 2003; 318–30.

9. Dimitry ES, Subak-Sharpe R, Mills M, et al. Nine cases of heterotopic pregnancies in 4 years of in-vitro fertilization. *Fertil Steril* 1990; **53**: 107–10.

10. Rizk B, Morcos S, Avery S, et al. Rare ectopic pregnancies after *in-vitro* fertilization: one unilateral twin and four bilateral tubal pregnancies. *Hum Reprod* 1990; **5**(8): 1025–8.

11. Rizk B, Tan SL, Morcos S, et al. Heterotopic pregnancies following in-vitro fertilization and embryo transfer. *Am J Ob Gyn* 1991; **164**(1): 161–4.

12. Dimitry ES, Rizk B. Ectopic pregnancy: epidemiology, advances in diagnosis and management. *Brit J Clin Pract* 1992; **46**(1): 52–4.

13. Rizk B, Brinsden PR. Total abdominal and pelvic ultrasound: incidental findings and the comparison between out-patient and general practice referrals in 1000 cases. *Br J Radiol* 1990; **63**: 501–2.

14. Rizk B, Dimitry ES, Morcos S, et al. A multicentre study on combined intrauterine and extrauterine pregnancy after IVF. *II European Society*

for *Human Reproduction and Embryology*, 1990; Milan, Italy.

15. Marcus SF, Macnamee M, Brinsden P. Heterotopic pregnancies after in vitro fertilization and embryo transfer. *Hum Reprod* 1995; **10**(5): 1232–6.

16. Marcus SF, Brinsden PR. Analysis of the incidence and risk factors associated with ectopic pregnancy following in-vitro fertilization and embryo transfer. *Hum Reprod* 1995; **10**(1): 199–20.

17. Rizk B. The impact of pelvic inflammatory disease and tubal damage on heterotopic pregnancy following in vitro fertilization and embryo transfer. *J Clin Pract Sexuality* 1996; **11** (3/4): 46–51.

18. Marcus S, Rizk B, Fountain S, Brinsden PR. Tuberculous infertility and in vitro fertilization *Am J Obstet Gynecol* 1994; **171**(6): 1593–6.

19. Stiller RJ, de Regt RH, Blair E. Transvaginal ultrasonography in patients at risk for ectopic pregnancy. *Am J Obstet Gynecol* 1989; **161**: 930–3.

20. Fleischer AC, Pennell RG, McKee MS, et al. Ectopic pregnancy: Features at transvaginal sonography. *Radiology* 1990; **174**: 375–8.

21. Rizk B, Steer C, Tan SL, et al. Vaginal versus abdominal ultrasound guided oocyte retrieval in IVF. *Br J Radiol* 1990; **63**: 638.

22. Steer C, Rizk B, Tan SL, et al. Vaginal versus abdominal ultrasound for obtaining uterine artery Doppler flow velocity waveforms. *Br J Radiol* 1990; **63**: 398–9.

23. Steer C, Rizk B, Tan SL, et al. Vaginal color Doppler assessment of uterine artery impedance in a subfertile population. *Br J Radiol* 1990; **63**: 638.

24. Brown DL, Doubilet PM. Transvaginal sonography for diagnosing ectopic pregnancy: positivity criteria and performance characteristics. *J Ultrasound Med* 1994; **13**: 259–66.

25. Kurjak A, Zalud I, Schulman H. Ectopic pregnancy: transvaginal color Doppler of trophoblastic flow in questionable adnexa. *J Ultrasound Med* 1991; **10**: 685–9.

26. Cacciatore B. Can the status of tubal pregnancy be predicted with transvaginal sonography? A prospective comparison of sonographic, surgical, and serum hCG findings. *Radiology* 1990; **177**: 481–4.

27. Kelly H. Treatment of ectopic pregnancy by vaginal puncture. *Johns Hopkins Medical Bulletin, Proceedings of Societies, The Johns Hopkins Medical Society Meeting*, 1896; 68–69(Nov–Dec); 209–10.

28. Mahfouz N. Ectopic pregnancy. *J Obstet Gynaecol Br Emp* 1938; **45**(2): 201–30.

29. Feichtinger W, Kemeter P. Treatment of unruptured ectopic pregnancy by needling of sac and injection of methotrexate or PG E2 under transvaginal sonography control. *Arch Gynecol Obstet* 1989; **246**: 85–9.

30. Timor-Tritch IE, Baxi L, Peisner DB. Transvaginal salpingocentesis: a new technique for treating ectopic pregnancy. *Am J Obstet Gynecol* 1989; **160**: 459–61.

31. Milanowski A, Bates SK. Semantics and pitfalls in the diagnosis of cornual/interstitial pregnancy *Fertil Steril* 2006; **89**(6): 1764. e11–e14.

32. Tulandi T, Al-Jaroudi D. Interstitial pregnancy: results generated from the Society of Reproductive Surgeons Registry. *Obstet Gynecol* 2004; **103**: 47–50.

33. Timor-Tritch IE, Monteagudo A, Matera C, et al. Sonographic evolution of cornual pregnancies treated without surgery. *Obstet Gynecol* 1992; **79**: 1044–9.

34. Ackerman TE, Levi CS, Dashefky SC, et al. Interstitial line: sonographic finding in interstitial (cornual) ectopic pregnancy. *Radiology* 1993; **189**: 83–7.

35. Lawrence A, Jurdovic D. Three-dimensional ultrasound diagnosis of interstitial pregnancy. *Ultrasound Obstet Gynecol* 1999; **14**: 292–3.

36. Tanaka T, Hayashi H, Kutsuzawa T, et al. Treatment of interstitial ectopic pregnancy with methotrexate: report of a successful case. *Fertil Steril* 1982; **37**: 851–2.

37. Reich H, Johns DA, DeCaprio J, et al. Laparoscopic management of 109 ectopic pregnancies. *J Reprod Med* 1988; **33**: 885–90.

38. Meyer W, Mitchell DE Hysteroscopc removal of an interstitial ectopic gestation; a case report. *J Reprod Med* 1989; **34**: 928–9.

39. Kulkarni K, Ashraf M, Abuzeid M. Interstitial ectopic pregnancy: management and subsequent reproductive outcome. *American Association of Gynecologic Laparoscopists (AAGL) 37th Global Congress of Minimally Invasive Gynecology*, Las Vegas, NV, Oct 30–Nov 1, 2008.

40. Morito Y, Tsutsumi O, Momoeda M., Cornual pregnancy successfully treated laparoscopically with fibrin glue. *Obstet Gynecol* 1997; **90**: 685–90.

41. Choi Ys, Eun DS, Cho J, et al. Laparoscopic cornuotomy using a temporary tourniquet suture and a diluted vasopressin injection in interstitial pregnancy. *Fertil Steril* 2009; **91**(5): 193–7.

42. Aboulghar M, Rizk B. Ultrasonography of the cervix. In: Rizk B, Garcia-Velasco JA, Sallam H, Makrigiannakis A, eds. *Infertility and Assisted Reproduction*. New York: Cambridge University Press, 2008; 143–51.

43. Honey L, Leader A, Claman P. Uterine artery embolization-a successful treatment to control bleeding cervical pregnancy with a simultaneous intrauterine gestation. *Hum Reprod* 1999; **14**(2): 553–5.

44. Nappi C, D'Elia A, Di Carlo C, et al. Conservative treatment by angiographic uterine artery embolization of a 12 week cervical ectopic pregnancy. *Hum Reprod* 1999; **14**(4) 1118–21.

45. Mashiach S, Admon D, Oelsner G, et al. Cervical Shirodkar cerclage may be the treatment modality of choice for cervical pregnancy. *Hum Reprod* 2002; **17**(2): 493–6.

46. Ismail M., Ovarian pregnancy. *J Obstet Gynaecol Br Emp* 1950; **57**: 49–51.

47. Van Tussenbroek C. Un case de grossesse ovarienne. *Ann Gynecol* 1899; **52**: 537.

48. Spiegelberg O. Zur casuistik der ovaialschwangerschaft. *Arch Gynaekol* 1878; **13**: 73–6.

49. Boronow R, McElin TW, West RH, et al. Ovarian pregnancy; report of four cases and a thirteen-year

survey of the English literature *Obstet Gynecol* 1965; **143**: 55–60.

50. Grimes HG, Nosal RA, Gallagher JC., Ovarian pregnancy: a series of 24 cases. *Obstet Gynecol* 1983; **61**: 174–180.

51. Carter JE, Jacobsen A. Reimplantation of a human embryo with subsequent ovarian pregnancy. *Am J Obstet Gynecol* 1986; **155**: 282–3.

52. Rizk B, Lachelin GC, Davies MC, et al. Ovarian pregnancy following in vitro fertilization and embryo transfer. *Hum Reprod* 1990; **5**(6): 763–4.

53. Rizk B, Gorgy BA, West JD, et al. Calcified pelvic mass in a 75 year old woman. *Acad Radiol* 1996; **1**(1): 3–16.

Chapter 32

Heterotopic pregnancy and assisted reproduction

Samuel F. Marcus, Essam S. Dimitry, Maria Dimitry, Diana M. Marcus and Botros Rizk

Introduction

Heterotopic pregnancy (HP) is defined as combined intrauterine and ectopic pregnancy, wherever its location. Over 90% of ectopic pregnancies occur in the fallopian tubes; however, implantation can occur in the cervix, ovary, previous caesarean section scar, or abdomen [1,2]. The incidence of heterotopic pregnancy has increased drastically since the introduction of in-vitro fertilization (IVF) and gamete intrafallopian transfer (GIFT) [3,4,5,6,7]. This increase is attributed to the widespread use of ovulation induction and assisted reproduction techniques. This rising incidence poses a serious problem, as the diagnosis of this potentially life-threatening condition is often difficult.

Incidence

Dimitry, Rizk, and Marcus and their co-workers were pioneers in alerting clinicians to the increased incidence of HP with the widespread use of IVF [4,6,8]. Increased ovulation induction is also a factor [9]. Heterotopic pregnancy occurs in 0.75–2.90% of assisted reproductive technology (ART) pregnancies [4,5,6,10,11]. Indeed, HP accounts for up to 15–16% of all ectopic pregnancies that result from IVF [5,12].

The incidence of heterotopic pregnancy after IVF and GIFT would thus seem to be 30–80 times higher with ART than after spontaneous conception, where the incidence has been reported as 1 in 2600 to 1 in 30 000 [13].

Etiology

The etiology of HP after IVF is multifactorial, but tubal damage is considered the main factor. IVF was introduced to help patients with tubal disease conceive, but it has also increased tubal pregnancy conception. The first pregnancy reported after in-vitro fertilization and embryo transfer was ectopic [14]. Causes of tubal damage linked to ectopic pregnancy include chronic pelvic infection, appendicectomy [15], tubal surgery, previous ectopic pregnancy, sterilization, and reversal of sterilization. Subsequently, Steptoe and Edwards advocated tubal diathermy and division near the cornual ends to minimize the risk of ectopic pregnancy. Although bilateral salpingectomy reduces the risk of ectopic pregnancy, it does not prevent cornual ectopic pregnancy [3]. Dubuisson and colleagues reported the incidence of ectopic pregnancy in patients with bilateral salpingectomy as 4% compared with 14.2% in patients who had hydrosalpinx and 9.9% in patients with pathological but patent tubes [16]. These authors also reported 100% pathological lesions in their series of ectopic pregnancy, even when IVF had been done for endometriosis or unexplained infertility. Marcus et al. reported that tubal damage was present in 60% of their heterotopic pregnancy series [5], and Dimitry et al. reported that all of their nine cases had tubal damage [4].

Other risk factors associated with heterotopic pregnancy include ovarian stimulation. Marcus et al. reported ovulation stimulation in 90% of their series [5]. High numbers of transferred embryos are associated with heterotopic pregnancy [2,5,13], although HP has also been seen after the transfer of just two embryos [17].

The technique of embryo transfer may also contribute to the chance of extrauterine implantation by forcing the embryos through the tubal ostia by hydrostatic pressure. This may be due to the large volumes of culture medium injected [18]. However, Marcus et al. reported that reducing the volume of culture medium to 15 microliters did not prevent extrauterine implantation [5]. Other techniques of embryo transfer have been implicated as risk factors for HP, such as placing the embryo catheter beyond the midcavity or in the tube itself [7,18].

Retrograde migration of the embryos into the tubes has been implicated [18] and may be associated with high concentrations of estradiol after ovarian stimulation. It has been suggested that the patient's position at the time of embryo transfer, for example, dorsal position with the head tilted downward, could be a contributing factor. Lastly, it is also possible that extrauterine pregnancy might result from spontaneous fertilization of unrecovered oocytes if coitus occurred near the time of oocyte recovery.

Diagnosis

The clinical presentation of HP is variable, 45% of patients being asymptomatic, 30% having abdominal pain and vaginal bleeding, and about 25% presenting with abdominal pain but

Ultrasonography in Reproductive Medicine and Infertility, ed. Botros R. M. B. Rizk. Published by Cambridge University Press. © Cambridge University Press 2010.

Table 32.1. Clinical presentation and ultrasonographic diagnosis of 17 heterotopic pregnancies following IVF

Patient no.	Clinical presentation	Examination type	Ultrasonographic findings			Duration of pregnancy at time of diagnosis	
			Gestational sac in utero (*n*)	Fetal heart in utero (*n*)	Ectopic pregnancy (*n*)	Intrauterine	Ectopic
1	Abdominal pain	Abdominal	1	1	1	6	8
2	Abdominal pain	Abdominal	3	2	0	6	No
3	Abdominal pain	Abdominal	1	0	0	5	No
4	Abdominal pain	Abdominal	1	0	1	6	6
5	Abdominal pain	Abdominal	1	0	0	5	No
6	Abdominal pain	Abdominal	1	0	1	7	7
7	Abdominal pain and bleeding	Abdominal	2	1	1	7	7
8	Abdominal pain and bleeding	Abdominal	1	0	0	7	No
9	Abdominal pain and bleeding	Abdominal	1	0	1	8	8
10	Acute abdominal pain	Abdominal	1	0	0	5	No
11	Acute abdominal pain	Abdominal	2	2	0	8	No
12	Acute abdominal pain	Abdominal	1	1	0	6	No
13	Asymptomatic	Abdominal + vaginal	1	1	1	7	7
14	Asymptomatic	Abdominal + vaginal	2	2	1	7	7
15	Asymptomatic	Abdominal + vaginal	1	1	1	7	7
16	Asymptomatic	Abdominal + vaginal	1	1	1	7	7
17	Asymptomatic	Abdominal + vaginal	1	1	1	7	7

Reproduced with permission from Rizk B, et al. [6]

no vaginal bleeding [5]. Furthermore, suspicion of HP may be aroused in asymptomatic patients with ongoing intrauterine pregnancy if hCG levels are above singleton levels [4,19]. The symptoms of ectopic pregnancy may also be attributed to complications of intrauterine pregnancies, such as miscarriage, that delay the diagnosis of HP.

In symptomatic women the differential diagnosis includes acute appendicitis, ruptured corpus luteum cyst or ovarian follicle, spontaneous abortion, threatened miscarriage, ovarian torsion, urinary tract disease, and degenerating fibroids (see Chapter 22).

Rizk et al. highlighted that a high index of suspicion is important for making a diagnosis of heterotopic pregnancy [6,10]. Given the high potential for misdiagnosis, there is a high incidence of rupture at presentation [1]. Without timely diagnosis and treatment, heterotopic pregnancy can become a life-threatening condition. Fortunately, with the use of modern diagnostic techniques, most heterotopic pregnancies are diagnosed prior to rupturing.

The advent of rapid assay of the serum beta subunit of human chorionic gonadotropin (β-hCG), and the development of high-resolution vaginal ultrasound scanning, have improved the rate of early diagnosis of heterotopic pregnancy.

Measurement of β-hCG levels is very useful in the diagnosis of singleton tubal pregnancy, because β-hCG levels are significantly lower than those in an uncomplicated intrauterine pregnancy [20,21], although in heterotopic pregnancy β-hCG levels fall within the normal range for an uncomplicated intrauterine pregnancy and are therefore not helpful in the diagnosis. Marcus and colleagues reported that serial β-hCG values may predict fairly accurately the outcome of the intrauterine component of heterotopic pregnancy [5].

Ultrasound (US) scanning is the modality of choice for diagnosis of heterotopic pregnancy (Table 32.1). Transvaginal sonography, with its greater resolution, is superior to transabdominal ultrasound in early pregnancy (Figures 32.1, 32.2) and offers the opportunity of conservative treatment by

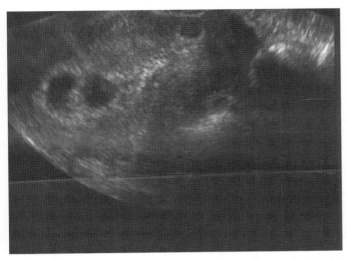

Figure 32.1. Ultrasonography of heterotopic pregnancy. (Courtesy MI Abuzeid.)

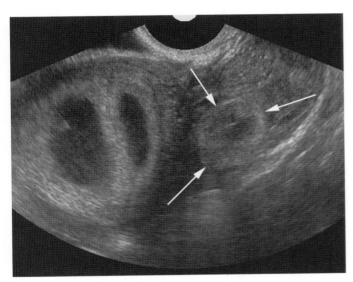

Figure 32.2. Heterotopic pregnancy in a patient with pelvic pain. (Courtesy A Eyvazzadeh and D Levine.)

ultrasound-guided aspiration of the gestational sac and injection of potassium chloride or laparoscopic surgery [5,10]. The reported efficacy of transvaginal ultrasonography in making the correct diagnosis of HP exceeds 90% [5,22].

Ultrasound scan findings include live extrauterine pregnancy, complex adnexal mass, free fluid in the pelvis, and extrauterine gestational sac with or without a fetal pole. The presence of free fluid in the pouch of Douglas and abdomen may be falsely labeled ascites associated with ovarian hyperstimulation syndrome. Color Doppler ultrasound has been demonstrated to improve the diagnostic sensitivity and specificity of transvaginal US, especially in cases where a gestational sac is questionable or absent.

The presence of an intrauterine pregnancy in an asymptomatic patient conceived by ovarian stimulation or IVF treatment should not exclude the diagnosis of a concurrent extrauterine pregnancy before careful ultrasonography of the pelvis, because of the 10-fold increased risk of heterotopic pregnancy in these patients. Failure to make a diagnosis early may not only lead to serious consequences for the mother, but may also jeopardize the intrauterine pregnancy [5].

Management

The management of heterotopic pregnancy is problematic, laparotomy during the first trimester may threaten the intrauterine pregnancy, and other modalities of treatment have their own limitations, although they are valuable in properly selected cases.

Treatment of HP should be tailored to the patient and is thus dependent on several factors, such as the location of the ectopic pregnancy, a previous ectopic in the same tube, the condition of the contralateral tube, and the general condition of the patient and the status of the pelvis. The aim of treatment is to preserve the concomitant intrauterine pregnancy.

Ultrasound-guided management

Ultrasound-guided management is becoming increasingly common. It can be performed safely in an outpatient setting and thereby obviates the need for laparoscopy or laparotomy, and eliminates the morbidity associated with both surgery and general anesthesia. Selection criteria include hemodynamically stable patients with unruptured ectopic pregnancy. Ultrasound-guided management involves aspiration of the gestational sac and injection of potassium chloride, or hyperosmolar glucose, or a hypertonic solution of sodium chloride into the fetal heart under transvaginal sonography [5,11,23]. Systemic or local methotrexate is contraindicated in the presence of a viable intrauterine pregnancy. Goldestein et al. reviewed the literature and reported that 55% of women who underwent potassium chloride injection for tubal heterotopic pregnancies required salpingectomy [2].

Expectant management

Expectant management of heterotopic pregnancy in hemodynamically stable patients with an intact ectopic pregnancy has been reported [5]. These patients should be carefully selected and followed up and should be made aware of the risks involved. To date, no selection criteria have been reported. In contrast to the expectant management of singleton tubal pregnancies, when initial and declining levels of β-hCG are the mainstay selection criteria, this is not applicable for heterotopic pregnancies with viable intrauterine pregnancies. Furthermore, there is a risk of tubal rupture, hemorrhage, and subsequent loss of the intrauterine pregnancy.

Surgical management

Laparoscopy is the recommended approach in most cases. Laparoscopy, in addition to making a diagnosis, allows the assessment of pelvic structures, presence of hemoperitoneum, and presence of other conditions, such as ovarian cysts and ovarian torsion. Laparoscopic salpingectomy is the gold standard surgical approach of coexistent tubal pregnancy. Many studies have demonstrated that laparoscopic treatment of ectopic pregnancy results in fewer postoperative adhesions compared with laparotomy. Furthermore, laparoscopy is associated with significantly less blood loss and a reduced need for analgesia. Finally, laparoscopy reduces cost, hospitalization time, and convalescence period.

Laparotomy is usually reserved for patients with cornual ectopic pregnancies and hemodynamically unstable patients. It is also the preferred method for a surgeon who is inexperienced in laparoscopy and in patients where the laparoscopic approach is difficult, such as in the presence of multiple, dense adhesions and obesity.

Surgical treatment in cases in which the pregnancy is located on the cervix, ovary, or in the interstitial or the cornual portion of the tube is often associated with increased risk of hemorrhage (see Chapters 31 and 33).

Cesarean section scar is managed by wedge resection of the ectopic pregnancy via laparotomy, laparoscopy, or hysteroscopy. Ultrasound-guided aspiration of the gestation sac with or without local injection of potassium chloride or hyperosmolar glucose is becoming increasingly common [11,24].

Approximately half to two-thirds of the coexistent intrauterine pregnancies miscarry [1,5,9]. Han et al. compared the clinical outcomes of tubal heterotopic pregnancy in assisted vs. spontaneous conceptions and reported that the assisted-conception group had a higher live birth rate than the spontaneous group (47.8% vs. 20%) [25].

References

1. BenNagi J, Helmy S, Ofili-Yebovi D, Yazbek J, Sawyer E, Jurkovic D. Reproductive outcome of women with a previous history of Caesarean scar ectopic pregnancies. *Hum Reprod* 2007; **22**(7): 2012–15.

2. Goldstein JS, Ratts VS, Philpott T, Dahan MH. Risk of surgery after use of potassium chloride for treatment of tubal heterotopic pregnancy. *J Obstet Gynecol* 2006; **107** (2): 506–8.

3. Blazar AS, Frishman GN, Winkler N. Heterotopic pregnancy after bilateral salpingectomy resulting in near-term delivery of a healthy infant. *Fertil Steril* 2007; **88**(6): 1676.e1–2.

4. Dimitry ES, Subak-Sharpe R, Mills M, Margara RA, Winston RML. Nine cases of heterotopic pregnancies in four years of in vitro fertilization. *Ferti Steril* 1990; **53**: 107–110.

5. Marcus SF, Macnamee M, Brinsden P. Heterotopic pregnancies after in vitro fertilization and embryo transfer. *Hum Reprod* 1995; **10**(5): 1232–6.

6. Rizk B, Tan SL, Marcus S, et al. Heterotopic pregnancies after in vitro fertilization and embryo transfer. *Am J Obstet Gynecol* 1991; **164**(1 pt 1): 161–4.

7. Yovich JL, McColm SC, Turner SR, Matson PL. Heterotopic pregnancy from in vitro fertilization. *J In Vitro Fert Embryo Transf* 1985; **2**(3): 143–50.

8. Marcus SF, Brinsden PR. Analysis of the incidence and risk factors associated with ectopic pregnancy following in-vitro fertilization and embryo transfer. *Hum Reprod* 1995; **10**(1): 199–203.

9. Tal J, Haddad S, Gordon N, Timor-Tritsch I. Heterotopic pregnancy after ovulation induction and assisted reproductive technologies: a literature review from 1971 to 1993. *Fertil Steril* 1996; **66**(1): 1–12.

10. Rizk B, Dimitry ES, Marcus SF A multi-centre study on combined intrauterine and extrauterine gestations after IVF. *Proc Eur Soc Hum Reprod Embryol*, Milan, Italy, 1990; Abstract 43.

11. Clayton HB, Schieve LA, Peterson HB, Jamieson DJ, Reynolds MA, Wright VC. A comparison of heterotopic and intrauterine-only pregnancy outcomes after assisted reproductive technologies in the United States from 1999 to 2002. *Fertil Steril* 2007; **87**(2): 303–9.

12. Ng EH, Yeung WS, So WW, Ho PC. An analysis of ectopic pregnancies following in vitro fertilization in a 10-year period. *J Obstet Gynecol* 1998 Jul; **18** (4): 359–64.

13. Habana A, Dokras A, Giraldo JL, Jones EE. Cornual heterotopic pregnancy: contemporary management options. *Am J Obstet Gynecol* 2000 May; **182**(5): 1264–70.

14. Steptoe PC, Edwards RG. Reimplantation of a human embryo with subsequent tubal pregnancy. *Lancet* 1976 Apr; **241**(7965): 880–2.

15. Dimitry, ES. Does previous appendectomy predispose to ectopic pregnancy? A retrospective case controlled study. *J Obstet Gynaecol*, 1987; 7: 221–4.

16. Dubuisson JB, Aubriot FX, Mathieu L, Foulot H, Mandelbrot L, de Jolière JB. Risk factors for ectopic pregnancy in 556 pregnancies after in vitro fertilization: implications for preventive management. *Fertil Steril* 1991 Oct; **56**(4): 686–90.

17. Knopman JM, Talebian S, Keegan DA, Grifo JA. Heterotopic abdominal pregnancy following two-blastocyst embryo transfer. *Fertil Steril* 2007 Nov; **88**(5): 1437.

18. Dor J, Seidman DS, Levran D, Ben-Rafael Z, Ben-Shlomo I, Mashiach S. The incidence of combined intrauterine and extrauterine pregnancy after in vitro fertilization and embryo transfer. *Fertil Steril* 1991; **55**(4): 833–4.

19. Dimitry ES, Soussis IS, Mastrominas M, Packham D, Margara R, Winston RML. Early diagnosis of asymptomatic heterotopic pregnancy after in vitro fertilisation (IVF) *Assist Reprod Technol/Androl J* 1991; (Suppl): 81–3.

20. Kadar N, Romero R. HCG assays and ectopic pregnancy. *Lancet* 1981; **30**: 1(8231): 1205–6.

21. Marcus SF, Macnamee M, Brinsden P. The prediction of ectopic pregnancy after in-vitro fertilization and embryo transfer. *Hum Reprod* 1995; **10**(8): 2165–8.

22. Soriano D, Shrim A, Seidman DS, Goldenberg M, Mashiach S, Oelsner G. Diagnosis and treatment of heterotopic pregnancy compared with ectopic pregnancy. *J Am Assoc Gyncol Laparos* 2002; **9**(3): 352–8.

23. Verma U, Goharkhay N. Conservative management of cervical ectopic

pregnancy. *Fertil Steril* 2009; **91**(3): 671–4.

24. Mitwally MFM, Albuarki H, Elhammady E, Diamond MP, Abuzeid M, Fakih MH. Gestational sac aspiration of ectopic

pregnancy in a caesarean section scar: case report of successful management of heterotopic pregnancy following in-vitro fertilization. 35th Annual Meeting of the American

Association of Gynecological Laparoscopists (AAGL), Las Vegas, Nevada, November, 2006. *J Minim Invasive Gynecol* **13**(Suppl 1): S–50.

25. Han SH, Jee BC, Suh CS, et al. Clinical outcomes of tubal heterotopic pregnancy: assisted vs. spontaneous conceptions. *Gynecol Obstet Invest* 2007; **64**(1): 49–54.

Chapter

33

Cervical pregnancy

Hany F. Moustafa, Botros Rizk, Nicole Brooks, Brad Steffler, Susan L. Baker and Elizabeth Puscheck

Cervical pregnancy (CP) is one of the rare forms of ectopic pregnancy [1]. It represents less than 1% of all ectopic pregnancies, with an incidence rate varying from 1/1000 to 1/18 000 live births [2,3]. It was first described in 1817 and first named as such in 1860. In 1911, Rubin tried to establish diagnostic criteria for cervical pregnancy [4]. Since this was before the era of ultrasonography, his criteria were mainly histoanatomic. These criteria were: (1) close attachment of placenta to the cervix, with the presence cervical glands opposite to the implantation site; (2) placental location below uterine vessel insertion or below the anterior reflection of the visceral peritoneum of the uterus; and (3) no fetal elements in the uterine corpus. Until the 1980s, the diagnosis of cervical pregnancy was usually made intraoperatively, when curettage for presumed incomplete spontaneous abortion resulted in severe uncontrollable hemorrhage leading to hysterectomy on many occasions [5].

In true cervical pregnancy the embryo implants in the cervical canal; thus both the fetus and the placenta will be situated in the cervix (Figure 33.1). In some cases, implantation can occur at the isthmico cervical junction, where the gestational sac mainly develops in the lower uterine segment with extension of the placenta into the cervix. This later condition should be considered as a variant of placenta previa and not CP. Some times it is difficult to differentiate the endocervical canal from the isthmic part of the uterus, and accordingly to differentiate pure CP from cases with cervico isthmic pregnancy. Generally, if there is an intact part of the cervical canal between the gestational sac and the endometrium of the uterus, this could be used as sonographic proof of an intracervical placentation. This criterion is valid only during the first trimester of CP [6].

Etiology

The exact etiology of CP is not fully understood. Most of the evidence is drawn from retrospective analysis of case series and case reports. One of the most commonly cited risk factors in the literature is cervical injury, which could be caused by prior cervical dilation, curettage, or surgery. Obviously this cannot explain the etiology in the 10% of cases that occur in primigravidas without any history of cervical procedures. Women undergoing in-vitro fertilization are at a higher risk than those with spontaneous conception to have CP [7].

Generally CP terminates spontaneously during the first trimester, leading to profuse, life-threatening hemorrhage from the site of cervical implantation. Less commonly, the pregnancy can progress to the second or even to the third trimester [8].

Clinical presentation

Painless first-trimester vaginal bleeding is invariably the first presenting symptom in women with cervical pregnancy. Patients may report some abdominal cramping, but usually it is described more as lower abdominal discomfort, increased pelvic pressure, or back pain. Urinary difficulties have been reported in patients with more advanced pregnancies [9].

Clinical diagnosis

On examination, the cervix appears cyanotic, hyperemic, and soft in consistency. The external os is usually open in more than half of the patients and may reveal bulging membranes. The cervix is usually diffusely enlarged, reaching the size of the uterus or even more if the pregnancy is advanced, but in 10% of patients the cervix will be normal in size. Without the use of ultrasound the clinical picture could be easily misdiagnosed as the cervical stage of inevitable abortion [5].

Ultrasonographic features

The use of transvaginal ultrasound has not only revolutionized the diagnosis of CP but also dramatically improved patient survival and allowed physicians to consider other fertility-sparing treatment options. Studies have shown that with the use of ultrasound, the proportion of cases diagnosed preoperatively rose from 35% between 1978 and 1982 to 87.5% between 1991 and 1994 [10].

During ultrasound examination it is important to document the exact location of the gestational sac in the cervix and to assess the uterine corpus (Figure 33.2). The location of the placenta, the extent of trophoblast invasion, and peritrophoblastic blood flow using color Doppler are also recorded [11]. Typically in women with CP, transvaginal scanning will show

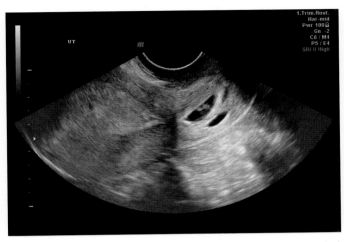

Figure 33.1. Cervical twin pregnancy; sagittal view of the uterus showing thick endometrium and two gestational sacs in the cervix below the internal os.

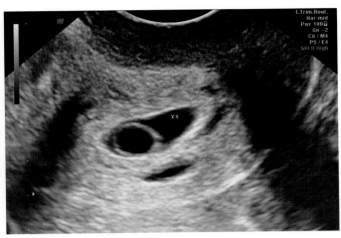

Figure 33.3. Cervical twin pregnancy; demonstrating a yolk sac in the larger gestational sac.

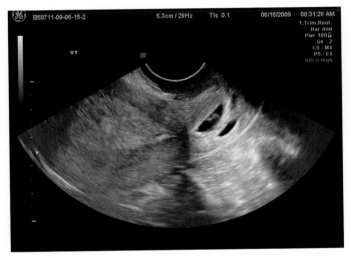

Figure 33.2. Assessing the uterine corpus.

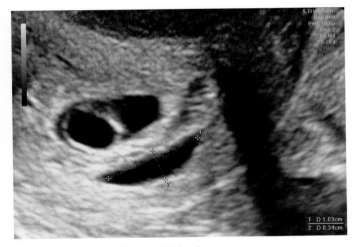

Figure 33.4. Diagnosis of cervical blighted ovum.

a gestational sac that lies entirely in the cervix below the level of the uterine corpus. Trophoblastic invasion of the cervix is an important component for the diagnosis of CP, and appears as a hyperechogenic trophoblastic thick ring around the implantation site [12]. Visualization of the endocervical canal extending above the margins of the gestational sac may be an additional sign of the trophoblastic invasion into the cervical wall, which is useful in early CP cases [13].

It is important to realize that, without the signs of trophoblastic invasion of the cervix the diagnosis of CP will be inadequate, because the mere presence of a gestational sac in the cervix may represent a cervical stage of abortion where the gestational sac is retained in the cervix before the dilatation of the external os [14]. Another sign that could help in differentiating both conditions is known as "the sliding sign," which was first described by Jurkovic et al. in 1996 [15]. To elicit this sign, the sonographer should apply gentle pressure on the cervix with the probe; if the gestational sac slides, this is more consistent with cervical abortion. This sliding motion will not be found in an implanted cervical pregnancy.

The use of Doppler can also help in differentiating the two conditions. The demonstration of peritrophoblastic blood flow from an active vascular supply to the gestational sac occurs only in CP, while if the sac is transiently passing through the cervix it will not have any peritrophoblastic flow as it is separated from its vascular supply [16].

Also, the internal os is invariably dilated in cervical abortion, while it is usually closed or at least snug in cases with early CP [5]. The uterus is characteristically empty, although in some cases a pseudogestational sac could be visualized. Also, there have been some case reports of simultaneous intrauterine and cervical pregnancies [17].

The appearance of the gestational sac is also variable. The sac may have a fetal pole and a yolk sac with or without fetal heart activity in more than three-quarters of cervical pregnancy cases (Figures 33.3, 33.4, 33.5, 33.6). Compared with tubal ectopic pregnancy, where the presence of fetal heart activity is limited to 5–10% of cases, the presence of fetal heart activity in cervical pregnancies is far more common (see Chapter 31) (Figure 33.7). This difference could be explained by the more

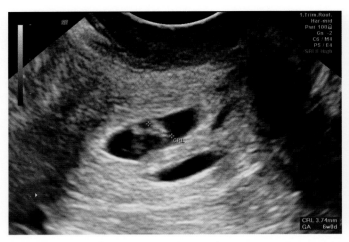

Figure 33.5. Cervical twin pregnancy showing the crown–rump length of the fetus of the first gestational sac.

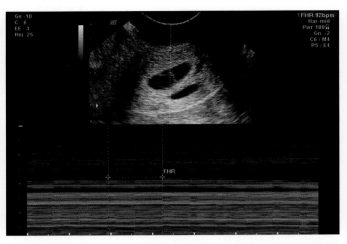

Figure 33.7. Transvaginal Doppler ultrasound demonstrating cardiac activity in the fetal pole.

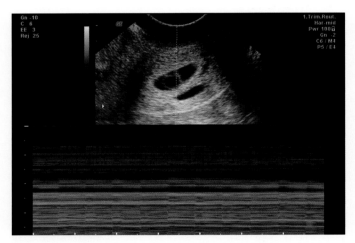

Figure 33.6. Doppler ultrasound confirming cardiac activity in cervical pregnancy.

favorable conditions for gestational sac development in CP (rich blood supply and the larger cervical tissue volume available for trophoblastic invasion) [10]. Less commonly a regular or an irregular cervical gestational sac is visualized without fetal structures or yolk sac, and in this case the diagnosis of cervical blighted ovum should be made, as visualized in the second gestational sac in Figure 33.4. In a minority of patients with CP, a cervical mass with an irregular hyper- or hypoechogenic structure has been reported. This form can easily be misdiagnosed as incomplete, missed, or inevitable abortion. Gestational trophoblastic disease or cervical tumors should also be considered in the differential diagnosis. Doppler sonography should be done in these cases as it will reveal a well-vascularized structure with low-resistance arterial flow in CP consistent with the peritrophoblastic flow. Unfortunately, a similar vascular flow pattern can also be seen in choriocarcinoma, although with the latter the vascularization pattern tends to be central, as opposed to peripheral in cases of CP. Beta-hCG, which is usually markedly elevated in gestational trophoblastic disease, can also be used to differentiate these conditions [5,10].

Management

Management of cervical pregnancy depends on a number of factors. These include the gestational age, patient stability, the desire to maintain future fertility, and the available resources and expertise where the patient is managed. Currently there are a number of treatment options that can be used either individually or in combination, depending on the clinical scenario. Patients who are hemodynamically stable and in whom the diagnosis has been confirmed by ultrasound should be managed conservatively [18]. Embarking on dilatation and curettage will frequently lead to severe hemorrhage, which requires hysterectomy in approximately 20% of these patients.

Systemic chemotherapy

Generally, if the gestational age is less than 9 weeks without fetal cardiac activity, systemic chemotherapy in the form of methotrexate alone is the first line of treatment. The use of methotrexate for the conservative management of CP was first reported in 1988 by Oyer et al. [19]. Although the successful use of other chemotherapeutic agents such as etoposide, actinomycin D, or a combination of actinomycin D, methotrexate, and cyclophosphamide has been reported, these are associated with greater toxicity and are less commonly used in clinical practice. Side effects of methotrexate include bone marrow depression, stomatitis, anorexia, nausea, vomiting, and diarrhea. Systemic methotrexate can be used in either a single-dose (50 mg/m^2) or multiple-dose regimen (1 mg/kg on days 1, 3, 5, 7). When multiple doses are used, folinic acid rescue (leucovorin 0.1 mg/kg) should be used on days 2, 4, 6, 8 to decrease the side effects [20].

Unlike tubal ectopic pregnancy, there is no contraindication to the use of systemic methotrexate if there is fetal heart activity and even with β-hCG levels more than 100 000, although the success rate tends to decrease and multiple courses may be needed. Also, multiple-dose regimens are more effective than single-dose regimens, but patients tend to exhibit more side effects. After the administration of methotrexate, serial β-hCG

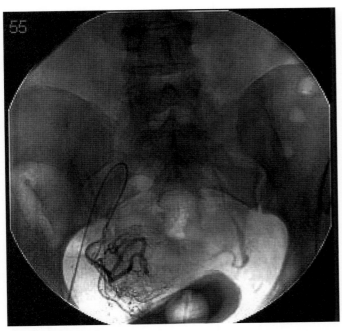

Figure 33.8. Right uterine artery embolization in a case of cervical twin pregnancy.

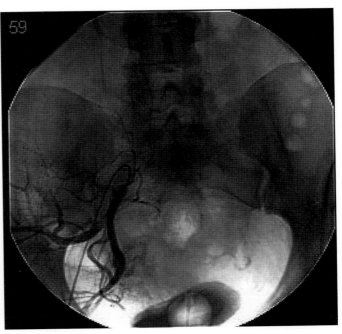

Figure 33.9. Right uterine artery embolization in a case of cervical twin pregnancy.

measurements should be done on days 4 and 7 [21]. It is not uncommon for β-hCG levels to rise or plateau on day 4, especially if fetal heart activity was present before treatment. This should not be considered as a sign of treatment failure, but if this persists through day 7, methotrexate injection should be repeated or another treatment option should be considered [22]. The average time needed to attain an undetectable β-hCG level depends on the pretreatment level of β-hCG and the presence of fetal heart activity. Generally, it takes about 6–8 weeks for a viable CP and 2–4 weeks for nonviable CP [5]. Spontaneous expulsion usually occurs during that time if D&C was not performed [23].

Intra-amniotic methotrexate injection

Intra-amniotic methotrexate injection is also an option, especially if the gestational age is less than 9 weeks and when there is no fetal heart activity. The usual dose is 50 mg [24]. Although it is injected into the gestational sac, patients can still report some side effects during treatment.

Intra-amniotic potassium chloride

If there is fetal heart activity and the gestational age is less than 12 weeks, intra-amniotic potassium chloride injection (3–5 ml of 2 mEq/ml) should be done first, followed by systemic methotrexate. The procedure can be performed without anesthesia using a 20-gauge needle and transvaginal US transducer. The fetal heart activity usually ceases immediately after injection. Potassium chloride can be also used as a primary treatment without methotrexate, but with lower success rates. This is the safest and probably the only option that can be used in case of

heterotopic cervical pregnancy if the intrauterine pregnancy needs to be conserved. When potassium chloride is used, the amniotic fluid should be withdrawn first to confirm needle location in the amniotic sac. It is important to realize that intra-amniotic injection may be complicated by gestational sac collapse during aspiration and profuse bleeding that requires surgical intervention [25,26].

Uterine artery embolization

Uterine artery embolization (UAE) has been used for many years in the treatment of symptomatic uterine fibroids and in acute obstetric hemorrhage. It is currently considered one of the important interventions in the conservative management of CP [27].

It was first reported as a possible conservative management option for CP by Pattinson and his colleagues in 1994 [28]. This was followed by many published case series that proved the efficacy of the procedure in reducing uterine bleeding and decreasing the risk of hysterectomy [26,27].

It can be performed in both the setting of acute bleeding and in stable patients who are managed conservatively using systemic methotrexate. UAE is usually performed by interventional radiologists using digital subtraction angiography with low-frequency pulsed fluoroscopy to reduce radiation exposure. After percutaneous catheterization of the femoral artery, a 4-French catheter is used to embolize both uterine arteries, usually using gelatin sponge particles that are injected under fluoroscopy until the distal descending portion of the uterine artery becomes completely blocked (Figures 33.8, 33.9, 33.10, 33.11). Other embolizing materials can be also used. Follow-up of such patients showed that most of them resumed menses

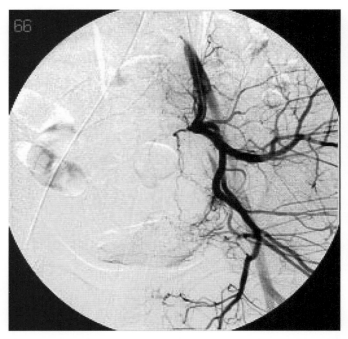

Figure 33.10. Left uterine artery embolization in a cervical twin pregnancy.

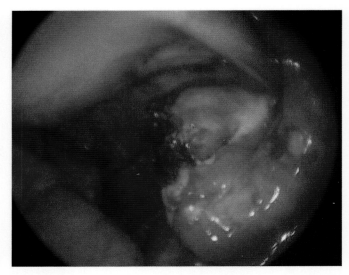

Figure 33.12. Cervical pregnancy at the time of dilatation and curettage.

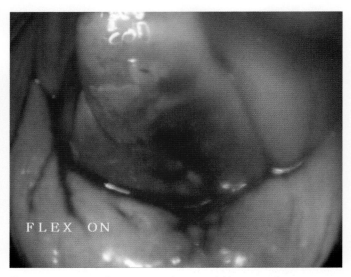

Figure 33.13. Cervical pregnancy at the time of dilatation and curettage.

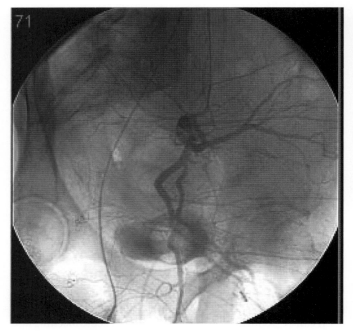

Figure 33.11. Left uterine artery embolization in a cervical twin pregnancy.

within 2 months after the procedure [29]. UAE is commonly performed after the administration of systemic methotrexate to reduce the blood loss after the expulsion of the gestational sac. It can also be used to before dilatation and curettage to decrease the risk of excessive bleeding during the procedure (Figures 33.12, 33.13, 33.14). UAE could also be performed in patients who present with acute hemorrhage to stop the bleeding in an attempt to avoid hysterectomy.

Other techniques to reduce blood loss

There are a number of techniques that can be used to decrease bleeding, either in patients who present with acute bleeding or in stable patients for whom D&C is planned. In patients with severe bleeding, general resuscitative measures should be taken first and bleeding should be controlled in an effort to spare the patient requiring hysterectomy. This can be achieved through Foley catheter tamponade, cervical and uterine packing, vaginal ligation of the cervical arteries, cervical cerclage, local injection of pressor agents such as vasopressin or prostaglandins, uterine artery ligation, or internal iliac artery ligation [5].

Foley catheter tamponade

The Foley catheter is an attractive option that has been used successfully in many cases. The bulb of the catheter is placed in

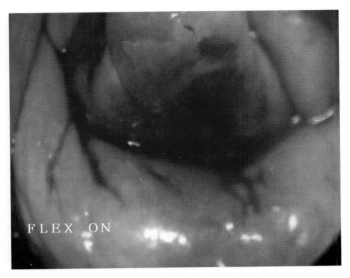

Figure 33.14. Cervical pregnancy after dilatation and curettage.

the cervix and inflated to as much as 90 ml to control hemorrhage. The central lumen of the catheter can be connected to a suction unit to drain the uterus and the balloon is left inflated for 24–48 hours. It is recommended to inflate the bulb under ultrasound guidance, especially in cases with advanced cervical pregnancy where there is marked thinning of the cervix, to avoid the possibility of cervical rupture [30,31].

Cervical cerclage

Cervical cerclage can be used as a way of controlling bleeding in the acute setting of CP or to reduce the chance of future bleeding in patients managed conservatively using systemic methotrexate [32]. Mashiach et al. reported the successful use of Shirodkar cerclage as a primary intervention in four cases of CP without the use of any systemic methotrexate. All patients showed resolution of their CP during follow-up. The disadvantages of using Shirodkar are that it requires surgical skill and general anesthesia, and carries the risk of bladder injury and significant bleeding [33].

Hysterectomy

Hysterectomy is still considered the most definitive management of CP if the patient does not wish to maintain her fertility. It is also the safest method of management in advanced pregnancy of more than 12 weeks. Hysterectomy should also be recommended for patients over 40 years, for those who have completed their family, or in those with other uterine pathology.

Fertility and pregnancy outcome after cervical pregnancy

Many case review reports have documented spontaneous pregnancy after conservative management of cervical pregnancy [25]. Some reports have shown increased incidence of cervical

insufficiency in these patients when they were scanned early in subsequent pregnancies that required cerclage. Reports also showed increased incidence of preterm labor. The effect of uterine artery embolization on future fertility is still controversial [21]. Although there have been numerous reports of spontaneous pregnancy after the use of uterine artery embolization in CP, patients should be counseled about the possibility of decreased fertility, increased incidence of adverse pregnancy outcome in the future, and even the chance of premature ovarian failure [29].

References

1. Dimitry ES, Rizk B. Ectopic pregnancy: Epidemiology, advances in diagnosis and management. *Br J Clin Pract* 1992; **46**(1): 52–4.

2. Rizk B, Dimitry ES, Morcos S, et al. A multicentre study on combined intrauterine and extrauterine pregnancy alter IVF. II European Society for Human Reproduction and Embryology, 1990; Milan, Italy. *Hum Reprod* 1990 (Suppl): Abstract 43.

3. Parente JT, Chau-su O, Levy J, Legatt E. Cervical pregnancy analysis. *Obstet Gynecol* 1983; **62**: 79–82.

4. Rubin IC. Cervical pregnancy. *Surg Gynecol Obstet* 1911; **13**: 625–33.

5. Ushakov FB, Elchalal U, Aceman PJ, Schenker J G. Cervical pregnancy: past and future. *Obstet Gynecol Surv* 1997; **52**(1): 45–59.

6. Sherer DM, Abramowicz JS, Thompson HO, Liberto L, Angel C, Woods JR Jr. Comparison of transabdominal and endovaginal sonographic approaches in the diagnosis of a case of cervical pregnancy successfully treated with methotrexate. *J Ultrasound Med* 1991; **10**(7): 409–11.

7. Rizk B, Tan SL, Morcos S, et al. Heterotopic pregnancies following in-vitro fertilization and embryo transfer. *Am J Obstet Gynecol* 1991; **164**(1): 161–4.

8. Shinagawa S, Nagayama M. Cervical pregnancy as a possible sequela of induced abortion. Report of 19 cases. *Am J Obstet Gynecol* 1969; **105**(2): 282–4.

9. Copas P, Semmer J. Cervical ectopic pregnancy: Sonographic demonstration at 28 weeks' gestation. *J Clin Ultrasound* 1983; **11**: 328–30.

10. Ushakov FB, Elchalal U, Aceman PJ, Schenker J G. Cervical pregnancy: past and future. *Obstet Gynecol Surv.* 1996; **52**: 45–59.

11. Lin EP, Bhatt S, Dogra V S. Diagnostic clues to ectopic pregnancy. *Radiographics.* 2008; **28**(6): 1661–71.

12. Timor-Tritsch IE, Monteagurdo A, Mandeville EO, et al. Successful management of viable cervical pregnancy by local injection of methotrexate guided by transvaginal ultrasonography. *Am J Obstet Gynecol* 1994; **17**: 737–9.

13. Bennett S, Waterstone J, Parsons J, Creighton S. Two cases of cervical pregnancy following in vitro fertilization and embryo transfer to the lower uterine cavity. *J Assist Reprod Genet* 1993; **10**(1): 100–3.

14. Vas W, Suresh PL, Tang-Barton P, et al. Ultrasonographic differentiation of cervical abortion from cervical pregnancy. *J Clin Ultrasound* 1984; **12**: 553–7.

15. Jurkovic D, Hacket E, Campbell S. Diagnosis and treatment of early cervical pregnancy. *Ultrasound*

Obstet Gynecol 1996; **8**: 373–80.

16. Pellerito J S, Taylor K J W, Quedens-Case C, et al. Ectopic pregnancy: Evaluation with endovaginal color flow imaging. *Radiology* 1992; 183: 407–11.

17. Dillon EH, Feyock AL, Taylor K J W . Pseudogestational sacs: Doppler US differentiation from normal or abnormal intrauterine pregnancies. *Radiology* 1990; 176: 359–64.

18. Mitra AG, Harris-Owens M. Conservative medical management of advanced cervical ectopic pregnancies. *Obstet Gynecol Surv* 2000; **55**(6): 385–9.

19. Oyer R, Tarakjian D, Lev-Toaff A, Friedman A, Chatwani A. Treatment of cervical pregnancy with methotrexate. *Obstet Gynecol* 1988; **71**(3 pt 2): 469–71.

20. Kirk E, Condous G, Haider Z, Syed A, Ojha K, Bourne T. The conservative management of cervical ectopic pregnancies.

21. Leeman LM, Wendland C L. Cervical ectopic pregnancy. Diagnosis with endovaginal ultrasound examination and successful treatment with methotrexate. *Arch Fam Med* 2000; **9**(1): 72–7.

22. Ferrara L, Belogolovkin V, Gandhi M, et al. Successful management of a consecutive cervical pregnancy by sonographically guided transvaginal local injection: case report and review of the literature. *J Ultrasound Med* 2007; **26**(7): 959–65.

23. Cipullo L, Cassese S, Fasolino L, Fasolino MC, Fasolino A. Cervical pregnancy: a case series and a review of current clinical practice. *Eur J Contracept Reprod Health Care* 2008; **13**(3): 313–19.

24. Jeng CJ, Ko ML, Shen J. Transvaginal ultrasound-guided treatment of cervical pregnancy. *Obstet Gynecol* 2007; **109**(5): 1076–82.

25. Marcovici I, Rosenzweig BA, Brill AI, Khan M,

Scommegna A. Cervical pregnancy. *Obstet Gynecol Surv* 1994; **49**: 49–55.

26. Frates MC, Benson CB, Doubilet PM, et al. Cervical ectopic pregnancy: Results of conservative treatment. *Radiology* 1994; **191**: 773–5.

27. Hirakawa M, Tajima T, Yoshimitsu K, et al. Uterine artery embolization along with the administration of methotrexate for cervical ectopic pregnancy: technical and clinical outcomes. *Am J Roentgenol* 2009; **192**(6): 1601–7.

28. Pattinson HA, Dunphy BC, Wood S, Saliken J. Cervical pregnancy following in vitro fertilization: evacuation after uterine artery embolization with subsequent successful intrauterine pregnancy. *Aust N Z J Obstet Gynaecol* 1994; **34**(4): 492–3.

29. Hirakawa M, Tajima T, Yoshimitsu K, et al. Uterine artery embolization along with the administration of methotrexate for cervical ectopic pregnancy: technical and clinical outcomes. *Am J*

Roentgenol 2009; **192**(6): 1601–7.

30. Kuppuswami N, Vindekilde J, Sethi CM, Seshadri M, Freese UE. Diagnosis and treatment of cervical pregnancy. *Obstet Gynecol* 1983; **61**(5): 651–3.

31. Hurley VA, Beischer NA. Cervical pregnancy: Hysterectomy avoided with the use of a large Foley catheter balloon. *Aust NZ J Obstet Gynaecol* 1988; **28**: 230–2.

32. Trojano G, Colafiglio G, Saliani N, Lanzillotti G, Cicinelli E. Successful management of a cervical twin pregnancy: neoadjuvant systemic methotrexate and prophylactic high cervical cerclage before curettage. *Fertil Steril* 2009; **91**(3): 935. e17–19.

33. Mashiach S, Admon D, Oelsner G, Paz B, Achiron R, Zalel Y. Cervical Shirodkar cerclage may be the treatment modality of choice for cervical pregnancy. *Hum Reprod* 2002; **17**(2): 493–6.

Chapter 34

Congenital anomalies and assisted reproductive technologies

Mona Aboulghar

Introduction

The population of children born after assisted reproductive technologies (ART) has increased dramatically around the world. An explicit example is Denmark, where 4% of infants are born after in-vitro fertilization (IVF) and intracytoplasmic sperm injection (ICSI) techniques, and 40% of these are twins [1]. There is naturally interest now in studying those children born regarding obstetric complications, congenital malformations, and long-term effects.

Risks associated with pregnancies following ART techniques

IVF pregnancies are associated with increased perinatal risks, of which multiple pregnancies are the most serious due to higher levels of obstetric complications [2,3,4].

Multiple pregnancies

Probably the highest risk result of IVF pregnancies is multiple pregnancy, which has been reported 27 times more frequently than in the general population [5].

The risks of multiple pregnancies include: perinatal mortality, preterm birth, low birth weight, gestational hypertension, placental abruption, and placenta previa [1,2]. The incidence of monozygotic twins is higher in ART pregnancies [6], and these are known to carry higher risks than dizygotic twins. Even when pregnancy starts with higher-order multiple pregnancy, the ongoing twins are still associated with a mild increased risk of premature delivery and low birth weight when compared with nonreduced twin pregnancies [7].

Increased perinatal morbidity is known to be higher in singleton ART pregnancies as well, which could be attributed to the underlying reproductive pathology [4].

Congenital malformations following IVF

Rizk and co-workers evaluated the congenital malformations in 961 babies conceived by IVF from Bourn Hall Clinic and the Hallam Medical Center between 1978 and 1987 [8]. The overall prevalence of congenital malformation was 3%, and 2.5% of the babies had at least one major malformation diagnosed during the first week of life (Table 34.1). The difference between the two proportions is due to multiple malformations in some babies: five babies had more than one malformation diagnosed under one week and two babies had more than one malformation diagnosed at any time. Although the malformation rates were higher in multiple births than with singleton births, the differences were not statistically significant (Table 34.1). Rizk et al. [8] compared the congenital malformations in IVF babies born and conceived in the United Kingdom with three sources of control data. Congenital malformations diagnosed during the first week of life were compared with the expected values from (1) the Office of Population Censuses and Surveys (OPCS), which is a voluntary scheme of reporting malformations diagnosed in the first week of life in England and Wales h (adjusted for maternal age and multiplicity); and (2) the Scottish Information Statistics Division, which routinely abstracts data on the prevalence of malformations in the live-born in Scotland diagnosed before one week of life (adjusted for maternal age) (Table 34.2). Congenital abnormalities diagnosed at any time (including terminations) were compared with the expected maternal age-adjusted values from the Liverpool Congenital Malformations Register, which contains data from many sources on malformations diagnosed at any age in the five health districts of the Liverpool region (UK) (Table 34.3). The information was presented system by system (Tables 34.2, 34.3). No specific malformations were significantly increased, but higher than expected numbers of central nervous system, chromosomal, urogenital, and limb malformations were observed (Table 34.3).

However, more recently published reports have suggested an increased risk of birth defects in both IVF and ICSI pregnancies (Tables 34.4, 34.5) [9] (Figures 34.1, 34.2, 34.3, 34.4, 34.5, 34.6, 34.7, 34.8, 34.9, 34.10). Buckett et al. reported on all ART procedures, as compared with naturally conceived children; IVF, IVM (in-vitro maturation), and ICSI were found to have slightly higher risks of congenital malformations. Odds ratios for any congenital abnormality were 1.42 (95% confidence interval [CI] 0.52–3.91) for IVM, 1.21 (95% CI 0.63–2.62) for IVF, and 1.69 (95% CI 0.88–3.26) for ICSI [3]. Olson et al.

Ultrasonography in Reproductive Medicine and Infertility, ed. Botros R. M. B. Rizk. Published by Cambridge University Press. © Cambridge University Press 2010.

Table 34.1. Major malformations diagnosed within the first week of life of IVF babies

	Singleton	Multiple	Total
Total *major* malformations (%)	2.9	3.3	3.0
Babies with at least one *major* malformation (%)	2.4	2.7	2.5

Reproduced with permission from Rizk B, et al. [8].

Table 34.2. Observed and expected malformations diagnosed under one week of age in IVF babies

	Observed	Expected
Central nervous system	3	2.2/2.2
Chromosomal	5	1.8/2.5
Urogenital system	13	3.2/12.4
Limb	16	6.8/53.0
Alimentary system	2	2.5/3.4
Respiratory system	1	0.1/1.0
Cardiovascular system	7	1.8/10.1
Eye and ear	4	1.0/2.4
Other musculoskeletal	7	1.8/6.5
Skin and integument	4	1.9/30.7
Other	2	–
Total *major* malformations	29	15.0/30.8
Total babies with at least one *major* malformation	24	12.4/25.8

Reproduced with permission from Rizk B, et al. [8].

Table 34.3. Observed and expected malformations diagnosed at any time (including termination) in IVF babies

	Observed	Expected
Central nervous system	5	2.8
Chromosomal	5	3.7
Urogenital system	3	1.9
Limb	8	5.4
Alimentary system	2	2.5
Respiratory system	1	0.4
Cardiovascular system	5	8.4
Eye and ear	1	1.4
Other musculoskeletal	2	2.0
Other	2	–
Total *major* malformations	34	29.0
Total babies with at least one *major* malformation	32	25.3

Reproduced with permission from Rizk B, et al. [8].

Reasons for concern after ICSI procedures

Concerns about ICSI are related to technical, biological, and genetic hazards. The link to increased incidence of chromosomal anomalies, congenital abnormalities, and perinatal hazards has been attributed to abnormal semen, to abnormal karyotyping, and to the technique of ICSI in which the oocyte membrane is pierced, bypassing the natural genetic selection that occurs in IVF [15].

Comparison of risks following IVF and ICSI

Because of the difference in technique used between ICSI and IVF where non-natural selection of the fertilizing sperm, and possible damage to the oocyte, occurs, there has been concern that ICSI could increase the risk of birth defects.

A follow-up study of 2059 neonates resulting from ICSI treatment [16], found 38 (1.8%) cases presenting with congenital abnormalities (22 major and 16 minor). Comparing the outcome of miscarriages and congenital malformations in terms of semen origin, ICSI and IVF were found not to differ.

A large prospective multicenter study including 59 centers in Germany compared the major malformation rate in ICSI pregnancies with that of naturally conceived controls [17]. A slight increase in malformations was reported, 8.6% versus 6.9%, resulting in a crude relative risk of 1.25 (95% CI 1.11–1.40). In their study they found no influence of sperm origin on major malformation rate in children born after ICSI.

Bonduelle et al. [18,19], in two large published studies, reported on major malformations (defined as those causing functional impairment or requiring surgical correction). The risk was similar in both ICSI and live-born IVF children: 3.4% versus 3.8% ($P = 0.538$). The malformation rate in ICSI was not found to be related to sperm origin or sperm quality. The number of

reported a 1.3-fold higher risk in IVF and one of 1.1 for IUI (intrauterine insemination) pregnancies for birth defects when compared with naturally conceived babies [10].

An Australian study found the odds ratio (OR) for multiple major defects to be 2.0 in IVF and ICSI, which was higher than that in the general population of naturally conceived infants [11]. This agrees with an Israeli study [12], in which the increase in congenital malformations was 2.3 and 1.75 times higher than in the spontaneously conceived group.

A Danish study included a large number of IVF/ICSI births (8602) between 1995 and 2000, of which 3438 were twins (40%) and 5164 were singletons (60%). The incidence of malformations was similar in ICSI compared with IVF babies; however, the total malformation rate was significantly higher in twins compared with singletons. A significant increase in hypospadias was observed in ICSI babies [1]. This has been reported in several other studies, when testicular sperm were used [13].

A study on cryopreserved ICSI embryos found a 2-fold increased incidence of congenital malformations [14].

Table 34.4. A summary of recent studies of IVF children and the risk of congenital anomalies

Author (year)	Number of IVF children	Type	Country	Risk of congenital anomaly in IVF vs. naturally conceived children ± odds ratio (OR)
Zhu (2006)	1483	Population-based study	Denmark	6.6% (hazard ratio 1.20)
Bonduelle (2005)	540	Population-based study	Belgium	OR 1.80
Kallen (2005)	16 280	Population-based registry	Sweden	5% vs 4% (relative risk 1.26)
Klemetti (2005)	4559	Population-based registry	Finland	OR 1.3
Merlob (2005)	278	Population-based registry	Israel	9.35% vs 4.05%
Olson (2005)	1462	Population-based registry	USA	6.2% vs 4.4%
Anthony (2002)	4224	Population-based registry	The Netherlands	OR 1.20
Hansen (2002)	837	Population-based registry	Australia	9% vs 4.2% (OR 2.0)
Isaksson (2002)	92	Case–control study	Finland	7.2% vs 3.5% in singletons.
Koivurova (2002)	304	Population-based registry	Finland	6.6% vs 4.4% (OR 1.53)
Ericson (2001)	9111 (estimated)	Population-based study	Sweden	OR 0.89
Koudstaal (2000)	307	Clinic	The Netherlands	2.3% (OR 1.0)
Bergh (1999)	5856	Population-based study	Sweden	5.4% vs 3.9%
Bowen (1998)	84	Case–control study	Australia	3.6% vs 5% (no significant difference)
D'souza (1997)	278	Case–control study	USA	2.5% vs 0%
Sutcliffe (1995)	91	Clinic	UK	OR 1.4

Reproduced with permission from Anpananthar A, Sutcliffe A. [9].

Table 34.5. A summary of recent studies of ICSI children and the risk of congenital anomalies

Author (year)	Number of ICSI children	Type	Country	Risk of congenital anomaly in ICSI vs. naturally conceived children ± odds ratio (OR)
Zhu (2006)	398	Population-based study	Denmark	8.8% (hazard ratio 1.39)
Bonduelle (2005)	540	Population-based study	Belgium	4.6% (OR 2.7)
Katalinic (2004)	3372	Tertiary infertility center	Germany	8.7% vs 6.1% (OR 1.24%)
Hansen (2002)	301	Population-based study	Australia	8.6% vs 4.2% (OR 2)
Ludwig (2002)	3372	Population-based study	Germany	8.6% vs 6.9% (RR 1.25)
Sutcliffe (2001)	208	Case-control-study	UK	4.8% vs 4.5% (OR 1.06)
Wennerholm (2000)	1139	Population-based study	Sweden	7.6% (OR 1.75)
Bowen (1998)	89	Case-control study	Australia	4.5% vs 5% (no significant difference)
Bonduelle (1996)	877	Population-based study	Belgium	2.6% (within normal range)
Sutcliffe (1995)	56	Fertility center	Australia	OR 0.67

Reproduced with permission from Anpananthar A, Sutcliffe A. [9].

stillbirths was similar in both groups (1.69% in the ICSI group versus 1.31% in the IVF). The total malformation rate taking into account major malformations in stillbirths, in terminations, and in live-born children was again similar (4.2% versus 4.6%, $P = 0.482$).

A meta-analysis of 19 studies reported an OR of 1.29 for congenital malformations, being similar in children born from IVF and ICSI [20].

Knoester et al. [21] compared singleton ICSI, IVF, and naturally conceived children as regards congenital malformations and fetal growth, general health, and medical consumption,

excluding preterm deliveries. ICSI pregnancies were comparable to those from IVF, and both had worse perinatal outcomes than naturally conceived pregnancies. No long-term effects were observed in children up to the age of 5–8 years.

Chromosomal abnormalities

Chromosomal study of abortuses following ART techniques showed no increase in the incidence of anomalies when compared with naturally conceived pregnancies, or between IVF (54.5%) and ICSI (61.5%), but there was an increase in ICSI

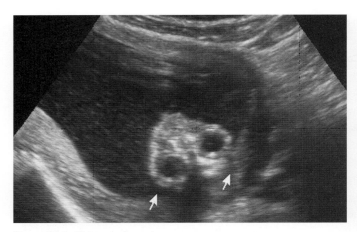

Figure 34.1. 2D image of acrania.

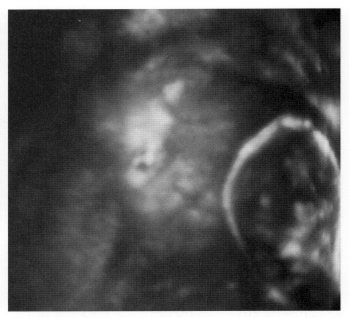

Figure 34.3. 3D image of median facial cleft.

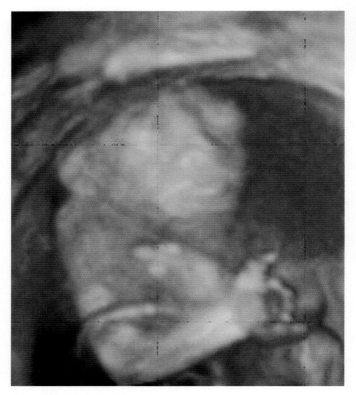

Figure 34.2. 3D image of acrania.

TESE (testicular sperm extraction), and in cryo-oocytes and IUI pregnancies [22]. However, in another study [23], ICSI pregnancies had a significantly higher rate of chromosomal aberrations than IVF.

First-trimester screening using nuchal translucency (NT) thickness, biochemical marker assessment, pregnancy-associated plasma protein A (PAPP-A), and free beta human chorionic gonadotropin (β-hCG) is now routine practice in many countries. Since the numbers of pregnancies following ART procedures are increasing around the world, it became necessary to determine whether any difference could be detected in the first-trimester screening among the naturally conceived population compared with the assisted-conception

population. A Danish study [24] compared 1000 pregnancies achieved after ART with a control group of 2543 pregnancies conceived spontaneously, as regards NT thickness, PAPP-A, and free β-hCG. In chromosomally normal pregnancies conceived after IVF and ICSI, the PAPP-A MOMs (multiples of the median) values were significantly decreased when compared with those of pregnancies conceived spontaneously (0.78 and 0.79 vs. 0.98), while there was no difference in the group treated by frozen embryo replacement. There was no difference in the level of free β-hCG between groups. The median nuchal translucency thickness was smaller in the overall ART group than in controls. The false-positive rate of first-trimester combined screening in the overall ART group, adjusted for maternal age, was significantly higher than in controls (9.0% vs. 6.0%). This stresses the importance of including data of mode of conception while calculating the risk for Down syndrome in patients following ART procedures.

Reported anomalies following ART procedures

Specific anomalies reported with IVF include the extrophy epispadius complex, which showed a 7.3-fold relative increase in incidence in IVF infants ($P = 0.0021$) [25]. Reported anomalies having higher prevalence in ART techniques include gastrointestinal (GI) (OR 9.85; 95% CI 3.44–28.44), cardiovascular (OR 2.30; 95% CI 1.11–4.77), and skeletal (OR 1.54; 95% CI 0.48–4.94) [9].

A review of our own data based on mid-trimester ultrasound examination of 1690 ICSI pregnancies showed 1018 singletons, 621 twins, 10 triplets, and 41 cases of anomalies representing 2.4%, of which 90.2% (37) were major and 9.7% minor [4]. This was compared with a control group of 3396 spontaneously pregnant patients: 3200 singletons, 99 twins, and 11 triplets, and 86 cases of anomalies (2.5%). Of those, 87.2% (75) were

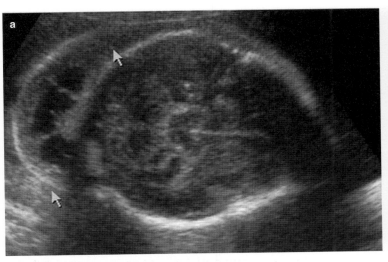

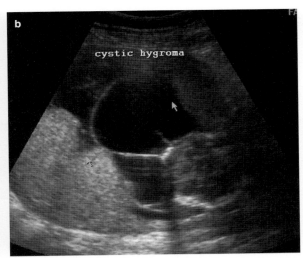

Figure 34.4. (a) Septated cystic hygroma, 2D image. (b) Cystic hygroma.

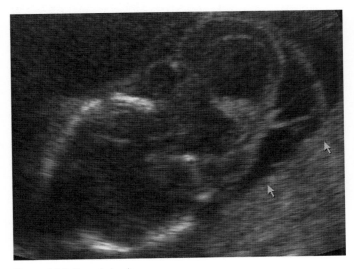

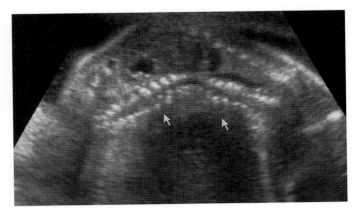

Figure 34.6. Kyphosoliosis.

Figure 34.5. Encephalocele.

major and 12.7% minor [11]. The odds ratio for incidence of anomalies in ICSI pregnancies was 1.04 (CI 0.71–1.52). These results were similar in twin ICSI and spontaneous groups: 2.5% and 3.5%, respectively ($P = 0.50$). (MMA Aboulghar, unpublished data). The most common anomalies were CNS –31% of the ICSI group compared with 37% in the spontaneous group; similarly, 31% renal anomalies compared with 18.6%, GI anomalies 31.7% and 12.7%, followed by skeletal 12.9% and 12.7%, heart anomalies 7.3% and 5.8%; no difference was found in the type of anomalies. The incidence of anomalies agrees with several Egyptian studies. The incidence of congenital malformations in live-born infants ranged from 1.16% to 3.17% [26].

Examples of detected anomalies are shown in Figures 34.1, 34.2, 34.3, 34.4, 34.5, 34.6, 34.7, 34.8, 34.9, and 34.10.

Intrauterine insemination (IUI) pregnancies

The rate of congenital malformations is not increased and no effect of frozen semen or donated semen has been confirmed

from the literature. Reported incidence of malformations is 1.4% in singletons and 1.7% in twins; there was a slightly higher incidence of trisomy 21, possibly related to higher maternal age. The commonest malformations were cardiovascular, similar to the general population [27].

In the French registry, a higher rate of congenital malformations was found among IVF pregnancies compared with IUI, 2.7% compared with 1.9% ($P = 0.009$). However, this rate did not differ using husband semen or donor semen. The rate of trisomy 21 increased with maternal age as well as donor age [28]. Other reports agreed with these results and, in addition, assessment of the psychosocial development of such infants up to the age of 8–10 years appeared to be reassuring [29].

Anomalies after testicular sperm extraction (TESE)

The incidence of hypospadias was significantly higher in the male offspring using epididymal or testicular sperm [13]. These findings are supported by another study including IVF pregnancies and was attributed to the high incidence of maternal progesterone administration [30]. Other malformations were

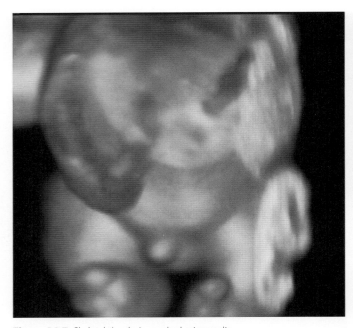

Figure 34.7. Skeletal dysplasia, marked micromelia.

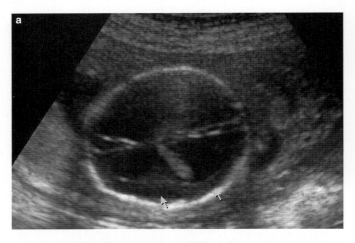

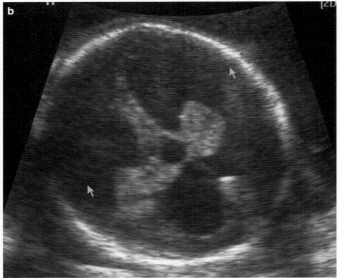

Figure 34.8a, b. Ventriculomegaly.

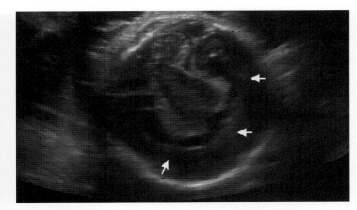

Figure 34.9. Holoprosencephaly.

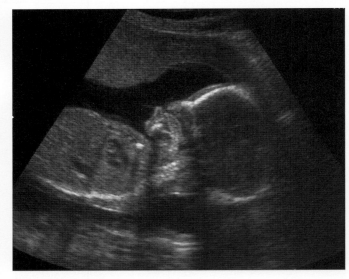

Figure 34.10. Facial cleft.

not found to be increased in ICSI children conceived with epididymal or testicular sperm when compared with malformation rates for IVF or spontaneously conceived children [13]. The data published did not show any differences between non-obstructive azoospermia (NOA) and obstructive azoospermia pregnancies, except for a strong tendency toward a lower gestational age in singletons and a higher percentage of premature twins in the NOA group [31].

Congenital malformations in infertile patients conceiving naturally

Compared with singletons born of fertile couples, singletons born of infertile couples who had conceived naturally or after treatment had a higher prevalence of congenital malformation: hazard ratios – 1.20 (95% CI 1.07–1.35) and 1.39 (1.23–1.57). The overall prevalence of congenital malformations increased with increasing time to pregnancy [32]. It is suggested that the hormonal treatment used for infertility management may explain the occurrence of genital organ malformations.

However, the increased prevalence of congenital malformations seen in singletons born after ART is partly due to underlying infertility or its determinants [32].

Conclusion

The population of children born after ART has increased dramatically worldwide, and a literature search has shown increased perinatal risks with IVF pregnancies. Multiple pregnancies are the most serious due to higher obstetric complications. These include perinatal mortality, preterm birth, low birth weight, gestational hypertension, placental abruption, and placenta previa. The risks are higher with singleton pregnancies as well. Congenital malformations are reported to be higher in IVF and ICSI pregnancies, reaching an OR of 2.0 in some studies. These were significantly higher in twins. Concern exists with the ICSI procedure, as it produces a non-natural selection of sperm and piercing of oocyte cytoplasm; however, studies comparing congenital malformations in ICSI with those in IVF showed no difference in incidence.

First-trimester screening for chromosomal anomalies using PAPP-A and β-hCG, as well as NT thickness measurement, showed differences between spontaneous and IVF pregnancies as well as a higher false-positive rate.

Some congenital malformations are more common following ART pregnancies, including hypospadias, especially after testicular sperm extraction, and the extrophy–epispadius complex.

In our own data of ultrasound-detected anomalies, the incidence of congenital malformations was similar between ICSI and spontaneous pregnancies.

Anomalies are not increased in IUI pregnancies.

The incidence of congenital malformations is higher in spontaneous pregnancies of infertile couples.

References

1. Pinborg A, Loft A, Nyboe Andersen A, Neonatal outcome in a Danish national cohort of 8602 children born after in vitro fertilization or intracytoplasmic sperm injection: the role of twin pregnancy. *Acta Obstet Gynecol Scand.* 2004; **83**(11): 1071–8.

2. Allen VM, Wilson RD, Cheung A. Pregnancy outcomes after assisted reproductive technology. *J Obstet Gynaecol Can.* 2006 **28**(3): 220–50.

3. Buckett WM, Chian RC, Holzer H, Dean N, Usher R, Tan SL. Obstetric outcomes and congenital abnormalities after in vitro maturation, in vitro fertilization, and intracytoplasmic sperm injection. *Obstet Gynecol* 2007; **110**(4): 885–91.

4. Reddy UM, Wapner RJ, Rebar RW, Tasca RJ. Infertility, assisted reproductive technology, and adverse pregnancy outcomes: executive summary of a National Institute of Child Health and Human Development workshop. *Obstet Gynecol* 2007; **109**(4): 967–77.

5. Bergh T, Ericson A, Hillensjö T, Nygren KG, Wennerholm UB. Deliveries and children born after in-vitro fertilization in Sweden 1982–95: a retrospective cohort study. *Lancet* 1999; **354**(9190): 1579–85.

6. Vitthala S, Gelbaya TA, Brison DR, Fitzgerald CT, Nardo LG. The risk of monozygotic twins after assisted reproductive technology: a systematic review and meta-analysis, *Hum Reprod Update* 2009; **15**(1): 45–55.

7. Cheang CU, Huang LS, Lee TH, Liu CH, Shih YT, Lee MS. A comparison of the outcomes between twin and reduced twin pregnancies produced through assisted reproduction, *Fertil Steril* 2007; **88**(1): 47–52.

8. Rizk B, Doyle P, Tan SL, et al. Perinatal outcome and congenital malformations in in-vitro fertilization babies from Bourn-Hallam group. *Human Reprod* 1991; **6**(9): 1259–64.

9. Anpananthar A, Sutcliffe A. Congenital anomalies and assisted reproductive technology. In: Rizk B, Garcia-Velasco JA, Sallam HN, Makrigiannakis A, eds. *Infertility and Assisted Reproduction*, chapter 68. Cambridge: Cambridge University Press, 2008; 684–94.

10. Olson CK, Keppler-Noreuil KM, Romitti PA, et al. In vitro fertilization is associated with an increase in major birth defects. *Fertil Steril* 2005; **84**(5): 1308–15.

11. Hansen M, Kurinczuk JJ, Bower C, Webb S. The risk of major birth defects after intracytoplasmic sperm injection and in vitro fertilization. *N Engl J Med* 2002; **346**(10): 725–30.

12. Merlob P, Sapir O, Sulkes J, Fisch B. The prevalence of major congenital malformations during two periods of time, 1986–1994 and 1995–2002 in newborns conceived by assisted reproduction technology. *Eur J Med Genet* 2005; **48**(1): 5–11.

13. Fedder J, Gabrielsen A, Humaidan P, Erb K, Ernst E, Loft A. Malformation rate and sex ratio in 412 children conceived with epididymal or testicular sperm. *Hum Reprod* 2007; **22**(4): 1080–5.

14. Belva F, Henriet S, Van den Abbeel E, et al. Neonatal outcome of 937 children born after transfer of cryopreserved embryos obtained by ICSI and IVF and comparison with outcome data of fresh ICSI and IVF cycles. *Hum Reprod* 2008; **23**(10): 2227–38.

15. Verpoest W, Tournaye H. ICSI: hype or hazard? *Hum Fertil (Camb)* 2006; **9**(2): 81–92.

16. Palermo GD, Neri QV, Hariprashad JJ, Davis OK, Veeck LL, Rosenwaks Z. ICSI and its outcome. *Semin Reprod Med* 2000; **18**(2): 161–9.

17. Ludwig M, Katalinic A. Malformation rate in fetuses and children conceived after ICSI: results of a prospective cohort study. *Reprod Biomed Online* 2002; **5**(2): 171–8.

18. Bonduelle M, Liebaers I, Deketelaere V, et al. Neonatal data on a cohort of 2889 infants born after ICSI (1991–1999) and of 2995 infants born after IVF (1983–1999). *Hum Reprod* 2002; **17**(3): 671–94.

19. Bonduelle M, Bergh C, Niklasson A, Palermo GD, Wennerholm UB. York Medical follow-up of study of 5-year-old ICSI children. *Reprod Biomed Online* 2004; **9**(1): 91–101.

20. Rimm AA, Katayama AC, Diaz M, Katayama KP. A meta-analysis of controlled studies comparing major malformation rates in IVF and ICSI infants with naturally conceived children. *J Assist Reprod Genet* 2004; **21**(12): 437–43.

21. Knoester M, Helmerhorst FM, Vandenbroucke JP, van der Westerlaken LA, Walther FJ, Veen S. Leiden Artificial Reproductive Techniques Follow-up Project (L-art-FUP), Perinatal outcome, health, growth, and medical care utilization of 5- to 8-year-old intracytoplasmic sperm injection singletons. *Fertil Steril* 2008; **89**(5): 1133–46.

22. Bettio D, Venci A, Levi Setti PE. Chromosomal abnormalities in miscarriages after different assisted reproduction procedures. *Placenta* 2008; **29**(Suppl B): 126–8.

23. Gjerris AC, Loft A, Pinborg A, Christiansen M, Tabor A. Prenatal testing among women pregnant after assisted reproductive techniques in Denmark 1995–2000: a national cohort study. *Hum Reprod* 2008; **23**(7): 1545–52.

24. Gjerris AC, Loft A, Pinborg A, Christiansen M, Tabor A. First-trimester screening markers are altered in pregnancies conceived after IVF/ICSI. *Ultrasound Obstet Gynecol* 2009; **33**(1): 8–17.

25. Wood HM, Trock BJ, Gearhart JP. In vitro fertilization and the cloacal-bladder exstrophy-epispadias complex: is there an association? *J Urol* 2003; **169**(4): 1512–15.

26. Temtamy SA, Abdel Meguid N, Mazen I, Ismail SR, Kassem NS, Bassiouni RI. A genetic epidemiological study of malformations at birth in Egypt. *Eastern Medit Health J* 1998; **4**: 252–9.

27. Thepot F, Mayaux MJ, Czyglick F, Wack T, Selva J, Jalbert P., Incidence of birth defects after artificial insemination with frozen donor spermatozoa: a collaborative study of the French CECOS Federation on 11,535 pregnancies. *Hum Reprod* 1996; **11**(10): 2319–23.

28. Lansac J, Thepot F, Mayaux MJ, et al. Pregnancy outcome after artificial insemination or IVF with frozen semen donor: a collaborative study of the French CECOS Federation on 21,597 pregnancies. *Eur J Obstet Gynecol Reprod Biol* 1997; **74**(2): 223–8.

29. Lansac J, Royere D. Follow-up studies of children born after frozen sperm donation, *Hum Reprod Update* 2001; **7**(1): 33–7.

30. Silver RI, Rodriguez R, Chang TS, Gearhart JP. In vitro fertilization is associated with an increased risk of hypospadias. *J Urol* 1999; **161**(6): 1954–7.

31. Vernaeve V, Bonduelle M, Tournaye H, Camus M, Van Steirteghem A, Devroey P. Pregnancy outcome and neonatal data of children born after ICSI using testicular sperm in obstructive and non-obstructive azoospermia. *Hum Reprod* 2003; **18**(10): 2093–7.

32. Zhu JL, Basso O, Obel C, Bille C, Olsen J. Infertility, infertility treatment, and congenital malformations: Danish national birth cohort. *BMJ* 2006; **333**(7570): 679.

Chapter
35
Multiple pregnancy following IVF

James Hole, Kathy B. Porter, Sherri K. Taylor, Vicki Arguello, Robin Brown, Tiffany Driver and Willie Cotten

Introduction

The diagnosis of multiple gestation is frequently met with joy and excitement by families who have undergone assisted reproduction; however, the happiness is tempered when the realization occurs that this diagnosis places the mother and the gestation at significantly increased risk for morbidity and mortality. The incidence of twin pregnancies in the United States has been increasing at an alarming rate from both delay of childbearing until later in life and, more importantly, the use of assisted reproductive techniques. The classically reported rate for spontaneous twinning is 1:80 and for triplets 1:6000 to 1:8000 [1,2]. When compared with natural ovulation, assisted reproduction significantly increases the chance of multiple gestation: 20-fold for twin gestation and 40-fold for triplets or quadruplets [3].

Twinning can be classified as either monozygotic (when a single fertilized ovum divides into two embryos) or dizygotic (when two separate ova are fertilized and implant in the same cycle). Monozygosity occurs in 31% of spontaneous twins, whereas dizygosity accounts for 69%. Most monozygotic twins are dichorionic/diamniotic (when division occurs within 3 days post fertilization) or monochorionic/diamniotic (division on days 4–8); however, when division occurs on days 8–12, the result will be a monochorionic/monoamniotic twin (approximately 1:10 000 pregnancies). If division is delayed until 13 days, the result is a conjoined twin. The incidence of monozygotic twinning has consistently reported to be stable at 4–5 per 1000 births. The incidence of dizygotic twinning continues to vary depending on race and ethnicity, ranging from 1.3 per 1000 in Japan to 49 per 1000 in certain Nigerian tribes. The increase in twins has typically been from dizygotic gestations, with no consistent increase in the rate of monozygosity. Higher-order multiple gestations (triplets or above) are usually combinations of multiple (di-, tri-, and higher) zygosity and monozygotic divisions within these (Figures 35.1, 35.2, 35.3, 35.4, 35.5).

Diagnosis

The diagnosis of spontaneous multiple gestation is often made when the clinical examination suggests size greater than dates or during routine first- or second-trimester dating or anatomical ultrasound evaluation. Multiple gestation in assisted reproduction is generally diagnosed very early during the post-therapy ultrasound evaluation. Ultrasound can usually delineate chorionicity, which should always be ascertained as early as possible in gestation. Monochorionicity has been shown to be a more important predictor of adverse outcome than zygosity [4]. The "twin peak" (also called lambda) sign is a very reliable marker for dichorionicity. The lack of this finding and the presence of the so-called "T" sign strongly suggest monochorionicity (Figures 35.6, 35.7). Other useful sonographic tools include the number of yolk sacs, placental locations and apparent number, and fetal sex.

Complications

There is significant increase in both maternal and fetal morbidity and mortality with multifetal pregnancies. Congenital anomalies, preterm birth, low birth weight, cerebral palsy, intracranial hemorrhage, blindness, and chronic pulmonary disease are among the more common known complications of twin gestations that occur either directly from the twinning or from prematurity [5]. From 1978 to 1987 at the Bourn Hall clinic and the Hallam Medical Center, Rizk et al. reported a 23% multiple pregnancy rate in 961 babies conceived by in-vitro fertilization [6]. Twins were present in 19% and triplets in 4% with no quadruplet or high-order multiple pregnancy. Overall, 32% were categorized as low birth weight and 6% as very low birth weight (Tables 35.1, 35.2). The perinatal mortality rate was 2- to 3-fold higher than that of infants born in England and Wales; this is attributed to multiple pregnancy (Tables 35.3, 35.4, 35.5). The congenital malformations were within expected range (2.5%), as discussed in Chapter 34. Tan et al. reported the obstetric outcome from the same series and highlighted the increased incidence of preeclampsia, placenta previa, and cesarean section [7]. Increased maternal morbidities included hypertension, gestational diabetes, anemia, preeclampsia, antepartum and postpartum hemorrhage, abnormal placentation, polyhydramnios and cesarean section [8,9]. Less frequently considered, but of significant consequence, is the

Ultrasonography in Reproductive Medicine and Infertility, ed. Botros R. M. B. Rizk. Published by Cambridge University Press. © Cambridge University Press 2010.

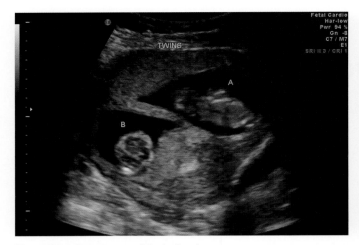

Figure 35.1. First-trimester dichorionic twins.

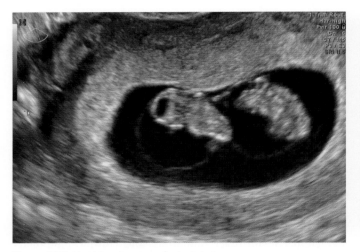

Figure 35.2. First-trimester monochorionic twins.

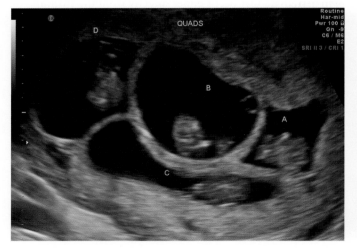

Figure 35.3. Quadruplet gestation.

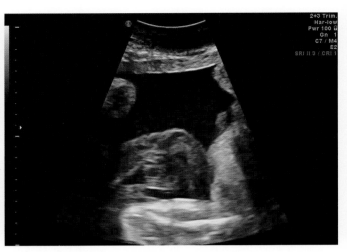

Figure 35.4. Monochorionic/monoamniotic cord knot.

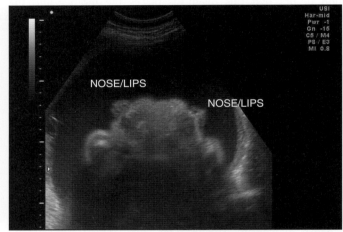

Figure 35.5. Conjoined twins.

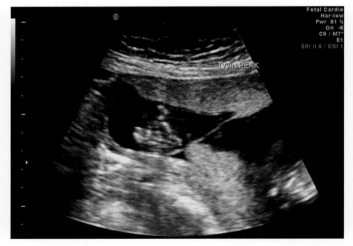

Figure 35.6. Dichorionic twins, "lambda" sign.

parenting stress sustained by the mothers and families of multiple gestations. A study of scores evaluating "severe parental stress" in IVF pregnancies gave results of 22% for multiples as compared with 5% for singletons [10].

Aneuploidy screening

Assessment for aneuploidy is an important aspect in the evaluation of abnormalities in any pregnancy, singleton or multiple. As

Table 35.1. Gestational age according to multiplicity in 961 IVF babies (1978–1987)

Gestational age (weeks)	Deliveries			
	Singleton % (n)	Twin % (n)	Triplet % (n)	Total % (n)
Preterm (< 37)	14 (67)	58 (72)	95 (19)	25 (158)
Term	86 (427)	42 (53)	5 (1)	75 (481)
Total	100 (494)	100 (125)	100 (20)	100 (639)
Mean	38.7	36.0	33.5	38.0
(± SE)	(0.12)	(0.24)	(0.57)	(0.12)

Reproduced with permission from Rizk B, et al. [6].

Table 35.2. Birth weight categories according to multiplicity in 961 IVF babies (1978–1987)

Birth weight (g)	Singleton % (n)	Twin % (n)	Triplet % (n)	Total babies % (n)
<1000	2 (8)	3 (9)	4 (3)	2 (20)
1000–1499	2 (8)	5 (12)	18 (14)	4 (34)
1500–2499	10 (52)	45 (119)	70 (53)	26 (224)
2500–3499	58 (304)	45 (118)	8 (6)	50 (428)
3500	29 (155)	2 (4)	- (0)	18 (159)
Total	100 (527)	100 (262)	100 (76)	100 (865)
Mean	3124	2389	1895	2793
(± SE)	(29.2)	(36.3)	(53.9)	(26.1)

Reproduced with permission from Rizk B, et al. [6].

Table 35.3. Stillbirth and perinatal death rate per 1000 total births and infant mortality rate per 1000 live births in IVF babies compared with mortality rates in England and Wales

Outcome	Bourn-Hallam IVF babies	England and Wales
Stillbirth	11.4	5.5
Perinatal mortality rate	22.9	9.8
Neonatal deaths	15.8	5.3
Early	11.6	4.3
Late	4.2	1.0
Postneonatal mortality	5.3	3.9
Infant mortality	21.1	9.4

Reproduced with permission from Rizk B, et al. [6].

Table 35.4. Observed and expected deaths

	Singleton babies		Twin and triplet babies	
	Observed deaths	Expected deaths	Observed deaths	Expected deaths
Stillbirths	3	3.2	8	5.6
Deaths 0–7 days	5	2.4	6	6.8
Deaths 8–27 days	2	0.6	2	1.3
Deaths 28 days to 1 year	1	1.9	4	2.9

Reproduced with permission from Rizk B, et al. [6].

Table 35.5. Stillbirth and death rates for IVF babies

Rate	Singleton	Twin	Triplet	Total
Stillbirth rate per 1000 births	5.07	20.8	24.7	11.4
Perinatal death rate per 1000 births	13.5	38.2	37.0	22.9
Neonatal death rate per 1000 live births (0–27 days)	11.9	21.3	25.3	15.8
Infant death rate per 1000 live births (<1 year)	13.7	28.4	50.6	21.1

Reproduced with permission from Rizk B, et al. [6]

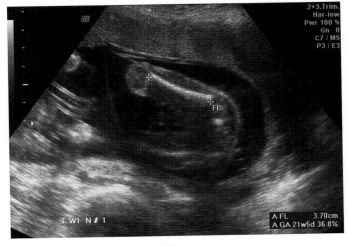

Figure 35.7. Monochorionic twins, "T" sign.

with advancing maternal age, this assumes even greater importance in assisted reproduction and multiple gestations.

Nuchal translucency (NT) measurement has become an integral part of singleton pregnancy evaluation. In addition to aneuploidy, abnormal NT measurements have been shown to be associated with fetal congenital heart disease and other

there is further increase in aneuploid risk for dizygotic (or greater) gestations as well as the known increase associated

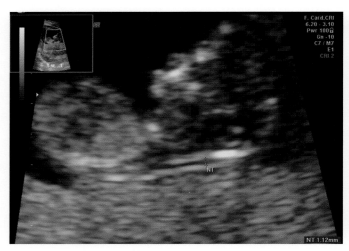

Figure 35.8. Nuchal translucency, twin A.

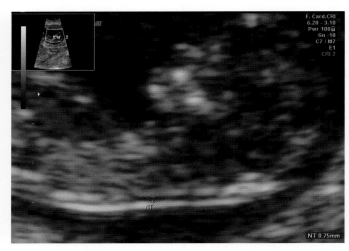

Figure 35.9. Nuchal translucency, twin B.

anatomic abnormalities. Studies evaluating the quality of NT measurements in multiple gestations have shown that there is no significant difference between image quality in singleton versus multiple gestations (Figures 35.8, 35.9).

However, as would not be unexpected, the fetuses that are located farthest from the uterine wall in multiple gestations are more difficult to evaluate and have poorer image scores [11]. Importantly, NT distributions and cut-off values do not differ between singleton and multiple gestations and can therefore be used for evaluation with the same sensitivity [12]. Abnormal NT evaluation in twin gestations has been shown to be associated with future development of twin–twin transfusion and discordance for anomalies.

Maternal serum analyte (marker) interpretation in conjunction with NT measurement is commonly used in singleton gestations, with free beta human chorionic gonadotropin (β-hCG) and pregnancy-associated plasma protein A (PAPP-A) and NT having a 90% detection rate with a 5% false-positive rate. However, the Fetal Medicine Foundation found a decrease to 75% in dizygotic pregnancies discordant for trisomy 21 [13]. Second-trimester serum analyte (most commonly maternal serum alpha-fetoprotein, β-hCG, serum estriol, and inhibin) has also been shown to have a decreased detection rate in multiple gestation as compared with singletons [14]. In conclusion, serum screening tests in multiple pregnancy have not been found to be as sensitive in singletons. Nuchal translucency alone offers a better detection rate and can be followed up with early diagnostic testing [15].

Invasive procedures

As in singleton pregnancies, when there are maternal age-related risks, abnormal first- or second-trimester screening, or the finding of congenital anomalies, definitive fetal karyotype assessment is often requested in multiple gestations. Both amniocentesis and chorionic villus sampling can be safely accomplished in multiple gestations.

Amniocentesis is generally performed after 15 weeks. Ultrasound evaluation should always be performed with care to accurately determine the location of each fetus and sac in order to be able to distinguish which specimen was from which fetus in case the results return discordance for aneuploidy. Unless there is discordance for an anomaly, in general both twins need to be sampled. There is some question whether both need to be sampled in a monozygotic gestation. As there have been reports of postzygotic mutations and discordance for abnormalities, however, most authorities recommend that both be sampled. Continuous ultrasound guidance is used during the procedure and single- and double-needle techniques can be utilized. Indigo carmine dye is injected into the sac of the tested fetus so that when the next sac is sampled clear fluid confirms that the same sac is not being inadvertently re-sampled. When high-order gestations are sampled, each successively tested sac is injected with dye. Methylene blue is not to be used because of significant associated fetal risks. There are limited data on the risks of procedure-associated loss rates in multiple gestations, with a reported range from 2.3% to 8.1%. As the background loss rate for twins prior to 24 weeks is 6%, it is unclear whether the loss rate is attributable to the procedure or to the twin pregnancy [16]. Amniocentesis is also used frequently in multiple gestations for assessment of fetal lung maturity or intra-amniotic infection. Continuous ultrasound guidance during the procedure is again used to improve the success rate and safety.

Chorionic villus sampling (CVS) can also be performed in multiple gestations, and is usually performed at 10–12 weeks' gestation using either a transabdominal or transcervical approach. Each placenta can usually be biopsied using the transabdominal technique due to a variety of procedural "windows." However, because of placental/cervical orientation, only one placenta in a multifetal gestation is typically able to be sampled transcervically. Continuous ultrasound guidance is used for these procedures. As with amniocentesis, care is needed to determine the location of each placenta in relation to each sac and fetus. Also as with amniocentesis, there are limited data on the procedural loss rate for CVS in multiple gestations. The reported studies show acceptable loss rates (0.6–4.2%) in relation to the background loss rate [16]. In both multifetal amniocentesis and CVS, operator experience is of paramount importance in determining loss rates.

Multifetal reduction

Because of the significant increase in risk associated with multiple gestations, especially high-order ones, reduction of the number of fetuses has been used in an attempt to decrease overall morbidity and mortality. Multifetal pregnancy reduction (MPR) and selective termination (ST) are techniques developed in an attempt to decrease specific risks from multiple gestation. Ultrasound is essential in the performance of MPR and ST for use in identifying chorionicity, in diagnosis of anomalies, and for guidance during the procedure itself. The most commonly used technique for MPR and ST involves injection of potassium chloride into the fetus(es) to be reduced. This can be done safely in multichorionic gestations as there are no interfetal vascular anastamoses. However, virtually all monochorionic gestations have some degree of vascular communication and this allows passage of the toxin used between gestations. Further, adverse hemodynamic changes can occur in the survivor due to blood loss into the dead fetus. As discussed previously, early assessment of chorionicity can generally be established by ultrasound assessment of membrane status.

MPR is usually done at 10–13 weeks. This is beyond the time when most spontaneous losses will have occurred, and allows for ease in technical performance of the reduction procedure and use of CVS (if desired) prior to reduction. The fetus(es) reduced are usually those that are most easily accessible (usually those closest to the anterior uterine wall). If possible, the fetus nearest the cervix is avoided for the reason of theoretical concerns about infection and uterine irritability. The unintended loss rate (loss of the entire pregnancy before 24 weeks) from the procedure was 9.6% in the largest reported series [17]. However, this is weighed against the reported benefits, with one study of triplet gestations reduced to twins compared with expectant management showing a decrease in the rate of preterm delivery (less than 31 weeks) from 26.7% to 10.4% [18]. Most reductions are to twins, although some now advocate consideration of reduction to singleton.

Selective termination has been shown to be feasible and to help improve perinatal outcomes. It involves early diagnosis of abnormalities to allow selective reduction of the affected fetus. This can be accomplished as early as 11–14 weeks. A large series involving triplet gestations found that ST resulted in significantly longer gestations than with expectant management (35.6 versus 31.1 weeks), higher mean birth weight, and more liveborn fetuses (97.4% versus 85.6%) [19]. A common situation for ST would be one fetus of a multiple gestation with anencephaly. The anomaly can result in polyhydramnios of the affected fetus due to impaired swallowing, with increased risk for preterm labor and delivery (Figure 35.10). The technique for

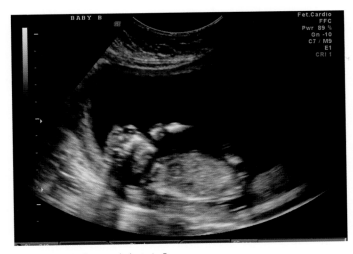

Figure 35.10. Anencephaly, twin B.

ST usually involves the injection of potassium chloride into the thorax or heart of the affected fetus under ultrasound guidance.

Monochorionic fetal reduction involves specific procedures to avoid the risks due to interfetal placental vascular communications. It is most commonly done by cord occlusion via ultrasound guidance followed by fetoscopy with cord ligation, bipolar coagulation, or laser occlusion. Because of technical limitations, it is generally only performed in the second trimester and is reserved for reductions indicated for reasons of discordance for anomalies, twin–twin transfusion, and monochorionicity.

Pregnancy surveillance

Ultrasound plays an integral role in the surveillance of multiple gestations and improvements in the outcomes of these pregnancies and would not be possible without advances in the technology. The use of ultrasound in pregnancy can be divided into four main categories:

1. Growth evaluation
2. Doppler velocimetry
3. Cervical length evaluation
4. Antenatal testing

Growth evaluation

Multiple gestations have a significantly increased risk of fetal growth abnormalities compared with singletons and also are at risk for discordant growth between fetuses. Growth abnormalities in twin and triplet gestations have been shown to be related to the increase in morbidity and mortality, second only to prematurity [20]. The finding of intrauterine growth restriction (IUGR) in a fetus from a twin or triplet gestation, or the development of significant birth weight discordance between fetuses, results in higher perinatal mortality, most likely due to placental dysfunction/insufficiency [21,22]. Most management protocols for twins recommend growth evaluation every 4 weeks after 18–20 weeks when dichorionic and every 2–4 weeks when monochorionic (due to the further increased risk for twin–twin transfusion). In trichorionic triplet gestations, growth evaluation is generally recommended every 3–4 weeks, and every 2–3 weeks when the triplets are monochorionic. A special note should be made when there is a finding of a velamentous cord insertion of one or more of the fetuses. This has been reported to occur in as many as 28.2% of triplet gestations and is significantly associated with small-for-gestational age fetuses [23].

Doppler velocimetry

Pulsed-wave Doppler assessment of velocity in the fetal umbilical and middle cerebral arteries is commonly performed during ultrasound evaluation of multiple gestations; however, the available data do not support a benefit for the routine assessment of these in uncomplicated twin and triplet gestations. In contrast, studies do show that Doppler evaluation can result in a significant improvement in the accuracy of ultrasound in the prediction of fetal growth restriction in both twins and triplets.

Cervical length evaluation

A relatively recent advance in the management of multiple gestation has been the use of endovaginal assessment of cervical length in the prediction of risk for preterm birth (generally defined as prior to 35 weeks). The finding of a cervix that is normal in length (25 mm or more) is very reassuring that the risk of preterm delivery is not high. One study of twins found that in women who were actively contracting, none of the 21 women with a cervical length of 25 mm or higher delivered within the next 7 days. In contrast, in 66 women with contractions and a length less than 25 mm, 16 delivered within this interval [24]. In a study of triplet gestations, a length of less than or equal to 25 mm between 15 and 20 weeks had a specificity and positive predictive value of 100% for delivery prior to 28 weeks. This length found at 21–24 weeks' gestation had a sensitivity of 86% for prediction of delivery prior to 28 weeks [25]. Identification of risk for preterm delivery can allow for timely

administration of antenatal corticosteroids and consideration of tocolysis.

Cervical length evaluation can also be used to assess for risk of early second-trimester delivery due to cervical insufficiency. The risk of early second-trimester delivery is known to be increased in multiple gestations and this is felt to be due to biochemical changes and mechanical forces on the cervix from overdistension. The sonographic findings of a shortened cervical length, dilatation of the internal os, and/or funneling of the membranes into the endocervical canal are the earliest identifiable manifestations of cervical insufficiency [26]. Findings that are concerning for cervical insufficiency may allow for identification of women who need more intense follow-up or possible placement of a cervical cerclage (Figures 35.11, 35.12, 35.13).

Antenatal testing

Because of the increased rates of perinatal mortality in multiple gestations, antenatal assessment of fetal well-being is used in essentially all of these pregnancies. However, regarding the

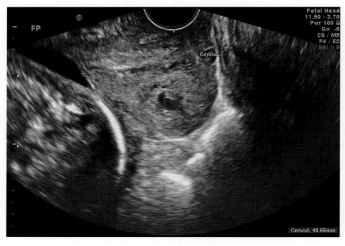

Figure 35.11. Quadruplet gestation, normal cervix.

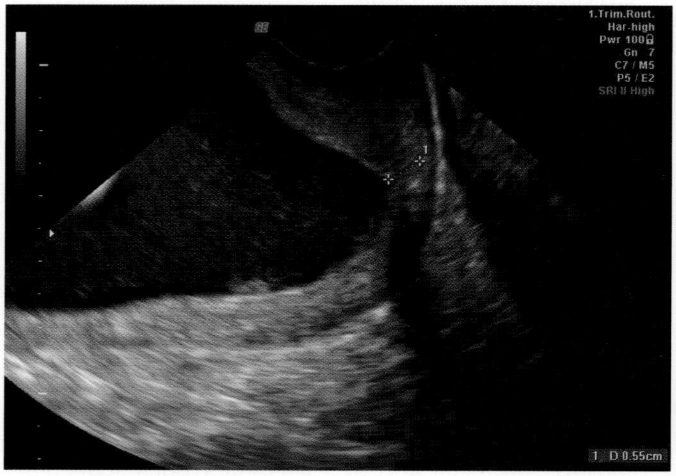

Figure 35.12. Twin gestation cervix with funneling and shortening.

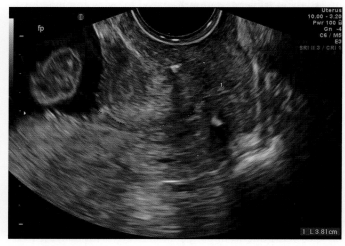

Figure 35.13. Twin gestation, cervix with cerclage.

efficacy in uncomplicated multiple gestations, prospective data are lacking. Assessment of well-being has been shown to decrease mortality in higher-risk settings including IUGR, growth discordance, amniotic fluid volume abnormalities, monochorionicity/monoamnionicity, and preeclampsia [27]. Initiation of antenatal testing is recommended when any significant maternal or fetal complication arises after viability. In uncomplicated twin and triplet gestations, testing is usually started at 32 weeks and continued weekly until delivery. Biophysical profile (BPP) and nonstress test (NST)/amniotic fluid volume (AFV) assessment have been shown to be equivalent predictors of well-being in twin gestations. As continuous and identifiable NST monitoring of each fetus in a triplet or higher gestation cannot be assured, BPP is the testing method of choice.

Intrapartum assessment

At the time of labor and/or delivery, multiple gestations pose multiple problems for the delivery team. Ultrasound assessment is considered an essential component in the intrapartum management of these pregnancies. The management of premature labor, abnormal fetal lie, abnormal placentation, cord presentation/accidents, and retained placental tissue are all improved by the use of ultrasound. In twin gestations with planned vaginal delivery, assessment of presentation is paramount both for initial assessment and also after delivery of the first twin. If a nonvertex second twin version is needed, ultrasound monitoring enhances the safety of the procedure. If there is consideration of breech extraction, estimation of fetal weight and head extension of the second twin is necessary (Figure 35.14). When cesarean delivery is needed, ultrasound evaluation of a transverse back-down presentation of the presenting fetus allows planning for a vertical uterine incision to allow safe delivery of the fetus. If there is persistent hemorrhage in the third stage of labor or placental examination suggests incomplete removal, ultrasound evaluation can be used to assess for retained tissue and guide curettage, if needed [28].

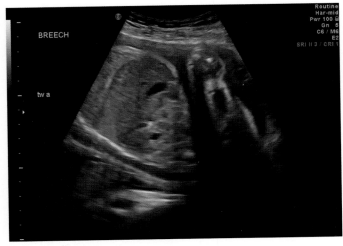

Figure 35.14. Breech presentation, twin A.

References

1. Benirschke K, Kim CK. Multiple pregnancy. *N Engl J Med* 1973; **288**: 1276–84.

2. Benirschke K, Kim CK. Multiple pregnancy. *N Engl J Med* 1973; **288**: 1329–36.

3. Brinsden PR. Controlling the high order multiple birth rate: the European perspective. *Reprod Biomed Onliine* 2003; **6**: 339–44.

4. Dube J, Dodds L, Armson BA. Does chorionicity or zygosity predict adverse perinatal outcome in twins?. *Am J Obstet Gynecol* 2002; **186**: 579–83.

5. Scholtz T, Bartholomaus S, Grimmer I. Problems of multiple births after ARTT: medical, psychological, social and financial aspects. *Hum Reprod* 1999; **14**: 2932–7.

6. Rizk B, Doyle P, Tan SL, et al. Perinatal outcome and congenital malformations in in-vitro fertilization babies from the Bourn-Hallam group. *Human Reprod* 1991; **6**(9): 1259–64.

7. Tan SL, Doyle P, Campbell S, et al. Obstetric outcome of in-vitro fertilization pregnancies compared to naturally conceived pregnancies. *Am J Obstet and Gynecol* 1992; **167**(3): 778–84.

8. Kinzler WL, Ananth CV, Vintzileos AM. Medical and economic effects of twin gestations. *J Soc Gynecol Invest* 2000; **7**: 321–7.

9. Nowak E, Blickstein I, Papiernik E. Iatrogenic multiple pregnancies: do they complicate perinatal care?. *J Reprod Med* 2003; **48**: 601–9.

10. Glazebrook C, Sheard C, Cox S. Parenting stress in first-time mothers of twins and triplets conceived after in vitro fertilization. *Fertil Steril* 2004; **81**: 505–11.

11. Zohav E. Quality of nuchal translucency measurements in multifetal pregnancies.

J Matern Fetal Neonatal Med 2006; **19**(10): 663–6.

12. Maslovitz S. Feasibility of nuchal translucency in triplet pregnancies. *J Ultrasound Med* 2004; **23**(4): 501–4.

13. Avgidou K, Papgeorghious A, Bindra R, et al. Prospective first-trimester screening for trisomy 21 in 30,564 pregnancies. *Am J Obstet Gynecol* 2005; **192**: 1761–7.

14. Wald NJ, Rish S. Prenatal screening for Down syndrome and neural tube defects in twin pregnancies. *Prenat Diagn* 2005; **25**: 740–5.

15. American College of Obstetricians and Gynecologists. Screening for fetal chromosomal abnormalities. *ACOG Practice Bulletin 77.* Washington, DC, American College of Obstetricians and Gynecologists, 2007.

16. Rochon M, Eddleman K, Stone J. Invasive procedures in multifetal pregnancies. *Clin Perinatol* 2005; **32**(2): 355–371.

17. Evans MI, Berkowitz RL, Wapner RJ, et al. Improvement in outcomes of multifetal pregnancy reduction with increased experience. *Am J Obstet Gynecol* 2001; **184**: 97–103.

18. Papgeorghiou AT, Avgidou K, Bakoulas V, et al. Risks of miscarriage and early preterm birth in trichorionic triplet pregnancies with embryo reduction versus expectant management: new data and systematic review. *Hum Reprod* 2006; **21**: 1912–17.

19. Geipel A. Targeted first-trimester penatal diagnosis before fetal reduction in triplet gestations and subsequent outcome. *Ultrasound Obstet Gynecol* 2004; **24**(7): 724–9.

20. Garite TJ, Clark RH, Elliot JP, et al. Twins and triplets:

The effect of plurality and growth on neonatal outcome compared to singleton infants. *Am J Obstet Gynecol* 2004; **191**: 700–7.

21. Hamilton EF, Platt RW, Morin L, et al. How small is too small in a twin pregnancy?. *Am J Obstet Gynecol* 1998; **179**: 682–5.

22. Rodis JF, Arky L, Egan JF, et al. Comprehensive fetal ultrasonic growth measurements in triplet gestations. *Am J Obstet Gynecol* 1999; **181**: 1128–32.

23. Feldman DM, Borgida AF, Trymbulak WP, et al. Clinical complications of velamentous cord insertion in triplet gestations. *Am J Obstet Gynecol* 2002; **186**(4): 809–11.

24. Fuchs I, Tsoi E, Henrich W, et al. Sonographic measurement of cervical length in pregnancies in threatened preterm labor. *Ultrasound Obstet Gynecol* 2004; **23**: 42–6.

25. Guzman ER, Walters C, O'Reilly-Green C, et al. Use of cervical ultrasonography in prediction of spontaneous preterm birth in triplet gestations. *Am J Obstet Gynecol* 2000; **183**(5): 1108–13.

26. Marder SJ, Jackson M. Sonographic assessment of incompetent cervix during pregnancy. *Semin Roentgenol* 1999; **34**: 35–40.

27. American College of Obstetricians and Gynecologists. Special problems of multiple gestation. *ACOG Educational Bulletin 253.* Washington, DC, American College of Obstetricians and Gynecologists, 1998.

28. Egan JF, Borgida AF. Multiple gestations: the importance of ultrasound. *Obstet Gynecol Clin North Am* 2004; **31**(1): 141–58.

Chapter 36

Ultrasonography in the prediction and management of ovarian hyperstimulation syndrome

Botros Rizk, Christopher B. Rizk, Mary G. Nawar, Juan A. Garcia-Velasco and Hassan N. Sallam

Ovarian hyperstimulation syndrome

Ovarian hyperstimulation syndrome (OHSS) is a serious iatrogenic complication of ovarian stimulation. It is characterized by bilateral multiple follicular and thecal lutein ovarian cysts (Figures 36.1, 36.2, 36.3) and in acute shift in body fluid distribution, resulting in ascites (Figure 36.4) and pleural effusion (Figure 36.5) [1,2,3,4,5,6,7,8]. OHSS may present in its mild form, with the patient complaining of discomfort and distension. However, the severe form may be complicated by hemoconcentration, thromboembolism, renal failure, and adult respiratory distress syndrome [9,10].

Ovarian hyperstimulation can be early or late in onset [Figure 36.6], spontaneous or iatrogenic in etiology [Figure 36.7], moderate or severe in clinical manifestations. OHSS can present 3–7 days after the ovulatory dose of human chorionic gonadotropin (hCG) (early onset) or 12–17 days after hCG administration (late onset) (Figure 36.6). Early-onset OHSS relates to excessive preovulatory response to stimulation, whereas late-onset OHSS relates to the occurrence of pregnancy, particularly multiple pregnancy [11,12]. Most cases of OHSS are iatrogenic as a result of gonadotropin ovarian stimulation. Rarely, spontaneous cases of OHSS can occur due to the presence of FSH receptor mutations [13].

Classification of ovarian hyperstimulation syndrome

The objectives of OHSS classification according to its severity are threefold [14]. The first objective is to compare the incidence of OHSS; the second is to evaluate the efficacy of the different approaches for the prevention of the syndrome; and the final objective is to plan the management of OHSS depending on its severity and the presence or absence of complications. Aboulghar and Mansour [14] reviewed the classifications of OHSS over the last four decades (see Table 36.1). Rabau et al. presented the first classification of OHSS (1), and this was reorganized by Schenker and Weinstein into mild, moderate, and severe [2]. Golan et al. were the first to use ultrasonography in the classification of OHSS [3]. Patients with ascitic fluid that is detected by ultrasound but have no clinical manifestations of

ascites are classified as "moderate OHSS" to distinguish them from "mild OHSS," which is very common, and "severe OHSS," which could be associated with complications. Navot et al. suggested making a distinction between severe and life-threatening OHSS by dividing it into two subgroups [4].

The most recent classification with further modifications was introduced by Rizk and Aboulghar [15]. They classified the syndrome into moderate and severe [15]. The purpose of the classification is to categorize patients with OHSS into more defined clinical groups that correlate with the prognosis of the syndrome. Treatment may be advised depending on the group to which the patient belongs. The great majority of cases of OHSS presenting with symptoms belong to the moderate degrees of OHSS. In addition to the presence of ascites on ultrasound, the patient's complaints are usually limited, so mild abdominal pain and distension and their hematological and biochemical findings are normal. Severe OHSS is divided into three grades according to the clinical manifestations. Patients with severe OHSS of grade C have life-threatening complications such as adult respiratory distress syndrome, and would require intensive-care treatment.

- **Moderate OHSS**
  Discomfort, pain, nausea, abdominal distension, no clinical evidence of ascites, but ultrasonic evidence of ascites and enlarged ovaries; normal hematological and biological profiles; can be treated on an outpatient basis with extreme vigilance.

- **Severe OHSS**
  - **Grade A**: Dyspnea, oliguria, nausea, vomiting, diarrhea, abdominal pain; clinical evidence of ascites plus marked distension of abdomen or hydrothorax; ultrasound scan showing large ovaries and marked ascites. Normal biochemical profiles can be treated as in patient or out patient depending on the physician's comfort, the patient's compliance, and medical facilities.
  - **Grade B**: All symptoms of grade A, plus massive tension ascites, markedly enlarged ovaries, severe dyspnea, and marked oliguria; biochemical changes in the form of increased hematocrit, elevated serum creatinine, and liver dysfunction; would be treated in an inpatient hospital setting with expert supervision.

Ultrasonography in Reproductive Medicine and Infertility, ed. Botros R. M. B. Rizk. Published by Cambridge University Press. © Cambridge University Press 2010.

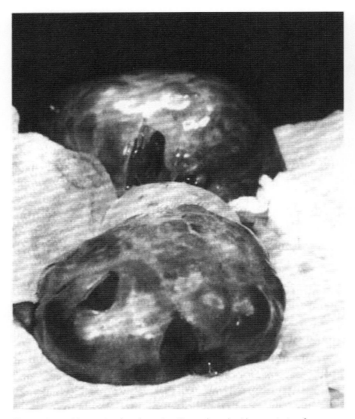

Figure 36.1. Hyperstimulated ovaries. Reproduced with permission from reference [8].

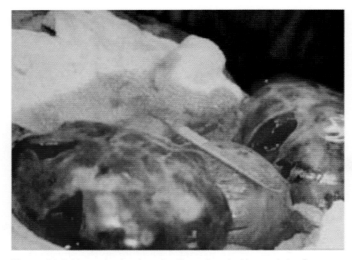

Figure 36.2. Hyperstimulated ovaries. Reproduced with permission from reference [7].

- **Grade C:** OHSS complicated by respiratory distress syndrome, renal shut-down, or venous thrombosis, which is critical; would be treated in an intensive-care setting.

Pathophysiology of OHSS

The pathophysiology of OHSS involves the explanation of two phenomena. The first is the presence of multiple hemorrhagic

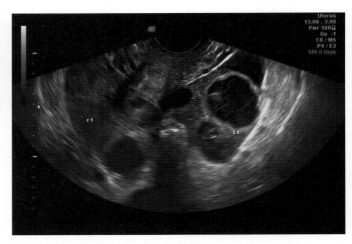

Figure 36.3. Bilateral enlarged cystic ovaries.

follicular and theca lutein cysts. The second is acute body fluid shifts resulting in ascites and pleural effusion. The fluid shifts appear to be the end result of increased capillary permeability.

Rizk et al. [16] and Pellicer et al. [17] investigated the role of vascular endothelial growth factor (VEGF) and interleukins in the pathogenesis of OHSS. While many mediators have been investigated, VEGF production by the granulosa cells and the endothelial cells is responsible for the majority of the fluid leakage (Figure 36.8). The VEGF family includes four different dimeric forms (A–D) and placental growth factors, which all bind differently to the three receptors (VEGF-R1 to R3) that are expressed on endothelial cells. It appears that VEGF-A stimulating VEGF-R2 is responsible for the increased capillary permeability and fluid leakage (Figures 36.9, 36.10).

Factors predicting ovarian hyperstimulation syndrome

The cornerstone of successful prevention of OHSS is accurate prediction (Table 36.2). Rizk and Smitz reviewed their experience in the prediction of OHSS [18]. Prediction of OHSS depends on identification of factors prior to ovarian stimulation, such as the history of previous OHSS or polycystic ovary syndrome [18,19]. Other personal factors are age, body mass index, allergies, and hyperinsulinism [19]. Rizk [13] investigated the role of follicle-stimulating hormone (FSH)-receptor mutations and polymorphisms in the development of OHSS. Mutations in the FSH-receptors could be activating, leading to predisposition to OHSS, or conversely, inactivating, resulting in sterility. Polymorphisms of FSH receptors have also been investigated and, to date, 744 single-nucleotide polymorphisms have been identified in the FSH receptor gene. Genetic studies of FSH-receptor mutations have increased the expectations that OHSS may be predicted in advance on the basis of FSH-R genotype [13]. The potential association of the S^{680} allele with poor responders to ovarian stimulation for IVF [20,21] led to the hypothesis that the N^{680} allele could be associated with hyper-responders, i.e., patients at risk of iatrogenic OHSS. In an elegant study published by Daelemans et al. [22], no statistically significant differences

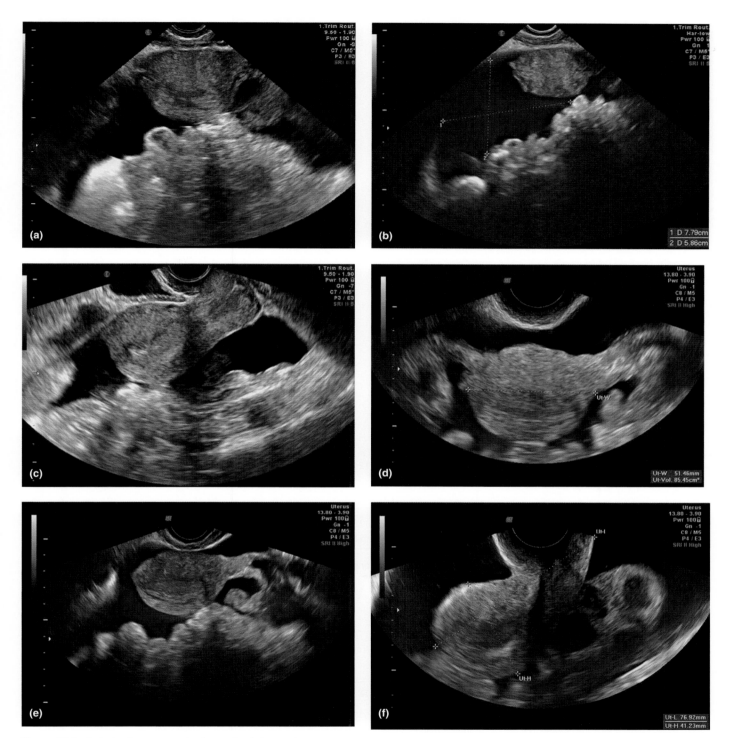

Figure 36.4a–f. Ascites in severe ovarian hyperstimulation syndrome.

between the IVF control population and the OHSS patients in allelic or genotypic frequencies were found. However, Daelemans et al. observed a significant enrichment in allele 680 as the severity of OHSS increased ($P = 0.034$). The authors suggested that the genotype in position 680 of the FSH receptor cannot predict which patients will develop OHSS, but could be a predictor of severity of OHSS symptoms among OHSS patients [22].

During ovarian stimulation, a sharp rise in estradiol or high levels in the presence of a large number of follicles is the best predictor (Figure 36.11). Increased blood flow to the ovaries and increased ovarian stromal blood flow are also useful predictors of OHSS (Figures 36.12, 36.13, 36.14). The occurrence of pregnancy (Figure 36.15), particularly multiple pregnancies, adds to the risk of developing OHSS (Figure 36.16).

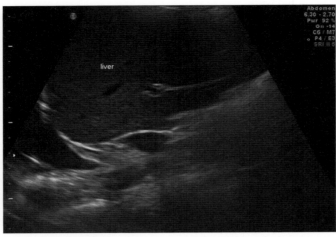

Figure 36.5. Right pleural effusion in ovarian hyperstimulation syndrome.

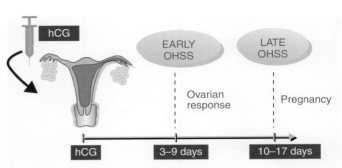

Figure 36.6. Classification of ovarian hyperstimulation syndrome: early and late.

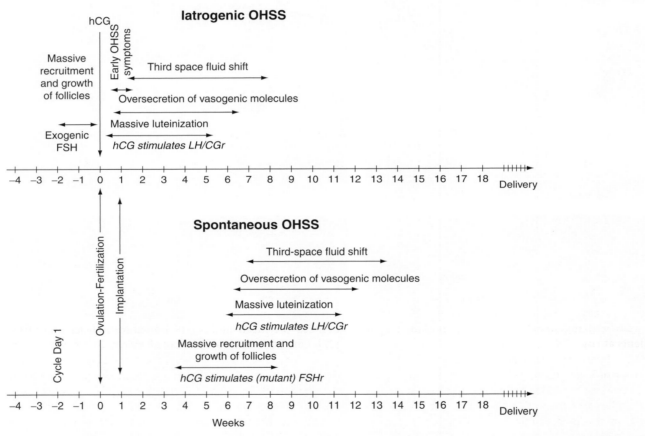

Figure 36.7. Chronological development of iatrogenic and spontaneous ovarian hyperstimulation syndrome. Reproduced with permission from reference [48].

Ultrasonography in prediction of OHSS

Baseline necklace sign appearance

The diagnosis of polycystic ovaries at ultrasound examination (the necklace sign) is crucial in the prediction of OHSS [18,19]. It improved the prediction of OHSS to 79% in a Belgian multi-center study [19].

Baseline ovarian volume and the prediction of OHSS

Danninger et al. studied the baseline ovarian volume prior to stimulation, to investigate whether it would be a suitable predictor for the risk of OHSS [23]. They performed three-dimensional volumetric ultrasound assessment of the ovaries prior to ovarian stimulation and on the day of hCG injection.

Table 36.1. Classifications of ovarian hyperstimulation syndrome (1967–1999)

Study	Mild	Moderate	Severe	
Rabau et al. [1]	Grade 1: estrogen >150 µg and pregnanediol >10 mg/24 h Grade 2: + enlarged ovaries and possibly palpable cysts Grade 1 and 2 were not included under the title of mild OHSS	Grade 3: grade 2 + confirmed palpable cysts and distended abdomen Grade 4: grade 3 + vomiting and possibly diarrhea	Grade 5: grade 4 + ascites and possibly hydrothorax	Grade 6: grade 5 + changes in blood volume, viscosity, and coagulation time
Schenker and Weinstein [2]	Grade 1: estrogen >150 µg/24 h and pregnanediol >10 mg/24 h Grade 2: grade 1+ enlarged ovaries, sometimes small cysts	Grade 3: grade 2+ abdominal distension Grade 4: grade 3 + nausea, vomiting and/or diarrhea	Grade 5: grade 4 + large ovarian cysts, ascites and/or hydrothorax	Grade 6: marked hemoconcentration + increased blood viscosity, and possibly coagulation abnormalities
Golan et al. [3]	Grade 1: abdominal distension and discomfort Grade 2: grade 1 + nausea, vomiting, and/or diarrhea, enlarged ovaries 5–12 cm	Grade 3: grade 2 + ultrasound evidence of ascites	Grade 4: grade 3 + clinical evidence of ascites and/or hydrothorax and breathing difficulties	Grade 5: grade 4 + hemoconcentration, increased blood viscosity, coagulation abnormality, and diminished renal perfusion
Navot et al. [4]			Severe OHSS: variable enlarged ovary; massive ascites ± hydrothorax; Hct >45%; WBC >15 000; oliguria; creatinine 1.0–1.5; creatinine clearance ≥50ml/min; liver dysfunction; anasarca	Critical OHSS: variably enlarged ovary; tense ascites ± hydrothorax; Hct >55%; WBC ≥25 000; oliguria; creatinine ≥1.6; creatinine clearance <50 ml/min; renal failure; thromboembolic phenomena; ARDS
Rizk and Aboulghar [15]	Discomfort, pain, nausea, abdominal distension, ultrasonic evidence of ascites and enlarged ovaries; normal hematological and biological profiles	Grade A: dyspnea, oliguria, nausea, vomiting, diarrhea, abdominal pain, clinical evidence of ascites, marked distension of abdomen or hydrothorax; US showing large ovaries and marked ascites; normal biochemical profile	Grade B: Grade A plus massive tension ascites, markedly enlarged ovaries, severe dyspnea and marked oliguria, increased hematocrit, elevated serum creatinine and liver dysfunction	Grade C: Complications as respiratory distress syndrome, renal shutdown, or venous thrombosis

Reproduced with permission from Aboulghar and Mansour [14].

There was a significant correlation between the baseline ovarian volume and the subsequent occurrence of OHSS. The authors suggested that volumetry of the ovaries could help to detect patients at risk.

Lass et al. [24] studied whether ovarian volume in the early follicular phase of WHO group II anovulatory patients would predict the response to ovulation induction with gonadotropins. They analyzed retrospective data from two prospective randomized multicenter studies, including 465 patients undergoing ovulation induction, and found that WHO Group II anovulatory women with medium-sized or large ovaries undergoing low-dose gonadotropin stimulation for ovulation induction have a higher risk for OHSS than women with small ovaries.

Number and size of follicles during ovarian stimulation

Ultrasound is widely used for monitoring follicular development in assisted conception [25,26]. The number, size, and pattern of distribution of the follicles are important in the prediction of OHSS. Tal et al. found a positive correlation between the mean number of immature follicles and OHSS [27]. One of the most often quoted articles in reference to the prediction is that by Blankstein et al. (1987), who stated that a decrease in the fraction of the mature follicles and an increase in the fraction of the very small follicles correlated with an augmented risk for the development of severe OHSS [28]. More recently, Kwee et al. found that women with an antral follicle count of 15 or more are at a higher risk of developing OHSS (Table 36.3) [29].

Low intravascular ovarian resistance

Moohan et al. [30] assessed the intraovarian blood flow in relation to the severity of OHSS in 30 patients with OHSS after embryo transfer who also had sonographic evidence of ascites. The authors measured the resistance to blood flow within the ovaries of 11 patients with severe OHSS and 19 patients with mild OHSS using transabdominal

Table 36.2. Prediction of OHSS

History and physical

1. OHSS in a previous cycle
2. Polycystic syndrome
3. Young patient
4. Low body mass index
5. Hyperinsulinism
6. Allergies

During ovarian stimulation

1. High serum estradiol, rapid slope of E_2, and absolute value
2. Ultrasonography

   a. Baseline PCO pattern
   b. PCO pattern of response to GnRH before gonadotropins
   c. Large number of follicles, >20, in each ovary

3. Doppler: low intraovarian vascular resistance

Outcome of ART cycles

1. Conception cycles
2. Multiple pregnancy

(a) **Pathophysiology:**

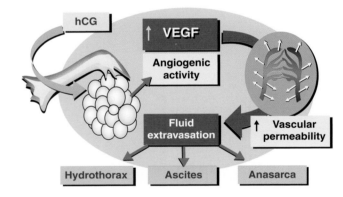

(b)

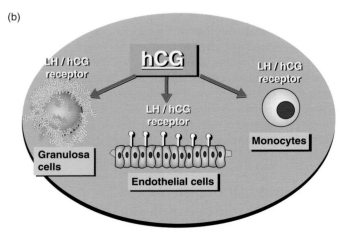

Figure 36.8a,b. Pathophysiology of ovarian hyperstimulation syndrome.

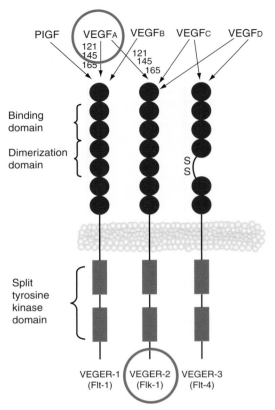

Figure 36.9. Vascular endothelial growth factor receptors.

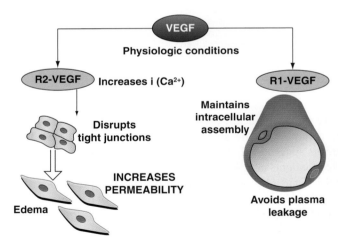

Figure 36.10. Vascular endothelial growth factor receptors and vascular permeability.

ultrasonography with color flow and pulsed Doppler imaging. The pulsatility index (PI), the resistance index (RI), and the S-D ratio, all measures of downstream vascular impedance, were significantly lower in severe OHSS patients. More than two-thirds of the patients with RI <0.48 had pleural effusion. In patients with either PI <0.75 or S-D <1.92, pleural effusion was observed in more than one-half. The blood flow velocity did not differ significantly between the two groups despite the fact that

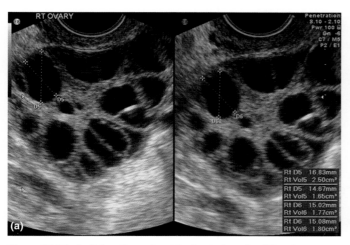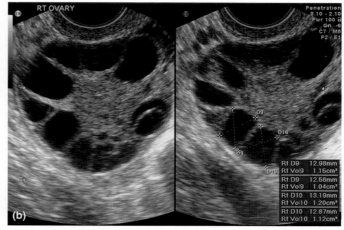

Figure 36.11a,b. Polycystic ovaries at the beginning of an IVF cycle.

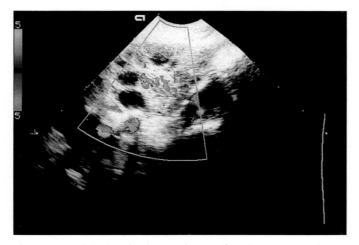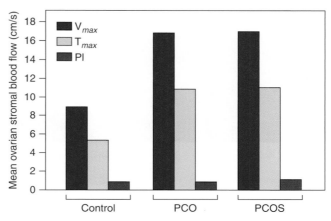

Figure 36.12. Color Doppler ultrasound image of a polycystic ovary indicating active blood flow. Reproduced with permission from reference [49].

Figure 36.13. Increased ovarian stromal blood flow in PCOS. Reproduced with permission from reference [50], figure 5–4

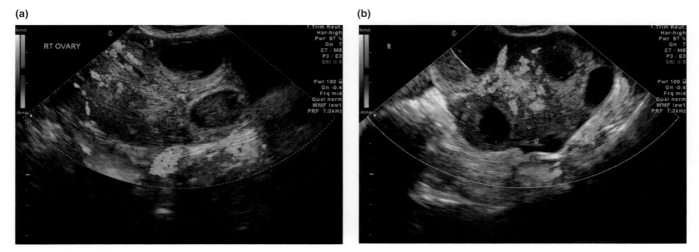

Figure 36.14a,b. Increased ovarian blood flow by Doppler in severe ovarian hyperstimulation syndrome.

Table 36.3. Antral follicle count and prediction of OHSS

Total AFC	Sensitivity	Specificity	PPV	Accuracy
<10	0.94	0.71	0.36	0.76
<12	0.88	0.80	0.44	0.81
<14	0.82	0.89	0.58	0.88
<16	0.47	0.96	0.67	0.88
<18	0.29	0.98	0.71	0.87

Reproduced with permission from Kwee. et al. [29].
PPV = positive predictive value.

Table 36.4. Primary prevention of OHSS

The ten commandments
1. Prediction of OHSS from history, examination, and ultrasound
2. Laparoscopic ovarian drilling in PCOS patients
3. Metformin in PCOS patients
4. Octreotide in PCOS patients
5. Low-dose gonadotropins in PCOS patients
6. GnRH antagonist protocol
7. Recombinant LH to trigger ovulation
8. GnRH agonist to trigger ovulation'
9. In-vitro maturation of oocytes
10. Replacement of only one embryo

Reproduced with permission from Rizk [6].

Table 36.5. Secondary prevention of OHSS

The ten commandments
1. Withholding hCG +/− continuation of GnRH-a/GnRH antagonist
2. Coasting or delaying hCG: currently most popular method
3. Use of GnRH-a to trigger ovulation
4. Follicular aspiration
5. Progesterone for luteal phase
6. Cryopreservation and replacement of frozen-thawed embryos at a subsequent cycle
7. Dopamine agonist
8. Albumin, administration at time of retrieval
9. Glucocorticoid administration
10. Aromatase inhibitors

Reproduced with permission from Rizk [6].

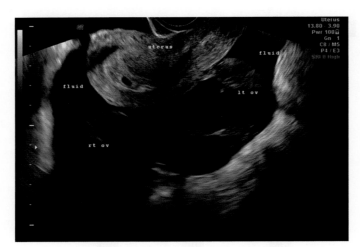

Figure 36.15. Ascites in moderate ovarian hyperstimulation syndrome in early pregnancy.

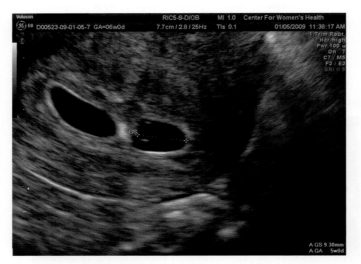

Figure 36.16. Twins associated with ovarian hyperstimulation syndrome.

there were changes in vascular impedance. A close correlation was observed between the OHSS severity and the intraovarian blood flow resistance. The authors suggested that measurements of intraovarian vascular resistance in patients undergoing controlled ovarian hyperstimulation may help in predicting those patients at particular risk of developing OHSS.

The combination of estradiol and ultrasonography offers the best chance for the prediction of OHSS. Ultrasonographic follow-up of the leading follicles should be used for the determination of the hCG administration and serum estradiol measurement, and sonographic visualization of small and intermediate follicles should be used to determine the likelihood of OHSS.

Prevention of OHSS

Rizk in 1993 suggested the "Ten Commandments" for the prevention of OHSS [31]. Today the list has expanded to two lists of "Ten Commandments" [32]. The first list addresses the primary prevention of OHSS, which includes options before stimulation such as ovarian diathermy, and during stimulation such as the use of low-dosage gonadotropins [32] (Table 36.4). The second list addresses the secondary prevention of OHSS, which includes withholding or delaying hCG, use of luteinizing hormone or gonadotropin-releasing hormone (GnRH) agonist (GnRh-a) in place of hCG for triggering ovulation, and progesterone for luteal phase support (Figure 36.17; Table 36.5).

Rizk has recently noted that among the options available for the prevention of OHSS, "coasting", or delaying hCG administration until the estradiol levels drop to below 3000 pg/ml, is currently the most popular method [26]. When estradiol levels increase rapidly in women undergoing controlled ovarian hyperstimulation (COH) with the concomitant administration of gonadotropins and GnRH-a, if gonadotropins and not

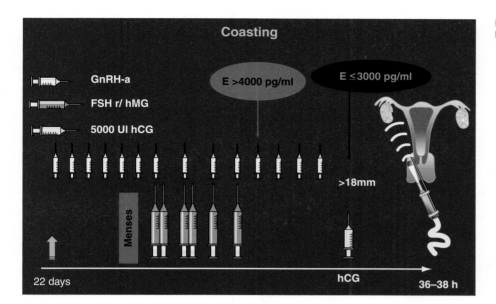

Figure 36.17. Coasting for prevention of ovarian hyperstimulation syndrome.

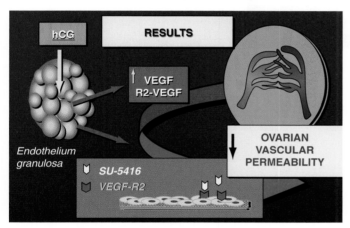

Figure 36.18. VEGF receptor blockade in prevention of ovarian hyperstimulation syndrome.

GnRH-a are withheld, as there is no endogenous gonadotropin secretion to sustain follicular growth, a rapid decline in estradiol levels will occur (Figure 36.17). Healthy developing follicles tolerate a brief period of gonadotropin deprivation, but granulosa cells of smaller follicles are less tolerant of withholding of gonadotropin stimulus [33,34,35]. Further evidence that could explain the coasting physiology is that VEGF expression and secretion are significantly decreased in coasted patients [33]. This is the rationale for coasting to reduce the risk/severity of OHSS in a high-risk population [33,34,35].

In women who develop OHSS, VEGF is overexpressed and produced by granulosa-lutein cells and released into the follicular fluid in response to hCG, inducing increased capillary permeability. hCG induces the expression of VEGF in cultured granulosa-lutein cells of women developing OHSS [16]. Similarly, hCG stimulates the release of VEGF in human endothelial cells, which in turn act in an autocrine manner, increasing vascular permeability (VP). Thus, both the granulosa and endothelial cells may be involved in the production and release

of VEGF in women who develop OHSS, although the concept that granulosa-lutein cells behave as actual endothelial cells has also been proposed [33,34,35]. The ability to reverse hCG action on VP by targeting the VEGF-R2 employing SU5416 was not only reassuring of the key role of VEGF in OHSS but also provided new insights into the development of strategies to prevent and treat the syndrome based on its pathophysiological mechanism [36], rather than using empirical approaches as we do today (Figures 36.18, 36.19, 36.20).

Dopamine receptor 2 agonists inhibit VEGF-R2-dependent VP and angiogenesis when administered at high doses in animal cancer models. To test whether VEGF-R2-dependent VP and angiogenesis could be segregated in a dose-dependent fashion with cabergoline, a well-established OHSS rat model supplemented with prolactin was used [37]. Low-dose cabergoline at 100 µg/kg reversed VEGF-R2-dependent VP without affecting luteal angiogenesis through partial inhibition of ovarian VEGF-R2 phosphorylation levels. No luteolytic effects (serum progesterone levels and luteal apoptosis unaffected) were observed. Cabergoline administration also did not affect VEGF/VEGF-R2 ovarian mRNA levels (Figures 36.18, 36.19, 36.20) [37,38,39,40]. In a recent prospective, randomized, controlled trial, Carizza et al. found that, in humans, cabergoline was beneficial in the prevention of early-onset but not late-onset OHSS [41]. The authors studied 166 patients with estradiol concentrations of greater than 4000 pg/ml on the day of hCG administration. They all received 20 g of intravenous human albumin on the day of oocyte retrieval. The patients were randomized into two groups: group A ($n = 83$) received 0.5 mg. oral cabergoline per day for 3 weeks beginning on the day after oocyte retrieval, and group B ($n = 83$) received no medication. In group A, no patients progressed to early OHSS and 9 patients developed late OHSS. In group B, 12 patients progressed to early OHSS and 3 to late OHSS. The authors concluded that cabergoline decreased the risk of early OHSS significantly ($P < 0.001$), but not late-onset OHSS.

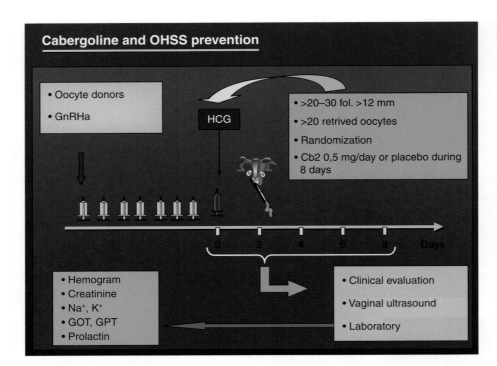

Figure 36.19. Cabergoline and prevention of ovarian hyperstimulation syndrome.

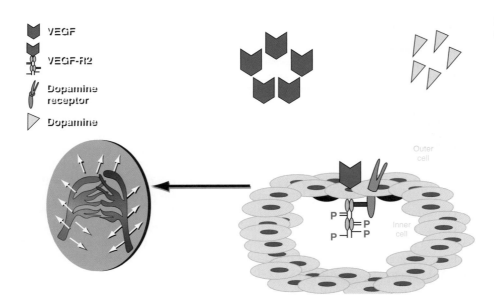

Figure 36.20. Molecular mechanism of dopamine agonist on vascular permeability.

Treatment of OHSS

The management of OHSS depends on the severity and the presence or absence of complications [42]. Most patients with mild or moderate OHSS are treated as outpatients. The comfort of the physician and the reliability of the patient are crucial determinants. Patients with severe OHSS (grade C) are treated in the hospital, while patients with grades A and B may be treated in the IVF unit or the hospital depending on the presence or absence of complications. The indications for hospitalization are listed in Table 36.6.

Medical treatment in the hospital consists of correction of circulatory volume and electrolyte imbalance (Figure 36.21). Anticoagulation is given in patients who have developed thromboembolism or to those who are at risk of developing thromboembolism. Today, we have a more liberal approach to anticoagulating these patients. Diuretics should not be administered in patients with severe OHSS, except for the treatment of pulmonary edema. Navot and colleagues have the largest experience of the management of patients with severe OHSS using albumin and Lasix, and their experience should be consulted in the management of these critical patients [4].

Ultrasonography is also essential in the management of severe OHSS. Rizk and Aboulghar in 1991 recommended that aspiration of ascitic fluid be performed transvaginally or trans-abdominally under ultrasonographic guidance in the presence of tense ascites [42]. Aboulghar et al. demonstrated that trans-vaginal aspiration improves patients' symptoms and renal function (43). The increased intra-abdominal pressure may compromise venous return and, consequently, cardiac output as well as threaten renal edema and possibly thrombosis. In the presence of tense ascites and oliguria, increasing levels of crea-tinine, or hemoconcentration that is unresponsive to medical therapy, ultrasound-guided aspiration of ascitic fluid must be performed. The dramatic improvement in clinical symptoms (rise in urine output and creatinine clearance, decrease in hematocrit, alleviation of dyspnea and abdominal discomfort) supports this treatment modality as safe and exceptionally beneficial [44]. Repeated transabdominal aspiration can also be safely performed [45]. Chen et al. investigated the effects of paracentesis on uterine and intraovarian hemodynamics by color Doppler ultrasound to determine the influence of

repeated paracentesis on pregnancy outcome in severe OHSS [45]. In their study, 41 abdominal paracenteses were performed on 7 pregnant women with tense ascites, and thoracocenteses were performed on 3 pregnant women with pleural effusion. Pulsatility index and maximum peak systolic velocity of uterine and intraovarian arteries were measured before and after each intervention. The mean pulsatility index of uterine arteries was decreased significantly after paracentesis but not after thoraco-centesis. Interestingly, the authors observed a decrease in the uterine pulsatility index in 13 out of 14 paracenteses (93%) with less than 2500 ml of ascites removed compared with 8 out of 13 (62%) with more than 2500 ml of ascites removed. After para-centesis, there were no significant changes in the intraovarian pulsatility index and mean peak systolic velocity in either group. The authors observed no difference in miscarriage rates between the two groups and concluded that repeated abdominal paracentesis increased uterine perfusion without adverse effects on pregnancy outcome in patients with severe OHSS [43]. Al-Ramahi et al. reported three cases where an indwelling peritoneal catheter was used to decrease the need for paracentesis. Under ultrasound guidance, a closed-system Dawson–Mueller catheter with "simp-loc" locking design was inserted to allow continuous drainage of the ascitic fluid [46]. The authors concluded that continuous drainage of the ascitic fluid is preferable to multiple abdominal paracenteses in the management of severe OHSS. Abuzeid et al. studied the efficacy and safety of percutaneous pigtail catheter drainage for the management of ascites complicating severe OHSS [47]. A pig-tail catheter was inserted under ultrasound guidance and kept in place until drainage ceased. Surgery should be avoided in most patients with OHSS, except in the cases of ovarian torsion or hemorrhage.

Table 36.6. Indications for hospitalization of patients with severe OHSS

1. Severe abdominal pain or peritoneal signs
2. Intractable nausea and vomiting that prevents ingestion of food and adequate fluids
3. Severe oliguria or anuria
4. Tense ascites
5. Dyspnea or tachypnea
6. Hypotension (relative to baseline), dizziness, or syncope
7. Severe electrolyte imbalance (hypernatremia, hyperkalemia)

Reproduced with permission from Rizk [6].

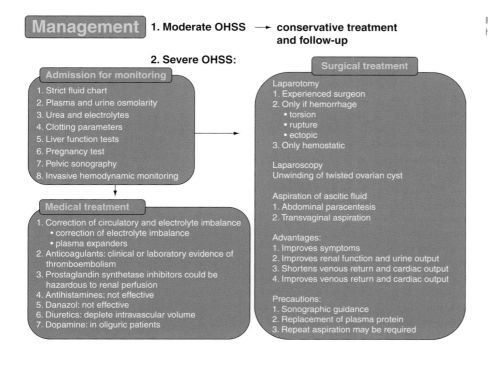

Figure 36.21. Management of ovarian hyperstimulation syndrome.

Key points in clinical practice

- Ovarian hyperstimulation syndrome is characterized by bilateral cystic ovarian enlargement and third-space fluid shift resulting in ascites and pleural effusion.

- Severe ovarian hyperstimulation syndrome might be associated with serious complications such as thromboembolism, adult respiratory distress syndrome, and kidney failure.

- Human chorionic gonadotropin increases VEGF production by granulosa cells and endothelial cells, which results in increased vascular permeability.

- The cornerstone of successful prevention of OHSS is accurate prediction.

- Previous history of OHSS or polycystic ovary syndrome is highly predictive of the development of OHSS during ovarian stimulation.

- Ultrasound is essential for the prediction of OHSS before, during, and after the treatment cycle.

- Baseline antral follicle count and ovarian volume are strongly associated with OHSS.

- The presence of a large number of follicles (>20 per ovary) and increase in the small and intermediate follicles are associated with an increased risk for the development of severe OHSS.

- Increased intraovarian blood flow and low intravascular ovarian resistance are correlated with the severity of OHSS in patients who develop the syndrome.

- The presence of multiple pregnancy increases the risk of the severity and duration of OHSS.

- The primary prevention of OHSS can be achieved by the use of low-dose gonadotropins and, in some cases, ovarian drilling prior to IVF.

- The secondary prevention of OHSS involves delaying the hCG, known as "coasting," and, in some cases, cancellation of the hCG.

- The medical treatment of OHSS consists of correction of circulatory volume and electrolyte imbalance.

- Ultrasonographic guidance of transvaginal or transabdominal aspiration of ascites improves the symptoms of patients with OHSS.

References

1. Rabau E, Serr DM, David A, et al. Human menopausal gonadotrophin for anovulation and sterility. *Am J Obstet Gynecol* 1967; **98**: 92–8.

2. Schenker JG, Weinstein D. Ovarian hyperstimulation syndrome: a current survey. *Fertil Steril* 1978; **30**: 255–68.

3. Golan A, Ron-El R, Herman A, et al. Ovarian hyperstimulation syndrome: an update review. *Obstet Gynecol Surv* 1989; **44**: 430–40.

4. Navot D, Bergh PA, Laufer N. Ovarian hyperstimulation syndrome in novel reproductive technologies: prevention and treatment. *Fertil Steril* 1992; **58**: 249–61.

5. Mozes M, Bogowsky H, Anteby E, et al. Thrombo-embolic phenomena after ovarian stimulation with human menopausal gonadotrophins. *Lancet* 1965; **2**: 1213–15.

6. Rizk B. Classification of ovarian hyperstimulation syndrome. In: Rizk B, ed. *Ovarian Hyperstimulation Syndrome: Epidemiology, Pathophysiology, Prevention and Management.* Chapter 1. New York and Cambridge: Cambridge University Press, 2006; 1–9.

7. Serour G. Ovarian hyperstimulation syndrome In: Gerris J, Olivennes F, Delvigne A, eds. *Ovarian Hyperstimulation Syndrome.* London: Taylor and Francis, 2006.

8. Schenker JG. Ovarian hyperstimulation syndrome. In: Wallach EE, Zacur HA, eds. *Reproductive Medicine and Surgery.* Chapter 35. St. Louis: Mosby, 1996; 654.

9. Rizk B, Meagher S, Fisher AM. Ovarian hyperstimulation syndrome and cerebrovascular accidents. *Hum Reprod* 1990; **5**: 697–8.

10. Rizk B. Ovarian hyperstimulation syndrome. In: Studd J, ed. *Progress in Obstetrics and Gynecology.* Vol 11, Chapter 18. Edinburgh: Churchill Livingstone, 1995; 311–49.

11. Dahl-Lyons CA, Wheeler CA, Frishman GN, et al. Early and late presentation of the ovarian hyperstimulation syndrome: two distinct entities with different risk factors. *Hum Reprod* 1994; **9**: 792–9.

12. Mathur RS, Akande AV, Keay SD, et al. Distinction between early and late ovarian hyperstimulation syndrome. *Fertil Steril* 2000; **73**(5): 901–7.

13. Rizk B. Genetics of ovarian hyperstimulation syndrome. *Reprod Biomed Online.* 2009; **19**(1): 14–27.

14. Aboulghar MA, Mansour RT. Ovarian hyperstimulation syndrome: classifications and critical analysis of preventive measures. *Hum Reprod Update* 2003; **9**: 275–89.

15. Rizk B, Aboulghar MA. Classification, pathophysiology and management of ovarian hyperstimulation syndrome. In: Brinsden P, ed. *A Textbook of In Vitro Fertilization and Assisted Reproduction.* 2nd edn. Chapter 9. Carnforth, UK: Parthenon, 1999, Chapter 11, 131–55.

16. Rizk B, Aboulghar MA, Smitz J, Ron-El R. The role of vascular endothelial growth factor and interleukins in the pathogenesis of severe ovarian hyperstimulation syndrome. *Hum Reprod Update* 1997; **3**: 255–66.

17. Pellicer A, Albert C, Mercader A, et al. The pathogenensis of ovarian hyperstimulation syndrome: in vivo studies investigating the role of interleukin 1-β, interleukin-6 and vascular endothelial growth factor. *Fertil Steril* 1999; **71**: 482–9.

18. Rizk B, Smitz J. Ovarian hyperstimulation syndrome after superovulation for IVF and related procedures. *Hum Reprod* 1992; **7**: 320–7.

19. Delvigne A, Dubois M, Batteu B, et al. The ovarian hyperstimulation syndrome in in-vitro fertilization: a Belgian multicenter study. II. Multiple discriminant analytes for risk prediction. *Hum Reprod* 1993; **8**: 1361–6.

20. Perez Mayorga M, Gromoll J, Behre M, et al. Ovarian response to follicle stimulating hormona (FSH) stimulation depends on the FSH receptor genotype.

J Clin Endocrinol Metab
2000; **85**: 3365–9.

21. De Castro R, Ruiz R, Montoro L, et al. Role of follicle stimulating hormone receptor ser680Asn polymorphism in the efficacy of follicle stimulating hormone. *Fertil Steril* 2003; **80**: 571–6.

22. Daelemans C, Smits G, de Maerlelaer V, et al. Prediction of severity of symptoms in iatrogenic ovarian hyperstimulation syndrome by follicle stimulating hormone receptor Ser680Asn polymorphism. *J Clin Endocrinol Metab* 2004; **89**: 6310–15.

23. Danninger B, Brunner M, Obruca A, et al. Prediction of ovarian hyperstimulation syndrome of baseline ovarian volume prior to stimulation. *Hum Reprod* 1996; **11**: 1597–9

24. Lass A, Vassiliev A, Decosterd G, et al. Relationship of baseline ovarian volume to ovarian response in World Health Organization Group II anovulatory patients who underwent ovulation induction with gonadotropins. *Fertil Steril* 2002; **78**: 265–9.

25. Rizk B, Nawar MG. Ovarian hyperstimulation syndrome. In: Serhal P, Overton C, eds. *Good Clinical Practice in Assisted Reproduction.* Chapter 8. Cambridge: Cambridge University Press, 2004; 146–66.

26. Rizk B. Complications of ovulation induction. II Ovarian hyperstimulation syndrome, ovarian torsion. In: Dickey RP, Brinsden PR, Pyrzak R, eds. *Manual of Intrauterine Insemination and Ovulation Induction.* Chapter 15. Cambridge: Cambridge University Press, 2010; 152–60.

27. Tal J, Faz B, Samberg I, et al. Ultrasonographic and clinical correlates of menotrophin versus sequential clomiphene citrate: menotrophin therapy for induction of ovulation. *Fertil Steril* 1985; **4**: 342–9.

28. Blankstein J, Shalev J, Saadon T, et al. Ovarian hyperstimulation syndrome prediction by number and size of preovulatory ovarian follicles. *Fertil Steril* 1987; **47**: 597–602.

29. Kwee J, Elting M, Schats R, et al. Ovarian volume and antral follicle count for the prediction of low and hyper responders with in vitro fertilization. *Reprod Biol Endocrinol* 2007, **5**: 9.

30. Moohan JM, Curcio K, Leoni M, et al. Low intraovarian vascular resistance: a marker for severe ovarian hyperstimulation syndrome. *Fertil Steril* 1997; **57**: 728–32.

31. Rizk B. Prevention of ovarian hyperstimulation syndrome: the Ten Commandments. Presented at the *European Society of Human Reproduction and Embryology Symposium,* Tel Aviv, Israel, 1993; 1–2.

32. Rizk B. Prevention of ovarian hyperstimulation syndrome. In: Rizk B, ed. *Ovarian Hyperstimulation Syndrome.* Chapter 7. Cambridge: Cambridge University Press, 2006; 130–99.

33. Busso CE, Garcia-Velasco JA, Gomez R, et al. Ovarian hyperstimulation syndrome. In: Rizk B, Garcia-Velasco JA, Sallam H, Madrigiannakis A, eds. *Infertility and Assisted Reproduction.* Chapter 27. Cambridge: Cambridge University Press, 2008; 243–57.

34. Garcia-Velasco JA, Zuniga A, Pacheco A, et al. Coasting acts through downregulation of VEGF gene expression and protein secretion. *Hum Reprod* 2004; **19**: 1530–8.

35. Garcia-Velasco JA, Isaza B, Quea G, et al. Coasting for the prevention of ovarian hyperstimulation syndrome: much to do about nothing? *Fertil Steril* 2006; **85**: 547–54.

36. Gomez R, Simon C, Remohi J, et al. Vascular endothelial growth factor receptor-2 activation induces vascular permeability in hyperstimulated rate, and this effect is prevented by receptor blockade. *Endocrinology* 2002; **143**(11): 4339–48.

37. Gomez R, Gonzalez-Izquierdo M, Zimmermann RC, et al. Low dose dopamine agonist administration blocks vascular endothelial growth factor (VEGF)-mediated vascular hyperpermeability without altering VEGF receptor 2-dependent luteal angiogenesis in a rat ovarian hyperstimulation model. *Endocrinology* 2006; **147**: 5400–11.

38. Alvarez C, Marti-Bonmati L, Novella-Maestre E, et al. Dopamine agonist cabergoline reduces hemoconcentration and ascites in hyperstimulated women undergoing assisted reproduction. *J Clin Endocrinol Metab* 2007; **92**: 2931–7.

39. Alvarez C, Alonso-Muriel A, Garcia G, et al. Implantation is apparently unaffected by the dopamine agonist cagergoline when administered to prevent ovarian hyperstimulation in women undergoing assisted reproduction treatment: a pilot study. *Hum Reprod* 2007; **22**(12): 3210–14.

40. Garcia-Velasco JA. How to avoid ovarian hyperstimulation syndrome: a new indication for dopamine agonists. *RBM Online* 2009; **18**(2): 71–5.

41. Carizza C, Abdelmassih VG, Abdelmassih S, et al. Cabergoline reduces the early onset of ovarian hyperstimulation syndrome: a prospective randomized study. *RBM Online* 2008; **17**(6): 751–5.

42. Rizk B, Aboulghar MA. Modern magagement of ovarian hyperstimulation syndrome. *Hum Reprod* 1991; **6**: 1082–7.

43. Aboulghar MA, Mansour RT, Serour GI, et al. Ultrasonically guided vaginal aspiration of ascites in the treatment of ovarian hyperstimulation syndrome. *Fertil Steril* 1990; **53**: 933–5.

44. Rizk B, Aboulghar MA. Ovarian hyperstimulation syndrome. In: Aboulghar MA, Rizk, B, eds. *Ovarian Stimulation.* Cambridge: Cambridge University Press, 2010.

45. Chen DC, Yang J, Chao, K, et al. Effects of repeated abdominal paracentesis on uterine and intraovarian haemodynamics and pregnancy outcome in severe ovarian hyperstimulation syndrome. *Hum Reprod* 1998; **13**(8): 2077–81.

46. Al-Ramahi M, Leader A, Claman P, et al. A novel approach to the treatment of ascites associated with ovarian hyperstimulation syndrome. *Hum Reprod* 1997; **12**: 2614–16.

47. Abuzeid MI, Nassar Z, Massaad Z, et al. Pigtail catheter for the treatment of ascites associated with ovarian hyperstimulation syndrome. *Hum Reprod* 2003; **18**: 370–3.

48. Delbaere A, Smits G, Olatunbosun O, Pierson R, Vassart G, Costagliola S. New insights into the pathophysiology of ovarian hyperstimulation syndrome. What makes the difference between spontaneous and iatrogenic syndrome? *Hum Reprod* 2004; **19**(3):486–9.

49. Zaidi J, Campbell S, Pittrof R, et al. Ovarian stromal blood flow in women with polycystic ovaries – a possible new marker for diagnosis? *Hum Reprod* 1995; **10**(8):1992–6.

50. Jacobs HS. Polycystic ovary syndrome. In: Stenchever M, Mishell D, eds. *Atlas of Clinical Gynecology*. Volume III, Reproductive Endocrinology. Chapter 5. Philadelphia: Current Medicine, 1999; 53.

Index

Note: Page numbers in *italics* refer to figures and tables